Dictionary of
Medical
Acronyms &
Abbreviations

Third Edition

Dictionary of
Medical
Acronyms &
Abbreviations

Third Edition

Compiled and edited by
Stanley Jablonski

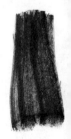

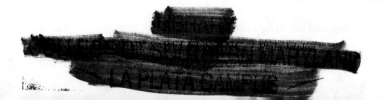

Publisher: HANLEY & BELFUS, INC.
Medical Publishers
210 South 13th Street
Philadelphia, PA 19107
(215) 546-7293; 800-962-1892
FAX (215) 790-9330
Web site: http://www.hanleyandbelfus.com

**Dictionary of Medical Acronyms
& Abbreviations, 3rd edition**
ISBN 1-56053-264-5

Library of Congress Catalog card number 97-80820.

Last digit is the print number: 9 8 7 6 5 4 3 2

Other Books of Interest from HANLEY & BELFUS, INC.

Rx SHORTHAND, by Stanley Jablonski

A LITTLE BOOK OF DOCTORS' RULES, by Clifton K. Meador, MD

A LITTLE BOOK OF NURSES' RULES, by Rosalie Hammerschmidt, RN, and Clifton K. Meador, MD

A LITTLE BOOK OF DENTAL HYGIENISTS' RULES, by Esther M. Wilkins, RDH, DMD

THE BEST OF MEDICAL HUMOR, 2nd ed., by Howard J. Bennett, MD

THE BEST OF NURSING HUMOR, by Colleen Kenefick and Amy Young

THE BEST OF DENTAL HUMOR, by Stephen T. Sonis, DMD, DMSc

THE SECRETS SERIES®
   These mini-textbooks in question-and-answer format help students, residents, and practitioners hone their skills for practice and board exams.

THE PEARLS SERIES®
   Using an efficient problem solving, self-study approach, books in The Pearls Series® challenge the reader by using 75–100 actual case studies. A brief clinical vignette, accompanied by a chest radiograph, is presented. The reader is encouraged to consider a differential diagnosis and formulate a plan for diagnosis and treatment. The subsequent page discloses the diagnosis, followed by a discussion of the case, clinical pearls, and two or three key references.

HANLEY & BELFUS, INC., 210 South 13th Street, Philadelphia, PA 19107
Orders/Customer Service 800-962-1892; 215-546-7293; fax 215-790-9330; web site www.hanleyandbelfus.com

Preface to the First Edition

Acronyms and abbreviations are used extensively in medicine, science and technology for good reason—they are more essential in such fields. It would be difficult to imagine how one could write down chemical and mathematical formulas and equations without using abbreviations or symbols. In medicine, they are used as a convenient shorthand in writing medical records, instructions, and prescriptions, and as space-saving devices in printed literature. It is easier and more economical to write down the acronyms HETE and RAAS than their full names 12-*L*-hydroxy-5,8,10,14-eicosatetraenoic acid and renin-angiotensin-aldosterone system, respectively.

The main reason for abbreviations is said to be economy. Some actually save space in print, such as acronyms for the names of institutions and organizational units, as well as being convenient to use. Many are used for other reasons, as for instance, when trying to be delicate, we may euphemistically refer to bowel movement as BM, an unprincipled individual as SOB, and body odor as BO. Also, it is sometimes difficult to fathom the reasoning of bureaucratic acronym makers, who have created some tongue-twisting monstrosities, such as ADCOMSUBORDCOMPHIBSPAC (for Administrative Command, Amphibious Forces, Pacific Fleet, Subordinate Command).

Abbreviations and acronyms used in medicine can be grouped into two broad categories. The first consists of official abbreviations and symbols used in chemistry, mathematics, and other sciences, and those designating weights and measures, whose exact form, capitalization, and punctuation have been determined by official governing bodies. In this category, they mean only one thing (e.g., kg is the symbol for kilogram and Hz for hertz), and their form, capitalization, and punctuation have been established by the International System of Units (Système International d'Unités). Abbreviations in the second group, on the other hand, may appear in a variety of forms, the same abbreviation having a different number of letters, sometimes capitalized, at other times not, with or without punctuation. Moreover, they may also have numerous meanings. The abbreviation AP may mean alkaline phosphatase, acid phosphatase, action potential, angina pectoris, and many other things.

Editors of individual scientific publications make an effort to standardize the form of abbreviations and symbols in their journals and books, but they generally vary from one publication to another.

This dictionary lists acronyms and abbreviations occurring with a reasonable frequency in the medical literature that were identified by a systematic scanning of collections of books and periodicals at the National Library of Medicine. Except as they take the form of Greek letters, pure geometric symbols are not included. Although we have attempted to be as inclusive as possible, a book such as this one can never be complete, in spite of the most diligent effort, and it is expected that some abbreviations and acronyms may have escaped detection and others may have been introduced since completion of the manuscript.

Stanley Jablonski
Bethesda, Maryland

Preface to the Second Edition

It is a reality of medicine and science that the number of acronyms and abbreviations is increasing dramatically. Despite the efforts of teachers and editors to contain them, clinicians and researchers constantly introduce new ones, as perusal of any current journal demonstrates. This growth attests to the fact that acronyms and abbreviations are necessary and useful in medical writing and speaking, conserving space and preventing needless repetition.

This edition, like its predecessor, is a selective collection of the most frequently used acronyms and abbreviations. Over 2,000 entries have been added. We trust you will find it to be a handy reference to be kept within easy reach.

Stanley Jablonski

The purpose of this edition, like that of the previous two editions, is to provide a compact, useful, and affordable collection of the most frequently used acronyms and abbreviations in medicine and the health care professions. As in previous editions, the goal was not to be comprehensive but rather to focus on acronyms and abbreviations that occur with reasonable frequency in the health care literature.

Approximately 5,000 entries have been added to reflect new material related to burgeoning fields such as health care management, long-term care, outcomes research, medical informatics, molecular biology, and outpatient care, to name just a few. The symbol section in the front of the book has also been expanded and now includes genetic symbols as well as the Greek alphabet.

We welcome feedback and suggestions from readers, which can be sent to me in care of the publisher, Hanley & Belfus in Philadelphia. I hope you find this new edition user friendly and helpful.

Stanley Jablonski

Symbols

°	degree		∡	angle of entry
′	foot		∡	angle of exit
″	inch		└	right lower quadrant
/	per		┌	right upper quadrant
%	per cent		┐	left upper quadrant
:	ratio		┘	left lower quadrant
∞	infinity		>	greater than
+	positive		<	less than
−	negative		Δ	change
±	positive or negative		√	root; square root
#	number; fracture; pound		χ^2	chi square (test)
÷	divided by		σ	1/1000 of a second standard deviation
×	multiplied by; magnification		Σ	sum of
=	equals		π	3.1415—ratio of circumference of a circle to its diameter
≠	does not equal			
~	approximate			
↓	decreased		τ	life (time)
↑	increased		τ½	half-life (time)
→	to (in direction of)		λ	wavelength
∅	normal		@	at
V	systolic blood pressure		ā	before
Λ	diastolic blood pressure		c̄	with
∠	angle		√c̄	check with

$\bar{p}$	after	†	deceased
$\bar{s}$	without	◊	lozenge; sex unknown or unspecified
24°	24 hours	Ⓐ , (ax)	axilla (temperature)
Δt	time interval	Ⓗ , (h)	hypodermically
2d	second	(IM)	intramuscularly
1°	primary	(IV)	intravenously
2°	secondary to	(L)	left
♀	female	(M)	murmur
♂	male	(m)	by mouth, murmur
ℨ	dram	(O)	by mouth, orally
℥	ounce	(R)	rectally, registered trademark, right
–ve	negative	(X)	end of anesthesia, end of operation
+ve	positive		
D_x	diagnosis		
R_x	treatment or therapy		

Genetic Symbols

□	male	(□)(○)	adopted
○	female	half siblings	half siblings
◇	sex unspecified	stillbirth or abortion	stillbirth or abortion
□—○	mating or marriage	no offspring	no offspring
□—○	consanguinity	■ ●	affected offspring
□¦○	illegitimate offspring	proband, propositus, or index case	proband, propositus, or index case
□⫻○	divorce		
□—○—□	multiple marriage	◫ ◖	heterozygotes for autosomal recessive
dizygotic twins	dizygotic twins		
monozygotic twins	monozygotic twins	⊙	carrier of sex-linked recessive
4 ③	number of children of sex indicated	⊘ ∅	death

Greek Alphabet and Symbols

α	A	alpha
β	B	beta
χ	X	chi
δ	Δ	delta (diagnosis; change)
ε	E	epsilon
η	H	eta
γ	Γ	gamma
ι	I	iota
κ	K	kappa
λ	Λ	lambda
μ	M	mu
ν	N	nu

ω	Ω	omega
o	O	omicron
φ	Φ	phi
π	Π	pi
ψ	Ψ	psi
ρ	P	rho
σ	Σ	sigma
τ	T	tau
θ	Θ	theta
υ	Y	upsilon
ξ	Ξ	xi
ζ	Z	zeta

A abnormal; abortion; absolute temperature; absorbance; acceptor; accommodation; acetone; acetum; acid; acidophil; acidophilic; acromion; actin; *Actinomyces*; activity [radiation]; adenine; adenoma; adenosine; admittance; adrenalin; adriamycin; adult; age; akinetic; alanine; albino [guinea pig]; albumin; allergologist, allergy; alpha [cell]; alveolar gas; ambulation; ampere; amphetamine; ampicillin; anaphylaxis; androsterone; anesthetic; angstrom, Ångström unit; anode; *Anopheles*; antagonism; anterior; antibody; antrectomy; apical; aqueous; area; argon; artery [Lat. *arteria*]; atomic weight; atrium; atropine; auricle; auscultation; axial; axilla, axillary; before [Lat. *ante*] blood group A; ear [Lat. *auris*]; mass number; subspinale; total acidity; water [Lat. *aqua*]; year [Lat. *annum*]

A [band] the dark-staining zone of a striated muscle

Å Ångström unit

Ã cumulated activity; antinuclear antibody

A₁ aortic first sound

A₂ aortic second sound

A₂₋ₒₛ aortic second sound, opening snap

A₂ P₂ aortic second sound; pulmonary second sound

AI, AII, AIII angiotensin I, II, III

a absorptivity; acceleration; accommodation; acidity; activated; ampere; anode; ante [before]; anterior; area; arterial blood; artery [Lat. *arteria*]; atto-; thermodynamic activity; total acidity; water [Lat. *aqua*]

ā before [Lat. *ante*]

A see *alpha*

α see *alpha*

AA abdominal aorta; acetic acid; achievement age; active alcoholic; active assistive [range of motion]; active avoidance; acupuncture analgesia; adenine arabinoside; adenylic acid; adjuvant arthritis; adrenal androgen; agranulocytic angina; Alcoholics Anonymous; allergic alveolitis; alopecia areata; alveolo-arterial; amino acid; aminoacyl; amyloid A; anticipatory avoidance; antigen aerosol; aortic arch; aplastic anemia; arachidonic acid; arteries; ascending aorta; atlanto-axial; atomic absorption; Australia antigen; autoanalyzer; automobile accident; axonal arborization

A-a alveolar-atrial

aa arteries [Lat. *arteriae*]

A&A aid and attendance; awake and aware

aA abampere

AAA abdominal aortic aneurysm/aneurysmectomy; acne-associated arthritis; acquired aplastic anemia; acute anxiety attack; alacrimia-achalasia-addisonianism [syndrome]; American Academy of Addictionology; American Academy of Allergy; American Association of Anatomists; androgenic anabolic agent; aneurysm of ascending aorta; Area Agency on Aging; aromatic amino acid; arrest after arrival

AAAD aromatic amino acid decarboxylase

AA/AD alcohol abuse/alcohol dependence

AAAE amino acid activating enzyme

AAAHE American Association for the Advancement of Health Education

AAAI American Academy of Allergy and Immunology

AAALAC American Association for Accreditation of Laboratory Animal Care

1

AAAS American Association for the Advancement of Science

AAB American Association of Bioanalysts; aminoazobenzene

AABB American Association of Blood Banks

AABCC alertness (consciousness), airway, breathing, circulation, cervical spine

AABS automobile accident, broadside

AAC antibiotic-associated [pseudomembranous] colitis; antimicrobial agent-induced colitis; augmentative and alternative communication

AACA acylaminocephalosporanic acid

AACC American Association for Clinical Chemistry

AACCN American Association of Critical Care Nurses

AACG acute angle closure glaucoma

AACHP American Association for Comprehensive Health Planning

AACIA American Association for Clinical Immunology and Allergy

AACN American Association of Colleges of Nursing; American Association of Critical-Care Nurses

AACP American Academy of Cerebral Palsy; American Association of Colleges of Pharmacy

AACPDM American Academy for Cerebral Palsy and Developmental Medicine

AACSH adrenal androgen corticotropic stimulating hormone

AACT American Academy of Clinical Toxicology

AAD acute agitated delirium; alloxazine adenine dinucleotide; alpha-1-antitrypsin deficiency; American Academy of Dermatology; antibiotic-associated diarrhea; aromatic acid decarboxylase

AADC amino acid decarboxylase

AADE American Association of Dental Editors; American Association of Dental Examiners

AADGP American Academy of Dental Group Practice

AADH alopecia-anosmia-deafness-hypogonadism [syndrome]

(A-a)D_{N2} alveolo-arterial nitrogen tension difference

AAD$_{O2}$, (a-A) D_{O2} arterio-alveolar oxygen tension difference

AADP American Academy of Denture Prosthetics; amyloid A-degrading protease

AADPA American Academy of Dental Practice Administration

AADR American Academy of Dental Radiology

AADS American Academy of Dental Schools

AAE active assistive exercise; acute allergic encephalitis; American Association of Endodontists; annuloaortic ectasia

AAEE American Association of Electromyography and Electrodiagnosis

AAEM American Academy of Environmental Medicine; American Association of Electrodiagnostic Medicine

AA ex active assistive exercise

AAF acetylaminofluorene; ascorbic acid factor

AAFP American Academy of Family Physicians; American Academy of Family Practice

AAG 3-alkaladenine deoxyribonucleic acid glycosylase; allergic angiitis and granulomatosis; alpha-1-acid glycoprotein; alveolar arterial gradient; autoantigen

AAGL American Academy of Gynecologic Laparoscopists

AAGP American Academy of General Practice; American Association for Geriatric Psychiatry

AAHA American Academy of Hospital Attorneys; American Association of Homes for the Aging

AAHC American Academy of Healthcare Consultants; Association of Academic Health Centers

AAHD American Association of Hospital Dentists

AAHE Association for the Advancement of Health Education

AAHP American Association of Health Plans

AAHPER American Association for Health, Physical Education, and Recreation

AAHS American Association for Hand Surgery

AAHSLD Association of Academic Health Sciences Library Directors

AAI acute alveolar injury; Adolescent Alienation Index; American Association of Immunologists; atrial inhibited [pacemaker]

AAIB alpha-1-aminoisobutyrate

AAID American Academy of Implant Dentures

AAIN American Association of Industrial Nurses

AAK allo-activated killer

AAL anterior axillary line

AALAS American Association of Laboratory Animal Science

AALL American Association for Labor Legislation

AAM acute aseptic meningitis; American Academy of Microbiology; amino acid mixture

AAMA American Academy of Medical Administrators; American Association of Medical Assistants

AAMC American Association of Medical Clinics; Association of American Medical Colleges

AAMD American Academy of Medical Directors; American Association of Mental Deficiency

AAME acetylarginine methyl ester

AAMFT American Association for Marriage and Family Therapy

AAMI Association for the Advancement of Medical Instrumentation

AAMIH American Association for Maternal and Infant Health

AAMMC American Association of Medical Milk Commissioners

AAMP American Academy of Maxillofacial Prosthetics; American Academy of Medical Prevention

AAMR American Academy of Mental Retardation

AAMRL American Association of Medical Record Librarians

AAMRS automated ambulatory medical record system

AAMS acute aseptic meningitis syndrome

AAMSI American Association for Medical Systems and Informatics

AAMT American Association for Medical Transcription

AAN AIDS-associated nephropathy; alpha-amino nitrogen; American Academy of Neurology; American Academy of Nursing; American Academy of Nutrition; American Association of Neuropathologists; amino acid nitrogen; analgesic-associated nephropathy; attending's admission notes

AANA American Association of Nurse Anesthetists

AANE American Association of Nurse Executives

AANM American Association of Nurse-Midwives

AANPI American Association of Nurses Practicing Independently

AAO American Academy of Ophthalmology; American Academy of Optometry; American Academy of Osteopathy; American Academy of Otolaryngology; American Association of Ophthalmologists; American Association of Orthodontists; amino acid oxidase; ascending aorta; awake, alert, and oriented

AAo ascending aorta

A-a O$_2$ alveolo-arterial oxygen tension

AAOC antacid of choice

AAofA Ambulance Association of America

AAOHN American Association of Occupational Health Nurses

AAOM American Academy of Oral Medicine

AAOO American Academy of Ophthalmology and Otolaryngology

AAOP American Academy of Oral Pathology

AAOPP American Association of Osteopathic Postgraduate Physicians

AAOS American Academy of Orthopedic Surgeons

AAP air at atmospheric pressure; American Academy of Pediatrics; American Academy of Pedodontics; American Academy of Periodontology; American Academy of Psychoanalysts; American Academy of Psychotherapists; American Association of Pathologists; Association for the Advancement of Psychoanalysis; Association for the Advancement of Psychotherapy; Association of Academic Physiatrists; Association of American Physicians

AAPA American Academy of Physician Assistants; American Association of Pathologist Assistants

AAPB American Association of Pathologists and Bacteriologists

AAPC antibiotic-associated pseudomembranous colitis

AAPCC adjusted annual per capita cost; adjusted average per capita cost; American Association of Poison Control Centers

AaP$_{CO2}$, (A-a)P$_{CO2}$ alveolo-arterial carbon dioxide tension difference

AAPF anti-arteriosclerosis polysaccharide factor

AAPHD American Association of Public Health Dentists

AAPHP American Association of Public Health Physicians

AAPL American Academy of Psychiatry and the Law

AAPM American Association of Physicists in Medicine

AAPMC antibiotic-associated pseudomembranous colitis

AAPM&R American Academy of Physical Medicine and Rehabilitation

AaP$_{O2}$, (A-a) P$_{O2}$ alveolo-arterial oxygen tension difference

AAPP American Academy on Physician and Patient

AAPPO American Association of Preferred Provider Organizations

AAPS American Association of Plastic Surgeons; Arizona Articulation Proficiency Scale; Association of American Physicians and Surgeons

AAR active avoidance reaction; acute articular rheumatism; antigen-antiglobulin reaction

aar against all risks

AARE automobile accident, rear end

AAROM active assertive range of motion; active-assisted range of motion

AARP American Association of Retired Persons

AART American Association for Rehabilitation Therapy; American Association for Respiratory Therapy

AAS Aarskog-Scott [syndrome]; acid aspiration syndrome; alcoholic abstinence syndrome; American Academy of Sanitarians; American Analgesia Society; aneurysm of atrial septum; anthrax antiserum; aortic arch syndrome; atomic absorption spectrophotometry

AASD American Academy of Stress Disorders

aa seq amino acid sequence

AASH adrenal androgen stimulating hormone; American Association for the Study of Headache

AASK African American Study of Kidney Diseases and Hypertension Pilot Study

AASP acute atrophic spinal paralysis; American Association of Senior Physicians; ascending aorta synchronized pulsation

AASS American Association for Social Security

AAT Aachen Aphasia Test; academic aptitude test; alanine aminotransferase; alkylating agent therapy; alpha-1-antitrypsin; atrial triggered [pacemaker]; auditory apperception test; automatic atrial tachycardia

α_1AT alpha-1-antitrypsin

AATS American Association for Thoracic Surgery

AAU acute anterior uveitis

AAV adeno-associated virus

AAVMC Association of American Veterinary Medical Colleges

AAVP American Association of Veterinary Parasitologists

AAVP American Association of Veterinary Parasitologists

AAW anterior aortic wall

AB abdominal; abnormal; abortion; Ace bandage; active bilaterally; aid to the blind; alcian blue; alertness behavior; antibiotic; antibody; antigen binding; apex beat; asbestos body; asthmatic bronchitis; axiobuccal; Bachelor of Arts [Lat. *Artium Baccalaureus*]; blood group AB

A/B acid-base ratio

A&B apnea and bradycardia

A>B air greater than bone [conduction]

Ab abortion; antibiotic; antibody

aB azure B

ab abortion; antibody; from [Lat.]

3AB 3-aminobenzamide

ABA abscissic acid; allergic bronchopulmonary aspergillosis; American Board of Anesthesiologists; antibacterial activity; arrest before arrival

ABAT American Board of Applied Toxicology

ABB Albright-Butler-Bloomberg [syndrome]; American Board of Bioanalysis

ABBQ Acquired Immunodeficiency Syndrome Beliefs and Behavior Questionnaire

abbr abbreviation, abbreviated

ABC absolute basophil count; absolute bone conduction; acalculous biliary colic; acid balance control; aconite-belladonna-chloroform; airway, breathing, and circulation; alignment, blue, calcium [synovial fluid pearls in gout and pseudogout]; alternative birth center; alum, blood, and charcoal [purification and deodorizing method]; alum, blood, and clay [sludge deodorizing method]; American Blood Commission; aneurysmal bone cyst; antigen-binding capacity; apnea, bradycardia, cyanosis; aspiration biopsy cytology; assessment of basic competency; atomic, biological, and chemical [warfare]; axiobuccocervical

A&BC air and bone conduction

ABCC Atomic Bomb Casualty Commission

ABCD airway, breathing, circulation, differential diagnosis (or defibrillate) [in cardiopulmonary resuscitation]; asymmetry, borders are irregular, color variegated, diameter > 6 mm [biopsy in melanoma]

ABCDE airway, breathing, circulation, disability, exposure [in trauma patients]; botulism toxin pentavalent

ABCDES abnormal alignment, bones—periarticular osteoporosis, cartilage—joint space loss, deformities, marginal erosions, soft tissue swelling [x-ray features in rheumatoid arthritis]; adjust medication, bacterial prophylaxis, cervical spine disease, deep vein thrombosis prophylaxis, evaluate extent and activity of disease, stress-dose steroid coverage [preoperative evaluation in rheumatoid diseases]; alignment, bone mineralization, calcifications, distribution of joints, erosions, soft tissue and nails [x-ray features in arthritis]; ankylosis, bone osteoporosis, cartilage destruction, deformity of joints, erosions, swelling of soft tissues [x-ray features of septic arthritis]

ABCIC airway, breathing, circulation, intravenous crystalloid

ABCIL antibody-mediated cell-dependent immunolympholysis

ABCN American Board of Clinical Neuropsychology

ABD abdomen; aged, blind, and disabled; aggressive behavioral disturbance; average body dose

Abd, abd abdomen, abdominal; abduct, abduction, abductor

abdom abdomen, abdominal

ABDPH American Board of Dental Public Health

ABE acute bacterial endocarditis; American Board of Endodontics; botulism equine trivalent antitoxin

ABEM American Board of Emergency Medicine

ABEPP American Board of Examiners in Professional Psychology

ABER auditory brainstem evoked response

aber aberrant

ABF aortic blood flow; aortobifemoral

ABG arterial blood gas; axiobucco-gingival

ABI ankle/brachial index; atherothrombotic brain infarct

ABIC Adaptive Behavior Inventory for Children

ABIM American Board of Internal Medicine

ABIMCE American Board of Internal Medicine certifying examination

ABIT assertive behavior inventory tool

ABK aphakic bullous keratopathy

ABL abetalipoproteinemia; acceptable blood loss; African Burkitt lymphoma; Albright-Butler-Lightwood [syndrome]; angioblastic lymphadenopathy; antigen-binding lymphocyte; Army Biological Laboratory; automated biological laboratory; axiobuccolingual

ABLB alternate binaural loudness balance

ABM adjusted body mass; alveolar basement membrane; autologous bone marrow

ABMI autologous bone marrow transplantation

AbMLV Abelson murine leukemia virus

ABMM American Board of Medical Management

ABMS American Board of Medical Specialties

ABMT American Board of Medical Toxicology; autologous bone marrow transplantation

AbN antibody nitrogen

Abn, abn abnormal; abnormality(ies)

ABNMP alpha-benzyl-N-methyl phenethylamine

abnor abnormal

ABO abortion; absent bed occupancy; American Board of Orthodontists; blood group system consisting of groups A, AB, B, and O

ABOHN American Board for Occupational Health Nurses

ABOMS American Board of Oral and Maxillofacial Surgery

ABOP American Board of Oral Pathology

Abor, abor abortion

ABP actin-binding protein; ambulatory blood pressure; American Board of Pedodontics; American Board of Periodontology; American Board of Prosthodontists; antigen-binding protein; androgen-binding protein; arterial blood pressure; avidin-biotin peroxidase

aBP arterial blood pressure

ABPA actin-binding protein, autosomal form; allergic bronchopulmonary aspergillosis

ABPC antibody-producing cell

ABPE acute bovine pulmonary edema

ABPM&R American Board of Physical Medicine and Rehabilitation

ABR abortus Bang ring [test]; absolute bed rest; auditory brainstem response

ABr agglutination test for brucellosis

Abr, Abras abrasion

ABS abdominal surgery; acute brain syndrome; Adaptive Behavior Scale; admitting blood sugar; adult bovine serum; aging brain syndrome; alkylbenzene sulfonate; aloin, belladonna, strychnine; American Board of Surgery; amniotic band sequence; amniotic band syndrome; anti-B serum; Antley-Bixler syndrome; arterial blood sample; at bed side

Abs absorption

abs absent; absolute

AB-SAAP autologous blood selective aortic arch perfusion

absc abscess; abscissa

abs conf absolute configuration

ABSe ascending bladder septum

abs feb while fever is absent

ABSITE American Board of Surgery In-Training Examination

absorp absorption

AbSR abnormal skin reflex

abst, abstr abstract

ABT autologous blood transfusion

abt about

ABU asymptomatic bacteriuria

ABV actinomycin D–bleomycin–vincristine; arthropod-borne virus

ABVD Adriamycin, bleomycin, vinblastine, and dacarbazine

ABW average body weight

ABY acid bismuth yeast [medium]

AC abdominal circumference; abdominal compression; absorption coefficient; abuse case; acetate; acetylcholine; acidified complement; *Acinetobacter calcoaceticus;* acromioclavicular; activated charcoal; acupuncture clinic; acute; acute cholecystitis; adenocarcinoma; adenylate cyclase; adherent cell; adrenal cortex; adrenocorticoid; air chamber; air conditioning; air conduction; alcoholic cirrhosis; alternating current; alveolar crest; ambulatory care; anesthesia circuit; angiocellular; anodal closure; antecubital; anterior chamber; anterior column; anterior commissure; antibiotic concentrate; anticoagulant; anticomplement; antiphlogistic corticoid; aortic closure; aortocoronary; arm circumference; ascending colon; atriocarotid; axiocervical

A-C acromioclavicular; adult-versus-child; aortocoronary bypass

A/C albumin/coagulin [ratio]; anterior chamber of eye; assist control [ventilation]

A2C apical two-chamber [view]

A4C apical four-chamber [view]

Ac accelerator [globulin]; acetate; acetyl; actinium; arabinosyl cytosine

aC abcoulomb; arabinsyl cytosine

ac acceleration; acetyl; acid; acromioclavicular; acute; alternating current; antecubital; anterior chamber; atrial contraction; axiocervical

5-AC azacitidine

ACA abnormal coronary artery; acrodermatitis chronica atrophicans; acute cerebellar ataxia; adenocarcinoma; adult child of an alcoholic; American Chiropractic Association; American College of Allergists; American College of Anesthesiologists; American College of Angiology; American College of Apothecaries; American Council on Alcoholism; aminocephalosporanic acid; ammonia, copper, and acetate; amyotrophic choreo-acanthocytosis; anterior cerebral artery; anterior communicating aneurysm [or artery]; anticardiolipin antibody; anticentromere antibody; anticollagen antibody; anticomplement activity; anticytoplasmic antibody; Automatic Clinical Analyzer

AC/A accommodative convergence/accommodation [ratio]

ACAAI American College of Allergy, Asthma and Immunology

ACAC acetyl-coenzyme A cocarboxylase; activated charcoal artificial cell

ACACN American Council of Applied Clinical Nutrition

ACACT acyl-coenzyme A:cholesterol acyl transferase

ACAD asymptomatic coronary artery disease

Acad academy

A-CAH autoimmune chronic active hepatitis

ACAO acyl coenzyme A oxidase

ACAT acetocoenzyme A acetyltransferase; automated computerized axial tomography

ACB antibody-coated bacteria; aortocoronary bypass; arterialized capillary blood; asymptomatic carotid bruit

ACBaE air contrast barium enema

AC/BC air conduction/bone conduction [time ratio]

ACBE air contrast barium enema

ACBG aortocoronary bypass graft

ACC accommodation; acetyl coenzyme A carboxylase; acinic cell carcinoma; acute care center; adenoid cystic carcinoma; administrative control center; adrenocortical carcinoma; alveolar cell carcinoma; ambulatory care center; American College of Cardiology; anodal closure contraction; anterior cingulate cortex; antitoxin-containing cell; aplasia cutis congenita; articular chondrocalcinosis; automated cell count; automated cell counter

Acc adenoid cystic carcinoma; acceleration

acc acceleration, accelerator; accident; accommodation

ACCA American College of Cardiovascular Administrators

ACCE American College of Clinical Engineering

ACCESS Ambulatory Care Clinic Effectiveness Systems Study; automated cervical cell screening system

ACCH Association for the Care of Children's Health

AcCh acetylcholine

AcChR acetylcholine receptor

AcCHS acetylcholinesterase

accid accident, accidental

acc insuff accommodation insufficiency

ACCL, Accl anodal closure clonus

ACCME Accreditation Council for Continuing Medical Education

AcCoA acetyl coenzyme A

accom accommodation

ACCP American College of Chest Physicians; American College of Clinical Pharmacology; American College of Clinical Pharmacy

ACCR amylase-creatinine clearance ratio

accum accumulation

accur accurately [lat. *accuratissime*]

ACD absolute cardiac dullness; absolute claudication distance; acid-citrate-dextrose [solution]; actinomycin D; active compression-decompression; adult celiac disease; advanced care directive; allergic contact dermatitis; American College of Dentists; angiokeratoma corporis diffusum; anterior chest diameter; anticoagulant citrate dextrose; area of cardiac dullness

AC-DC, ac/dc alternating current or direct current

ACD-CPR active compression-decompression cardiopulmonary resuscitation

ACD-PCR active compression-decompression post-compression remodeling

ACE acetonitrile; acetylcholine esterase; acute cerebral encephalopathy; acute coronary event; adrenocortical extract; alcohol, chloroform, and ether; angiotensin-converting enzyme

ace acentric; acetone

ACED anhydrotic congenital ectodermal dysplasia

ACEDS angiotensin-converting enzyme dysfunction syndrome

ACEH acid cholesterol ester hydrolase

ACEI angiotensin-converting enzyme inhibitor

ACEP American College of Emergency Physicians

AcEst acetyl esterase

ACET, acet acetone; vinegar [*Lat.* acetum]

acetab acetabular, acetabulum

acetyl-CoA acetyl coenzyme A

ACF accessory clinical findings; acute care facility; anterior cervical fusion; area correction factor; asymmetric crying facies

ACFAO American College of Foot and Ankle Orthopedics and Medicine

ACFAS American College of Foot and Ankle Surgeons

ACET Advisory Committee for the Elimination of Tuberculosis

ACG accelerator globulin; alternative care grant; ambulatory care group; American College of Gastroenterology; angiocardiography, angiocardiogram; aortocoronary graft; apexcardiogram

AC-G, AcG, ac-g accelerator globulin

ACGIH American Conference of Governmental Industrial Hygienists

ACGME Accreditation Council for Graduate Medical Education

ACGP American College of General Practitioners

ACGPOMS American College of General Practitioners in Osteopathic Medicine and Surgery

ACGT antibody-coated grid technique

ACH acetylcholine; achalasia; active chronic hepatitis; adrenocortical hormone; amyotrophic cerebellar hypoplasia; arm girth, chest depth, and hip width [nutritional index]

ACh acetylcholine

ACHA American College of Hospital Administrators

AChA anterior choroidal artery

ACHE American College of Healthcare Executives; American Council for Headache Education

AChE acetylcholinesterase

ACHOO autosomal dominant compelling helio-ophthalmic outburst [syndrome]

ACHPR Agency for Health Care Policy and Research

AChR acetylcholine receptor

AChRAb acetylcholine receptor antibody

AChRP acetylcholine receptor protein

ACI acceleration index; acoustic comfort index; acute cardiac ischemia; acute coronary infarction; acute coronary insufficiency; adenylate cyclase inhibitor; adrenocortical insufficiency; anticlonus index

ACID Arithmetic, Coding, Information, and Digit Span; automatic implantable cardioverter defibrillator

ACIF anticomplement immunofluorescence

ACIP acute canine idiopathic polyneuropathy; Advisory Committee on Immunization Practices [CDC]

ACIR Automotive Crash Injury Research

ACI-TIPI acute cardiac ischemia-time insensitive predictive instrument

AcK francium [actinium K]

ACKD acquired cystic kidney disease

ACL Achievement Check List; acromegaloid features, cutis verticis gyrata, corneal leukoma [syndrome]; anterior cruciate ligament

ACl aspiryl chloride

aCL anticardiolipin [antibody]

ACLA American Clinical Laboratory Association

ACLC Assessment of Children's Language Comprehension

ACLD Association for Children with Learning Disabilities

ACLF adult congregate living facility

ACLI American Council on Life Insurance

ACLM American College of Legal Medicine

ACLPS Academy of Clinical Laboratory Physicians and Scientists

ACLR anterior capsulolabral reconstruction

ACLS advanced cardiac life support; Assessment of Children's Language Comprehension

AcLV avian acute leukemia virus

ACM acetaminophen; acute cerebrospinal meningitis; Adriamycin, cyclophosphamide, methotrexate; albumin-calcium-magnesium; alveolar capillary membrane; anticardiac myosin; Arnold-Chiari malformation

ACMA American Occupational Medical Association

ACMC Association of Canadian Medical Colleges

ACMD associate chief medical director

ACME Advisory Council on Medical Education; Automated Classification of Medical Entities

ACMF arachnoid cyst of the middle fossa

ACMI American College of Medical Informatics

ACML atypical chronic myeloid leukemia

ACMP alveolar-capillary membrane permeability

ACMR Advisory Committee on Medical Research

ACMS American Chinese Medical Society

ACMT artificial circus movement tachycardia

ACMV assist-controlled mechanical ventilation

ACN acute conditioned neurosis; Ambulatory Care Network; American College of Neuropsychiatrists; American College of Nutrition

ACNM American College of Nuclear Medicine; American College of Nurse-Midwives

ACNP acute care nurse practitioner; American College of Nuclear Physicians

ACO acute coronary occlusion; alert, cooperative, and oriented; anodal closure odor

ACOA adult children of alcoholics

ACoA anterior communicating artery

ACOEM American College of Occupational and Environmental Medicine

ACOEP American College of Osteopathic Emergency Physicians

ACOG American College of Obstetricians and Gynecologists

ACOHA American College of Osteopathic Hospital Administrators

ACO-HNS American Council of Otolaryngology-Head and Neck Surgery

ACOI American College of Osteopathic Internists

ACOM American College of Occupational Medicine; anterior communicating [artery]

AComA anterior communicating artery

ACOMS American College of Oral and Maxillofacial Surgeons

ACOOG American College of Osteopathic Obstetricians and Gynecologists

ACOP American College of Osteopathic Pediatricians; approved code of practice

ACORDE A Corsortium on Restorative Dentistry Education

ACOS American College of Osteopathic Surgeons; associate chief of staff

ACOS/AC associate chief of staff for ambulatory care

Acous acoustics, acoustic

ACP accessory conduction pathway; acid phosphatase; acyl carrier protein; American College of Pathologists; American College of Pharmacists; American College of Physicians; American College of Prosthodontists; American College of Psychiatrists; Animal Care Panel; anodal closure picture; aspirin-caffeine-phenacetin; Association for Child Psychiatrists; Association of Clinical Pathologists; Association of Correctional Psychologists

ACPA American Cleft Palate Association

ACPC aminocyclopentane carboxylic [acid]

ACPE American College of Physician Executives

AC-PH, ac phos acid phosphatase

ACPM American College of Preventive Medicine

ACPP adrenocortical polypeptide; prostate-specific acid phosphatase

ACPS acrocephalopolysyndactyly

ACR abnormally contracting region; absolute catabolic rate; acriflavine; adenomatosis of colon and rectum; adjusted community rate; ambulance call report; American College of Radiology; American College of Rheumatology; anticonstipation regimen; axillary count rate

Acr acrylic

ACRF ambulatory care research facility

ACRM American Congress of Rehabilitation Medicine

ACS acrocallosal syndrome; acrocephalosyndactyly; acute chest syndrome; acute confusional state; Alcon Closure System; American Cancer Society; American Chemical Society; American College of Surgeons; anodal closure sound; antireticular cytotoxic serum; aperture current setting; Association of Clinical Scientists

ACSA adenylate cyclase-stimulating activity

ACS AO ascending aorta

ACSE association control service element

ACSF artificial cerebrospinal fluid

ACSM American College of Sports Medicine

ACSP adenylate cyclase-stimulating protein

AC/SIUG ambulatory care special-interest user group

ACSV aortocoronary saphenous vein

ACSVBG aortocoronary saphenous vein bypass graft

ACT achievement through counseling and treatment; actin; actinomycin; activated clotting time; advanced coronary treatment; anterocolic transposition; antichymotrypsin; anticoagulant therapy; anxiety control training; asthma care training; atropine coma therapy

AcT acceleration time

act actinomycin; activity, active

ACTA American Cardiology Technologists Association; automatic computerized transverse axial [scanning]

Act-C actinomycin C

Act-D actinomycin D

ACTe anodal closure tetanus

ACTG AIDS Clinical Trial Group

ACTH adrenocorticotropic hormone

ACTH-LI adrenocorticotropin-like immunoreactivity

ACTHR adrenocorticotropic hormone receptor

ACTH-RF adrenocorticotropic hormone releasing factor

activ active, activity

ACTN adrenocorticotropin

ACTP adrenocorticotropic polypeptide

ACT/PD actual nursing hours per patient/day

ACTS acute cervical traumatic sprain or syndrome; advanced communication technology satellite; American College Testing Services; Auditory Comprehension Test for Sentences

ACU acquired cold urticaria; acute care unit; agar colony-forming unit; ambulatory care unit

ACURP American College of Utilization Review Physicians

ACV acute cardiovascular [disease]; acyclovir; assisted controlled ventilation; atrial/carotid/ventricular

ACVB aortocoronary venous bypass

ACVD acute cardiovascular disease, atherosclerotic cardiovascular disease

ACx anomalous circumflex [coronary artery]

AD accident dispensary; acetate dialysis; active disease; acute dermatomyositis; addict, addiction; adenoid degeneration [agent]; adjuvant disease; admitting diagnosis; adrenostenedione; adult disease; advanced directive; aerosol deposition; affective disorder; after discharge; alcohol dehydrogenase; Aleutian disease; alveolar diffusion; alveolar duct; Alzheimer dementia; Alzheimer disease; analgesic dose; anodal duration; anterior division; antigenic determinant; appropriate disability; arthritic dose; associate degree; atopic dermatitis; attentional disturbance; Aujeszky disease; autonomic dysreflexia; autosomal dominant; average deviation; axiodistal; axis deviation; right ear [Lat. *auris dextra*]

A/D analog-to-digital [converter]

A&D admission and discharge; ascending and descending

Ad adenovirus; adrenal; anisotropic disk

ad add [Lat. *adde*] let there be added [up to a specified amount] [Lat. *addetur*]; axiodistal; right ear [Lat. *auris dextra*]

ADA adenosine deaminase; American Dental Association; American Dermatological Association; American Diabetes Association; American Dietetic Association; Americans with Disabilities Act; anterior descending artery; antideoxyribonucleic acid antibody; approved dietary allowance

ADAA American Dental Assistants Association

ADAM amniotic deformity, adhesion, mutilation [syndrome]

ADAMHA Alcohol, Drug Abuse, and Mental Health Administration

ADAP American Dental Assistant's Program; Assistant Director of Army Psychiatry

ADAPT American Disabled for Attendant Programs Today [organization]

ADAS Alzheimer disease assessment scale

ADAS-COG cognitive portion of the Alzheimer's Disease Assessment Scale

ADase adenosine deaminase

ADAU adolescent drug abuse unit

ADB accidental death benefit

ADC adult day care [facility]; affective disorders clinic; Aid to [Families with] Dependent Children; AIDS-dementia complex; albumin, dextrose, and catalase [medium]; ambulance design criteria; analog-to-digital converter; anodal duration contraction; apparent diffusion coefficient; average daily census; axiodistocervical

AdC adenylate cyclase; adrenal cortex

ADCC acute disorder of cerebral circulation; antibody-dependent cell-mediated cytotoxicity

ADCP adenosine deaminase complexing protein

ADCS Argonz del Castillo syndrome

ADCY adenyl cyclase

ADD acceptable daily dose; adduction; adenosine deaminase; attentional deficit disorder; average daily dose

add addition; adductor, adduction; let there be added [Lat. *addatur*]

ADDH attention deficit disorder with hyperactivity

ADD/HA attention deficit disorder/hyperactivity

addict addiction, addictive

add poll adductor pollicis

ADDS American Digestive Disease Society

ADDU alcohol and drug dependence unit

ADE acute disseminated encephalitis; adverse drug event; antibody-dependent enhancement; apparent digestible energy

Ade adenine

AdeCbl adenosyl cobalamine

ADEE age-dependent epileptic encephalopathy

ADEM academic department of emergency medicine; acute disseminated encephalomyelitis

AdenCa adenocarcinoma

adeq adequate

ADF administrative determination of fault

ADFN albinism-deafness [syndrome]; albinism-deafness syndrome

ADFR activate, depress, free, repeat [coherence therapy]

ADFS alternative delivery and financing system

ADG ambulatory diagnostic group; atrial diastolic gallop; axiodistogingival

ADH Academy of Dentistry for the Handicapped; adhesion; alcohol dehydrogenase; antidiuretic hormone; arginine dihydrolase

adh adhesion, adhesive; antidiuretic hormone

ADHA American Dental Hygienists Association

ADHD attention deficit-hyperactivity disorder

ADI Academy of Dentistry International; acceptable daily intake; AIDS-defining illness; allowable daily intake; artificial diverticulum of the ileum; atlas-dens interval; axiodistoincisal

adj adjacent; adjoining; adjuvant

ADK adenosine kinase

ADKC atopic dermatitis with keratoconjunctivitis

ADL activities of daily living; Amsterdam Depression List; annual dose limit

ADLAR advanced design linear accelerator radiosurgery

ADLC antibody-dependent lymphocyte-mediated cytotoxicity

ad lib as desired [Lat. *ad libitum*]

ADM abductor digiti minimi; administrative medicine; admission; Adriamycin; Alcohol, Drug Abuse and Mental Health [grant of US Department of Health and Human Services]

AdM adrenal medulla

adm administration; admission; apply [Lat. *admove*]

Adm Dr admitting doctor

ADME [drug] absorption, distribution, metabolism, and excretion

Admin administration

Adm Ph admitting physician

ADMR average daily metabolic rate

ADMX adrenal medullectomy

ADN antideoxyribonuclease; aortic depressor nerve; associate degree in nursing

ad naus to the point of producing nausea [Lat. *ad nauseam*]

ADN-B antideoxyribonuclease B

ADO adolescent medicine; axiodistoocclusal

Ado adenosine

AdoCbl 5'-adenosylcobalamin
ADOD arthrodentosteodysplasia
AdoDABA adenosyldiaminobutyric acid
AdoHcy S-adenosylhomocysteine
adol adolescence, adolescent
AdoMet S-adenosylmethionine
Adox oxidized adenosine
ADP adenopathy; adenosine diphosphate; administrative psychiatry; approved drug product; area diastolic pressure; automatic data processing
AdP adductor pollicis
ADPase adenosine diphosphatase
ADPKD autosomal dominant polycystic kidney disease
ADPL average daily patient load
ADPR adenosine diphosphate ribose
ADPRT adenosine diphosphate ribosyltransferase
ADQ abductor digite quinte
ADR activation, depression, repetition [in bone remodeling]; adrenodoxin reductase; Adriamycin; adverse drug reaction; airway dilation reflex; alternative dispute resolution; arrested development of righting response; ataxia-deafness-retardation [syndrome]
Adr adrenalin; Adriamycin
adr adrenal, adrenalectomy
ADRA1C alpha-1C-adrenergic receptor
ADRBK beta-1-adrenergic receptor kinase
ADRBR adrenergic beta-receptor
ADRDA Alzheimer Disease and Related Disorders Association
ADRP adipose differentiation-related protein
ADS acute death syndrome; acute diarrheal syndrome; Alcohol Dependence Scale; alternative delivery system; anatomical dead space; anonymous donor's sperm; antibody deficiency syndrome; antidiuretic substance; Army Dental Service
ADSL asymmetrical digital single line

ADSS adenylsuccinate synthetase
ADT Accepted Dental Therapeutics; adenosine triphosphate; admission, discharge, transfer; agar-gel diffusion test; alternate day therapy; any, what you desire, thing (a placebo); Alzheimer-type dementia; asphyxiating thoracic dystrophy; Auditory Discrimination Test
ADTA American Dental Trade Association
ADTe anodal duration tetanus
AD&U acid dissociation and ultrafiltration
ADV adenovirus; adventitia; Aleutian disease virus; Aujeszky disease virus
Adv adenovirus
adv advanced; against [Lat. *adversum*]
ADVIRC autosomal dominant vitreoretinochoroidopathy
ADW assault with deadly weapon
A5D5W alcohol 5%, dextrose 5%, in water
ADX adrenalectomized; adrenodoxin
AE above-elbow [amputation]; acrodermatitis enteropathica; activation energy; adult erythrocyte; adverse event; aftereffect; agarose electrophoresis; air embolism; air entry; alcoholic embryopathy; anion exchange; anoxic encephalopathy; autiepileptic; antitoxic unit [Ger. *Antitoxineinheit*]; apoenzyme; aryepiglottic; atherosclerotic encephalopathy; atrial ectopic [heart beat]; avian encephalomyelitis
A+E accident and emergency [department]; analysis and evaluation
A/E above elbow [amputation]
AEA alcohol, ether, and acetone [solution]; apocrine membrane antigen
AEB acute erythroblastopenia; avian erythroblastosis
AEC ankyloblepharon, ectodermal defects, and cleft lip [syndrome]; at earliest convenience; Atomic Energy Commission

AECD allergic eczematous contact dermatitis

AED antiepileptic drug; antihidrotic ectodermal dysplasia; automatic external defibrillator

AEDP automated external defibrillator pacemaker

AEE atomic energy establishment

AEF allogenic effect factor; amyloid enhancing factor; aorto-enteric fistula

AEG air encephalography, air encephalogram; atrial electrogram

AEGIS Aid for the Elderly in Government Institutions

AEI arbitrary evolution index; atrial emptying index

AEL acute erythroleukemia

AEM Academic Emergency Medicine [journal]; analytical electron microscopy; ambulatory electrocardiographic monitoring; ataxia episodica with myokymia; avian encephalomyelitis

AEMIS Aerospace and Environmental Medicine Information System

AEMK ataxia episodica with myokymia

A-EMT advanced emergency medical technician

AEN aseptic epiphyseal necrosis

AEP acute edematous pancreatitis; artificial endocrine pancreas; auditory evoked potential; average evoked potential

AEq age equivalent

AER abduction/external rotation; acoustic evoked response; acute exertional rhabdomyolysis; agranular endoplasmic reticulum; albumin excretion rate; aldosterone excretion rate; apical ectodermal ridge; auditory evoked response; average electroencephalic response; average evoked response

AERE Atomic Energy Research Establishment

Aero Aerobacter

AERP antegrade effective refractory period; atrial effective refractory period

AERPAP antegrade effective refractory period accessory pathway

AES acetone-extracted serum; American Electroencephalographic Society; American Encephalographic Society; American Endocrine Society; American Endodontic Society; American Epidemiological Society; American Equilibration Society; anterior esophageal sensor; anti-embolic stockings; antral ethmoidal sphenoidectomy; aortic ejection sound; Auger's electron spectroscopy; auto-erythrocyte sensitization

AEST aeromedical evacuation support team

AET absorption-equivalent thickness;S-(2-aminoethyl) isothiuronium

AEV avian erythroblastosis virus

AEZ acrodermatitis enteropathica, zinc deficient

AF abnormal frequency; acid-fast; adult female; afebrile; aflatoxin; albumin-free; albumose-free; aldehyde fuchsin; amaurosis fugax; aminophylline; amniotic fluid; angiogenesis factor; anteflexion; anterior fontanelle; antibody-forming; anti-fog; aortic flow; Arthritis Foundation; artificial feeding; ascitic fluid; atrial fibrillation; atrial flutter; atrial fusion; attenuation factor; attributable fraction; audio frequency

aF abfarad

af audio frequency

AFA acromegaloid facial syndrome; advanced first aid; alcohol-formaldehyde-acetic [fixative]

AFAFP amniotic fluid alpha-fetoprotein

AFAR American Foundation for Aging Research

AFB acid-fast bacillus; aflatoxin B; air fluidized bed; aortofemoral bypass

AFBG aortofemoral bypass graft

AFC adult foster care; antibody-forming cell
AFCI acute focal cerebral ischemia
AFCR American Federation for Clinical Research
AFD accelerated freeze drying; acrofacial dysostosis
AFDC Aid to Families with Dependent Children
AFDH American Fund for Dental Health
AFDW ash-free dry weight
AFE amniotic fluid embolism
afeb afebrile
AFF atrial fibrillation; atrial filling fraction; atrial flutter
aff afferent
AFFN acrofrontofacionasal [dysostosis]
AFG aflatoxin G; amniotic fluid glucose
aFGF acidic fibroblast growth factor
AFH angiofollicular hyperplasia; anterior facial height
AFI amaurotic familial idiocy
AFib atrial fibrillation
AFIP Armed Forces Institute of Pathology
AFIS amniotic fluid infection syndrome
AFL antifibrinolysin; artificial limb; atrial flutter
AFLNH angiofollicular lymph node hyperplasia
AFLP acute fatty liver of pregnancy
AFM aflatoxin M; after fatty meal; American Federation of Musicians
AFMA automated fabrication of modality aids
AFN afunctional neutrophil
AFNC Air Force Nurse Corps
AFND acute febrile neutrophilic dermatosis
AFO ankle/foot orthotic [brace or cast]; ankle-foot orthosis
AFORMED alternating failure of response, mechanical, [to] electrical depolarization

AFP alpha-fetoprotein; anterior faucial pillar; atypical facial pain
AFPP acute fibropurulent pneumonia
AFQ aflatoxin Q
AFR aqueous flare response; ascorbic free radical
AFRAX autism-fragile X [syndrome]
AFRD acute febrile respiratory disease
AFRI acute febrile respiratory illness
AFS acquired or adult Fanconi syndrome; alternative financing system; American Fertility Society; antifibroblast serum
AFSAM Air Force School of Aviation Medicine
AFSCME American Federation of State, County and Municipal Employees
AFSP acute fibrinoserous pneumonia
AFT aflatoxin; agglutination-flocculation test
AFTA American Family Therapy Association
AFTN autonomously functioning thyroid nodule
AFV amniotic fluid volume; aortic flow velocity
AG abdominal girth; agarose; aminoglutethimide; analytical grade; anion gap; antigen; antiglobulin; antigravity; atrial gallop; attached gingiva; axiogingival; azurophilic granule
AG, A/G albumin-globulin [ratio]
Ag antigen; silver [Lat. *argentum*]
ag antigen
AGA accelerated growth area; allergic granulomatosis and angiitis; American Gastroenterological Association; American Genetic Association; American Geriatrics Association; American Goiter Association; anti-IgG autoantibody; anti-glomerular antibody; appropriate for gestational age
Ag-Ab antigen-antibody complex
AGAG acidic glycosaminoglycans
AGBAD Alexander Graham Bell Association for the Deaf

AGC absolute granulocyte count; automatic gain control

AGCT antiglobulin consumption test; Army General Classification Test

AGD agar gel diffusion; agarose diffusion; alpha-ketoglutarate dehydrogenase

AGDD agar gel double diffusion

AGE acrylamide gel; acute gastroenteritis; advanced glycation end product; agarose gel electrophoresis; angle of greatest extension; arterial gas embolism

AGED automated general experimental device

AGEPC acetyl glyceryl ether phosphorylcholine

AGF adrenal growth factor; angle of greatest flexion

AGG agammaglobulinemia

agg agglutination; aggravation; aggregation

aggl, agglut agglutination

aggrav aggravated, aggravation

aggreg aggregated, aggregation

AGGS anti-gas gangrene serum

AGI adjusted gross income

agit agitated, agitation; shake [Lat. *agita*]

AGL acute granulocytic leukemia; agglutination; aminoglutethimide

AGMK African green monkey kidney [cell]

AGMkK African green monkey kidney [cell]

AGN acute glomerulonephritis; agnosia

VIII$_{AGN}$ factor VIII antigen

agn agnosia

AgNOR silver-staining nucleolar organizer region

AGOS American Gynecological and Obstetrical Society

AGP acid glycoprotein; agar gel precipitation; azurophil granule protein

AGPA American Group Practice Association; American Group Psychotherapy Association

AGPI agar gel precipitin inhibition

AGPT agar-gel precipitation test

AGR aniridia, genitourinary abnormalities, and mental retardation; anticipatory goal response

agri agriculture

AGS adrenogenital syndrome; Alagille syndrome; American Geriatrics Society; audiogenic seizures

AGT abnormal glucose tolerance; activity group therapy; acute generalized tuberculosis; angiotensin; antiglobulin test

agt agent

AGTH adrenoglomerulotropic hormone

AGTr adrenoglomerulotropin

AGTT abnormal glucose tolerance test

AGU aspartylglucosaminuria

AGV aniline gentian violet

AH abdominal hysterectomy; absorptive hypercalciuria; accidental hypothermia; acetohexamide; acid hydrolysis; acute hepatitis; adrenal hypoplasia; after hyperpolarization; agnathia-holoprosencephaly; alcoholic hepatitis; amenorrhea and hirsutism; aminohippurate; anterior hypothalamus; antihyaluronidase; arcuate hypothalamus; Army Hospital; arterial hypertension; artificial heart; ascites hepatoma; astigmatic hypermetropia; ataxic hemiparesis; autoimmune hepatitis; autonomic hyperreflexia; axillary hair

A/H amenorrhea-hyperprolactinemia

A + H accident & health [policy]

A·h ampere hour

aH abhenry

ah hyperopic astigmatism

AHA acetohydroxamic acid; acquired hemolytic anemia; acute hemolytic anemia; American Heart Association; American Hospital Association; anterior hypothalamic area; anti-heart antibody; antihistone antibody; area health authority; arthritis-hives-angioedema [syndrome]; aspartyl-hydroxamic acid; Associate, Institute of Hospital Administrators; autoimmune hemolytic anemia

AHB alpha-hydroxybutyric acid

AHC academic health care; academic health center; acute hemorrhagic conjunctivitis; acute hemorrhagic cystitis; antihemophilic factor C

AHCA Agency for Health Care Administration; American Health Care Association

AHCD acquired hepatocellular degeneration

AHCPR Agency for Health Care Policy and Research

AHCy adenosyl homocysteine

AHD acquired hepatocerebral degeneration; acute heart disease; antihyaluronidase; antihypertensive drug; arteriohepatic dysplasia; arteriosclerotic heart disease; atherosclerotic heart disease; autoimmune hemolytic disease

AHDMS automated hospital data management system

AHDP azacycloheptane diphosphonate

AHDS Allan-Herndon-Dudley syndrome

AHE acute hazardous events [database]; acute hemorrhagic encephalomyelitis

AHEA area health education activity

AHEC area health education center

AHES artificial heart energy system

AHF acute heart failure; American Health Foundation; American Hepatic Foundation; American Hospital Formulary; antihemolytic factor; antihemophilic factor; Argentinian hemorrhagic fever; Associated Health Foundation

AHFS American Hospital Formulary Service

AHG aggregated human globulin; antihemophilic globulin; antihuman globulin

AHGG antihuman gammaglobulin; aggregated human gammaglobulin

AHGS acute herpetic gingival stomatitis

AHH alpha-hydrazine analog of histidine; anosmia and hypogonadotropic hypogonadism [syndrome]; arylhydro-

carbon hydroxylase; Association for Holistic Health

AHI active hostility index; Animal Health Institute; apnea-plus-hypopnea index

AHIMA American Health Information Management Association

AHIP assisted health insurance plan

AHIS automated hospital information system

AHJ artificial hip joint

AHL apparent half-life

AHLE acute hemorrhagic leukoencephalitis

AHLG antihuman lymphocyte globulin

AHLS antihuman lymphocyte serum

AHM Allied health manpower; ambulatory Holter monitor

AHMA American Holistic Medicine Association; antiheart muscle autoantibody

AHMC Association of Hospital Management Committees

AHMC Association of Hospital Management Committees

AHN Army Head Nurse; assistant head nurse

AHO Albright hereditary osteodystrophy

AHP accountable health plan or partnership; acute hemorrhagic pancreatitis; after hyperpolarization; air at high pressure; analytic hierarchy process; approved health plan; Assistant House Physician

AHPA American Health Planning Association

AHPO anterior hypothalamic preoptic [area]

AHR antihyaluronidase reaction; Association for Health Records; atrial heart rate

AHRA American Hospital Radiology Administration

AHRF acute hypoxemic respiratory failure; American Hearing Research Foundation

AHS Academy of Health Sciences; African horse sickness; alveolar hypoventilation syndrome; American Hearing Society; American Hospital Society; area health service; assistant house surgeon

AHSA American Health Security Act

AHSDF area health service development fund

AHSG alpha-2HS-glycoprotein

AHSN Assembly of Hospital Schools of Nursing

AHSP AIDS Health Services Program [of the Robert Wood Johnson Foundation]

AHSR Association for Health Services Research

AHT aggregation half time; antihyaluronidase titer; augmented histamine test; autogenous hamster tumor

AHTG antihuman thymocyte globulin

AHTP antihuman thymocyte plasma

AHTS antihuman thymus serum

AHU acute hemolytic uremic [syndrome]; arginine, hypoxanthine, and uracil

AHuG aggregated human IgG

AHV avian herpes virus

AI accidental injury; accidentally incurred; adiposity index; aggregation index; allergy and immunology; amylogenesis imperfecta; anaphylatoxin inactivator; angiogenesis inhibitor; angiotensin I; anxiety index; aortic incompetence; aortic insufficiency; apical impulse; articulation index; artificial insemination; artificial intelligence; atherogenic index; atrial insufficiency; autoimmune, autoimmunity; axio-incisal; first meiotic anaphase

A&I allergy and immunology

aI active ingredient

AIA allylisopropylacetamide; amylase inhibitor activity; anti-immunoglobulin antibody; anti-insulin antibody; aspirin-induced asthma; automated image analysis

AIB aminoisobutyrate; avian infectious bronchitis

AIBA aminoisobutyric acid

AIBS American Institute of Biological Sciences

AIC Akaike's information criterion [a goodness-of-fit measure]; aminoimidazole carboxamide; Association des Infirmières Canadiennes

A-IC average integrated concentration

AICA anterior inferior cerebellar artery; anterior inferior communicating artery

AI-CAH autoimmune-type chronic active hepatitis

AICAR aminoimidazole carboxamide ribonucleotide

AICD automatic implantable cardioverter defibrillator

AICE angiotensin I converting enzyme

AICF autoimmune complement fixation

AI/COAG artificial intelligence hemostasis consultant system

AID acquired immunodeficiency disease; acute infectious disease; acute ionization detector; Agency for International Development; argon ionization detector; artificial insemination by donor; autoimmune deficiency; autoimmune disease; automatic implantable defibrillator; average interocular difference

AIDP acute idiopathic demyelinating polyneuropathy

AIDS acquired immune deficiency syndrome

AIDSDRUGS clinical trials of acquired immunodeficiency drugs [MEDLARS data base]

AIDS-KS acquired immune deficiency syndrome with Kaposi's sarcoma

AIDSLINE on-line information on acquired immunodeficiency syndrome [MEDLARS data base]

AIDSTRIALS clinical trials of acquired immunodeficiency syndrome drugs [MEDLARS data base]

AIE acute inclusion-body encephalitis; acute infectious encephalitis; acute infective endocarditis

AIEP amount of insulin extractable from pancreas

AIF anemia-inducing factor; anti-inflammatory; anti-invasion factor

AIFD acute intrapartum fetal distress

AIG anti-immunoglobulin

AIH amelogenesis imperfecta, hypomaturation type; American Institute of Homeopathy; artificial insemination, homologous; artificial insemination by husband

AIHA American Industrial Hygiene Association; autoimmune hemolytic anemia

AIHC American Industrial Health Conference

AIHD acquired immune hemolytic disease

AII acute intestinal infection; second meiotic anaphase

AIIS anterior inferior iliac spine

AIIT amiodarone-iodine-induced thyrotoxicosis

AIL acute infectious lymphocytosis; angiocentric immunoproliferative lesion; angioimmunoblastic lymphadenopathy

AILD alveolar interstitial lung disease; angioimmunoblastic lymphadenopathy

AIM Abridged Index Medicus; acute transverse myelopathy; area of interest magnification; artificial intelligence in medicine

AIMD abnormal involuntary movement disorder

AIMS abnormal involuntary movement scale; aid for the impaired medical student; arthritis impact measurement scale

AIN acute interstitial nephritis; American Institute of Nutrition; anterior interosseous nerve

AINA automated immunonephelometric assay

AINS anti-inflammatory nonsteroidal

AION anterior ischemic optic neuropathy

AIOS acute illness observation scale

AIP acute idiopathic pericarditis; acute infectious polyneuritis; acute intermittent porphyria; aldosterone-induced protein; automated immunoprecipitation; average intravascular pressure; integral anatuberculin, Petragnani

AIPE acute interstitial pulmonary emphysema; alcoholism intervention performance evaluation

AIPFP acute idiopathic peripheral facial nerve palsy

AIPS American Institute of Pathologic Science

AIR amino-imidazole ribonucleotide; average impairment rating

AIRA anti-insulin receptor antibody

AIRE Acute Infarction Ramipril Efficacy [trial]

AIRF alterations in respiratory function

AI/RHEUM artificial intelligence rheumatology consultant system

AIRS Amphetamine Interview Rating Scale

AIS Abbreviated Injury Scale; amniotic infection syndrome; androgen insensitivity syndrome; anterior interosseous nerve syndrome; anti-insulin serum; automotive injury score

AISA acquired idiopathic sideroblastic anemia

AIS/MR Alternative Intermediate Services for the Mentally Retarded

AIT acute intensive treatment

AITP autoimmune idiopathic thrombocytopenic purpura

AITT arginine insulin tolerance test; augmented insulin tolerance test

AIU absolute iodine uptake; antigen-inducing unit

AIUM American Institute of Ultrasound in Medicine

AIVR accelerated idioventricular rhythm

AIVV anterior informal vertebral vein

AJ, A/J ankle jerk

AJCC American Joint Commission for Cancer

AJCCS American Joint Committee on Cancer Staging

AJDL arteriojugular venous lactate content difference

AJDO₂ arteriojugular venous oxygen content difference

AJR abdominojugular reflux maneuver

AJS acute joint syndrome

AK above knee; acetate kinase; adenosine kinase; adenylate kinase; artificial kidney

A/K, ak above knee [amputation]

A→K ankle to knee

AKA above-knee amputation; alcoholic ketoacidosis; also known as; antikeratin antibody

aka also known as

AK amp above-knee amputation

AKE acrokeratoelastoidosis

A/kg amperes per kilogram

AKP alkaline phosphatase

AKS alcoholic Korsakoff syndrome; auditory and kinesthetic sensation

AKU alkaptonuria

AL absolute latency; acinar lumen; acute leukemia; adaptation level; albumin; alcoholism [and other drug dependence services]; alignment; amyloid L; amyloidosis; anterior leaflet; antihuman lymphocytic [globulin]; avian leukosis; axial length; axillary loop; axiolingual; left ear [Lat. *auris laeva*]

A_L angiographic area of lateral projection

Al allantoic; allergic, allergy; aluminum

al left ear [Lat. *auris laeva*]

ALA American Laryngological Association; American Lung Association; aminolevulinic acid; axiolabial

ALa axiolabial

Ala alanine

AL-Ab antilymphocyte antibody

ALAD abnormal left axis deviation

ALAD, ALA-D aminolevulinic acid dehydrase

ALADH delta-aminolevulinate dehydratase

ALAG, ALaG axiolabiogingival

A-LAK adherent lymphokine-activated killer [cell]

ALAL, ALaL axiolabiolingual

A_LAO angiographic area of left anterior oblique projection

AlaP, ala-P alafosfalin

ALARA as low as reasonably achievable [radiation exposure]

ALARM adjustable leg and ankle repositioning mechanism

ALAS delta-aminolevulinate synthase

ALASH delta-aminolevulinate synthase, housekeeping type

ALAT alanine aminotransferase

ALB albumin; avian lymphoblastosis

alb albumin; white [Lat. *albus*]

ALBC albumin clearance

ALB/GLOB albumin/globulin [ratio]

ALC absolute lymphocyte count; acute lethal catatonia; aided living center; Alternative Lifestyle Checklist; approximate lethal concentration; avian leukosis complex; axiolinguocervical

alc alcohol, alcoholism, alcoholic

ALCA anomalous left coronary artery

ALCAPA anomalous origin of left coronary artery from pulmonary artery

ALCAR acetyl-L-carnitine

ALCEQ Adolescent Life Change Event Questionnaire

alcoh alcohol, alcoholic, alcoholism

AlcR, alcR alcohol rub

AlCr aluminum crown

ALD adrenoleukodystrophy; alcoholic liver disease; aldolase; anterior latissimus dorsi; Appraisal of Language Disturbance; assistive listening device

Ald aldolase
ALDA aldolase A
ALDB aldolase B
ALDC aldolase C
ALDH aldehyde dehydrogenase
Aldo, ALDOST aldosterone
ALDOA aldolase A
ALDOC aldolase C
ALDP adrenoleukodystrophy protein
ALDR aldose reductase
ALDS albinism-deafness syndrome
ALE active life expectancy; allowable limits of error; amputated lower extremity
ALEC artificial lung-expanding compound
ALEP atypical lymphoepithelioid cell proliferation
ALF acute liver failure; American Liver Foundation; assisted living facilities
ALFT abnormal liver function test
ALG antilymphocytic globulin; axiolinguogingival
alg allergy
ALGOL algorithmic oriented language
ALH angiolymphoid hyperplasia; anterior lobe hormone; anterior lobe of hypophysis
ALHE angiolymphoid hyperplasia with eosinophilia
ALI acute lung injury; annual limit of intake; average lobe index
ALIP abnormal localized immature mye-loid precursor
ALK, alk alkaline; alkylating
ALK-P alkaline phosphatase
ALL acute lymphoblastic leukemia; acute lymphocytic leukemia
all allergy, allergic
ALLHAT Antihypertensive and Lipid Lowering Treatment to Prevent Heart Attack Trial
ALLA acute lymphocytic leukemia antigen
ALLO atypical *Legionella*-like organism

ALM aerial lentiginous melanoma; alveolar living material
ALME acetyl-lysine methyl ester
ALMI anterior lateral myocardial infarct
ALMV anterior leaflet of the mitral valve
ALN allylnitrile; anterior lymph node
ALO average lymphocyte output; axiolinguo-occlusal
ALOS average length of stay
ALOSH Appalachian Laboratory for Occupational Safety and Health
ALOX aluminum oxide
ALP acute leukemia protocol; acute lupus pericarditis; alkaline phosphatase; alveolar proteinosis; anterior lobe of pituitary; antileukoproteinase; antilymphocytic plasma; argon laser photocoagulation
AlPase alkaline phosphatase
ALPG alkaline phosphatase, germ-cell
α Greek letter alpha; angular acceleration; first [carbon atom next to the carbon atom bearing the active group in organic compounds]; optical rotation; probability of type I error; solubility coefficient
alpha$_2$-AP alpha 2-antiplasmin
alpha-GLUC alpha-glucosidase
alpha$_2$M alpha$_2$-macroglobulin
ALPL alkaline phosphatase, liver
ALPP alkaline phosphatase, placental
ALPPL alkaline phosphatase-like, placental
ALPS angiolymphoproliferative syndrome; Aphasia Language Performance Scale; attitudinal listening profile system
ALR aldehyde reductase
ALRI anterolateral rotatory instability
ALROS American Laryngological, Rhinological, and Otological Society
ALS acute lateral sclerosis; advanced life support; afferent loop syndrome; amyotrophic lateral sclerosis; angiotensin-like

substance; anterolateral sclerosis; anticipated life span; antilymphocyte serum

ALSD Alzheimer-like senile dementia

ALS-PD amyotrophic lateral sclerosis-parkinsonism-dementia [complex]

AL-SV avian leukosis sarcoma virus

ALT alanine aminotransferase; argon laser trabeculoplasty; avian laryngotracheitis

Alt, alt aluminum tartrate; alternate; altitude

AlT aluminum tartrate

ALTB acute laryngotracheobronchitis

ALTE apparent life-threatening event

ALTEE acetyl-*L*-tyrosine ethyl ester

ALTS acute lumbar traumatic sprain [or syndrome]

ALU arithmetic and logic unit

ALV Abelson leukemia virus; adeno-like virus; alveolar, alveolus; ascending lumbar vein; avian leukosis virus

Alv alveolus, alveolar

ALVAD abdominal left ventricular assist device

ALVF acute left ventricular failure

ALV M alveolar mucosa

ALVT aortic and left ventricular tunnel

alv vent alveolar ventilation

ALVX alveolectomy

ALW arch-loop whorl

ALWMI anterolateral wall myocardial infarct

AM Academic Medicine [journal]; actomyosin; acute myelofibrosis; adult male; adult monocyte; aerospace medicine; akinetic mutism; alveolar macrophage; alveolar mucosa; amacrine cell; ambulatory; amethopterin; ametropia; ammeter; amperemeter; ampicillin; amplitude modulation; amyl; anovular menstruation; arithmetic mean; arousal mechanism; articular manipulation; aviation medicine; axiomesial; before noon [Lat. *ante meridiem*]; Master of Arts [Lat. *artium magister*]; meter angle; myopic astigmatism

Am americium; amnion; amyl

A/m amperes per meter

A-m² ampere-square meter

am ametropia; amyl; amplitude; before noon [Lat. *ante meridiem*]; meter angle; myopic astigmatism

AMA against medical advice; alkaline membrane assay; American Management Association; American Medical Association; antimitochondrial antibody; antimyosin antibody; antithyroid microsomal antibody; arm muscle area; Australian Medical Association

AMA-DE American Medical Association Drug Evaluation

AMAL Aero-Medical Acceleration Laboratory

AMAP as much as possible

A-MAT amorphous material

AMB avian myeloblastosis; amphotericin B; anomalous muscle bundle

Amb ambulance; ambulatory, ambulation

amb ambient; ambiguous; ambulance; ambulatory

AMBER advanced multiple-beam equalization radiography

ambig ambiguous

AMBL acute megakaryoblastic leukemia

AMbL acute myeloblastic leukemia

ambul ambulatory

AMC academic medical center; acetylmethyl carbinol; Animal Medical Center; antibody-mediated cytotoxicity; antimalaria campaign; arm muscle circumference; Army Medical Corps; arthrogryposis multiplex congenita; ataxia-microcephaly-retardation [syndrome]; automated mixture control; axiomesiocervical

AMCAS American Medical College Application Service

AMCHA aminomethylcyclohexanecarboxylic acid

AMCN anteromedial caudate nucleus

AMCRA American Managed Care and Review Association

AMD acid maltase deficiency; acromandibular dysplasia; actinomycin D; adrenomyelodystrophy; age-related macular degeneration; Aleutian mink disease; alpha-methyldopa; Association for Macular Diseases; axiomesiodistal; S-adenosylmethionine decarboxylase

AMDGF alveolar macrophage-derived growth factor

AMDS Association of Military Dental Surgeons

AME amphotericin methyl ester; apparent minerallocorticoid excess; aseptic meningoencephalitis

AMEA American Medical Electroencephalographic Association

AMEAE acute monophasic experimental autoimmune encephalomyelitis

AMEDS Army Medical Service

AMEGL, AMegL acute megakaryoblastic leukemia

AMet adenosyl-*L*-methionine

AMF antimuscle factor

AMFAR American Foundation for AIDS Research

AMG amyloglucosidase; antimacrophage globulin; axiomesiogingival

A₂MG alpha-2-macroglobulin

AMH Accreditation Manual for Hospitals; anti-müllerian hormone; automated medical history

Amh mixed astigmatism with myopia predominating

AMHA Association of Mental Health Administrators

AMHT automated multiphasic health testing

AMI acquired monosaccharide intolerance; acute myocardial infarction; amitriptyline; anterior myocardial infarction; Association of Medical Illustrators; Athletic Motivation Inventory; axiomesioincisal

AMIA American Medical Informatics Association

AMKL acute megakaryoblastic leukemia

AML acute monocytic leukemia; acute mucosal lesion; acute myeloblastic leukemia; acute myelocytic leukemia; acute myelogenous leukemia; anatomic medullary locking; angiomyolipoma; anterior mitral leaflet; automated multitest laboratory

AMLB alternate monoaural loudness balance

AMLC adherent macrophage-like cell; autologous mixed lymphocyte culture

AMLR autologous mixed lymphocyte reaction

AMLS antimouse lymphocyte serum

AMLSGA acute myeloblastic leukemia surface glycoprotein antigen

AMM agnogenic myeloid metaplasia; ammonia; antibody to murine cardiac myosin; World Medical Association [Fr. *Association Médicale Mondiale*]

amm, ammonia

AMML acute myelomonocytic leukemia

AMMoL acute myelomonoblastic leukemia

ammon ammonia

AMN adrenomyeloneuropathy; alloxazine mononucleotide; aminonucleoside; anterior median nucleus

AMNS aminonucleoside

AMO assistant medical officer; axiomesio-occlusal

A-mode amplitude mode; amplitude modulation

AMOG adhesion molecule on glia

AMOL acute monoblastic leukemia

amo, amor amorphous

AMP accelerated mental processes; acid mucopolysaccharide; adenosine monophosphate; amphetamine; ampicillin; ampule; amputation; average mean pressure

amp ampere; amplification; ampule; amputation, amputee

AMPA alpha-amino-3-hydroxy-5-methyl-4-isoxazolepropionate; American Medical Publishers Association

AMPAC American Medical Political Action Committee

AMP-c cyclic adenosine monophosphate

AMPH, amphet amphetamine

amp-hr ampere-hour

ampl large [Lat. *amplus*]

AMPLE allergies, medications, past medical history, last meal, events preceding present condition

A-M pr Austin-Moore prosthesis

AMPS abnormal mucopolysacchariduria; acid mucopolysaccharide

AMPT alpha-methylparatyrosine

ampul ampule

AMR acoustic muscle reflex; activity metabolic rate; acute mitral stenosis; alopecia-mental retardation [syndrome]; alternate motion rate; alternating motion reflex

AMRA American Medical Record Association

AMRF American Medical Resources Foundation

AMRI anteromedial rotatory instability

AMRL Aerospace Medical Research Laboratories

AMRNL Army Medical Research and Nutrition Laboratory

AMRS automated medical record system

AMS ablepharon-microstomia syndrome; acute mountain sickness; adenosylmethionine synthetase; aggravated in military service; altered mental status; American Microscopical Society; amount of substance; amylase; antimacrophage serum; Army Medical Service; aseptic meningitis syndrome; Association of Military Surgeons; auditory memory span; automated multiphasic screening

ams amount of a substance

AMSA acridinylamine methanesulfon-m-anisidide; American Medical Society on Alcoholism; American Medical Students Association; amsacrine

AMSAODD American Medical Society on Alcoholism and Other Drug Dependencies

AMSC Army Medical Specialist Corps

AMSP Association of Medical School Pharmacology

AMSRDC Army Medical Service Research and Development Command

AMSU ambulatory minor surgery unit

AMT acute miliary tuberculosis; alpha-methyltyrosine; American Medical Technologists; amethopterin; amitriptyline; amphetamine; anxiety management training

amt amount

AMU Army Medical Unit

amu atomic mass unit

AmuLV Abelson murine leukemia virus; amphotrophic murine leukemia virus

AMV assisted mechanical ventilation; avian myeloblastosis virus

AMVI acute mesenteric vascular insufficiency

aMVL anterior mitral valve leaflet

AMWA American Medical Women's Association; American Medical Writers' Association

AMX amoxicillin

AMY, amy amylase

AN acanthosis nigricans; acne neonatorum; acoustic neuroma; adult, normal; ala nasi; amyl nitrate; aneurysm; anisometropia; anode; anorexia nervosa; antenatal; anterior; antineuraminidase; aseptic necrosis; atmosphere normal; atrionodal; autonomic neuropathy; avascular necrosis

A/N antenatal; as needed

An actinon; anisometropia; anode, anodal; atmosphere normal

A$_n$ atmosphere normal

ANA acetylneuraminic acid; American Narcolepsy Association; American Neurological Association; American Nurses Association; anesthesia [*anaesthesia*]; antibody to nuclear antigens; antinuclear antibody; aspartyl naphthylamide

Ana anaplastic

ANAD anorexia nervosa with associated disorders

ANAE alpha-naphthyl acetate esterase

anal analgesia, analgesic; analysis, analytic

ANAG acute narrow angle glaucoma

ANAL, anal analgesia, analgesic; analysis, analytic

ANAP agglutination negative, absorption positive [reaction]

ANAS anastomosis; auditory nerve activating substance

anast anastomosis

Anat, anat anatomy, anatomist

ANB avascular necrosis of bone

ANC absolute neutrophil count; acid neutralization capacity; antigen-neutralizing capacity; Army Nurse Corps

ANCA antineutrophil cytoplasm antibody

ANCC, AnCC anodal closure contraction

ANCOVA analysis of covariance

AND algoneurodystrophy; anterior nasal discharge

ANDA Abbreviated New Drug Application

ANDRO, andro androsterone

ANDTE, AnDTe anodal duration tetanus

anes, anesth anesthesia, anesthetic

ANESR apparent norepinephrine secretion rate

AnEx, an ex anodal excitation

ANF alpha-naphthoflavone; American Nurses' Foundation; antineuritic factor; antinuclear factor; atrial natriuretic factor

ANG angiogenin; angiogram; angiography; angiotension

ang angiogram; angiography, angle, angular

Ang GR angiotensin generation rate

Angio angiography, angiogram, angiographic

ang pect angina pectoris

ANH academic nursing home

anh anhydrous

ANI acute nerve irritation

ANIA automated nephelometric immunoassay

ANIS Anorexia Nervosa Inventory for Self-rating

aniso anisocytosis

ANIT alpha-naphthyl-isothiocyanate

ANK, Ank ankyrin

ank ankle

ANL acute nonlymphoblastic leukemia

ANLI antibody-negative with latent infection

ANLL acute nonlymphocytic leukemia

ANN artificial neural network

Ann annual

ann fib annulus fibrosus

ANOC, AnOC anodal opening contraction

ANOCL anodal opening clonus

ANOP anophthalmia

ANOV, ANOVA analysis of variance

ANP acute necrotizing pancreatitis; adult nurse practitioner; ancillary nursing personnel; A-norprogesterone; atrial natriuretic peptide

A-NPP absorbed normal pooled plasma

ANRC American National Red Cross

ANRL antihypertensive neutral renomedullary lipid

ANS acanthion; American Nutrition Society; 8-anilino-1-naphthalene-sulfonic acid; anterior nasal spine; antineutrophilic serum; antirat neutrophil serum; Army Nursing Service; arterionephrosclerosis; Associate in Nursing Science; autonomic nervous system

ANSCII American National Standard Code for Information Interchange

ANSI American National Standards Institute

ANSWER Agency for Toxic Substances and Disease Registry/National Library of Medicine's Workstation for Emergency Response

ANT acoustic noise test; adenine nucleotide translocator; aminonitrothiazole; anterior

ant anterior; antimycin

ANT3Y adenine nucleotide translocator 3 Y

AntA antimycin A

antag antagonist

anti-HB$_c$ antibody to hepatitis B core antigen

anti-HB$_e$ antibody to hepatitis B early antigen

anti-HB$_s$ antibody to hepatitis B surface antigen

anti-PNM Ab anti-peripheral nerve myelin antibody

ANTR apparent net transfer rate

ANTU alpha-naphthylthiourea

ANuA antinuclear antibody

ANUG acute necrotizing ulcerative gingivitis

ANV avian nephritis virus

ANX annexin

anx anxiety

AO abdominal aorta; achievement orientation; acid output; acridine orange; ankle orthosis; anodal opening; anterior oblique; aorta; aortic opening; atelosteogenesis; atomic orbital; atrioventricular valve opening; average optical [density]; axio-occlusal

Ao aorta

A$_o$ orifice area

A&O, A/O alert and oriented

AOA Administration on Aging; Alpha Omega Alpha Honor Society; American Optometric Association; American Orthopedic Association; American Orthopsychiatric Association; American Osteopathic Association

AOAA amino-oxyacetic acid

AOAC Association of Official Agricultural Chemists

AOAP as often as possible

AoArE aortic arch epinephrine

AOAS American Osteopathic Academy of Sclerotherapy

AOB accessory olfactory bulb; alcohol on breath

AOBS acute organic brain syndrome

AOC abridged ocular chart; amyloxycarbonyl; anodal opening contraction; area of concern

AOCA American Osteopathic College of Anesthesiologists

AOCD American Osteopathic College of Dermatology

AOCl anodal opening clonus

AOCN advanced oncology certified nurse

AOCPA American Osteopathic College of Pathologists

AOCPR American Osteopathic College of Proctology

AOCR American Osteopathic College of Radiology; American Osteopathic College of Rheumatology

AOD Academy of Operative Dentistry; Academy of Oral Dynamics; adult onset diabetes; anesthesiologist-on-duty; arterial oxygen desaturation; arteriosclerotic occlusive disease; auriculo-osteodysplasia

AODM adult onset diabetes mellitus

AODME Academy of Osteopathic Directors of Medical Education

AODP alcohol and other drug problems

AOE admission order entry

AoE aortic epinephrine

AOHA American Osteopathic Hospital Association

AOIVM angiographically occult intracranial vascular malformation

AOL acro-osteolysis

AOM acute otitis media; alternatives of management; arthroophthalmopathy; azoxymethane

AOMA American Occupational Medical Association

AOMP, AoMP aortic mean pressure

AOO anodal opening odor; atrial asynchronous (competitive, fixed-rate) [pacemaker]

AOP anodal opening picture; aortic pressure

AoP aortic pressure

AOPA American Orthotics and Prosthetics Association

AOPC adult outpatient psychotherapy clinic

AOPW, AoPW aortic posterior wall

AOR Alvarado Orthopedic Research [instruments]; auditory oculogyric reflex

AORN Association of Operating Room Nurses

AOS American Ophthalmological Society; American Otological Society; anodal opening sound; anterior [o]esophageal sensor

AOSSM American Orthopedic Society for Sports Medicine

AOT accessory optic tract; Anderson Olsson table; anodal opening tetanus; Association of Occupational Therapists

AOTA American Occupational Therapy Association

AOTe anodal opening tetanus

AOTF American Occupational Therapy Foundation

AOU apparent oxygen utilization

AOV, AoV aortic valve

AP accessory pathway; accounts payable; acid phosphatase; acinar parenchyma; action potential; active pepsin; acute pancreatitis; acute phase; acute pneumonia; acute proliferative; adenomatous polyposis; adolescent psychiatry; alkaline phosphatase; alum precipitated; aminopeptidase; aminopurine; amyloid P-component; angina pectoris; antepartal [Lat. *ante partum*]; anterior pituitary; anteroposterior; antidromic potential; antipyrine; antral peristalsis; aortic pressure; aortopulmonary; apical pulse; apothecary; appendectomy; appendicitis; appendix; apurinic acid; area postrema; arithmetic progression; arterial pressure; artificial pneumothorax; aspiration pneumonia; assessment and plans; association period; atherosclerotic plaque; atrial pacing; atrioventricular pathway; axiopulpal; before parturition [Lat. *ante partum*]

A-P anteroposterior

A/P abdominal/perineal; antepartum; ascites/plasma [ratio]

A&P anterior and posterior; assessment and plans; auscultation and percussion

Ap apex

ap anteroposterior; attachment point

APA action potential amplitude; aldosterone-producing adenoma; Ambulatory Pediatric Association; American Pancreatic Association; American Pharmaceutic Association; American Physiotherapy Association; American Podiatric Association; American Psychiatric Association; American Psychoanalytic Association; American Psychological Association; American Psychopathological Association; American Psychotherapy Association; aminopenicillanic acid; anterior margin of pulmonary artery; antipernicious anemia [factor]; antiphospholipid antibody; antiproliferative antibody; arcuate premotor area

APAAP alkaline phosphatase-antialkaline phosphatase [labeling]

APAB antiphospholipid antibody

APACHE Acute Physiology and Chronic Health Evaluation [severity-of-illness index]

APAF antipernicious anemia factor

APAP acetaminophen

APB abductor pollicis brevis; atrial premature beat

APBD adult polyglucosan body disease

APC acetylsalicylic acid, phenacetin, and caffeine; activated protein C; adenoidal-pharyngeal-conjunctival [agent]; adenomatous polyposis coli; all-purpose capsule; antigen-presenting cell; antiphlogistic corticoid; aperture current; apneustic center; aspirin-phenacetin-caffeine; atrial premature contraction

APCC aspirin-phenacetin-caffeine-codeine

APCD acquired prothrombin complex deficiency [syndrome]; adult polycystic kidney disease

APCF acute pharyngoconjunctival fever

APCG apex cardiogram

Ap4CH apical four-chamber plane

APCKD adult-type polycystic kidney disease

APD action potential duration; acute polycystic disease; advanced physical diagnosis; anteroposterior diameter; antipsychotic drug; atrial premature depolarization; autoimmune progesterone dermatitis; automated peritoneal dialysis

A-PD anteroposterior diameter

APDER anterior-posterior dual energy radiography

APDI Adult Personal Data Inventory

APDIM Association of Program Directors in Internal Medicine

APE acetone powder extract; acute polioencephalitis; acute psychotic episode; airway pressure excursion; aminophylline, phenobarbital, and ephedrine; anterior pituitary extract; asthma of physical effort; avian pneumoencephalitis

APECED autoimmune polyendocrinopathy-candidosis-ectodermal dystrophy

APF acidulated phosphofluoride; American Psychological Foundation; anabolism-promoting factor; animal protein factor; antiperinuclear factor

APG acid-precipitated globulin; ambulatory patient group; animal pituitary gonadotropin; antegrade pyelography

APGAR American Pediatric Gross Assessment Record

APGL alkaline phosphatase activity of granular leukocytes

APGO Association of Professors of Gynecology and Obstetrics

APH alcohol-positive history; alternative pathway hemolysis; aminoglycoside phosphotransferase; antepartum hemorrhage; anterior pituitary hormone; Association of Private Hospitals

Aph aphasia

APHA American Protestant Hospital Association; American Public Health Association

APhA American Pharmaceutical Association

APHIS Animal and Plant Health Inspection Service

APHP anti-Pseudomonas human plasma

API alkaline protease inhibitor; Analytical Profile Index; arterial pressure index; atmospheric pressure ionization; Autonomy Preference Index

APIC Association for Practitioners in Infection Control

APIE assessment, plan, implementation, and evaluation

APIM Association Professionnelle Internationale des Médecins

APIP additional personal injury protection

APIVR artificial pacemaker-induced ventricular rhythm

APKD adult-onset polycystic kidney disease

APL abductor pollicis longus; accelerated painless labor; acute promyelocytic leukemia; animal placenta lactogen; anterior pituitary-like; anterior pulmonary leaflet

aPL antiphospholipid

A-P&L anteroposterior and lateral

APLA, aPLA antiphospholipid antibody

APLP amyloid precursor-like protein

APM Academy of Parapsychology and Medicine; Academy of Physical Medicine; Academy of Psychosomatic Medicine; acid precipitable material; admission pattern monitoring; alternating pressure mattress; anteroposterior movement; aspartame; Association of Professors of Medicine

APMOMS Advisory Panel on the Mission and Organization of Medical Schools

APMR Association for Physical and Mental Retardation

APN acute pyelonephritis; advanced practice nurse; average peak noise

APNH antiporter sodium-hydrogen ion

APO abductor pollicis obliguus; acquired pendular oscillation; adriamycin, prednisone, vincristine; adverse patient occurrence; aphoxide; apolipoprotein; apomorphine; apoprotein

Apo, apo apolipoprotein

APOA, apoA apolipoprotein A

APOB, apoB apolipoprotein B

APOC, apoC apolipoprotein C

APOE, apoE apolipoprotein E

APOJ, apoJ apolipoprotein J

APORF acute postoperative renal failure

apoth apothecary

APP acute phase protein; alum-precipitated pyridine; aminopyrazolopyrimidine; amyloid peptide precursor; amyloid precursor protein; antiplatelet plasma; aqueous procaine penicillin; automated physiologic profile; avian pancreatic polypeptide

App, app appendix

APPA American Psychopathological Association

appar apparatus

APPG aqueous procaine penicillin G

appl appliance; application, applied

approp appropriate

approx approximate

APPS amyloid precursor protein secretase

appt appointment

appx appendix

appy appendectomy

APR abdominoperineal resection; absolute proximal reabsorption; acute phase reaction or reactant; amebic prevalence rate; anatomic porous replacement; anterior pituitary reaction; average payment rate

aprax apraxia

APRL American Prosthetic Research Laboratory

AProL acute promyelocytic leukemia

APRP acidic proline-rich protein; acute phase reactant protein

APRT adenine phosphoribosyl transferase

APRV airway pressure release ventilation

APS adenosine phosphosulfate; American Pain Society; American Pediatric Society; American Physiological Society; American Proctologic Society; American Prosthodontic Society; American Psychological Society; American Psychosomatic Society; ammonium persulfate; antiphospholipid antibody syndrome; attending physician's statement; autoimmune polyglandular syndrome; automated patent system; prostate-specific antigen

APSAC acylated plasminogen-streptokinase activator complex; anisoylated plasminogen streptokinase activator complex

APSD aorticopulmonary septal defect

APSGN acute poststreptococcal glomerulonephritis

APSQ Abbreviated Parent Symptom Questionnaire

APSS Association for the Psycho-physiological Study of Sleep

APT alum-precipitated toxoid; amino-phenylthioether

APTA American Physical Therapy Association

APTD Aid to Permanently and Totally Disabled

APTF American Physical Therapy Foundation

APTI airway pressure time index

APTT, aPTT activated partial thromboplastin time

APUD amine precursor uptake and decarboxylation

APV abnormal posterior vector

APVC anomalous pulmonary venous connection

APW alkaline peptone water

APWS attending physician work station

AQ achievement quotient; any quantity; aphasia quotient

aq aqueous; water [Lat. *aqua*]

AQS additional qualifying symptoms

aqu aqueous

AR absolute risk; accounts receivable; achievement ratio; actinic reticuloid [syndrome]; active resistance; acute rejection; adherence ratio; admitting room; airway resistance; alarm reaction; alcohol related; alkali reserve; allergic rhinitis; alloy restoration; amplitude ratio; analytical reagent; androgen receptor; anterior root; aortic regurgitation; apical-radial; Argyll Robertson [pupil]; aromatase; arsphenamine; articulare; artificial respiration; ascorbate reductase; assisted respiration; at risk; atrial rate; atrophic rhinitis; autoradiography; autoregressive; autosomal recessive

Ar argon; articulare

ar aromatic

A/R apical/radial

A&R advised and released

ARA Academy of Rehabilitative Audiometry; acetylene reduction activity; American Rheumatism Association; anorectal agenesis; antireticulin antibody; aortic root angiogram; arabinose; Associate of the Royal Academy

ara arabinose

ara-A adenine arabinoside

ara-C acytosine arabinose; cytosine arabinoside

ARAL adjustment reaction to adult life

ARAM antigen recognition activation motif

ARAMIS American Rheumatism Association Medical Information System

A$_{RAO}$ angiographic area of right anterior oblique projection

ARAS ascending reticular activating system

ara-U arabinosyluracil

ARB adrenergic receptor binder

arb arbitrary unit

ARBD alcohol-related birth defects

ARC accelerating rate calorimetry; acquired immunodeficiency syndrome-related complex; active renin concentration; AIDS-related complex; American Red Cross; anomalous retinal correspondence; antigen reactive cell; arcuate; Arthritis Rehabilitation Center; arthrogryposis-renal dysfunction-cholestasis [syndrome]; Association for Retarded Children

ARCA acquired red cell aplasia

ARCI Addiction Research Center Inventory

ARCS Associate of the Royal College of Science

ARC-ST Accreditation Review Council for Educational Programs in Surgical Technology

ARD absolute reaction of degeneration; acute radiation disease; acute respiratory disease; adult respiratory distress; allergic respiratory disease; anorectal dressing;

arthritis and rheumatic diseases; atopic respiratory disease

ARDMS American Registry of Diagnostic Medical Sonographers

ARDS acute respiratory distress syndrome; adult respiratory distress syndrome

ARE active-resistive exercises; AIDS-related encephalitis

AREDYLD acrorenal field defect, ectodermal dysplasia, lipoatrophic diabetes [syndrome]

AREPA acetazolamide-responsive familial paroxysmal ataxia

ARES antireticulo-endothelial serum

ARF acute renal failure; acute respiratory failure; acute rheumatic fever; Addiction Research Foundation; ambulance report form; area resource file

ARFC active rosette-forming T-cell; autologous rosette-forming cell

ARG, Arg arginine

arg arginine; silver [Lat. *argentum*]

ARGS antitrypsin-related gene sequence

ARI acute respiratory illness; airway reactivity index; anxiety reaction, intense

ARIA acetylcholine receptor-inducing activity; automated radioimmunoassay

ARIMA autoregressive integrated moving average

ARIS auto-regulated inspiratory support

Ar Kr argon-krypton [laser]

ARL Association of Research Libraries; average remaining lifetime

ARLD alcohol related liver disease

ARM adrenergic receptor material; aerosol rebreathing method; ambulatory renal monitor; anorectal manometry; anxiety reaction, mild; Armenian [hamster]; artificial rupture of membranes; atomic resolution microscopy

ARMS adverse reaction monitoring system; amplification refractory mutation system

ARN acute renal necrosis; acute retinal necrosis; arcuate nucleus; Association of Rehabilitation Nurses

ARNMD Association for Research in Nervous and Mental Diseases

ARNP Advanced Registered Nurse Practitioner

ARO Associate for Research in Ophthalmology

AROA autosomal recessive ocular albinism

AROM active range of motion; artificial rupture of membranes

arom aromatic

ARP absolute refractory period; American Registry of Pathologists; anticipated recovery path; apolipoprotein regulatory protein; assay reference plasma; assimilation regulatory protein; at risk period; automaticity recovery phase

ARPANET Advanced Research Projects Agency Network

ARPD autosomal recessive polycystic disease

ARPES angular resolved photoelectron spectroscopy

ARPKD autosomal recessive polycystic kidney disease

ARPT American Registry of Physical Therapists

ARR aortic root replacement

arr arrest, arrested

ARRC Associate of the Royal Red Cross

ARRS American Roentgen Ray Society

ARRT American Registry of Radiologic Technologists

ARS acquiescence response scale; adult Reye's syndrome; alcohol-related seizures; alizarin red S; American Radium Society; American Rhinologic Society; antirabies serum; arsphenamine; arylsulfatase; autonomously replicating sequence

Ars arsphenamine

ARSA American Reye's Syndrome Association; arylsulfatase A

ARSACS autosomal recessive spastic ataxia of Charlevoix-Saguenay

ARSC arylsulfatase C; Associate of the Royal Society of Chemistry

ARSM acute respiratory system malfunction

ARSPH Associate of the Royal Society for the Promotion of Health

ART absolute retention time; Accredited Record Technician; acoustic reflex test; algebraic reconstruction technique; algebraic reconstructive technique; artery; assisted reproductive technique; automated reagin test; automaticity recovery time

art artery, arterial; articulation; artificial

arth arthritis

artic articulation, articulated

artif artificial

ARV acquired immunodeficiency syndrome-related virus; anterior right ventricle; avian reovirus

ARVD arrhythmogenic right ventricular dysplasia

ARVP arginine-vasopressin

AS acetylstrophanthidin; acidified serum; acoustic schwannoma; acoustic stimulation; active sarcoidosis; active sleep; Adams-Stokes [disease]; Alport syndrome; alveolar sac; amyloid substance; anal sphincter; androsterone sulfate; Angelman syndrome; ankylosing spondylitis; anovulatory syndrome; antiserum; antisocial; antistreptolysin; antral spasm; anxiety state; aortic sound; aortic stenosis; approaching significance [statistical]; aqueous solution; aqueous suspension; arteriosclerosis; artificial sweetener; aseptic meningitis; asparagine synthetase; astigmatism; asymmetric; atrial septum; atrial stenosis; atropine sulfate; audiogenic seizure; Auto-Suture; left ear [Lat. *auris sinistra*]

As arsenic; astigmatism; asymptomatic

A(s) asplenia syndrome

A·s ampere second

A x s ampere per second

aS absiemens

as left ear [Lat. *auris sinistra*]

ASA acetylsalicylic acid; active systemic anaphylaxis; Adams-Stokes attack; American Society of Anesthesiologists; American Standards Association; American Surgical Association; aminosalicylic acid; anterior spinal artery; antibody to surface antigen; argininosuccinic acid; arylsulfatase-A; aspirin-sensitive asthma; asthma-nasal polyps-aspirin intolerance [triad]

ASAAD American Society for the Advancement of Anesthesia in Dentistry

ASAC acidified serum-acidified complement

ASAH antibiotic sterilized aortic valve homograft

ASAHP American Society of Allied Health Professions

ASAIO American Society for Artificial Internal Organs

ASAL arginosuccinic acid lyase

ASAP American Society for Adolescent Psychology; as soon as possible

ASAS argininosuccinate synthetase

ASAT aspartate aminotransferase

ASB American Society of Bacteriologists; anencephaly–spina bifida [syndrome]; anesthesia standby; Anxiety Scale for the Blind; asymptomatic bacteriuria

ASBS American Society for Bariatric Surgery

ASBV avocado sunblotch viroid

ASC acetylsulfanilyl chloride; altered state of consciousness; ambulatory surgical center; American Society of Cytology; antigen-sensitive cell; ascorbate, ascorbic acid; asthma symptom checklist

asc ascending; anterior subcapsular

ASCAD atherosclerotic coronary artery disease

ASCAo ascending aorta

ASCH American Society of Clinical Hypnosis

ASCI acute spinal cord injury; American Society for Clinical Investigation

ASCII American Standard Code for Information Interchange

ASCLT American Society of Clinical Laboratory Technicians

ASCMS American Society of Contemporary Medicine and Surgery

ASCO American Society of Clinical Oncology; American Society of Contemporary Ophthalmology

ASCOT a severity characterization of trauma

ASCP American Society of Clinical Pathologists; American Society of Consulting Pharmacists

ASCR American Society of Chiropodical Roentgenology

ASCS admissions scheduling system

ASCT autologous stem cell transplantation

ASCVD arteriosclerotic cardiovascular disease; atherosclerotic cardiovascular disease

ASD aldosterone secretion defect; Alzheimer senile dementia; antisiphon device; arthritis syphilitica deformans; arthroscopic subacromial decompression; atrial septal defect

ASDC American Society of Dentistry for Children; Association of Sleep Disorders Centers

ASDH acute subdural hemorrhage or hematoma

ASDP anal sphincter dysplasia

ASE acute stress erosion; American Society of Electrocardiography; axilla, shoulder, and elbow

ASF African swine fever; aniline-sulfur-formaldehyde [resin]

ASFR age-specific fertility rate

ASG advanced cell group; American Society for Genetics; Army Surgeon General; aspermiogenesis

ASGBI Association of Surgeons of Great Britain and Ireland

ASGE American Society for Gastrointestinal Endoscopy

AS/GP antiserum, guinea pig

ASGR asialoglycoprotein receptor

ASH aldosterone-stimulating hormone; American Society of Hematology; alkylosing spinal hyperostosis; antistreptococcal hyaluronidase; asymmetric septal hypertrophy

AsH astigmatism, hypermetropic

A&Sh arm and shoulder

ASHA American School Health Association; American Social Health Association; American Speech and Hearing Association

ASHAC acquired immunodeficiency syndrome self-help and care

ASHBM Associate Scottish Hospital Bureau of Management

ASHCRM American Society of Health Care Risk Managers

ASHCSP American Society for Hospital Central Service Personnel [of AHA]

ASHCVD atherosclerotic hypertensive cardiovascular disease

ASHD arteriosclerotic heart disease; atrioseptal heart disease

ASHE American Society for Hospital Engineering

ASHET American Society for Health Manpower Education and Training

ASHFSA American Society for Hospital Food Service Administrators

ASHG American Society for Human Genetics

ASHI Association for the Study of Human Infertility

ASHN acute sclerosing hyaline necrosis

AS/Ho antiserum, horse

ASHP American Society of Hospital Pharmacists; American Society for Hospital Planning

ASHPA American Society for Hospital Personnel Administration

ASHT American Society of Hand Therapists

ASI addiction severity index; anxiety state inventory; anxiety status inventory; arthroscopic screw installation

ASIA American Spinal Injury Association

ASIF Association for Study of Internal Fixation

ASII American Science Information Institute

ASIM American Society of Internal Medicine

ASIS anterior superior iliac spine

ASK antistreptokinase

ASL antistreptolysin; argininosuccinate lyase

ASLIB Association of Special Libraries and Information Bureau

ASLM American Society of Law and Medicine

ASLN Alport syndrome-like hereditary nephritis

ASLO antistreptolysin O

ASLT antistreptolysin test

ASM acid sphingomyelinase; airway smooth muscle; American Society for Microbiology; anterior scalenus muscle

AsM astigmatism, myopic

ASMA antismooth muscle antibody

ASMC arterial smooth muscle cell

ASMD anterior segment mesenchymal dysgenesis; atonic sclerotic muscle dystrophy

ASME Association for the Study of Medical Education

ASMI anteroseptal myocardial infarct

As/Mk antiserum, monkey

ASMPA Armed Services Medical Procurement Agency

ASMR age-standardized mortality ratio

ASMT American Society for Medical Technology

ASMTY acetylserotonin methyltransferase Y

ASN abstract syntax notation; alkali-soluble nitrogen; American Society of Nephrology; American Society of Neurochemistry; arteriosclerotic nephritis; asparagine; Associate in Nursing

Asn asparagine

ASO administrative services only; allele-specific oligonucleoside; antistreptolysin O; arteriosclerosis obliterans

ASOD anterior segmental ocular dysgenesis

ASOS American Society of Oral Surgeons

ASOT antistreptolysin-O test

ASP abnormal spinal posture; acute symmetric polyarthritis; African swine pox; aged substrate plasma; alkali-stable pepsin; American Society of Parasitology; ankylosing spondylitis; anorectal malformation, sacral bony abnormality, presacral mass [association]; antisocial personality; aortic systolic pressure; area systolic pressure; asparaginase; aspartic acid

Asp aspartic acid; asparaginase

asp aspartate, aspartic acid; aspiration

ASPA American Society of Physician Analysts; American Society of Podiatric Assistants; aspartoacylase

ASPAT antistreptococcal polysaccharide test

ASPDM American Society of Psychosomatic Dentistry and Medicine

ASPEN American Society for Parenteral and Enteral Nutrition

ASPG antispleen globulin

ASPM American Society of Paramedics

ASPO American Society for Psychoprophylaxis in Obstetrics

ASPP Association for Sane Psychiatric Practices

ASPRS American Society of Plastic and Reconstructive Surgeons

ASPS advanced sleep phase syndrome

ASPVD atherosclerotic peripheral vascular disease

ASQ Abbreviated Symptom Questionnaire; Anxiety Scale Questionnaire

ASR aldosterone secretion rate; antistreptolysin reaction

AS/Rab antiserum, rabbit

ASRT American Society of Radiologic Technologists

ASS acute serum sickness; acute spinal stenosis; anterior superior spine; argininosuccinate synthetase

ASSA, ASSAS aminopterin-like syndrome sine aminopterin

ASSC acute splenic sequestration crisis

AS-SCORE age, stage of disease, physiological system involved, complications, response to therapy

ASSERT improving Alcohol and Substance abuse Services and Educating providings to Refer patients to Treatment

ASSH American Society for Surgery of the Hand

ASSI Accurate Surgical and Scientific Instruments

assim assiimilate, assimilation

ASSO American Society for the Study of Orthodontics

Assoc association, associate

ASSP argininosuccinate synthetase pseudogene

ASSR adult situation stress reaction

ASSX argininosuccinate synthetase pseudogene

AST allergy serum transfer; angiotensin sensitivity test; anterior spinothalamic tract; antistreptolysin test; aspartate aminotransferase (SGOT); Association of Surgical Technologists; astigmatism;

atrial overdrive stimulation rate; audiometry sweep test

Ast astigmatism

ASTA anti-alpha-staphylolysin

ASTH, Asth asthenopia

ASTHO Association of State and Territorial Health Officers

ASTI antispasticity index

ASTM American Society for Testing and Materials

ASTMH American Society of Tropical Medicine and Hygiene

ASTO antistreptolysin O

as tol as tolerated

ASTRO American Society for Therapeutic Radiology and Oncology

ASTZ antistreptozyme

ASV anodic stripping voltammetry; antisiphon valve; antisnake venom; avian sarcoma virus

ASVO American Society of Veterinary Ophthalmology

ASVPP American Society of Veterinary Physiologists and Pharmacologists

ASW artificial sweetener

Asx amino acid that gives aspartic acid after hydrolysis; asymptomatic

asym asymmetry, asymmetric

AT abdominal thrusts; achievement test; Achilles tendon; Achard-Thiers [syndrome]; adaptive thermogenesis; adenine-thyronine; adipose tissue; adjunctive therapy; adnexal torsion; air temperature; allergy treatment; aminotransferase; amitriptyline; anaerobic threshold; anaphylotoxin; anterior tibia; antithrombin; antitrypsin; antral transplantation; applanation tonometry; ataxia-telangi-ectasia; atmosphere; atraumatic; atresia, tricuspid; atrial tachycardia; atropine; attenuate, attenuation; axonal terminal; old tuberculin [Gr. *alt Tuberkulin*]

A-T ataxia telangiectasia

AT$_{10}$ dihydrotachysterol

AT I angiotensin I

AT II angiotensin II
AT III angiotensin III; antithrombin III
At acidity, total; astatine; atrium, atrial
at air tight; atom, atomic
ATA alimentary toxic aleukia; American Thyroid Association; aminotriazole; antithymic activity; antithyroglobulin antibody; anti-Toxoplasma antibody; atmosphere absolute; aurintricarboxylic acid
ATB at the time of the bomb [A-bomb in Japan]; atrial tachycardia with block
Atb antibiotic
ATC activated thymus cell; around the clock
ATCase aspartate transcarbomoylase
ATCC American Type Culture Collection
ATCL adult T-cell leukemia or lymphoma
ATCS anterior tibial compartment syndrome
ATD Alzheimer-type dementia; androstatrienedione; anthropomorphic test dummy; antithyroid drug; aqueous tear deficiency; asphyxiating thoracic dystrophy
ATDC Association of Thalidomide Damaged Children
ADTP attitude toward disabled persons [scale]
ATE acute toxic encephalopathy; adipose tissue extract; autologous tumor extract
ATEE N-acetyl-1-tyrosyl-ethyl ester
ATEM analytic transmission electron microscopy
Aten atenolol
ATF activating transcription factor; anterior talofibular [ligament]; ascites tumor fluid
At fib atrial fibrillation
ATG adenine-thymidine-guanine anti-human thymocyte globulin; antithrombocyte globulin; antithymocyte globulin; antithyroglobulin

ATGAM antithymocyte gamma-globulin
AT/GC adenine-thymine/guanine-cytosine [ratio]
ATH acetyl-tyrosine hydrazide
ATh Associate in Therapy
Athsc atherosclerosis
ATI abdominal trauma index
ATL Achilles tendon lengthening; acute T-cell leukemia; adult T-cell leukemia; anterior tricuspid leaflet; antitension line; atypical lymphocyte
ATLA adult T-cell leukemia virus-associated antigen; alternatives to laboratory animals
ATLL adult T-cell leukemia/lymphoma
ATLS acute tumor lysis syndrome; advanced trauma life support
ATLV adult T-cell leukemia virus
ATM abnormal tubular myelin; acute transverse myelopathy; asynchronous transfer mode; atmosphere
atm standard atmosphere
ATMA antithyroid plasma membrane antibody
atmos atmospheric
ATN acute tubular necrosis; augmented transition network
ATNC atraumatic normocephalic
at no atomic number
ATNR asymmetric tonic neck reflex
A-to-D analog-to-digital
ATP adenosine triphosphate; ambient temperature and pressure; autoimmune thrombocytopenic purpura
A-TP adsorbed test plasma
AT-P antitrypsin-Pittsburgh
AtP attending physician
AT-PAS aldehyde-thionine-periodic acid Schiff [test]
ATPase adenosine triphosphatase
ATPD dried at ambient temperature and pressure
ATP-2Na adenosine triphosphate disodium

ATPS ambient temperature and pressure, saturated

ATR Achilles tendon reflex; alpha-thalassemia-mental retardation [syndrome]

atr atrophy

Atr fib atrial fibrillation

ATRX, ATR-X X-linked alpha-thalassemia mental retardation [syndrome]

ATS Achard-Thiers syndrome; acid test solution; alpha-D-tocopherol acid succinate; American Thoracic Society; American Trudeau Society; American Trauma Society; antirat thymocyte serum; antitetanus serum; antithymocyte serum; anxiety tension state; arteriosclerosis

ATSDR Agency for Toxic Substances and Disease Registry

ATT arginine tolerance test; aspirin tolerance time

att attending

ATV Abelson virus transformed; avian tumor virus

at vol atomic volume

at wt atomic weight

ATx adult thymectomy

atyp atypical

ATZ atypical transformation zone

AU according to custom [Lat. *ad usum*]; allergenic unit; Ångström unit; antitoxin unit; arbitrary unit; Australia antigen; azauridine

Au Australia [antigen]; authorization; gold [Lat. *aurum*]

AUA American Urological Association; asymptomatic urinary abnormalities

Au Ag Australia antigen

AUB abnormal uterine bleeding

AUC area under the curve

AUD arthritis of unknown diagnosis

aud auditory

AUDIT alcohol use disorders identification test

aud-vis audiovisual

AUG acute ulcerative gingivitis; adenosine-uracil-guanine

AUGH acute upper gastrointestinal hemorrhage

AuHAA Australia hepatitis-associated antigen

AUI Alcohol Use Inventory

AUL acute undifferentiated leukemia

AUO amyloid of unknown origin

AuP Australian antigen protein

AUPHA Association of University Programs in Health Administration

aur, auric auricle, auricular

AUS acute urethral syndrome

AuS Australia serum hepatitis

aus, ausc auscultation

AuSH Australia serum hepatitis

Auto-PEEP self-controlled positive end-expiratory pressure

AUV anterior urethral valve

aux auxiliary

AV Adriamycin and vincristine; air velocity; allergic vasculitis; anteroventral; anteversion; anticipatory vomiting; antivirin; aortic valve; arteriovenous; artificial ventilation; assisted ventilation; atrioventricular; audiovisual; augmented vector; average; aviation medicine; avoirdupois

A-V arteriovenous; atrioventricular

A/V ampere/volt; arteriovenous

Av average; avoirdupois

aV abvolt

av air velocity; average; avulsion

AVA activity vector analysis; antiviral antibody; aortic valve area; aortic valve atresia; arteriovenous anastomosis

AV/AF anteverted, anteflexed

AVB atrioventricular block

AVC aberrant ventricular conduction; Academy of Veterinary Cardiology; aortic valve closure; associative visual cortex; Association of Vitamin Chemists; associative visual cortex; atrioventricular canal; automatic volume control

AVCN anteroventral cochlear nucleus

AVCS atrioventricular conduction system

AVCx atrioventricular circumflex branch

AVD aortic valvular disease; apparent volume of distribution; atrioventricular dissociation; Army Veterinary Department

AVDO$_2$ arteriovenous oxygen saturation difference

AVDO$_2$B arteriovenous oxygen saturation difference, basal

AVDP average diastolic pressure

avdp avoirdupois

AVE aortic valve echocardiogram

ave, aver average

AVF antiviral factor; arteriovenous fistula

aVF automated volt foot

aV$_F$ unipolar limb lead on the left leg in electrocardiography

AVG ambulatory visit group

avg average

AVH acute viral hepatitis

AVHD acquired valvular heart disease

AVHS acquired valvular heart syndrome

AVI air velocity index; Association of Veterinary Inspectors

AVJ atrioventricular junction

AVJR atrioventricular junction rhythm

AVJRe atrioventricular junctional reentrant

aVL automated volt left

aV$_L$ unipolar limb lead on the left arm in electrocardiography

AVLINE Audiovisuals On-Line [data base]

AVM arteriovenous malformation; atrioventricular malformation; aviation medicine

AVMA American Veterinary Medical Association

AVN acute vasomotor nephropathy; atrioventricular nodal [conduction]; atrioventricular node; avascular necrosis

AVND atrioventricular node dysfunction

AVNFH avascular necrosis of the femoral head

AVNFRP atrioventricular node functional refractory period

AVNR atrioventricular nodal reentry

AVNRT atrioventricular node reentry tachycardia

AVO aortic valve opening; aortic valve orifice; atrioventricular opening

AVO$_2$ arteriovenous oxygen ratio

AVP abnormal vasopressin; actinomycin-vincristine-Platinol; ambulatory venous pressure; antiviral protein; aqueous vasopressin; arginine–vasopressin; arteriovenous passage time

AVPU alert, verbal, painful, unresponsive [neurologic test]

AVR accelerated ventricular rhythm; antiviral regulator; aortic valve replacement

aVR automated volt right

aV$_R$ unipolar limb lead on the right arm in electrocardiography

AVRI acute viral respiratory infection

AVRP atrioventricular refractory period

AVRR antiviral repressor regulator

AVRT atrioventricular reentrant tachycardia; atrioventricular reciprocating tachycardia

AVS aortic valve stenosis; arteriovenous shunt; auditory vocal sequencing

AVSD atrioventricular septal defect

AVSV aortic valve stroke volume

AVT Allen vision test; arginine vasotocin; Aviation Medicine Technician

Av3V anteroventral third ventricle

AVZ avascular zone

AW able to work; above waist; abrupt withdrawal; alcohol withdrawal; alveolar wall; anterior wall; atomic warfare; atomic weight

A&W alive and well

aw airway; water activity

AWAR anterior wall of aortic root

AWBM alveolar wall basement membrane

AWG American Wire Gauge

AWI anterior wall infarction

AWM abnormal wall motion

AWMI anterior wall myocardial infarction

AWMV amplitude-weighted mean velocity

AWOL absent without official leave

AWP airway pressure; any willing provider; average of the wholesale prices; average wholesale price

AWRS anti-whole rabbit serum

AWRU active wrist rotation unit

AWS Alagille-Watson syndrome; alcohol withdrawal syndrome

AWTA aniridia-Wilms tumor association

awu atomic weight unit

ax axillary; axis, axial

AXD axillary dissection

AXF advanced x-ray facility

AXG adult xanthogranuloma

AXL anexelekto [oncogene]; axillary lymphoscintigraphy

AXR abdominal x-ray [examination]

AXT alternating exotropia

AYA acute yellow atrophy

AYF antiyeast factor

AYP autolyzed yeast protein

AYV aster yellow virus

AZ Aschheim-Zondek [test]; 5-azacytidine; azathioprine

Az nitrogen [Fr. *azote*]

AZA azathioprine

AzC azacytosine

AZF azospermia factor

AzG; azg azaguanine

AZGP zinc-alpha-2-glycoprotein

AZO [indicates presence of the group –N:N–]

AZQ diaziquone

AZR alizarin

AZT Aschheim-Zondek test; azidothymidine; 3'-azido-3'-deoxythymidine; zidovudine (azidothymidine)

AZT-TP 3'azido-3'-dexythymidine triphosphate

AZU azauracil; azurodicin

AzUr 6-azauridine

B bacillus; bands; barometric; base; basophil, basophilic; bath [Lat. *balneum*]; Baumé scale; behavior; bel; Benoist scale; benzoate; beta; biscuspid; black; blood, bloody; blue; body; boils at; Bolton point; bone marrow-derived [cell or lymphocyte]; born; boron; bound; bovine; break; bregma; bronchial, bronchus; brother; *Brucella*; bruit; buccal; Bucky [film in cassette in Potter-Bucky diaphragm]; Bucky factor; bursa cells; bypass; byte; magnetic induction; minimal detectable blurring; supramentale [point]

b barn; base; boils at; born; brain; [chromosome] break; supramentale [point]; twice [Lat. *bis*]

B_0 constant magnetic field in nuclear magnetic resonance

B_1 induced field in magnetic resonance imaging; radiofrequency magnetic field in nuclear magnetic resonance; thiamine

B_2 riboflavin

B_6 pyridoxine

B_7 biotin

B_8 adenosine phosphate

B_{12} cyanocobalamin

β see beta

BA Bachelor of Arts; backache; bacterial agglutination; basilar artery; basion; benzyladenine; best amplitude; betamethasone acetate; bilateral asymmetrical; bile acid; biliary atresia; biological activity; blocking antibody; blood agar; blood alcohol; bone age; boric acid; bovine albumin; brachial artery; breathing apparatus; bronchial asthma; buccoaxial; buffered acetone

Ba barium; barium enema; basion

ba basion

BAA benzoylarginine amide; branched amino acid

BAB blood agar base

Bab Babinski's reflex; baboon

BabK baboon kidney

BAC bacterial adherent colony; bacterial antigen complex; blood alcohol concentration; British Association of Chemists; bronchoalveolar cells; buccoaxiocervical

Bac, bac *Bacillus*, bacillary

Bact, bact *Bacterium*; bacterium, bacteria

BAD biological aerosol detection; British Association of Dermatologists

BADS black locks-albinism-deafness syndrome

BAE bovine aortic endothelium; bronchial artery embolization

BaE barium enema

BAEC bovine aortic endothelial cells

BAEE benzoylarginine ethyl ester

BaEn barium enema

BAEP brainstem auditory evoked potential

BAER brainstem auditory evoked response

BaEV baboon endogenous virus

BaFBr:Eu europium-activated barium fluorohalide

BAG buccoaxiogingival

BAGG buffered azide glucose glycerol

BAHS butoctamide hydrogen succinate

BAI basilar artery insufficiency; beta-aminoisobutyrate

BAIB beta-aminoisobutyric [acid]

BAIF bile acid independent flow

BAIT bacterial automated identification technique

BAL blood alcohol level; British antilewisite; bronchoalveolar lavage

bal balance; balsam

BALB binaural alternate loudness balance

BALF broncho-alveolar lavage fluid
bals balsam
BALT broncho-alveolar lavage fluid; bronchus-associated lymphoid tissue
BAM basilar artery migraine; bilateral augmentation mammoplasty; brachial artery mean [pressure];
BaM barium meal
Bam benzamide
BAME benzoylarginine methyl ester
BAN British Approved Name; British Association of Neurologists
BANS back, arms, neck, and scalp
BAO basal acid output; brachial artery output
BAO-MAO basal acid output to maximal acid output [ratio]
BAP bacterial alkaline phosphatase; Behavior Activity Profile; beta-amyloid peptide; blood-agar plate; bovine albumin in phosphate buffer; brachial artery pressure
BAPhysMed British Association of Physical Medicine
BAPI barley alkaline protease inhibitor
BAPN beta-aminoproprionitrile fumarate
BAPP beta amyloid precursor protein
BAPS biomechanical ankle platform system; bovine albumin phosphate saline; British Association of Paediatric Surgeons; British Association of Plastic Surgeons
BAPT British Association of Physical Training
BAPTA 1,2-bis (aminophenoxy) ethane-N,N,N',N'-tetraacetic acid
BAPV bovine alimentary papilloma virus
BAQ brain-age quotient
BAR bariatrics; barometer, barometric; beta-adrenergic receptor
bar barometric
Barb, barb barbiturate, barbituric
BARK beta-adrenergic receptor kinase
BARN bilateral acute retinal necrosis
BARS behaviorally anchored rating scale

BART blood-activated recalcification time
BAS balloon atrial septostomy; benzyl anti-serotinin; beta-adrenergic stimulation; boric acid solution
BaS barium swallow
bas basilar; basophil, basophilic
BASA Boston Assessment of Severe Aphasia
BASE B27-arthritis-sacroiliitis-extra-articular features [syndrome]
BASH body acceleration synchronous with heart rate
BASIC Beginner's All-Purpose Symbolic Introduction Code
baso basophil
BAT basic aid training; best available technology; blunt abdominal trauma; brown adipose tissue
BAUP Bovie-assisted uvulopalatoplasty
BAUS British Association of Urological Surgeons
BAV bicuspid aortic valve
BAVCP bilateral abductor vocal cord paralysis
BAVFO bradycardia after arteriovenous fistula occlusion
BAW bronchoalveolar washing
BB bad breath; bed bath; beta blockade, beta blocker; BioBreeding [rat]; blanket bath; blood bank; blood buffer; blow bottle; blue bloaters [emphysema]; borderline; both bones; breakthrough bleeding; breast biopsy; brush border; buffer base; bundle branch; isoenzyme of creatine kinase containing two B subunits
bb Bolton point; both bones
BBA born before arrival
BBB blood-brain barrier; blood buffer base; bundle-branch block
BBBB bilateral bundle-branch block
BBBD blood brain barrier disruption
BBC bromobenzycyanide
BBD benign breast disease
BBE *Bacteroides* bile esculin [agar]

BBEP brush border endopeptidase
BBF bronchial blood flow
BBI Biomedical Business International; Bowman-Birk soybean inhibitor
BBM brush border membrane
BBMV brush border membrane vesicle
BBN broad band noise
BBRS Burks' Behavior Rating Scale
BBS Barolet-Biedl syndrome; bashful bladder syndrome; benign breast syndrome; bilateral breath sounds; bombesin; borate-buffered saline; brown bowel syndrome
BBT basal body temperature
BB/W BioBreeding/Worcester [rat]
BC Bachelor of Surgery [Lat. *Baccalaureus Chirurgiae*]; back care; bactericidal concentration; basal cell; basket cell; battle casualty; bicarbonate; biliary colic; bipolar cell; birth control; blastic crisis; blood count; blood culture; Blue Cross [plan]; board certified; bone conduction; brachiocephalic; breast cancer; bronchial carcinoma; buccal cartilage; buccocervical; buffy coat
B&C biopsy and curettage
b/c benefit/cost [ratio]
BCA balloon catheter angioplasty; bicinchoninic acid; blood color analyzer; Blue Cross Association; branchial cleft anomaly; breast cancer antigen
BCAA branched chain amino acid
BCAT brachiocephalic arterial trunk
BCB blood-cerebrospinal fluid barrier; brilliant cresyl blue
BCBR bilateral carotid body resection
BC/BS Blue Cross/Blue Shield [plan]
BCBSA Blue Cross and Blue Shield Association
BCC basal-cell carcinoma; biliary cholesterol concentration; birth control clinic
bcc body-centered-cubic
BCCG British Cooperative Clinical Group
BCCP biotin carboxyl carrier protein

BCD binary-coded decimal; bleomycin, cyclophosphamide, dactinomycin
BCDDP Breast Cancer Detection Demonstration Project
BCDF B-cell differentiation factor
BCDL Brachmann-Cornelia de Lange [syndrome]
BCDRS brief Carroll depression rating scale
BCDS bulimia cognitive distortions scale
BCDSP Boston Collaborative Drug Surveillance Program
BCE basal cell epithelioma; benign childhood epilepsy; bubble chamber equipment
BCEI breast cancer estrogen-inducible
BCF basophil chemotactic factor; bioconcentration factor; breast cyst fluid
BCFP breast cyst fluid protein
BCG bacille Calmette-Guérin [vaccine]; ballistocardiography, ballistocardiogram; bicolor guaiac test; bromcresol green
BCGF B-cell growth factor
BCH basal cell hyperplasia
BCh Bachelor of Surgery [Lat. *Baccalaureus Chirurgiae*]
BChD Bachelor of Dental Surgery
BCHE butyrylcholinesterase
BChir Bachelor of Surgery [Lat. *Baccalaureus Chirurgiae*]
Bchl, bChl bacterial chlorophyll
BCHS Bureau of Community Health Services
BCI behavioral cues index; brain-computer interface
BCIA Biomedical Clinical Instrumentation Association
BCIP 5-bromo-4-chloro-3-inodolyl phosphate
BCKA branched-chain keto acid
BCKD branched-chain alpha-keto acid dehydrogenase
BCL basic cycle length; B-cell leukemia/lymphoma

BCLL B-cell chronic lymphocytic leukemia

BCLP bilateral cleft of lip and palate

BCLS basic cardiac life support

BCM B-cell maturation; birth control medication; blood-clotting mechanism effects; body cell mass; body control and movement

BCME bis-chloromethyl ether

BCMF B-cell maturation factor

BCMS Bioethic Citation Maintenance System

BCN basal cell nevus; bilateral cortical necrosis

BCNS basal cell nevus syndrome

BCNU 1,3-bis-(2-chloroethyl)-1-nitrosourea; bleomycin and camustine

BCO biliary cholesterol output

BCOC bowel care of choice

BCP basic calcium phosphate; birth control pill; blue cone pigment; Blue Cross Plan; bromcresol purple

BCPD bromcresol purple deoxylate

BCPT breast cancer prevention trial

BCPV bovine cutaneous papilloma virus

BCQ breast cancer questionnaire

BCR B-cell reactivity; birth control regimen; breakpoint cluster region; bromocriptine; bulbocavernous reflex

BCRS brief cognitive rating scale

BCRx birth control drug

BCS battered child syndrome; blood cell separator; British Cardiac Society; Budd-Chiari syndrome

BCSI breast cancer screening indicator

BCT brachiocephalic trunk; branched-chain amino acid transferase

BCTF Breast Cancer Task Force

BCtg bovine chymotrypsinogen

BCtr bovine chymotrypsin

BCW biological and chemical warfare

BCYE buffered charcoal-yeast extract [agar]

BD barbital-dependent; barbiturate dependence; base deficit; base of prism down; basophilic degeneration; Batten disease; behavioral disorder; Behçet disease; belladonna; bicarbonate dialysis; bile duct; binocular deprivation; birth date; black death; block design [test]; blood donor; blue diaper [syndrome]; borderline dull; bound; brain damage; brain dead, brain death; Briquet disorder; bronchodilation, bronchodilator; buccodistal; Byler disease

B-D Becton-Dickinson

Bd board; buoyant density

bd band; bundle; twice a day [Lat. *bis die*]

BDA balloon dilation angioplasty; British Dental Association

BDAC Bureau of Drug Abuse Control

BDAE Boston Diagnostic Aphasia Examination

BDC Bazex-Dupré-Christol [syndrome]; burn-dressing change

BDE bile duct examination

BDentSci Bachelor of Dental Science

BDG buccal developmental groove; buffered desoxycholate glucose

BDI Beck Depression Inventory

BDIP biomedical digital image processing

BDIS Becton-Dickinson immunocytometry system

BDL behaviors of daily living; below detectable limits; bile duct ligation

BDLS Brachmann-de Lange syndrome

BDM Becker's muscular dystrophy

BDMS Bureau of Data Management and Strategy [of HCFA]

BDNF brain-derived neurotrophic factor

BDP beclomethasone dipropionate; benzodiazepine; bilateral diaphragmatic paralysis; bronchopulmonary dysplasia

BDR background diabetic retinopathy

BDRS Blessed Dementia Rating Scale

BDS Bachelor of Dental Surgery; biological detection system; Blessed Dementia Scale

bds to be taken twice a day [Lat. *bid in die summendus*]

BDSc Bachelor of Dental Science

BDUR bromodeoxyuridine

BDW buffered distilled water

BE bacillary emulsion; bacterial endocarditis; barium enema; Barrett's esophagus; base excess; below-elbow; bile-esculin [test]; bovine enteritis; brain edema; bread equivalent; breast examination; bronchoesophagology

B/E below-elbow

B&E brisk and equal

Be beryllium

Bé Baumé scale

BEA below-elbow amputation; bioelectrical activity; bromoethylamine

BEAM brain electrical activity monitoring

BEAP bronchiectasis, eosinophilia, asthma, pneumonia

BEAR biological effects of atomic radiation

BEB Biomedical Engineering Branch [of US Army]

BEC bacterial endocarditis; behavioral emergency committee; blood ethyl alcohol; bromo-ergocryptine

BECF blood extracellular fluid

BEE basal energy expenditure

beg begin, beginning

BEH benign exertional headache

beh behavior, behavioral

BEI back-scattered electron imaging; biological exposure indexes; butanol-extractable iodine

BEIR biological effects of ionizing radiation

BEK bovine embryonic kidney [cells]

BEL blood ethanol level; bovine embryonic lung

BELIR beta-endorphin-like immunoreactivity

BENAR blood eosinophilic non-allergic rhinitis

Benz, benz benzene; benzidine; benzoate

BEP brain evoked potential; basic element of performance

B-EP β-endorphin

BER basic electrical rhythm

BERA brainstem evoked response audiometry

BES balanced electrolyte solution; Baltimore Eye Study

BESM bovine embryonic skeletal muscle

BESP bovine embryonic spleen [cells]

BET benign epithelial tumor; bleeding esophageal varix; Brunauer-Emmet-Teller [method]

BETA Biomedical Electronics Technicians Association

β [Greek letter beta] an anomer of a carbohydrate; buffer capacity; carbon separated from a carboxyl by one other carbon in aliphatic compounds; a constituent of a plasma protein fraction; probability of Type II error; a substituent group of a steroid that projects above the plane of the ring

1–β power of statistical test

β₂m beta₂-microglobulin

BEV baboon endogenous virus; beam's eye view

BeV, Bev billion electron volts

bev beverage

BF bentonite flocculation; bile flow; black female; blastogenic factor; blister fluid; blood flow; body fat; bouillon filtrate [tuberculin] [Fr. *bouillon filtré*]; breakfast fed; breast feeding; buffered; burning feet [syndrome]; butter fat

bf black female; bouillon filtrate [tuberculin]

B3F band 3 cytoplasmic fragment

B/F black female; bound/free [antigen ratio]

BFB biological feedback; bronchial foreign body

BFDI bronchodilation following deep inspiration

BFEC benign focal epilepsy of childhood

BFC benign febrile convulsion

BFE blood flow energy

bFGF basic fibroblast growth factor

BFH benign familial hematuria

BFHD Beukes familial hip dysplasia

BFL bird fancier's lung; Börjeson-Forssman-Lehman [syndrome]

BFLS Börjeson-Forssman-Lehmann syndrome

BFO balanced forearm orthosis; ball-bearing forearm orthosis; blood-forming organ

BFP biologic false-positive

BFPR biologic false-positive reaction

BFPSTS biologic false-positive serological test for syphilis

BFR biologic false reaction; blood flow rate; bone formation rate; buffered Ringer [solution]

BFS blood fasting sugar

BFT bentonite flocculation test; biofeedback training

BFU burst-forming unit

BFU-E burst-forming unit, erythrocytes

BFU-ME burst-forming unit, myeloid/erythroid

BFV bovine feces virus

BG basal ganglion; basic gastrin; Bender Gestalt [test]; beta-galactosidase; beta-glucuronidase; bicolor guaiac [test]; Birbeck granule; blood glucose; bone graft; brilliant green; buccogingival

B-G Bordet-Gengou [agar, bacillus, phenomenon]

BGA blue-green algae

BGAg blood group antigen

BGAV blue-green algae virus

BGC basal ganglion calcification; blood group class

BGCA bronchogenic carcinoma

BGD blood group degradation

BGE butyl glycidyl ether

BGG bovine gamma-globulin

bGH bovine growth hormone

Bg^J beige [mouse]

BGLB brilliant green lactose broth

BGlu blood glucose

BGM bedside glucose monitoring

BGMR basal ganglion disorder with mental retardation

BGMV bean golden mosaic virus

BGO bismuth germanium oxide

BGP beta-glycerophosphatase

BGS balance, gait, and station; blood group substance; British Geriatrics Society

BGSA blood granulocyte-specific activity

BGTT borderline glucose tolerance test

BH base hospital; benzalkonium and heparin; bill of health; birth history; Bishop-Harman [instruments]; boarding home; board of health; Bolton-Hunter [reagent]; borderline hypertensive; both hands; brain hormone; Braxton-Hicks contractions; breathholding; bronchial hyperreactivity; Bryan high titer; bundle of His

BH$_4$ tetrahydrobiopterin

BHA bound hepatitis antibody; butylated hydroxyanisole

BHAT Beta Blocker Heart Attack Trial

BHB beta-hydroxybutyrate

bHb bovine hemoglobin

BHBA beta-hydroxybutyric acid

BHC benzene hexachloride

BHCDA Bureau of Health Care Delivery and Assistance

bHCG beta human chorionic gonadotropin

BHF Bolivian hemorrhagic fever

BHI biosynthetic human insulin; brain-heart infusion [broth]; British Humanities Index; Bureau of Health Insurance

BHIA brain-heart infusion agar

BHI-ac brain-heart infusion broth with acetone

BHIB brain-heart infusion broth

BHIBA brain-heart infusion blood agar

BHIRS brain-heart infusion and rabbit serum

BHIS beef heart infusion supplemented [broth]

BHK baby hamster kidney [cells]; type-B Hong Kong [influenza virus]

BHL bilateral hilar lymphadenopathy; biological half-life

bHLH basic helix-loop-helix

bHLH-ZIP basic helix-loop-helix-leucine zipper

BHM Bureau of Health Manpower

BHN bephenium hydroxynaphthoate; Brinell hardness number

BHP basic health profile

BHPr Bureau of Health Professions

BHR basal heart rate; benign hypertrophic prostatitis; bronchial hyperreactivity

BHS Bachelor of Health Science; beta-hemolytic streptococcus; breathholding spell

BHT beta-hydroxytheophylline; breath hydrogen test; butylated hydroxytoluene

BHU basic health unit

BHV bovine herpes virus

BH/VH body hematocrit-venous hematocrit [ratio]

BHyg Bachelor of Hygiene

BI background interval; bacterial or bactericidal index; base-in [prism]; basilar impression; Billroth I [operation]; biological indicator; biotehnology infomatics; bodily injury; bone injury; bowel impaction; brain injury; burn index

Bi bismuth

BIA biolectric impedance analysis; bioimmunoassay

BIAC Bioinstrumentation Advisory Council

BIB biliointestinal bypass; brought in by

biblio bibliography

BIBRA British Industrial Biological Research Association

BIBRA British Industrial Biological Research Association

B-IBS B-immunoblastic sarcoma

BIC blood isotope clearance

Bic biceps

BICAO bilateral internal carotid artery occlusion

bicarb bicarbonate

BICC Biomedical Information Communications Center

Bicnu 1,3-bis-(2-chloroethyl)-1-nitrosourea

BID bibliographic information and documentation; brought in dead

bid twice a day [Lat. *bis in die*]

BIDLB block in posteroinferior division of left branch

BIDS brittle hair, intellectual impairment, decreased fertility, and short stature [syndrome]

BIE bullous ichthyosiform erythroderma

BIG 6 analysis of 6 serum components

BIGGY bismuth glycine glucose yeast

BIH benign intracranial hypertension; Beth Israel Hospital

BII beat inclusion index; Billroth II [operation]; butanol-insoluble iodine

BIL basal insulin level; bilirubin

Bil bilirubin

bil bilateral

BILAG British Isles Lupus Assessment Group [Index]

BIL/ALB bilirubin/albumin [rate]

bilat bilateral

bili bilirubin

bili-c conjugated bilirubin

bilirub bilirubin

bili T&D bilirubin total and direct

BIMA bilateral internal mammary artery

BIN butylisonitrile

biochem biochemistry, biochemical

BIOD bony intraorbital distance

bioeng bioengineering

BIOETHICSLINE Bioethical Information Online

biol biology, biological

bioLH bioassay of luteinizing hormone

biophys biophysics, biophysical

BIOSIS BioScience Information Service

BIP bacterial intravenous protein; bi-parietal; bismuth iodoform paraffin; Blue Cross interim payment; brief infertility period

BIPAP bilevel positive airway pressure

BIPLED bilateral, independent, periodic, lateralized epileptiform discharge

BIPM International Bureau of Weights and Measures [Fr. *Bureau International des Poids et Mesures*]

BIPP bismuth iodoform paraffin paste

BIR basic incidence rate; British Institute of Radiology

BIS bone cement implantation syndrome; Brain Information Service; building illness syndrome

BiSP between ischial spines

bisp bispinous [diameter]

BIT binary digit; bitrochanteric

bit binary digit

BITE Bulimic Investigatory Test

BIU barrier isolation unit

BIVAS body image visual analogue scale

BJ Bence Jones [protein, proteinuria]; biceps jerk; Bielschowsky-Jansky [syndrome]; bones and joints

B&J bones and joints

BJE bones, joints, and examination

BJM bones, joints, and muscles

BJP Bence Jones protein or proteinuria

BK below the knee; bovine kidney [cells]; bradykinin

B-K initials of two patients after whom a multiple cutaneous nevus [mole] was named

B/K below knee [amputation]

Bk berkelium

bk back

BKA below-knee amputation

BK-A basophil kallikrein of anaphylaxis

BK amp below-knee amputation

bkf breakfast

Bkg background

BKS beekeeper serum

BKTT below knee to toe

BKWP below knee walking plaster

BL Barré-Lieou [syndrome]; basal lamina; baseline; Bessey-Lowry [unit]; black light; bladder; bleeding; blind loop; blood loss; bone marrow lymphocyte; borderline lepromatous; bronchial lavage; buccolingual; buffered lidocaine; Burkitt lymphoma

Bl black

B-l bursa-equivalent lymphocyte

bl black; blood, bleeding; blue

BLAD borderline left axis deviation

blad bladder

BLAT Blind Learning Aptitute Test

BLB Baker-Lima-Baker [mask]; Bessey-Lowry-Brock [method or unit]; black light bulb; Boothby-Lovelace-Bulbulian [oxygen mask]; bulb [syringe]

BL=BS bilateral equal breath sounds

BlC blood culture

BLCL Burkitt lymphoma cell line

B-LCL B-lymphocyte cell line

bl cult blood culture

BLD basal liquefactive degeneration; benign lymphoepithelial disease

bld blood

Bld Bnk blood bank

BLE both lower extremities; buffered lidocaine with epinephrine

BLEL benign lympho-epithelial lesion

BLEO bleomycin

bleph blepharitis

BLFD buccolinguofacial dyskinesia

BLG beta-lactoglobulin

blH biologically active luteinizing hormone

BLI bombesin-like immunoreactivity

blk black

BLL below lower limit

BLLD British Library Lending Division

BLM bilayer lipid membrane; bimolecular liquid membrane; bleomycin; buccolinguomasticatory

BLN bronchial lymph node

BLOBS bladder obstruction

BLOT British Library of Tape

BLP beta-lipoprotein

BlP blood pressure

B-LPH beta-lipoprotein hormone

B-LPN beta-lipotropin

bl pr blood pressure

BLQ both lower quadrants

BLRC Biomedical Library Review Committee

BLROA British Laryngological, Rhinological, and Otological Association

BLS bare lymphocyte syndrome; basic life support; blind loop syndrome; blood and lymphatic system; blood sugar; Bloom syndrome; Bureau of Labor Statistics

BlS blood sugar

BLSA basic life support ambulance

BLSD bovine lumpy skin disease

BLS-D Blessed scale-dementia

BLT bleeding time; blood-clot lysis time; blood test

BlT bleeding time; blood test; blood type, blood typing

BLU Bessey-Lowry unit

BLV blood volume; bovine leukemia virus

BlV blood viscosity; blood volume

BLVR biliverdin reductase

Blx bleeding time

BM Bachelor of Medicine; barium meal; basal medium; basal metabolism; basement membrane; basilar membrane; betamethasone; biomedical; black male; blood monitoring; body mass; Bohr magneton; bone marrow; bowel movement; breast milk; buccal mass; buccomesial

B/M black male

bm black male

B2M beta-2-microglobulin

BMA bone marrow arrest; British Medical Association

BmA Brugia malayi adult antigen

BMAD Medicare Part B Annual Data [file]

BMAP bone marrow acid phosphatase

B-MAST short Michigan Alcoholism Screening Test

BMB biomedical belt; bone marrow biopsy

BMBL benign monoclonal B cell lymphocytosis

BMC blood mononuclear cell; bone marrow cell; bone mineral content

BMCC beta-methylcrotonyl coenzyme A carboxylase

BMD Becker's muscular dystrophy; Boehringer Mannheim Diagnostics; bone marrow depression; bone mineral density; bovine mucosal disease

BMDC Biomedical Documentation Center

BME basal medium Eagle; biundulant meningoencephalitis; brief maximal effort

BMed Bachelor of Medicine

BMedBiol Bachelor of Medical Biology

BMedSci Bachelor of Medical Science

BMET biomedical equipment technician

BMF bone marrow failure

BMG benign monoclonal gammopathy

BMI body mass index

BMic Bachelor of Microbiology

BMJ bones, muscles, joints; British Medical Journal

bmk birthmark

BML bone marrow lymphocytosis

BMLS billowing mitral leaflet syndrome

BMMP benign mucous membrane pemphigoid

BMN bone marrow necrosis

BMNC blood mononuclear cell

BMOC Brinster's medium for ovum culture

Bmod behavior modification

B-mode brightness modulation

BMP bone morphogenetic protein

BMPI bronchial mucous proteinase inhibitor

BMPP benign mucous membrane pemphigus

BMQA Board of Medical Quality Assurance

BMR basal metabolic rate

BMS Bachelor of Medical Science; betamethasone; biomedical monitoring system; biomedical science; bleomycin sulfate; Bureau of Medical Services; Bureau of Medicine and Surgery; burning mouth syndrome

BMSA British Medical Students Association

BMSP biomedical sciences program

BMST Bruce maximum stress test

BMT Bachelor of Medical Technology; basement membrane thickening; benign mesenchymal tumor; bone marrow transplantation

BMU basic metabolic unit; basic multicellular unit

BMZ basement membrane zone

BN bladder neck; branchial neuritis; bronchial node; brown Norway [rat]; bulimia nervosa

BNA Basle Nomina Anatomica

BND barely noticeable difference

BNDD Bureau of Narcotics and Dangerous Drugs

BNEd Bachelor of Nursing Education

BNF British National Formulary

BNIST National Bureau of Scientific Information [Fr. *Bureau National d'Information Scientifique*]

BNO bladder neck obstruction; bowels not opened

bNOS brain nitric oxide synthase

BNPA binasal pharyngeal airway

BN/RN baccalaurate registered nurse

BNS benign nephrosclerosis

BNSc Bachelor of Nursing Science

BNT Boston Naming Test; brain neurotransmitter

BNYVV beet necrotic yellow vein virus

BO Bachelor of Osteopathy; base of prism out; behavior objective; belladonna and opium; body odor; bowel obstruction; bowels opened; bronchiolitis obliterans; bucco-occlusal

Bo Bolton point

bo bowels

B$_o$ constant magnetic field in a magnetic resonance scanner

B&O belladonna and opium

BOA born on arrival; British Orthopaedic Association

BOAT back pain outcome assessment team

BOBA beta-oxybutyric acid

BOC blood oxygen capacity; Bureau of Census; butyloxycarbonyl

BOD biochemical oxygen demand; brachymorphism-onychodysplasia-dysphalangism [syndrome]

Bod Bodansky [unit]

BOE benign occipital epilepsy

BOEA ethyl biscoumacetate

BOF branchio-oculofacial [syndrome]

BOFS branchio-oculofacial syndrome

BOH board of health

BOLD bleomycin, Oncovin, lomustin, dacarbazine; blood oxygenation level dependent

BOM bilateral otitis media

BOMA bilateral otitis media, acute

BOOP bronchiolitis obliterans-organizing pneumonia

BOP buffalo orphan prototype [virus]

BOR basal optic root; before time of operation; bowels open regularly; branchio-oto-renal [syndrome]

BORR blood oxygen release rate

BOSC Board of Scientific Counselors

BoSM Bolivian squirrel monkey

BOT botulinum toxin

bot bottle

BOU branchio-oto-ureteral [syndrome]
BOW bag of waters
BP Bachelor of Pharmacy; back pressure; barometric pressure; basic protein; bathroom privileges; bed pan; before present; behavior pattern; Bell palsy; benzpyrene; beta-protein; biotic potential; biparietal; biphenyl; bipolar; birth place; blood pressure; body plethysmography; boiling point; Bolton point; borderline personality; breech presentation; British Pharmacopoeia; bronchopleural; buccopulpal; bullous pemphigus; bypass
B/P blood pressure
BP II bipolar II disorder
bp base pair; bed pan; boiling point
BPA blood pressure assembly; bovine plasma albumin; British Paediatric Association; bronchopulmonary aspergillosis; burst-promoting activity
BPAEC bovine pulmonary artery endothelial cell
BPAG bullous pemphigoid antigen
BPB bromphenol blue; biliopancreatic bypass
BPC Behavior Problem Checklist; bile phospholipid concentration; blood pressure cuff; British Pharmaceutical Codex
BPCS back pain classification scale
BPD biparietal diameter; blood pressure decrease; borderline personality disorder; bronchopulmonary dysplasia
BPE bacterial phosphatidylethanolamine
BPEC benign partial epilepsy of childhood; bipolar electrocardiogram
BPEI blepharophimosis, ptosis, epicanthus inversus
BPES blepharophimosis-ptosis-epicanthus inversus syndrome
BPF bradykinin-potentiating factor; bronchopulmonary fistula; burst-promoting factor
BPG benzathine penicillin G; D-2,3-bisphosphoglycerate; blood pressure gauge; bypass graft

BPGM bisphosphoglyceromutase
BPH Bachelor of Public Health; benign prostatic hypertrophy
BPh British Pharmacopoeia; buccopharyngeal
Bph bacteriopheophytin
BPharm Bachelor of Pharmacy
BPHEng Bachelor of Public Health Engineering
BPheo bacteriopheophytin
BPHN Bachelor of Public Health Nursing
BPI bacterial permeability-increasing [protein]; Basic Personality Inventory; beef-pork insulin; blood pressure increase; blood pressure index; brief pain inventory
BPL benign proliferative lesion; benzyl penicilloyl-polylysine; beta-propiolactone
BPLA blood pressure, left arm
BPM beats per minute; biperidyl mustard; breaths per minute; brompheniramine maleate
bpm beats per minute
BPMF British Postgraduate Medical Federation
BPMS blood plasma measuring system
BPN bacitracin, polymyxin B, neomycin sulfate; brachial plexus neuropathy
BPO basal pepsin output; benzyl penicilloyl
BPP biophysical profile; bovine pancreatic polypeptide; bradykinin potentiating peptide
BP&P blood pressure and pulse
BPPN benign paroxysmal positioning nystagmus
BPPV benign paroxysmal positional vertigo; bovine paragenital papilloma virus
BPQ Berne pain questionnaire
BPR blood pressure recorder; blood production rate
BPRA blood pressure, right arm
BPRS brief psychiatric rating scale; brief psychiatric reacting scale

BPS beats per second; Behavioral Pharmacological Society; biophysical profile score; bits per second; bovine papular stomatitis; brain protein solvent; breaths per second

BPSA bronchopulmonary segmental artery

BPsTh Bachelor of Psychotherapy

BPT benign paroxysmal torticollis

BPTI basic pancreatic trypsin inhibitor; basic polyvalent trypsin inhibitor; bovine pancreatic trypsin inhibitor

BPV benign paroxysmal vertigo; benign positional vertigo; bioprosthetic valve; bovine papilloma virus

BP(Vet) British Pharmacopoeia (Veterinary)

Bq becquerel

BQA Bureau of Quality Assurance

BR barrier reared [experimental animals]; baseline recovery; bathroom; bed rest; bedside rounds; bilirubin; biologic response; branchial; breathing rate; bronchial, bronchitis, bronchus; *Brucella,* brucellosis

Br breech; bregma; bridge; bromine; bronchitis; brown; *Brucella;* brucellosis

br boiling range; brachial; branch; branchial; breath; brother

BRA bilateral renal agenesis; bone-resorbing activity; brain-reactive antibody

BRAC basic rest-activity cycle

Brach brachial

Brady, brady bradycardia

BRAMS Bech-Rafaelson melancholia scale

BRAO branch retinal artery occlusion

BRAP burst of rapid atrial pacing

BrAP brachial artery pressure

BRAT Baylor rapid autologous transfusion [system]

BRATT bananas, rice, applesauce, tea and toast

BRB bright red blood

BRBC bovine red blood cell

BRBN blue rubber bleb nevus

BRBNS blue rubber bleb nevus syndrome

BRBPR bright red blood per rectum

BRbx breast biopsy

Brc bromocriptine

BRCD breast cancer, ductal

BRCM below right costal margin

BRCS British Red Cross Society

BRD bladder retraining drill; bovine respiratory disease

BrdU bromodeoxyuridine

BrdUrd bromodeoxyuridine

BREASTS bronchopulmonary aspergillosis, radiotherapy, extrinsic allergic alveolitis, ankylosing spondylitis, sarcoidosis, tuberculosis, silicosis [x-ray findings in fibrotic pulmonary changes]

BRF bone-resorbing factor

BRH benign recurrent hematuria; Bureau of Radiological Health

BRIC benign recurrent intrahepatic cholestasis

BRIC benign recurrent intrahepatic cholestasis

BRIME brief repetitive isometric maximal exercise

Brkf breakfast

BRM biological response modifier; biuret reactive material

BRMS Bech-Rafaelsen melancholia scale

BRN Board of Registered Nursing

brn brown

BRO bronchiolitis obliterans; bronchoscopy

bro brother

brom bromide

Bron, Bronch bronchi, bronchial; bronchoscopy

Broncho bronchoscopy

BRP bathroom privileges; bilirubin production; bronchophony

Brph bronchophony

BRR Bannayan-Riley-Ruvalcaba [syndrome]; baroreceptor reflex response; breathing reserve ratio

BRS behavior rating scale; battered root syndrome; Bibliographic Retrieval Services; British Roentgen Society

BrSM Brazilian squirrel monkey

BRT Brook reaction test

brth breath

BRU bone remodeling unit

BrU bromouracil

Bruc Brucella

BRVO branch retinal vein occlusion

BRW Brown-Robert-Wells [stereotactic system]

BS Bachelor of Science; Bachelor of Surgery; *Bacillus subtilis*; Bartter syndrome; base strap; bedside; before sleep; Behçet syndrome; bilateral symmetrical; bile salt; Binet-Simon [test]; bismuth sulfite; blood sugar; Bloom syndrome; Blue Shield [plan]; body system; borderline schizophrenia; bowel sound; breaking strength; breath sound; British Standard; buffered saline; Bureau of Standards

B-S Bjork-Shiley [valve]

B&S Brown and Sharp [sutures]

bs bedside; bowel sound; breath sound

b x s brother x sister inbreeding

BSA benzenesulfonic acid; Biofeedback Society of America; bismuth-sulfite agar; bis-trimethylsilyl-acetamide; Blind Service Association; Blue Shield Association; body surface area; bovine serum albumin; bowel sounds active

bsa bovine serum albumin

BSAG Bristol Social Adjustment Guides

BSAM basic sequential access method

BSAP brief short-action potential; brief, small, abundant potentials

BSB body surface burned

BS=BL breath sounds equal bilaterally

BSC bedside commode; bedside care; bench scale calorimeter; bile salt con-

centration; Biological Stain Commission; Biomedical Science Corps

BSc Bachelor of Science

BSC-1, BS-C-1 *Cercopithecus* monkey kidney cells

BSCC British Society for Clinical Cytology

BSCP bovine spinal cord protein

BSD bedside drainage

BSDLB block in anterosuperior division of left branch

BSE behavior summarized evaluation; bilateral intranasal sphenoethmoiclectomy; bilateral symmetrical and equal; bovine spongiform encephalopathy; breast self-examination

BSEP brain stem evoked potential

BSER brain stem evoked response [audiometry]

BSF back scatter factor; B-cell stimulatory factor; busulfan

BSG basigin; branchio-skeleto-genital [syndrome]

BSH benign sexual headache

BSI behavior status inventory; blood stream infection; borderline syndrome index; bound serum iron; brainstem injury; brief symptom inventory; British Standards Institution

BSID Bayley scale of infant development

BSIF bile salt independent fraction

BSL benign symmetric lipomatosis; blood sugar level

BSM Bachelor of Science in Medicine

BSMC bronchial smooth muscle cell

BSN baccalaureate of science in nursing; Bachelor of Science in Nursing; bowel sounds normal

BSNA bowel sounds normal and active

BSO bilateral sagittal osteotomy; bilateral salpingo-oophorectomy; British School of Osteopathy; butathione sulfoximine

BSP bromsulphalein

BSp bronchospasm

BSPh bachelor of science in pharmacy

BSQ behavior style questionnaire

BSR basal skin resistance; blood sedimentation rate; bowel sounds regular; brain stimulation reinforcement; Buschke selective reminding [test]

BSS Bachelor of Sanitary Science; balanced salt solution; Bernard-Soulier syndrome; black silk suture; buffered salt solution; buffered single substrate

B-SS Bernard-Soulier syndrome

BSSE bile salt-stimulated esterase

BSSG sitogluside

BSSL bile salt-stimulated lipase

BST bacteriuria screening test; blood serologic test; brief stimulus therapy

BSTFA bis-trimethylsilyltrifluoroacetamide

BSU Bartholin, Skene, urethral [glands]; basic structural unit; British standard unit

BSV binocular single vision

BT base of tongue; bedtime; bitemporal; bitrochanteric; bladder tumor; Blalock-Taussig [shunt]; bleeding time; blood type, blood typing; blue tetrazolium; blue tongue; body temperature; borderline tuberculoid; bovine turbinate [cells]; brain tumor; breast tumor

BTA Blood Transfusion Association

BTB breakthrough bleeding; bromthymol blue

BTBL bromothymol blue lactose

BTC basal temperature chart; body temperature chart

BTCG Brain Tumor Cooperative Group

BTD biliary tract disease

BTDS benzoylthiamine disulfide

BTE behind the ear [hearing aid]; bovine thymus extract

BTFS breast tumor frozen section

BTG beta-thromboglobulin

BTg bovine trypsinogen

BThU British thermal unit

BTL bilateral tubal ligation

BTLS basic trauma life support

BTM benign tertian malaria; body or blood temperature monitor

BTMSA bis-trimethylsilacetylene

BTP biliary tract pain; biological treatment planning

BTPABA N-benzoyl-L-tyrosyl-p-aminobenzoic acid

BTPS at body temperature and ambient pressure, and saturated with water vapor [gas]

BTR Bezold-type reflex; biceps tendon reflex

BTr bovine trypsin

BTS blood transfusion service; blue toe syndrome; bradycardia-tachycardia syndrome

BTSG Brain Tumor Study Group

bTSH bovine thyroid-stimulating hormone

BTU British thermal unit

BTV blue tongue virus

BTX botulinum toxin; brevetoxin

BTx blood transfusion

BTX-B brevetoxin-B

BTZ benzothiazepine

BU base of prism up; Bethesda unit; blood urea; Bodansky unit; bromouracil; burn unit

Bu butyl

bu bushel

BUA blood uric acid; broadband ultrasonic attenuation

Buc, Bucc buccal

BUDR bromodeoxyuridine

BUDS bilateral upper dorsal sympathectomy

BUE both upper extremities

BUF buffalo [rat]

BUG buccal ganglion

BUI brain uptake index

BULIT bulimia test

BULL buccal or upper lingual of lower

BuMed Bureau of Medicine and Surgery

BUMP behavioral regression or upset in hospitalized medical patients [scale]

BUN blood urea nitrogen
bun br bundle branch
BUN/CR blood urea nitrogen/creatine ratio
BUO bleeding of undetermined origin, bruising of undetermined origin
BUQ both upper quadrants
BUR bilateral ureteral occlusion
Burd Burdick suction
BUS Bartholin, urethral, and Skene glands; busulfan
But, but butyrate, butyric
BV bacitracin V; bacterial vaginosis; biological value; blood vessel; blood volume; bronchovesicular
BVA Blind Veterans Association; British Veterinary Association
BVAD biventricular assist device
BVC British Veterinary Codex
BVD bovine viral diarrhea
BVDT brief vestibular disorientation test
BVDU bromovinyldeoxyuridine
BVDV bovine virus diarrhea virus
BVE binocular visual efficiency; blood vessel endothelium; blood volume expander
BVH biventricular hypertrophy
BVI blood vessel invasion
BVL bilateral vas ligation
BVM bag-valve-mask; bronchovascular markings; Bureau of Veterinary Medicine
BVMGT Bender Visual-Motor Gestalt Test
BVMOT Bender Visual-Motor Gestalt Test
BVMS Bachelor of Veterinary Medicine and Science

BVO branch vein occlusion
BVP blood vessel prosthesis; blood volume pulse; burst of ventricular pacing
BVR baboon virus replication
BVS blanked ventricular sense
BVSc Bachelor of Veterinary Science
BVU bromoisovalerylurea
BVV bovine vaginitis virus
BW bacteriological warfare; bed wetting; below waist; biological warfare; biological weapon; birth weight; bladder washout; blood Wasserman [reaction]; body water; body weight
B&W black and white [milk of magnesia and cascara extract]
bw body weight
BWD bacillary white diarrhea
BWFI bacteriostatic water for injection
BWS battered woman (or wife) syndrome; Beckwith-Wiedemann syndrome
BWST black widow spider toxin
BWSV black widow spider venom
BWt birth weight
Bwt body weight
BWYV beet western yellow virus
BX, bx bacitracin X; biopsy
BXO balanitis xerotica obliterans
ByCPR bystander cardiac pulmonary resuscitation
BYDV barley yellow dwarf virus
BYE Barila-Yaguchi-Eveland [medium]
BZ benzodiazepine
Bz, Bzl benzoyl
BZD benzodiazepine
BZQ benzquinamide
BZRP benzodiazepine receptor peripheral [type]
BZS Bannayan-Zonana syndrome

C about [Lat. *circa*]; ascorbic acid; bruised [Lat. *contusus*]; calcitonin-forming [cell]; calculus; calorie [large]; Campylobacter; Candida; canine tooth; capacitance; carbohydrate; carbon; cardiac; cardiovascular disease; carrier; cast; cathode; Caucasian; cell; Celsius; centigrade; central; central electrode placement in electroencephalography; centromeric or constitutive heterochromatic chromosome [banding]; cerebrospinal; certified; cervical; cesarean [section]; chest (precordial) lead in electrocardiography; chicken; *Chlamydia;* chloramphenicol; cholesterol; class; clearance; clonus; *Clostridium*; closure; clubbing; coarse [bacterial colonies]; cocaine; coefficient; color sense; colored [guinea pig]; complement; complex; compliance; component; compound [Lat. *compositus*]; concentration; conditioned, conditioning; condyle; constant; consultation; contraction; control; conventionally reared [experimental animal]; convergence; correct; cortex; coulomb; count; *Cryptococcus*; cubic; cubitus; curie; cyanosis; cylinder; cysteine; cytidine; cytochrome; cytosine; gallon [Lat. *congius*]; horn [Lat. *cornu*]; hundred [Lat. *centum*]; large calorie; molar heat capacity; rib [Lat. *costa*]; velocity of light; with [Lat. *cum*]

C1 first cervical nerve; first cervical vertebra; first component of complement

C_1 first rib

$\bar{C}1$ activated first component of complement

C1 INH inhibitor of first component of complement

CI first cranial nerve

C2 second cervical nerve; second cervical vertebra; second component of complement

C_2 second rib

$\bar{C}2$ activated second component of complement

CII second cranial nerve

C3 third cervical nerve; third cervical vertebra; third component of complement

C_3 Collins' solution; third rib

$\bar{C}3$ activated third component of complement

CIII third cranial nerve

C4 fourth cervical nerve; fourth cervical vertebra; fourth component of complement

$\bar{C}4$ activated fourth component of complement

CIV fourth cranial nerve

C5 fifth cervical nerve; fifth cervical vertebra; fifth component of complement

$\bar{C}5$ activated fifth component of complement

CV fifth cranial nerve

C6 sixth cervical nerve; sixth cervical vertebra; sixth component of complement

$\bar{C}6$ activated sixth component of complement

CVI sixth cranial nerve

C7 seventh cervical nerve; seventh cervical vertebra; seventh component of complement

$\bar{C}7$ activated seventh component of complement

CVII seventh cranial nerve

C8 eighth component of complement

$\bar{C}8$ activated eighth component of complement

CVIII eighth cranial nerve

C9 ninth component of complement

$\bar{C}9$ activated ninth component of complement

56

CIX-CXII ninth to twelfth cranial nerves

°C degree Celsius

C' complement

c about [Lat. *circa*]; calorie [small]; candle; canine tooth; capacity; carat; centi-; complementary [strand]; concentration; contact; cup; curie; cyclic; meal [Lat. *cibus*]; specific heat capacity; with [Lat. *cum*]

c' coefficient of portage

CA anterior commissure [Lat. *commissura anterior*]; calcium antagonist; California [rabbit]; cancer; *Candida albicans*; caproic acid; carbonic anhydrase; carcinoma; cardiac angiography; cardiac arrest; cardiac arrhythmia; carotid artery; cast; catecholamine, catecholaminergic; cathode; Caucasian adult; celiac axis; cerebral aqueduct; cerebral atrophy; cervicoaxial; Chemical Abstracts; chemotactic activity; child abuse; chloroamphetamine; cholic acid; chromosomal aberration; chronic anovulation; chronological age; citric acid; clotting assay; coagglutination; coarctation of the aorta; Cocaine Anonymous; coefficient of absorption; cold agglutinin; colloid antigen; common antigen; compressed air; conceptional age; coracoacromial; coronary artery; corpora alata; corpora amylacea; corpus albicans; corrected [echo] area; cortisone acetate; cricoarytenoid; cricoid arch; croup-associated [virus]; cytosine arabinoside; cytotoxic antibody

Ca calcium; cancer, carcinoma; *Candida albicans;* cathode

ca about [Lat. *circa*]; candle; carcinoma

C&A Clinitest and Acetest

CA-2 second colloid antigen

Ca²⁺-blocker calcium channel blocker

CAA carotid audiofrequency analysis; cerebral amyloid angiopathy; circulating anodic antigen; Clean Air Act; computer-assisted assessment; constitutional aplastic anemia; coronary artery aneurysm; crystalline amino acids

CAAH chronic active autoimmune hepatitis

CAAT computer-assisted axial tomography

CAAX [box] protein segment in which C is cysteine, A is usually but not always an aliphatic amino acid, and X is methionine or serine

CAB captive air bubble; cellulose acetate butyrate; coronary artery bypass

CABG coronary artery bypass grafting

CABGS coronary artery bypass graft surgery

CaBI calcium bone index

CABMET Colorado Association of Biomedical Engineering Technicians

CaBP calcium-binding protein

CABS coronary artery bypass surgery

CAC cardiac-accelerator center; cardiac arrest code; circulating anticoagulant

CaCC cathodal closure contraction

CAC/CIC chronic active/inactive cirrhosis

CACP cisplatin

CaCTe cathodal closure tetanus

CaCV calicivirus

CaCX cancer of cervix

CACY calcyclin

CAD cadaver, cadaveric; cold agglutinin disease; compressed air disease; computer-assisted design; computer-assisted diagnosis; congenital abduction deficiency; coronary artery disease; coronoradiographic documentation

Cad cadaver, cadaveric

CAD/CAM computer-aided design/computer-aided manufacturing

CADD computer-aided drug design

CADI coronary artery disease index

CADL Communicative Abilities in Daily Living

CaDTe cathodal-duration tetanus

CAE caprine arthritis-encephalitis; cellulose acetate electrophoresis; contingent after-effects; coronary artery embolism
CaE calcium excretion
CaEDTA calcium disodium ethylenediaminetetraacetate
CAEP cortical auditory evoked potential
CAEV caprine arthritis-encephalitis virus
CAF cell adhesion factor; citric acid fermentation
Caf caffeine
CAG cholangiogram, cholangiography; chronic atrophic gastritis; coronary angiography
CAGA calgranulin A
CAGB calgranulin B
CAGE *c*ut down, *a*nnoyed by criticism, *g*uilty about drinking, *e*ye-opener drinks (a test for alcoholism)
CAH chronic active hepatitis; chronic aggressive hepatitis; combined atrial hypertrophy; congenital adrenal hyperplasia; cyanacetic acid hydrazide
CAHD coronary arteriosclerotic heart disease
CAHEA Committee on Allied Health Education and Accreditation
CAHMR cataract-hypertrichosis-mental retardation [syndrome]
CAHS central alveolar hypoventilation syndrome
CAHV central alveolar hypoventilation
CAI cellular adaptive immunotherapy; complete androgen insensitivity; computer-assisted instruction
CAIS complete androgen insensitivity syndrome
CAL café au lait; calcium test; calculated average life; calories; chronic airflow limitation; computer-assisted learning; coracoacromial ligament
Cal caliber; large calorie
cal small calorie
C$_{alb}$ albumin clearance
Calc calcium

CALC calcitonin
calc calculation
calcif calcification
CALCR calcitonin receptor
CALD chronic active liver disease
CALGB cancer and leukemia group B
CALH chronic active lupoid hepatitis
cALL common null cell acute lymphocytic leukemia
cALLA common acute lymphoblastic leukemia antigen
CALM café-au-lait macules
CALP congenital absence of left pericardium
CAM calf aortic microsome; cell adhesion molecule; cell-associating molecule; chorioallantoic membrane; computer assisted myelography; confusion assessment method [rating for delirium]; contralateral axillary metastasis; cystic adenomatoid malformation
CaM calmodulin
C$_{am}$ amylase clearance
CAMAC computer automated measurement and control
CAMAK cataract-microcephaly-arthrogryposis-kyphosis [syndrome]
CAMCAM Center for Assessment and Management of Changes in Academic Medicine
CAMCOG Cambridge cognitive capacity scale
CAMDEX Cambridge mental disorders of the elderly examination
CAMF cyclophosphamide, Adriamycin, methotrexate, fluorouracil
CAMP Christie-Atkins-Munch-Petersen [test]; computer-assisted menu planning; concentration of adenosine monophosphate; cyclic adenosine monophosphote; cyclophosphamide, Adriamycin, methotrexate, and procarbazine
cAMP cyclic adenosine monophosphate
CAMS computer-assisted monitoring system

CaMV cauliflower mosaic virus
CAMVA chorioallantoic membrane vascular assay
Can cancer; Candida; *Cannabis*
CA/N child abuse and neglect
CANA circulating antineuronal antibody
CaNaEDTA calcium-disodium ethylenediamine tetraacetic acid
canc cancelled
C-ANCA cytoplasmic anti-neutrophilic cytoplasmic antibody
CANCERLIT Cancer Literature
CANCERPROJ Cancer Research Projects
CANP calcium-activated neutral protease
CANS central auditory nervous system
CAN'T LEAP cyclosporine, alcohol, nicotinic acid, thiazides, lasix, ethambutanol, aspirin, pyrazinamide [substances causing hyperuricemia]
CANX calnexin
CAO chronic airway obstruction; coronary artery obstruction
CAO$_2$ arterial oxygen content
CaOC cathodal opening contraction
CaOCL cathodal opening clonus
CAOD coronary artery occlusive disease
CAOM chronic adhesive otitis media
CAOT Canadian Association of Occupational Therapy
CaOTe cathodal opening tetanus
CAP camptodactyly-arthropathy-pericarditis [syndrome]; Canada Assistance Plan; capsule; captopril; catabolite gene activator protein; cell attachment protein; cellular acetate propionate; cellulose acetate phthalate; central apical part; chloramphenicol; chronic alcoholic pancreatitis; College of American Pathologists; complement-activated plasma; compound action potential; coupled atrial pacing; cyclosphosphamide, Adriamycin, and Platino [cisplatin]; cystine aminopeptidase

C$_{AP}$ cationic antimicrobial protein; circumference of apex
cap capacity; capsule
CAPA cancer-associated polypeptide antigen
CAPCC Canadian Association of Poison Control Centers
CAPD continuous ambulatory peritoneal dialysis
CAPE Clifton assessment procedures for the elderly; computer-assisted patient emulator
CAPERS Computer Assisted Psychiatric Evaluation and Review System
CAPP Captopril Prevention Project [study]
CAPPS Current and Past Psychopathology Scale
CAPRCA chronic, acquired, pure red cell aplasia
CAPRI Cardiopulmonary Research Institute
CAPS community adjustment profile system
caps capsule
CAR Canadian Association of Radiologists; cancer-associated retinopathy; cardiac ambulation routine; cell adhesion regulator; chronic articular rheumatism; computer-assisted radiology; computer-assisted research; conditioned avoidance response
car carotid
CARA chronic aspecific respiratory ailment
CARB carbohydrate; coronary artery bypass graft
carb carbohydrate; carbonate
carbo carbohydrate
CARD cardiac automatic resuscitative device
card cardiac
card insuff cardiac insufficiency
cardiol cardiology
CARE comprehensive assessment and

referral evaluation; computerized adult and records evaluation [system]

CARES cancer rehabilitation evaluation system

CARF Commission on Accreditation and Rehabilitation Facilities

CARP carbonic anhydrase-related polypeptide

CARS Childhood Autism Rating Scale; Children's Affective Rating Scale; cysteinyl-transfer ribonucleic acid synthetase

CART computer-assisted radiotherapy

cart cartilage

CAS calcarine sulcus; calcific aortic stenosis; Cancer Attitude Survey; carbohydrate-active steroid; cardiac adjustment scale; cardiac surgery; Celite-activated normal serum; Center for Alcohol Studies; central anticholinergic syndrome; cerebral atherosclerosis; Chemical Abstract Service; cognitive assessment scale; cold agglutinin syndrome; computer-assisted surgery; congenital alcoholic syndrome; control adjustment strap; coronary artery spasm; Council of Academic Societies

Cas casualty

cas castration, castrated

CASA computer-assisted self assessment

CASH Commission for Administrative Services in Hospitals; corticoadrenal stimulating hormone; cruciform anterior spinal hyperextension

CASHD coronary arteriosclerotic heart disease

CASI cognitive abilities screening instrument

CASMD congenital atonic sclerotic muscular dystrophy

CASPER computer-assisted pericardiac surgery

CASQ calsequestrin

CAS-REGN Chemical Abstracts Service Registry Number

CAS-REGN Chemical Abstracts Service Registry Number

CASRT corrected adjusted sinus node recovery time

CASS cataract-alopecia-sclerodactyly syndrome; Coronary Artery Surgery Study

CASSIS Classification and Search Support Information System [Patent Office]

CAST calpastatin; Cardiac Arrhythmia Suppression Trial; Children of Alcoholism Screening Test

CAT California Achievement Test; capillary agglutination test; catalase; cataract; catecholamine; Children's Apperception Test; chloramphenicol acetyltransferase; chlormerodrin accumulation test; choline acetyltransferase; chronic abdominal tympany; Cognitive Abilities Test; computed abdominal tomography; computed axial tomography; computer of average transients; critically appraised topic

cat catalysis, catalyst; cataract

CAT'ase catalase

CATB catalase B

CATCH Community Actions to Control High Blood Pressure

Cath cathartic; catheter, catheterize

cath catheterization

CATLINE Catalog On-Line

CATS Canadian American Ticlopidine Study

CAT-S Children's Apperception Test, Supplemental

CAT scan computed axial tomography scan

CATT calcium tolerance test

Cauc Caucasian

caud caudal

caut cauterization

CAV congenital absence of vagina; congenital adrenal virilism; constant angular velocity; croup-associated virus

cav cavity

CAVB complete atrioventricular block

CAVD complete atrioventricular dissociation; completion, arithmetic problems, vocabulary, following directions [test]; congenital aplasia of vas deferens

CAVG coronary artery vein graft

CAVH continuous arteriovenous hemofiltration

CAVHD continuous arteriovenous hemodialysis

CAVLT Children's Auditory Verbal Learning Test

CAVO common atrioventricular orifice

CAVS Conformance Assessment to Voluntary Standards

CAVU continuous arteriovenous ultrafiltration

CAW central airways

C_{AW} airway conductance

CB Bachelor of Surgery [Lat. *Chirurgiae Baccalaureus*]; calcium blocker; carbenicillin; carotid body; chocolate blood [agar]; chromatin body; chronic bronchitis; circumflex branch; code blue; color blind; compensated base; conus branch; Coomassie blue; coracobrachial

Cb cerebellum; niobium [columbium]

CBA chronic bronchitis and asthma; cost-benefit analysis

CBAB complement-binding antibody

CBADAA Certifying Board of the American Dental Assistants Association

CBAVD congenital bilateral absence of vas deferens

CBBM color blindness, blue monocone-monochromatic type

CBC capillary blood gases; carbenicillin; child behavior characteristics; complete blood cell count

cbc complete blood cell count

CBCL Child Behavior Checklist

CBCL/2-3 Child Behavior Checklist for ages 2-3

CBCN carbenicillin

CbCtx cerebellar cortex

CBD carotid body denervation; closed bladder drainage; common bile duct

CBDC chronic bullous disease of children

CBDE common bile duct exploration

CBE clinical breast examination

CBER Center for Biologic Evaluation and Research

CBET certified biomedical equipment technician

CBF capillary blood flow; cerebral blood flow; ciliary beat frequency; coronary blood flow; cortical blood flow

CBFB core binding factor, beta

CBG capillary blood gases; coronary bypass graft; corticosteroid-binding globulin; cortisol-binding globulin

CBGv corticosteroid-binding globulin variant

CBH chronic benign hepatitis; cutaneous basophilic hypersensitivity

CBI children's behavior inventory; continuous bladder irrigation

CBL circulating blood lymphocytes; chronic blood loss; cord blood leukocytes

Cbl cobalamin

CBM capillary basement membrane

CBMMP chronic benign mucous membrane pemphigus

CBN cannabinol; central benign neoplasm; Commission on Biological Nomenclature

CBO Congressional Budget Office

CBOC completion bed occupancy care

CBP calcium-binding protein; carbohydrate-binding protein; cardiopulmonary bypass; chlorobiphenyl; cobalamin-binding protein

C4BP complement 4 binding protein

CBPA competitive protein-binding assay

CBPS congenital bilateral perisylvian syndrome

CBR carbonyl reductase; chemical, biological, and radiological [warfare]; chemically-bound residue; chronic bed rest; complete bed rest; crude birth rate

CB3S Coxsackie B3 virus susceptibility

CBS cervicobrachial syndrome; chronic brain syndrome; clinical behavioral science; conjugated bile salts; culture-bound syndrome; cystathionine beta-synthase

CBT carotid body tumor; cognitive behavioral treatment/therapy; computed body tomography

CBV capillary blood cell velocity; catheter balloon valvuloplasty; central blood volume; cerebral blood volume; circulating blood volume; cortical blood volume; corrected blood volume; Coxsackie B virus

CBVD cerebrovascular disease

CBW chemical and biological warfare

CBX computer-based examination

CBZ carbamazepine

CC calcaneal-cuboid; calcium cyclamate; cardiac catheterization; cardiac contusion; cardiac cycle; cardiovascular clinic; cell culture; central compartment; cerebral commissure; cerebral cortex; chest circumference; cervical cancer; chief complaint; cholecalciferol; chondrocalcinosis; choriocarcinoma; chronic complainer; circulatory collapse; classical conditioning; clean catch [of urine]; Clinical Center [NIH]; clinical course; clomiphene citrate; closed cup; closing capacity; collagenous colitis; colony count; colorectal cancer; columnar cells; commission certified; common cold; complicating condition; compound cathartic; computer calculated; concordance; congenital cardiopathy; congenital cataract; consumptive coagulopathy; contrast cystogram; conversion complete; coracoclavicular; cord compression; corpus callosum; costochondral; Coulter counter; craniocaudal; craniocervical; creatinine clearance; critical care; critical condition; Crohn colitis; Cronkhite-Canada [syndrome]; crus

cerebri; cubic centimeter; current complaint; Current Contents

C-C convexo-concave

C&C cold and clammy

Cc concave

cc clean catch [urine]; concave; corrected; cubic centimeter

CCA cephalin cholesterol antigen; chick cell agglutination; chimpanzee coryza agent; choriocarcinoma; circulating cathodic antigen; circumflex coronary artery; common carotid artery; congenital contractural arachnodactyly; constitutional chromosome abnormality

CCAT chick cell agglutination test; conglutinating complement absorption test

CCB calcium channel blocker

CCBV central circulating blood volume

CCC care-cure coordination; cathodal closure contraction; chronic calculous cholecystitis; chronic catarrhal colitis; comprehensive care clinic; concurrent care concern; consecutive case conference; critical care complex; council on clinical classification; cylindrical confronting cisternae

CC&C colony count and culture

CCCC centrifugal countercurrent chromatography

cccDNA covalently closed circular deoxyribonucleic acid

CCCE cross-cultural cognitive examination

CCCl cathodal closure clonus

CCCP carbonyl cyanide m-chloro-phenyl-hydrazone

CCCR closed chest cardiac resuscitation

CCCS condom catheter collecting system

CCCT closed craniocerebral trauma

CCCU comprehensive cardiac care unit

CCD calibration curve data; central core disease; charge-coupled device; childhood celiac disease; cleidocranial dysplasia; countercurrent distribution; cumulative cardiotoxic dose

CCDC Canadian Communicable Disease Center

CCDN Central Council for District Nursing

ccDNA closed circle deoxyribonucleic acid

CCE carboline carboxylic acid ester; chamois contagious ecthyma; clear-cell endothelioma; clubbing, cyanosis, and edema; countercurrent electrophoresis

CCEHRP Committee to Coordinate Environmental Health and Related Programs

CCEI Crown-Crisp Experimental Index

CCF cancer coagulation factor; cardiolipin complement fixation; carotid-cavernous fistula; centrifuged culture fluid; cephalin-cholesterol flocculation; compound comminuted fracture; congestive heart failure; crystal-induced chemotactic factor

CCFA cefotoxin-cycloserine fructose agar

CCFAS compact colony-forming active substance

CCFE cyclophosphamide, cisplatin, fluorouracil, and extramustine

CCFMG Cooperating Committee on Foreign Medical Graduates

CCG Children's Cancer Study Group; cholecystogram, cholecystography; clinically coherent group

CCGC capillary column gas chromotography

CCH C-cell hyperplasia; chronic chloride hemagglutination; chronic cholestatic hepatitis

CCHA Canadian Council on Hospital Accreditation

CCHD cyanotic congenital heart disease

CCHE Central Council for Health Education

CCHFA Canadian Council on Health Facilities Accreditation

CCHMS Central Committee for Hospital Medical Services

CCHP Consumer Choice Health Plan

CCHS congenital central hypoventilation syndrome

CCI Cardiovascular Credentialing International; cholesterol crystallization inhibitor; chronic coronary insufficiency; common client interface; corrected count increment

CCK cholecystokinin

CCK-8 cholecystokinin octapeptide

CCKLI cholecystokinin-like immunoreactivity

CCK-OP cholecystokinin octapeptide

CCK-PZ cholecystokinin-pancreozymin

CCKRB cholecystokinin receptor B

CCL carcinoma cell line; certified cell line; Charcot-Leyden crystal; continuing care level; critical carbohydrate level

CCLI composite clinical and laboratory index

CCM cerebrocostomandibular [syndrome]; chemical cleavage of mismatch; congestive cardiomyopathy; craniocervical malformation; critical care medicine

c cm cubic centimeter

CCMC Committee on the Costs of Medical Care

CCME Coordinating Council on Medical Education

CCMS cerebrocostomandibular syndrome; clean catch midstream [urine]; clinical care management system

CCMSU clean catch midstream urine

CCMT catechol methyltransferase

CCMU critical care medical unit

CCN caudal central nucleus; community care network; coronary care nursing; critical care nursing

CCNHP community college nursing home project

CCNU N-(2-chloroethyl)-N'-cyclohexyl-N-nitrosourea

CCO cytochrome C oxidase

CCOT cervical compression overloading test

CCP cephalin-cholesterol flocculation; ciliocytophthoria; chronic calcifying pancreatitis; community care plan; cytidine cyclic phosphate

CCPD continuous cycling (cyclical) peritoneal dialysis

CCPDS Centralized Cancer Patient Data System

CCPR crypt cell production rate

CCR complete continuous remission

CCRC comprehensive care retirement community; continuing care retirement community

Ccr, C$_{cr}$ creatinine clearance

CCRG Cooperative Cataract Research Group (American)

CCRIS Chemical Carcinogenesis Research Information System

CCRN Critical Care Registered Nurse

CCRS Chemical Carcinogenesis Research Information System

CCRT computer-controlled radiation therapy

CCS Canadian Cardiovascular Society; casualty clearing station; cell cycle specific; cholecystosonography; chronic cerebellar stimulation; chronic compartment syndrome; cloudy cornea syndrome; composite cultured skin; concentration camp syndrome; costoclavicular syndrome

CCSCS central cervical spinal cord syndrome

CCSE Cognitive Capacity Screening Examination

CCSG Children's Cancer Study Group

CCSK clear cell sarcoma of the kidney

CCSP Clara cell-specific protein

CCT carotid compression tomography; central conduction time; cerebrocranial trauma; chocolate-coated tablet; coated compressed tablet; combined cortical thickness; composite cyclic therapy; computerized cranial tomography; contrast enhanced computed tomography; controlled cord traction; coronary care team; cranial computed tomography; cyclocarbothiamine

CCTe cathodal closure tetanus

CCTP coronary care training program

CCTV closed circuit television

CCU cardiac care unit; Cherry-Crandall unit; coronary care unit; critical care unit

ccua clean catch urinalysis

CCUP colpocystourethropexy

CCV channel catfish virus; conductivity cell volume

CCVD chronic cerebrovascular disease

CCVM congenital cardiovascular malformation

CCW critical care workstation; counterclockwise

CD cadaver donor; canine distemper; canine dose; carbohydrate dehydratase; carbon dioxide; cardiac disease; cardiac dullness; cardiac dysrhythmia; cardiovascular disease; Carrel-Dakin [fluid]; Castleman disease; caudad, caudal; celiac disease; cell dissociation; cervicodorsal; cesarean delivery; chemical dependency; circular dichroism; cluster of differentiation [antigens]; color Doppler; combination drug; common [bile] duct; communicable disease; compact disk; completely denatured; conduct disorder; conduction disorder; conjugata diagonalis; consanguineous donor; contact dermatitis; contagious disease; control diet; controlled drug; conventional dialysis; convulsive disorder; convulsive dose; corneal dystrophy; Cotrel-Dubousset [rod]; Crohn disease; crossed diagonal; curative dose; cutdown; cystic duct

C/D cigarettes per day; cup to disc ratio

C&D cystoscopy and dilatation

Cd cadmium; caudal; coccygeal; condylion

cd candela; caudal

c/d cigarettes per day

CD4 HIV helper cell count

CD8 HIV suppressor cell count

CD$_{50}$ median curative dose

CDA Canadian Dental Association; Certified Dental Assistant; chenodeoxycholic acid; ciliary dyskinesia activity; complement-dependent antibody; completely denatured alcohol; computer diagnostic assistant; congenital dyserythropoietic anemia

CDAC Clinical Data Abstraction Center

CDAI Crohn disease activity index

CDAP continuous distending airway pressure

C&DB cough and deep breath

CDC calculated date of confinement; cancer diagnosis center; capillary diffusion capacity; cell division control; cell division cycle; Centers for Disease Control and Prevention; chenodeoxycholate; children's diagnostic classification; Communicable Disease Center; complement-dependent cytotoxicity

CD-C controlled drinker-control

CDCA chenodeoxycholic acid

CDC-BRFS Centers for Disease Control Behavioral Risk Factor Survey

CDD certificate of disability for discharge; choledochoduodenostomy; chronic degenerative disease; chronic disabling dermatosis; craniodiaphyseal dysplasia

CDDP cis-diaminedichloroplatinum

CDE canine distemper encephalitis; chlordiazepoxide; color Doppler energy [imaging]; common duct exploration

CDEC Comprehensive Developmental Evaluation Chart

CDER Center for Drug Evaluation and Research; chronic granulomatous disease

CDF chondrodystrophia foetalis

CDG central developmental groove

CDGE constant denaturant gel electrophoresis

CDGG corneal dystrophy Groenouw type, granular

CDGS carbohydrate-deficient glycoprotein syndrome

cDGS complete form of DiGeorge syndrome

CDH ceramide dihexoside; congenital diaphragmatic hernia; congenital dislocation of hip; congenital dysplasia of hip

CDI cell-directed inhibitor; central or chronic diabetes insipidus; Children's Depression Inventory; color Doppler imaging; cranial diabetes insipidus; cyclin-dependent kinase interactor

CDILD chronic diffuse interstitial lung disease

CDK cell division kinase; climatic droplet keratopathy; cyclin-dependent kinase

CDL chlordeoxylincomycin; Cornelia de Lange [syndrome]

CDLE chronic discoid lupus erythematosus

CDLS Cornelia de Lange syndrome

CDM chemically-defined medium; clinical decision making

CDMNS clinical decision making in nursing scale

cDNA circular deoxyribonucleic acid; complementary deoxyribonucleic acid

CDNB 1-chloro-2,4-dinitrobenzene

CDP chondrodysplasia punctata; chronic destructive periodontitis; collagenase-digestible protein; continuous distending pressure; coronary drug project; cytidine diphosphate; cytosine diphosphate

CDPC cytidine diphosphate choline

CDPR chondrodysplasia punctata, rhizomelic

CDPS calcium-dependent protease small subunit

CDPX X-linked chondrodysplasia punctata

CDR calcium-dependent regulator; clinical dementia rating; complementary determining region; computerized digital radiography; cup/disk ratio

CDRH Center for Devices and Radiological Health

CD-ROM compact disk-read only memory

CDRS Children's Depression Rating Scale

CDS cardiovascular surgery; catechol-3, 5-disulfonate; caudal dysplasia syndrome; Chemical Data System; children's diagnostic scale; Christian Dental Society; cumulative duration of survival

CDSC Communicable Diseases Surveillance Centre [London]

CDSM Committee on Dental and Surgical Materials

cd-sr candela-steradian

CDSRF chronic disease and sociodemographic risk factors

CDSS clinical decision support system

CDT carbohydrate-deficient transferrin; carbon dioxide therapy; Certified Dental Technician; children's day treatment; *Clostridium difficile* toxin; combined diphtheria tetanus

CDTe cathode duration tetanus

CDV canine distemper virus

cDVH cumulative dose-volume histogram

Cdyn, C$_{dyn}$ dynamic compliance

CDZ chlordiazepoxide; conduction delay zone

CE California encephalitis; cardiac enlargement; cardioesophageal; carotid endarterectomy; catamenial epilepsy; cataract extraction; cell extract; central episiotomy; chemical energy; chick embryo; chloroform ether; cholesterol esters; chorioepithelioma; chromatoelectrophoresis; ciliated epithelium; columnar epithelium; conical elevation; conjugated estrogens; constant error; continuing education; contractile element; converting enzyme; crude extract; cytopathic effect

Ce cerium

C-E chloroform-ether

CEA carcinoembryonic antigen; carotid endarterectomy; cholesterol-esterifying activity; cost-effectiveness analysis; crystalline egg albumin

CEAC clinical education and assessment center

CEAL carcinoembryonic antigen-like [protein]

CEAP Clinical Efficacy Assessment Project [of ACP]

CEARP Continuing Education Approval and Recognition Program

CEAT chronic ectopic atrial tachycardia

CEB calcium entry blocker

cEBV chronic Epstein-Barr virus [infection]

CEC central echo complex; ciliated epithelial cell; Commission of the European Community

CECT contrast-enhanced computed tomography

CED chondroectodermal dysplasia

CEE Central European encephalitis; chick embryo extract

CEEA curved end-to-end anastomosis [stapler]

CEEF clinical evaluation encounter form

CEEG computer-analyzed electroencephalography

CEET chicken enucleated eye test

CEEV Central European encephalitis virus

CEF centrifugation extractable fluid; chick embryo fibroblast; constant electric field

CEFMG Council on Education for Foreign Medical Graduates

CEG chronic erosive gastritis

CEH cholesterol ester hydrolase

CEHC calf embryonic heart cell

CEI character education inquiry; converting enzyme inhibitor

CEID crossed electroimmunodiffusion

CEJ cement-enamel junction

CEK chick embryo kidney

CEL carboxyl-ester lipase

CELDIC Commission on Emotional and Learning Disorders in Children

Cell celluloid

CELO chick embryonal lethal orphan [virus]

Cels Celsius

CEM computerized electroencephalographic map; conventional transmission electron microscope

CEMC Clinical Engineering Management Committee [of AAMI]

CEN Certificate for Emergency Nursing; Comité European de Normalisation (standards); continuous enteral nutrition

cen centromere; central

CENP centromere protein

CENPA entromeric protein A

CENPB centromeric protein B

CENPC centromeric protein C

CENPD centromeric protein D

CENPE centromeric protein E

cent centigrade; central

CEO chick embryo origin; Chief Executive Officer

CEOT calcifying epithelial odontogenic tumor

CEP chronic eosinophilic pneumonia; chronic erythropoietic porphyria; congenital erythropoietic porphyria; continuing education program; cortical evoked potential; counter-electrophoresis

CEPA chloroethane phosphoric acid

CEPH cephalic; cephalosporin; Council on Education for Public Health

ceph cephalin

CEPH FLOC cephalin flocculation

CEQ Council on Environmental Quality

CER capital expenditure review; ceramide; conditioned emotional response; control electrical rhythm; cortical evoked response

CERAD Consortium to Establish a Registry for Alzheimer disease

CERCLA The Comprehensive Environmental Response, Compensation, and Liability Act

CERD chronic end-stage renal disease

CERP Continuing Education Recognition Program

Cert, cert certified

cerv cervix, cervical

CES carboxylesterase; cauda equina syndrome; cat's eye syndrome; central excitatory state; chronic electrophysiological study; clinical engineering services; conditioned escape response

CES-D Center for Epidemiological Studies of Depression [scale]

CESD cholesterol ester storage disease

CET capital expenditure threshold; congenital eyelid tetrad

CETE Central European tick-borne encephalitis

CETP cholesteryl ester transfer protein

CEU congenital ectropion uveae; continuing education unit

CEV California encephalitis virus; *Citrus exocortis* viroid

CEX clinical evaluation exercise

CEZ cefazolin

CF calcaneal fibular [ligament]; calcium leucovorin; calf blood flow; calibration factor; cancer-free; carbol-fuchsin; carbon filtered; cardiac failure; carotid foramen; carrier-free; cascade filtration; case file; Caucasian female; centrifugal force; characteristic frequency; chemotactic factor; chest and left leg [lead in electrocardiography]; Chiari-Frommel [syndrome]; chick fibroblast; Christmas factor; citrovorum factor; clotting factor; colicin factor; collected fluid; colonization factor; colony forming; complement fixation; computed fluoroscopy; constant frequency; contractile force; coronary flow; cough frequency; count fingers; counting finger; coupling factor; cycling fibroblast; cystic fibrosis

Cf californium

cf centrifugal force; bring together, compare [Lat. *confer*]

CFA colonization factor antigen; colony-forming assay; complement-fixing antibody; complete Freund's adjuvant; configuration frequency analysis; cryptogenic fibrosing alveolitis

CFAG cystic fibrosis antigen

CFB central fibrous body

CFC capillary filtration coefficient; colony-forming capacity; cardiofaciocutaneous [syndrome]; chlorofluorocarbon; colony-forming cell; continuous flow centrifugation

CFD cephalofacial deformity; craniofacial dysostosis

CFDS craniofacial dyssynostosis

CFDU color-flow Doppler ultrasonography; color flow Doppler ultrasound

CFF critical flicker fusion [test]; critical fusion frequency; cystic fibrosis factor; Cystic Fibrosis Foundation

cff critical flicker fusion; critical fusion frequency

CFFA cystic fibrosis factor activity

CFH complement factor H; Council on Family Health

CFHL complement factor H-like [protein]

CFHP Council on Federal Health Programs

CFI chemotactic-factor inactivator; closed-clenched fist injury; color flow imaging; complement fixation inhibition

CFM chlorofluoromethane; close-fitting mask; craniofacial microsomia

CFMA Council for Medical Affairs

CFMG Commission on Foreign Medical Graduates

CFND craniofrontonasal dysostosis

CFNS chills, fever, night sweats; craniofrontonasal syndrome

CFO chief financial officer

CFP chronic false positive; Clinical Fellowship Program; cyclophosphamide, fluorouracil, prednisone; cystic fibrosis of pancreas; cystic fibrosis protein

CFPC College of Family Physicians of Canada

CFPP craniofacial pattern profile

CFPR Canadian Familial Polyposis Registry

CFR case-fatality ratio; citrovorum-factor rescue; Code of Federal Regulations; complement-fixation reaction; correct fast reaction; cycloc flow reduction

CFS cancer family syndrome; Chiari-Frommel syndrome; chronic fatigue syndrome; craniofacial stenosis; crush fracture syndrome; culture fluid supernatant; Cystic Fibrosis Society

CFSE crystal field stabilization energy

CFSTI Clearinghouse for Federal Scientific and Technical Information

CFT cardiolipin flocculation test; clinical full time; complement-fixation test

CFTR cystic fibrosis transmembrane conductance regulator

CFU colony-forming unit

CFU-C CFU$_C$ colony-forming unit, culture

CFU-E, CFU$_E$ colony-forming unit, erythrocyte

CFU-EOS, CFU$_{EOS}$ colony-forming unit, eosinophil

CFU-F, CFU$_F$ colony-forming unit-fibroblastoid

CFU-G, CFU$_G$ colony-forming unit, granulocyte

CFU-GEMM, CFU$_{GEMM}$ colony forming unit, granulocyte, erythrocyte, macrophage, megakaryocyte

CFU-GM, CFU$_{GM}$ colony-forming unit, granulocyte macrophage

CFU-L, CFU$_L$ colony-forming unit, lymphocyte

CFU$_M$ colony-forming unit-megakaryocyte

CFU-MEG, CFU$_{MEG}$ colony-forming unit, megakaryocyte

CFU-NM, CFU$_{NM}$ colony-forming unit, neutrophil-monocyte

CFU-S, CFU$_S$ colony-forming unit, spleen; colony-forming unit, stem cells

CFV continuous flow ventilation

CFVS cerebrospinal fluid flow void sign

CFW Carworth farm [mouse], Webster strain

CFWM cancer-free white mouse

CFX cefoxitin; circumflex coronary artery

CFZ capillary free zone

CFZC continuous-flow zonal centrifugation

CG cardiography; cardiogreen; choking gas; choriogenic gynecomastia; chorionic gonadotropin; chromogranin; chronic glomerulonephritis; cingulate gyrus; colloidal gold; control group; cryoglobulin; cystine guanine; phosgene [choking gas]

cg center of gravity; centigram; chemoglobulin

CGA catabolite gene activator; color graphics adapter

CGAS Children's Global Assessment Scale

CGAT chromatin granule amine transformer

CGB chronic gonadotropin, beta-unit

CGD chronic granulomatous disease

CGDE contact glow discharge electrolysis

CGFH congenital fibrous histiocytoma

CGFNS Commission on Graduates of Foreign Nursing Schools

CGGE constant gradient gel electrophoresis

CGH chorionic gonadotropic hormone

CGI chronic granulomatous inflammation; Clinical Global Impression [scale]; common gateway interface [of the NCSA]; computer-generated imagery

CGKD complex glycerol kinase deficiency

CGL chronic granulocytic leukemia

c gl correction with glasses

CGM central gray matter

cgm centigram

CGMMV cucumber green mottle mosaic virus

cGMP cyclic guanosine monophosphate

CGN chronic glomerulonephritis

CGNB composite ganglioneuroblastoma

CG/OQ cerebral glucose-oxygen quotient

CGP N-carbobenzoxy-glycyl-L-phenylalanine; chorionic growth hormone-prolactin; choline glycerophosphatide; circulating granulocyte pool; circulatory gene pool

CGRP calcitonin gene-related peptide

cGRP calcitonin gene-related peptide

CGRPR calcitonin gene related peptide receptor

CGS cardiogenic shock; catgut suture

CGS, cgs centimeter-gram-second [system]

CGT chorionic gonadotropin; cyclodextrin glucanotransferase

CGTT cortisone glucose tolerance test

cGy centigray (1 rad)

CH case history; Chediak-Higashi [syndrome]; chiasma; Chinese hamster; chloral hydrate; cholesterol; Christchurch chromosome; chronic hepatitis; chronic hypertension; common hepatic [duct]; communicating hydrocele; community health; completely healed; Conradi-Hünermann [syndrome]; continuous heparin [infusion]; cortical hamartoma; crown-heel [length]; cycloheximide; cystic hygroma; wheelchair

CH$_{50}$ 50% hemolyzing dose of complement

C$_H$ constant domain of H chain

C&H cocaine and heroin; coarse and harsh [breathing]

Ch chest; Chido [antibody]; chief; child; choline; Christchurch [syndrome]; chromosome

cH⁺ hydrogen ion concentration

ch chest; child; chronic

CHA Canadian Hospital Association; Catholic Health Association; Chinese hamster; chronic hemolytic anemia; common hepatic artery; congenital hypoplasia of adrenal glands; congenital hypoplastic anemia; continuously heated aerosol; cyclohexyladenosine; cyclohexylamine

ChA choline acetylase

ChAC choline acetyltransferase

CHAD cold hemagglutinin disease; cyclophosphamide, hexamethylmelamine, Adriamycin (doxorubicin), and cisplatin

CHAF central hyperalimentation nutrition

CHAMP Children's Hospital Automated Medical Program

CHAMPUS Civilian Health and Medical Program of Uniformed Services

CHAMPVA Civilian Health and Medical Program of Veterans Administration

CHANDS curly hair–ankylobleph-aron–nail dysplasia syndrome

Chang C Chang conjunctiva cells

Chang L Chang liver cells

CHAP Certified Hospital Admission Program; Community Health Accreditation Program

CHAPS 3[3-cholaminopropyl diethyl-ammonio]-1-propane sulfonate

CHARGE coloboma, heart disease, atresia choanae, retarded growth and retarded development and/or CNS anomalies, genital hypoplasia, and ear anomalies and/or deafness [syndrome]

CHAS Center for Health Administration Studies

ChAT choline acetyltransferase

CHB chronic hepatitis B; complete heart block; congenital heart block

ChB Bachelor of Surgery [Lat. *Chirurgiae Baccalaureus*]

CHBA congenital Heinz body hemolytic anemia

CHBHA congenital Heinz body hemolytic anemia

CHC chromosome condensation; community health center; community health computing; community health council

CH₃ CCNU semustine

CHCP correctional health care program

CHCS composite health care system

CHD Chediak-Higashi disease; childhood disease; chronic hemodialysis; congenital or congestive heart disease; congenital hip dislocation; constitutional hepatic dysfunction; coronary heart disease; cyanotic heart disease

ChD Doctor of Surgery [Lat. *Chirurgiae Doctor*]

CHDM comprehensive hospital drug monitoring

ChE cholinesterase

che a gene involved in chemotaxis

CHEC community hypertension evaluation clinic

CHEF Chinese hamster embryo fibroblast

chem chemistry, chemical; chemotherapy

ChemID Chemical Identification; Chemical Identification File

CHEMLINE Chemical Dictionary On-Line

Chemo chemotherapy

CHEMTREC Chemical Transportation Emergency Center

CHERSS continuous high-amplitude EEG rhythmical synchronous slowing

CHESS chemical shift selective

CHF chick embryo fibroblast; chronic heart failure; congenital hepatic fibrosis; congestive heart failure; Crimean hemorrhagic fever

CHFD controlled high flux dialysis

CHFV combined high-frequency ventilation

chg change, changed

CHGA chromogranin A

CHGB chromogranin B

CHH cartilage-hair hypoplasia

CHHS congenital hypothalamic hamartoma syndrome

CHI closed head injury; creatinine height index

chi chimera

χ Greek letter *chi*

χ^2 chi-squared statistic; chi-squared [test, measure goodness of fit]

χ_m magnetic susceptibility

χ_s electric susceptibility

Chi-A chimpanzee leukocyte antigen

CHILD congenital hemidysplasia with ichthyosiform erythroderma and limb defects [syndrome]

CHIME coloboma, heart anomaly, ichthyosis, mental retardation, ear abnormality

CHINA chronic infectious neurotropic agent

CHIP comprehensive health insurance plan

CHIPASAT Children's Paced Auditory Serial Addition Task

CHIPPA community health planning agency

CHIPS catastrophic health insurance plans

Chir Doct Doctor of Surgery [Lat. *Chirurgiae Doctor*]

chirug surgical [Lat. *chirurgicalis*]

CHL Chinese hamster lung; chlorambucil; chloramphenicol

Chl chloroform; chlorophyll

CHLA cyclohexyl linoleic acid

Chlb chlorobutanol

CHLD chronic hypoxic lung disease

chlor chloride

ChlVPP chlorambucil, vinblastine, procarbazine, prednisone

ChM Master of Surgery [Lat. *Chirurgiae Magister*]

CHMD clinical hyaline membrane disease

CHN carbon, hydrogen, and nitrogen; child neurology; Chinese [hamster]; community health network; community health nurse

CHO carbohydrate; Chinese hamster ovary; chorea

Cho choline

C_{H_2O} water clearance

choc chocolate

CHOL, chol cholesterol

c hold withhold

CHOP cyclophosphamide, hydroxydaunomycin, Oncovin, and prednisone

CHP capillary hydrostatic pressure; charcoal hemoperfusion; Chemical Hygiene Plan; child psychiatry; community health plan; comprehensive health planning; coordinating hospital physician; cutaneous hepatic porphyria

ChP chest physician

CHPA community health planning agency; community health purchasing alliance

chpx chickenpox

CHQ chloroquinol

CHR cerebrohepatorenal [syndrome]

Chr *Chromobacterium*

chr chromosome; chronic

c hr candle hour

c-hr curie-hour

ChRBC chicken red blood cell

CHRIS Cancer Hazards Ranking and Information System

chron chronic

CHRONIC chronic disease, rheumatoid arthritis, neoplasms, infections, cryoglobulinemia [conditions in which rheumatoid factor is produced]

CHRPE congenital hypertrophy of the retinal pigment epithelium

CHRS cerebrohepatorenal syndrome; Christian syndrome

CHS central hypoventilation syndrome; Chediak-Higashi syndrome; cholinesterase; chondroitin sulfate; compression hip screw; congenital hypoventilation syndrome; contact hypersensitivity

CHSD Children's Health Services Division

CHSO total hemolytic serum C activity

CHSP Clinton Health Security Plan

CHSS cooperative health statistics system

CHT chemotherapy; combined hormone therapy; contralateral head turning

ChTg chymotrypsinogen

ChTK chicken thymidine kinase

CHU closed head unit

CHV canine herpes virus; centigrade heat unit

CI cardiac index; cardiac insufficiency; cell immunity; cell inhibition; cephalic index; cerebral infarction; chemotactic index; chemotherapeutic index; chromatid interchange; chronic infection; clinical investigator; clomipramine; clonus index; coefficient of intelligence; colloidal iron; color index; confidence interval; contamination index; continued insomnia; continuous infusion; contraindication or contraindicated; convergence insufficiency; coronary insufficiency; corrected count increment; crystalline insulin; cumulative incidence; cytotoxic index

Ci curie

CIA chemiluminescent immunoassay; chymotrypsin inhibitor activity; colony-inhibiting activity; congenital intestinal aganglionosis

CIBD chronic inflammatory bowel disease

CIBHA congenital inclusion-body hemolytic anemia

CIBP chronic intractable benign pain

CIBPS chronic intractable benign pain syndrome

CIC cardioinhibitor center; circulating immune complex; clean intermittent catheterization; completely in the canal [hearing aid]; constant initial concentration; crisis intervention center

CICA cervical internal carotid artery

CICU cardiac intensive care unit; cardiovascular inpatient care unit; coronary intensive care unit

CID cellular immunodeficiency; charge injection device; chick infective dose; combined immunodeficiency disease; Cosmetic Ingredient Dictionary; cytomegalic inclusion disease

CIDEMS Center for Information and Documentation

CIDEP chemically induced dynamic electron polarization

CIDNP chemically induced dynamic nuclear polarization

CIDP chronic idiopathic polyradiculopathy; chronic inflammatory demyelinating polyradiculoneuropathy

CIDS cellular immunity deficiency syndrome; circular intensity differential scattering; continuous insulin delivery system

CIE Canberra interview for the elderly; cellulose ion exchange; counter-current immunoelectrophoresis; counterimmunoelectrophoresis; crossed immunoelectrophoresis

CIEP counterimmunoelectrophoresis

CIF cloning inhibitory factor

CIFC Council for the Investigation of Fertility Control

CIG cold-insoluble globulin

CIg intracytoplasmic immunoglobulin

cIgM cytoplasmic immunoglobulin M

CIH carbohydrate-induced hyperglyceridemia; Certificate in Industrial Health; children in hospital

ci-hr curie-hour

CIHS central infantile hypotonic syndrome

CII Carnegie Interest Inventory

CIIA common internal iliac artery

CIIP chronic idiopathic intestinal pseudo-obstruction

CIM cimetidine; cortically induced movement; Cumulated Index Medicus

Ci/ml curies per milliliter

CIMS chemical ionization mass spectrometry

CIN central inhibition; cervical intraepithelial neoplasia; chronic interstitial nephritis

CIN1, CIN I cervical intraepithelial neoplasia, grade 1 (mild dysplasia)

CIN 2, CIN II cervical intraepithelial neoplasia, grade 2 (moderate-severe)

CIN 3, CIN III cervical intraepithelial neoplasia, grade 3 (severe dysplasia and carcinoma in situ)

C_{in} insulin clearance

CINCA chronic infantile neurological cutaneous and auricular [syndrome]

CINE chemotherapy-induced nausea and emesis

CIO chief information officer

CIOMS Council for International Organizations of Medical Sciences

CIP chronic idiopathic polyradiculoneuropathy; chronic intestinal pseudo-obstruction; Collection de l'Institut Pasteur

CIPF classic interstitial pneumonitis-fibrosis; clinical illness promoting factor

CIPN chronic inflammatory polyneuropathy

CIPSO chronic intestinal pseudo-obstruction

circ circuit; circular; circumcision; circumference

CIREN Crash Injury Research and Engineering Network

CIRSE Cardiovascular and Interventional Radiological Society of Europe

circ & sens circulation and sensation

CIS carcinoma in situ; catheter-induced spasm; central inhibitory state; Chemical Information Service; clinical information system; clinical interview schedule; continuous interleaved sampler; cumulative impairment score

CI-S calculus index, simplified

CiS cingulate sulcus

CISC complex-instructional-set computing

CISCA$_{II}$B$_{IV}$ Cytoxan, Adriamycin, platinum, vinblastine, bleomycin

cis-DPP cisplatin

CISH competitive in situ hybridization

CISP chronic intractable shoulder pain

CIS PT cisplatin

CISS Common Internet Scheme Syntax

CIT citrate; combined intermittent therapy; conjugated-immunoglobulin technique; crossed intrinsic transfer

cit citrate

CITS Carey infant temperament scale

CIVII continuous intravenous insulin infusion

CIXA constant infusion excretory urogram

CJ conjunctivitis

CJA Creutzfeldt-Jakob agent

CJD Creutzfeldt-Jakob disease

CJS Creutzfeldt-Jakob syndrome

CjvO$_2$ jugular venous oxygen content

CK calf kidney; casein kinase; chicken kidney; cholecystokinin; choline kinase; contralateral knee; creatine kinase; cyanogen chloride; cytokinin

ck check, checked

CKB creatine kinase, brain type

CKC cold-knife conization

CKG cardiokymography

CKI cyclin-dependent kinase inhibitor

CKM creatine kinase, muscle type

CKMB creatine kinase, myocardial bound

CKMM creatine kinase, muscle type

CK-PZ cholecystokinin-pancreozymin

CKS classic form of Kaposi sarcoma

CL capillary lumen; cardiolipin; cell line; centralis lateralis; chemiluminescence; chest and left arm [lead in electrocardiography]; cholelithiasis; cholesterol-lecithin; chronic leukemia; cirrhosis of liver; clavicle; clear liquid; clearance; cleft lip; clinical laboratory; clomipramine; complex loading; confidence limit or level; contact lens; corpus luteum; corrected [echo long axis] length; cricoid lamina; criterion level; critical list; cycle length; cytotoxic lymphocyte

C-L consultation-liaison [setting]

C$_L$ constant domain of L chain; lung compliance

Cl chloride; chlorine; clavicle; clear; clinic; *Clostridium*; closure; colistin

cl centiliter; clarified; clean; clear; cleft; clinic; clinical; clonus; clotting; cloudy

CLA cerebellar ataxia; Certified Laboratory Assistant; cervicolinguoaxial; contralateral local anesthesia; cutaneous lymphocyte antigen; cyclic lysine anhydride

ClAc chloroacetyl

CLAH congenital lipoid adrenal hyperplasia

CLam cervical laminectomy

CLAS congenital localized absence of skin

class, classif classification

clav clavicle

CLB chlorambucil; curvilinear body

CLBBB complete left bundle branch block

CLBP chronic low back pain

CLC Charcot-Leyden crystal; Clerc-Levy-Critesco [syndrome]

CLCD cleidocranial dysostosis

CLCN chloride channel

CL/CP cleft lip/cleft palate

CLCS colchicine sensitivity

CLD chloride diarrhea; chronic liver disease; chronic lung disease; congenital limb deficiency; crystal ligand field

CLDH choline dehydrogenase

cldy cloudy

CLE centrilobular emphysema; continuous lumbar epidural [anesthesia]

CLED cystine-lactose-electrolyte-deficient [agar]

CLF cardiolipin fluorescent [antibody]; ceroid lipofuscinosis; cholesterol-lecithin flocculation

CLH chronic lobular hepatitis; cleft limb-heart [syndrome]; corpus luteum hormone; cutaneous lymphoid hyperplasia

CLI complement lysis inhibitor; corpus luteum insufficiency

CLIA Clinical Laboratories Improvement Act

CLIF cloning inhibitory factor; *Crithidia luciliae* immunofluorescence

clin clinic, clinical

CLINPROT Clinical Cancer Protocols

CLIP capitolunate instability pattern; corticotropin-like intermediate lobe peptide

CLL cholesterol-lowering lipid; chronic lymphatic leukemia; chronic lymphocytic leukemia; cow lung lavage

CLMA Clinical Laboratory Management Association

CLMF cytotoxic lymphocyte maturation factor

CLML Current List of Medical Literature

CLMV cauliflower mosaic virus

CLO cod liver oil

clo "clothing"—a unit of thermal insulation

CLOF clofibrate

CLON clonidine

Clon *Clonorchis*

Clostr *Clostridium*

CLP chymotrypsin-like protein; cleft lip with cleft palate; paced cycle length

CL/P cleft lip with or without cleft palate

CL(P) cleft lip without cleft palate

ClP clinical pathology

CLS café-au-lait spot; Clinical Laboratory Scientist; Coffin-Lowry syndrome; Cornelia de Lange syndrome

CLSE calf lung surfactant extract

CLSH corpus luteum stimulating hormone

CLSL chronic lymphosarcoma (cell) leukemia

CLT Certified Laboratory Technician; chronic lymphocytic thyroiditis; Clinical Laboratory Technician; clot lysis time; clotting time; lung-thorax compliance

CL$_{TB}$ total body clearance

CLT(NCA) Laboratory Technician Certified by the National Certification Agency for Medical Laboratory Personnel

CLU clusterin

CLV cassava latent virus; constant linear velocity

CL VOID clean voided specimen [urine]

CLZ clozapine

CM California mastitis [test]; calmodulin; capreomycin; carboxymethyl; cardiac murmur; cardiac muscle; cardiomyopathy; carpometacarpal; castrated male; Caucasian male; cause of death [Lat. *causa mortis*]; cavernous malformation; cell membrane; center of mass; cerebral malaria; cerebral mantle; cervical mucosa or mucus; Chick-Martin [coefficient]; chloroquinemepacrine; chondromalacia; chopped meat [medium]; circular muscle; circulating monocyte; circumferential measurement; clindamycin; clinical medicine; clinical modification; coccidioidal meningitis; cochlear microphonic; combined modality; common migraine; complete medium; complications; condition median; conditioned medium; congenital malformation; congestive myocardiopathy; continuous murmur; contrast medium; copulatory mechanism; costal margin; cow's milk; cytometry; cytoplasmic membrane; Master of Surgery [Lat. *Chirurgiae Magister*]; narrow-diameter endosseous screw implant [Fr. *crête manche*]

C/M counts per minute

C&M cocaine and morphine

Cm curium; minimal concentration

C$_m$ maximum clearance

cM *centi-morgan*

cm centimeter

cm^2 square centimeter

cm^3 cubic centimeter

CMA Canadian Medical Association; Certified Medical Assistant; chronic metabolic acidosis; cow's milk allergy; cultured macrophages

CMAP compound muscle (or motor) action potential

CMAR cell matrix adhesion regulator

Cmax, C$_{max}$ maximum concentration

CMB carbolic methylene blue; Central Midwives' Board; chloromercuribenzoate

CMBES Canadian Medical and Biological Engineering Society

CMC carboxymethylcellulose; care management continuity; carpometacarpal; cell-mediated cytolysis or cytotoxicity; chloramphenicol; chronic mucocutaneous candidiasis; critical micellar concentration

CMCC chronic mucocutaneous candidiasis

CMCJ carpometacarpal joint

CMCt care management continuity across settings

CMD campomelic dysplasia; camptomelic dwarfism; cartilage matrix deficiency; chief medical director; childhood muscular dystrophy; comparative mean dose; congenital muscular dystrophy; count median diameter

cmDNA cytoplasmic membrane-associated deoxyribonucleic acid

CME cervical mediastinal exploration; continuing medical education; Council on Medical Education; crude marijuana extract; cystoid macular edema

CMF calcium-magnesium free; catabolite modular factor; chondromyxoid fibroma; Christian Medical Fellowship; cold mitten fraction; cortical magnification factor; craniomandibulofacial; cyclophosphamide, methotrexate, and fluorouracil

CMFT cardiolipin microflocculation test

CMFV cyclophosphamide, methotrexate, fluorouracil, and vincristine

CMFVP cyclophosphamide, methotrexate, fluorouracil, vincristine, prednisone

CMG canine or congenital myasthenia gravis; chopped meat glucose [medium]; cystometrography, cystometrogram

CMGN chronic membranous glomerulonephritis

CMGS chopped meat-glucose-starch [medium]; Clinical Molecular Genetics Society

CMGT chromosome-mediated gene transfer

CMH cardiomyopathy, hypertrophic; community mental health [services or program]; congenital malformation of the heart

CMHC community mental health center

C/MHC community/migrant health center

cmH₂O centimeters of water

CMI carbohydrate metabolism index; care management integration; case mix index; cell-mediated immunity; cell multiplication inhibition; chronic mesenteric ischemia; circulating microemboli index; colonic motility index; Commonwealth Mycological Institute; computed maxillofacial imaging; Cornell Medical Index

CMID cytomegalic inclusion disease

c/min cycles per minute

CMIR cell-mediated immune response

CMIT Current Medical Information and Terminology

CMJ carpometacarpal joint

CMK chloromethyl ketone; congenital multicystic kidney

CML carboxymethyl lysine; cell-mediated lymphocytotoxicity; cell-mediated lympholysis; central motor latency; chronic myelocytic leukemia; chronic myelogenous leukemia; clinical medical librarian

CMM cell-mediated mutagenesis; cutaneous malignant melanoma

cmm cubic millimeter

CMMC cervical myelomeningocele

CMME chloromethyl methyl ether

CMML chronic myelomonocytic leukemia

CMMoL chronic myelomonocytic leukemia

CMMS Columbia Mental Maturity Scale

CMN caudal mediastinal node; cystic medial necrosis

CMNA complement-mediated neutrophil activation

CMN-AA cystic medial necrosis of ascending aorta

CMO cardiac minute output; Chief Medical Officer; comfort measures only; competitive medical organization; corticosterone methyloxidase

cMO centimorgan

CMOL chronic monocytic leukemia

CMOS complementary metal-oxide semiconductor

CMP cardiomyopathy; cartilage matrix protein; chondromalacia patellae; collagen binding protein; competitive medical plan; comprehensive medical plan; cytidine monophosphate

CMPD chronic myeloproliferative disorder

cmpd compound, compounded

CMPGN chronic membranoproliferative glomerulonephritis

cmps centimeters per second

CMR cardiomodulorespirography; cerebral metabolic rate; chief medical resident; common medical record; common mode rejection; crude mortality ratio

CMRG cerebral metabolic rate of glucose

CMRGlc combined metabolic rate of glucose

CMRglu cerebral metabolic rate of glucose

CMRL cerebral metabolic rate of lactate

CMRO, CMRO$_2$ cerebral metabolic rate of oxygen consumption

CMRR common mode rejection ratio

CMS children's medical services; Christian Medical Society; chronic myelodysplastic syndrome; chromosome modification site; circulation, motion, sensation; clofibrate-induced muscular syndrome; Clyde Mood Scale; complement-mediated solubility; cortical magnetic stimulation

cm/s centimeters per second

CMSD congenital myocardial sympathetic dysinnervation

cm/sec centimeters per second

CMSS circulation, motor ability, sensation, and swelling; Council of Medical Specialty Societies

CMT California mastitis test; cancer multistep therapy; catechol methyltransferase; certified medical transcriptionist; cervical motion tenderness; Charcot-Marie-Tooth [syndrome]; chemotherapy; circus movement tachycardia; complex motor unit; continuous memory test; Council on Medical Television; Current Medical Terminology

CMTC cutis marmorata telangiectatica congenita

CMTD Charcot-Marie-Tooth disease

CMTS Charcot-Marie-Tooth syndrome

CMTX Charcot-Marie-Tooth [syndrome], X-linked

CMU chlorophenyldimethylurea

CMUA continuous motor unit activity

CMV continuous mandatory ventilation; controlled mechanical ventilation; conventional mechanical ventilation; cool mist vaporizer; cowpea mosaic virus; cucumber mosaic virus; cytomegalovirus

CMV-MN cytomegalovirus mononucleosis

CMX cefmenoxime

CN caudate nucleus; cellulose nitrate; charge nurse; child nutrition; chloroacetophenone; clinical nursing; cochlear nucleus; congenital nystagmus; cranial nerve; Crigler-Najjar [syndrome]; cyanogen; cyanosis neonatorum

C/N carbon/nitrogen [ratio]; carrier/noise [ratio]

CN⁻ cyanide anion

CN I to XII first to twelfth cranial nerves

CNA calcium nutrient agar; Canadian Nurses Association; certified nursing assistant

CNAF chronic nonvalvular atrial fibrillation

CNAG chronic narrow angle glaucoma

CNAP career nurse assistants' programs; compound nerve action potential

CNB cutting needle biopsy

CNBP cellular nucleic acid binding protein

CNC community nursing center

CNCbl cyanocobalamin

CNDC chronic nonspecific diarrhea of childhood; chronic nonsuppurative destructive cholangitis

CNE chief nurse executive; chronic nervous exhaustion; concentric needle electrode

CNES chronic nervous exhaustion syndrome

CNF chronic nodular fibrositis; congenital nephrotic syndrome of the Finnish [type]

CNGC cyclic nucleotide gated channel

CNH central neurogenic hyperpnea; community nursing home

CNHD congenital nonspherocytic hemolytic disease

CNI center of nuclear image; chronic nerve irritation

CNIDR Clearinghouse for Networked Information Discovery and Retrieval

CNK cortical necrosis of kidneys

CNL cardiolipin natural lecithin; chronic neutrophilic leukemia

CNM Certified Nurse-Midwife; computerized nuclear morphometry

CNMT Certified Nuclear Medicine Technologist

CNO community nursing organization

CNP community nurse practitioner; continuous negative pressure; cranial nerve palsy; 2',3'-cyclic nucleotide 3'-phosphodiesterase

CNPase 2',3'-cyclic nucleotide 3'-phosphohydrolase

CNPV continuous negative pressure ventilation

CNR cannabinoid receptor; Center for Nursing Research; contrast-to-noise ratio; Council of Nurse Researchers

CNRT corrected sinus node recovery time

CNS central nervous system; clinical nurse specialist; coagulase-negative staphylococci; congenital nephrotic syndrome; sulfocyanate

CNSHA congenital nonspherocytic hemolytic anemia

CNS-L central nervous system leukemia

CNSLD chronic nonspecific lung disease

CNST coagulase-negative staphylococci

CNTF ciliary neutrophilic factor

CNTFR ciliary neutrophilic factor receptor

CNV choroidal neovascularization; contingent negative variation; cutaneous necrotizing vasculitis

CO carbon monoxide; cardiac output; castor oil; casualty officer; centric occlusion; cervical orthosis; cervicoaxial; choline oxidase; coccygeal; coenzyme; compound; control; corneal opacity; cross over; cyclophosphamide and vincristine

C/O check out; complains of; in care of

c/o complains of

CO$_2$ carbon dioxide

Co cobalt

Co I coenzyme I

Co II coenzyme II

COA Canadian Ophthalmological Association; Canadian Orthopaedic Association; certificate of authority; cervico-oculo-acusticus [syndrome]; condition on admission

CoA coenzyme A

COACH cerebellar vermis hypoplasia/aplasia-oligophrenia-congenital ataxia-ocular colobomata-hepatic fibrosis [syndrome]

COAD chronic obstructive airway disease

COAG chronic open angle glaucoma

coag coagulation, coagulated

COAL chronic obstructive airflow limitation

COAP cyclophosphamide, cytosine arabinose, vincristine, prednisone

coarct coarctation

CoASH uncombined coenzyme A

CoA-SPC coenzyme A-synthetizing protein complex

COAT Children's Orientation and Amnesia Test

COB chronic obstructive bronchitis; coordination of benefits

coban cohesive bandage

COBOL common business oriented language

COBRA Consolidated Omnibus Reconciliation Act

COBS cesarean-obtained barrier-sustained; chronic organic brain syndrome

COBT chronic obstruction of the biliary tract

COC cathodal opening contraction; coccygeal; combination oral contraceptive

COCI Consortium on Chemical Information

COCl cathodal opening clonus

COCM congestive cardiomyopathy

COCP combined oral contraceptive pill

COD cause of death; cerebro-ocular dysplasia; chemical oxygen demand; codeine; condition on discharge

cod codeine

COD-MD cerebro-ocular dysplasia-muscular dystrophy [syndrome]

CODATA Committee on Data for Science and Technology

CODS Charnes organizational diagnosis survey

coeff coefficient

COEPS cortical originating extra-pyramidal system

COF cutoff frequency

CoF cobra factor; cofactor

C of A coarctation of the aorta

COFS cerebro-oculo-facial-skeletal [syndrome]

COG center of gravity; cognitive function tests

CoGME Council on Graduate Medical Education

COGTT cortisone oral glucose tolerance test

COH carbohydrate

CoHb carboxyhemoglobin

COHN Certified Occupational Health Nurse

COHSE Confederation of Health Service Employees

COI Central Obesity Index; certificate of insurance; cost of illness

COIF congenital onychodysplasia of the index finger

col collection; colicin; collagen; colony; colored; column; strain [Lat. *cola*]

COLD chronic obstructive lung disease

COLD A cold agglutinin titer

coll collateral; collection, collective; college; colloidal

collat collateral

COM chronic otitis media; College of Osteopathic Medicine; computer-output microfilm

com comminuted; commitment

COMAC/HRS/QA Community Concerted Action Programme on Quality Assurance in Health Care [European]

comb combination, combine

COMC carboxymethylcellulose

COME chronic otitis media with effusion

comf comfortable

comm, commun communicable

COMP cartilage oligomeric matrix protein; complication; cyclophosphamide, vincristine, methotrexate, prednisone

comp comparative; compensation, compensated; complaint; complete; composition; compound, compounded; comprehension; compress; computer

COMPASS Computerized Online Medicaid Pharmaceutical Analysis and Surveillance System

compd compound, compounded

compl complaint; complete, completed, completion; complication, complicated

complic complication, complicated

compn composition

compr compression

COMS cerebrooculomuscular syndrome

COMT catecholamine O-methyl transferase; certified ophthalmic medical technologist

COMTRAC computer-based case tracing

COMUL complement fixation murine leukosis [test]

CON certificate of need

Con concanavalin

con against [Lat. *contra*]; continuation, continue

Con A concanavalin A

Con A-HRP concanavalin A-horseradish peroxidase

c-onc cellular oncogene

conc, concentr concentrate, concentrated, concentration

cond condensation, condensed; condition, conditioned; conductivity; conductor

conf conference; confined; confinement; confusion

cong congested, congestion; gallon [Lat. *congius*]

congen congenital

coniz conization

conj conjunctiva, conjunctival

conjug conjugated, conjugation

CONPA-DRI I vincristine, doxorubicin, and melphalan

CONPA-DRI III conpa-dri I plus intensified doxorubicin

CONQUEST Computerized Needs-Oriented Quality Measurement Evaluation System

CONS coagulase-negative *Staphylococcus;* consultation; consultant

cons conservation; conservative; consultation

CONSENSUS Cooperative North Scandinavian Enalapril Survival Study

const constant

constit constituent

consult consultant, consultation

cont against [Lat. *contra*]; bruised [Lat. *contusus*]; contains, contents; continue, continuation

contag contagion, contagious

contr contracted, contraction

contra contraindicated

contralat contralateral

contrib contributory

conv convalescence, convalescent, convalescing; convergence, convergent; convulsions, convulsive

converg convergence, convergent

CONVINCE Controlled Onset Verapamil Investigation of Cardiovascular Endpoints

COO chief operating officer; cost of ownership [analysis]

COOD chronic obstruction outflow disease

COOH carboxy group; carboxy terminus

COOHTA Canadian Coordinating Office for Health Technology Assessment

COOP charts for primary care practices; cooperative

coord coordination, coordinated

COP capillary osmotic pressure; change of plaster; coefficient of performance; colloid oncotic pressure; colloid osmotic pressure; cryptogenic organizing pneumonitis; cyclophosphamide, Oncovin, and prednisone

COPA Council on Postsecondary Accreditation

COPAD cyclophosphamide, vincristine, Adriamycin, prednisone, cytarabine, asparagine, intrathecal methotrexate

COPC community oriented primary care

COPD chronic obstructive pulmonary disease

COPE chronic obstructive pulmonary emphysema

COP$_i$ colloid osmotic pressure in interstitial fluid

COPP cyclophosphamide, vincristine, procarbazine, prednisone; cyclophosphamide, Oncovin, procarbazine, prednisone

COP$_p$ colloid osmotic pressure in plasma

COPRO coproporphyrin

COPT circumoval precipitin reaction test

CoQ coenzyme Q

COR cardiac output recorder; comprehensive outpatient rehabilitation; conditioned orientation reflex; consensual ophthalmotonic reaction; corrosion, corrosive; cortisone; cortex; crude odds ratio; custodian of records

CoR Congo red

cor body [Lat. *corpus*]; coronary; correction, corrected;

CORA conditioned orientation reflex audiometry

CORD Commissioned Officer Residency Deferment; Council of Residency Directors

CORE comprehensive assessment and referral evaluation

CorPP coronary perfusion pressure

corr correspondence, corresponding

CORT corticosterone

cort bark [Lat. *cortex*]; cortex

COS cheiro-oral syndrome; chief of staff; Clinical Orthopaedic Society; clinically observed seizures

COSATI Committee on Scientific and Technical Information

COSMIS Computer System for Medical Information Systems

COSSMHO [National] Coalition of Hispanic Health and Human Services Organizations

COSTAR Computer-Stored Ambulatory Record

COSTEP Commissioned Officer Student Training and Extern Program

COSY correlated spectroscopy

COT colony overlay test; content of thought; contralateral optic tectum; critical off-time

COTA Certified Occupational Therapy Assistant

COTD cardiac output by thermodilution

COTe cathodal opening tetanus

COTH Council of Teaching Hospitals and Health Systems

COTRANS Coordinated Transfer Application System

coul coulomb

COV covariance; cross-over value

COVESDEM costovertebral segmentation defect with mesomelia [syndrome]

CoVF cobra venom factor

COWS cold to opposite and warm to same side

COX cytochrome c oxidase

CP candle power; capillary pressure; cardiac pacing; cardiac performance; cardiopulmonary; caudate putamen; cell passage; central pit; cephalic presentation; cerebellopontine; cerebral palsy; ceruloplasmin; chemically pure; chest pain; child psychiatry; child psychology; chloropurine; chloroquine-primaquine; chondrodysplasia punctata; chronic pain; chronic pancreatitis; chronic polyarthritis; chronic pyelonephritis; cicatricial pemphigoid; cleft palate; clinical pathology; clock pulse; closing pressure; cochlear potential; code of practice; cold pressor; color perception; combining power; compound; compressed; congenital porphyria; constant pressure; coproporphyrin; cor pulmonale; coracoid process; C peptide; creatine phosphate; creatine phosphokinase; cross-linked protein; crude protein; current practice; cyclophosphamide; cyclophosphamide and prednisone; cytosol protein

C&P compensation and pension; complete and pain free [joint movement]; cystoscopy and pyelography

C/P cholesterol-phospholipid [ratio]

C+P cryotherapy with pressure

Cp ceruloplasmin; chickenpox; *Corynebacterium parvum;* peak concentration

C_p constant pressure; phosphate clearance

cP centipoise

cp candle power; chemically pure; centipoise; compare

c_p constant pressure

CPA Canadian Physiotherapy Association; Canadian Psychiatric Association; carboxypeptidase A; cardiopulmonary arrest; carotid phonoangiography; cerebellopontine angle; chlorophenylalanine; circulating platelet aggregate; complement proactivator; control, preoccupation, and addiction; costophrenic angle; cyclophosphamide; cyproterone acetate

C3PA complement-3 proactivator

CPAF chlorpropamide-alcohol flushing

C$_{pah}$ para-aminohippurate clearance

CPAP continuous positive airway pressure

CPB carboxypeptidase B; cardiopulmonary bypass; cetylpyridinium bromide; competitive protein binding

CPBA competitive protein-binding analysis

CPBV cardiopulmonary blood volume

CPC central posterior curve; cerebellar Purkinje cell; cerebral palsy clinic; cerebral performance category; cetylpyridinium chloride; chest pain center; child protection center; chronic passive congestion; circumferential pneumatic compression; clinicopathological conference

CPCL congenital pulmonary cystic lymphangiectasia

CPCP chronic progressive coccidioidal pneumonitis

CPCR cardiopulmonary cerebral resuscitation

CPCS circumferential pneumatic compression suit

CPD calcium pyrophosphate deposition; cephalopelvic disproportion; cerebelloparenchymal disorder; childhood or congenital polycystic disease; chorioretinopathy and pituitary dysfunction; chronic peritoneal dialysis; chronic protein deprivation; citrate-phosphate-dextrose; contact potential difference; contagious pustular dermatitis; critical point drying; cyclopentadiene

cpd compound; cycles per degree

CPDA citrate-phosphate-dextrose-adenine

CPDD calcium pyrophosphate deposition disease; cis-platinum-diamine dichloride

cpd E compound E

cpd F compound F

CPDL cumulative population doubling level

CPDX cefpodoxime

CPDX-PR cefpodoxime proxetil

CPE cardiac pulmonary edema; chronic pulmonary emphysema; clinical progress exercise; compensation, pension, and education; complete physical examination; corona-penetrating enzyme; cytopathogenic effect

CPEO chronic progressive external ophthalmoplegia

CPF clot-promoting factor; complication probability factor; contraction peak force; current patient file

CPG capillary blood gases; cardiopneumographic recording; carotid phonoangiogram

CPGN chronic proliferative glomerulonephritis

CPGs clinical practice guidelines

CPH Certificate in Public Health; chronic paroxysmal hemicrania; chronic persistent hepatitis; chronic primary headache; corticotropin-releasing hormone

CPHA Canadian Public Health Association; Commission on Professional and Hospital Activities

CPHA-PAS Commission on Professional and Hospital Activities—Professional Activity Study

CPHQ certified professional in healthcare quality

CPI California Personality Inventory; Cancer Potential Index; congenital palatopharyngeal incompetence; constitutional psychopathic inferiority; coronary prognosis index; cysteine proteinase inhibitor

CPIB chlorophenoxyisobutyrate

CPIP chronic pulmonary insufficiency of prematurity

CPIJH compass proximal interphalangeal joint hinge

CPIR cephalic-phase insulin release

CPK cell population kinetic [model]; creatine phosphokinase

CPK-BB creatine phosphokinase, brain-type

CPKD childhood polycystic kidney disease

CPL caprine placental lactogen; conditioned pitch level; congenital pulmonary lymphangiectasia

C/PL cholesterol/phospholipid [ratio]

cpl complete, completed

CPLM cysteine-peptone-liver infusion medium

CPLS cleft palate-lateral synechia syndrome

CPM central pontine myelinosis; chlorpheniramine maleate; continuous passive motion; critical path method; cyclophosphamide

CP/M control program for microcomputers

C_{PM} circumference of papillary muscle

cpm counts per minute; cycles per minute

CPMC Columbia-Presbyterian Medical Center

CPMG Carr-Purcell-Meiboom-Gill [sequence]

CPMP complete patient management problems

CPMS chronic progressive multiple sclerosis

CPMV cowpea mosaic virus

CPN central parenteral nutrition; chronic polyneuropathy; chronic pyelonephritis

CPNE clinical performance nursing examination

CPNM corrected perinatal mortality

CPO contract provider organization; coproporphyrinogen oxidase

CPOTHA chest pain onset to hospital arrival

CPP cancer proneness phenotype; canine pancreatic polypeptide; cerebral perfusion pressure; chest pain policy; dl-2[3-(2'-chlorophenoxy)phenyl] propionic [acid]; chronic pigmented purpura; coronary perfusion pressure; cyclopentenophenanthrene

CPPB continuous positive pressure breathing

CPPD calcium pyrophosphate dihydrate deposition [syndrome]; cisplatin; cost per patient day

CPPV continuous positive pressure ventilation

CPQA certified professional in quality assurance

CPR cardiopulmonary reserve; cardiopulmonary resuscitation; centripetal rub; cerebral cortex perfusion rate; chlorophenyl red; computerized patient record; cortisol production rate; cumulative patency rate; customary, prevailing and reasonable [rate]

c-PR cyclopropyl

CPRAM controlled partial rebreathing anesthesia method

CPRCA constitutional pure red cell aplasia

CPRD Committee on Prosthetics Research and Development

CPRI Computerized Patient Record Institute

CPRO coproporphyrinogen oxidase

CPRS Children's Psychiatric Rating Scale; Comprehensive Psychopathological Rating Scale

CPS carbamoylphosphate synthetase; cardioplegic perfusion solution; centipoise; cervical pain syndrome; characters per second; chest pain syndrome; Child Personality Scale; Child Protective Services; chloroquine, pyrimethamine, and sulfisoxazole; chronic prostatitis syndrome; clinical performance score; Clinical Pharmacy Services; coagulase-positive *Staphylococcus*; complex partial seizures; concurrent planning system; constitutional psychopathic state; contagious pustular stomatitis; C-polysaccharide; cumulative probability of success; current population survey

cps counts per second; cycles per second

CPSC congenital paucity of secondary synaptic clefts [syndrome]; Consumer Products Safety Commission

CPSO College of Physicians and Surgeons of Ontario

CPSP central poststroke pain

CPT carnitine palmityl transferase; carotid pulse tracing; chest physiotherapy; child protection team; ciliary particle transport; cold pressor test; combining power test; complex physical therapy; continuous performance task; continuous performance test; Current Procedural Terminology

CPTH chronic post-traumatic headache

CPTN culture-positive toxin-negative

CPTP culture-positive toxin-positive

CPTX chronic parathyroidectomy

CPU caudate putamen; central processing unit

CPUE chest pain of unknown etiology

CPV canine parvovirus; cytoplasmic polyhedrosis virus

CPVC common pulmonary venous channel

CPVD congenital polyvalvular disease

CPX cleft palate, X-linked; clinical practice examination; complete physical examination

CPXD chondrodysplasia punctata, X-linked dominant

CPXR chondrodysplasia punctata, X-linked recessive

CPZ cefoperazone; chlorpromazine; Compazine

CQ chloroquine; chloroquine-quinine; circadian quotient; conceptual quotient

CQI continuous quality improvement

CQI/TQM continuous quality improvement/total quality management

CQM chloroquine mustard

CQMS cost quality management system

CR calculation rate; calculus removed; calorie-restricted; cardiac rehabilitation; cardiac resuscitation; cardiac rhythm; cardiorespiratory; cardiorrhexis; caries-resistant; cathode ray; cellular receptor; centric relation; chemoradiation; chest and right arm [lead in electrocardiography]; chest roentgenogram, chest roentgenography; chief resident; child-resistant [bottle top]; choice reaction; chromium; chronic rejection; clinical record; clinical remission; clinical research; clot retraction; coefficient of fat retention; colon resection; colonization resistance; colony reared [animal]; colorectal; complement receptor; complete remission; complete response; computed radiography; conditioned reflex, conditioned response; congenital rubella; Congo red; controlled release; controlled respiration; conversion rate; cooling rate; cortico-resistant; creatinine; cremaster reflex; cresyl red; critical ratio; crown-rump [measurement]

CR1 complement receptor type 1

C&R convalescence and rehabilitation

Cr chromium; cranium, cranial; creatinine; crown

CRA central retinal artery; Chinese restaurant asthma; chronic rheumatoid arthritis; constant relative alkalinity

CRABP cellular retinoic acid-binding protein

CRAD central retinal artery occlusion

CRAHCA Center for Research in Ambulatory Health Care Administration

CRAMS circulation, respiration, abdomen, motor, speech

cran cranium, cranial

CRAO central retinal artery occlusion

CRAW computed tomography acquisition workstation

CRB chemical, radiological, and biological; congenital retinal blindness

CRBBB complete right bundle branch block

CRBC chicken red blood cell

CRBP cellular retinol-binding protein

CRC cardiovascular reflex conditioning; clinical research center; colorectal carcinoma; concentrated red blood cells; cross-reacting cannabinoids; cyclic redundancy check

CrCl creatinine clearance

CRCS cardiovascular reflex conditioning system

CRD carbohydrate-recognition domain; chronic renal disease; chronic respiratory disease; child restraint device; childhood rheumatic disease; chorioretinal degeneration; chronic renal disease; chronic respiratory disease; complete reaction of degeneration; complex repetitive discharge; cone-rod retinal dystrophy; congenital rubella deafness; crown-rump distance

CR-DIP chronic relapsing demyelinating inflammatory polyneuropathy

CRDS client response documentation system

CRE cumulative radiation effect; cyclic adenosine monophosphate-response element

creat creatinine

CREM center for rural emergency medicine; cyclic adenosine monophosphate-response element modulator

crem cremaster

CREOG Council on Resident Education in Obstetrics and Gynecology

crep crepitation; crepitus

CREST calcinosis, Raynaud phenomenon, esophageal involvement, sclerodactyly, and telangiectasia [syndrome]

CRF case report form; chronic renal failure; chronic respiratory failure; coagulase-reacting factor; continuous reinforcement; corticotropin-releasing factor; cytokine receptor family

CRFK Crandell feline kidney cells

CRFR corticotropin-releasing factor receptor

CRG cardiorespirogram

CRH corticotropin-releasing hormone

CRHBP corticosterone-releasing hormone binding protein

CRHL Collaborative Radiological Health Laboratory

CRHV cottontail rabbit herpes virus

CRI Cardiac Risk Index; catheter-related infection; chronic renal insufficiency; chronic respiratory insufficiency; Composite Risk Index; congenital rubella infection; cross-reaction idiotype

CRIE crossed radioimmunoelectrophoresis

CRIP cysteine-rich intestinal protein

CRISP Computer Retrieval of Information on Scientific Projects; Consortium Research on Indicators of System Performance

Crit, crit critical; hematocrit

CRL cell repository line; Certified Record Librarian; complement receptor location; complement receptor lymphocyte; crown-rump length

CRM Certified Reference Materials; counting rate meter; cross-reacting material; crown-rump measurement

CRMO chronic recurrent multifocal osteomyelitis

CRN complement requiring neutralization

CRNA Certified Registered Nurse Anesthetist

cRNA chromosomal ribonucleic acid

CRNF chronic rheumatoid nodular fibrositis

Cr Nn, cr nn cranial nerves

CRO cathode ray oscilloscope; centric relation occlusion

CROM cervical range of motion

CROME congenital cataracts-epileptic fits-mental retardation [syndrome]

CROS contralateral routing of signals [hearing aid]

CRP chronic relapsing pancreatitis; corneal-retinal potential; coronary rehabilitation program; C-reactive protein; cross-reacting protein; cyclic AMP receptor protein

CrP creatine phosphate

CRPA C-reactive protein antiserum

CRPD chronic restrictive pulmonary disease

CRPF chloroquine-resistant *Plasmodium falciparum;* closed reduction and percutaneous fixation; contralateral renal plasma flow

CRPS complex regional pain syndrome [type I and II]

CRRN certified rehabilitation registered nurse

CrRT cranial radiotherapy

CRS Carroll rating scale for depression; catheter-related sepsis; caudal regression syndrome; cervical spine radiography; Chinese restaurant syndrome; colon and rectum surgery; compliance of the respiratory system; congenital rubella syndrome; craniosynostosis; cryptidin-related sequence

CRSM cherry red spot myoclonus

CRSP comprehensive renal scintillation procedure

CRST calcinosis, Raynaud phenomenon, sclerodactyly, telangiectasia [syndrome]; corrected sinus recovery time

CRT cadaveric renal transplant; cardiac resuscitation team; cathode-ray tube; certified; Certified Record Techniques; choice reaction time; chromium release test; complex reaction time; computerized renal tomography; copper reduction test; corrected; corrected retention time; cortisone resistant thymocyte; cranial radiation therapy

crt hematocrit

CRTM cartilage matrix protein

CRTP Consciousness Research and Training Project

CRTT Certified Respiratory Therapy Technician

CRU cardiac rehabilitation unit; clinical research unit

CRV central retinal vein

CRVF congestive right ventricular failure

CRVO central retinal vein occlusion

CRYG gamma crystallin gene

CRYM crystallin, MU

cryo cryogenic; cryoglobulin; cryoprecipitate; cryosurgery; cryotherapy

Cryoppt cryoprecipitate

crys, cryst crystal, crystaline

CS calf serum; campomelic syndrome; carcinoid syndrome; cardiogenic shock; caries-susceptible; carotid sheath; carotid sinus; cat scratch; celiac sprue; central service; central supply; cerebral scintigraphy; cerebrospinal; cervical spine; cervical stimulation; cesarean section; chest strap; chief of staff; cholesterol stone; chondroitin sulfate; chorionic somatomammotropin; chronic schizophrenia; cigarette smoker; citrate synthase; climacteric syndrome; clinical laboratory scientist; clinical stage; clinical status; clinic scheduling; Cockayne syndrome; complete stroke; compression syndrome; concentrated strength; conditioned stimulus; congenital syphilis; conjunctival secretion; conscious, consciousness; conscious sedation; conservative surgery; constant spring; contact sensitivity; continue same; contrast sensitivity; control serum; convalescence, convalescent; coronary sclerosis; coronary sinus; corpus striatum; corticoid-sensitive; corticosteroid; crush syndrome; current smoker;

current strength; Cushing syndrome; cycloserine; cyclosporine

C/S cesarean section; cycles per second

C&S calvarium and scalp; conjunctiva and sclera; culture and sensitivity

CS IV clinical stage 4

C4S chondroitin-4-sulfate

Cs case; cell surface; cesium; cyclosporine

C$_s$ standard clearance; static respiratory compliance

cS centistoke

cs chromosome; consciousness

CSA Canadian Standards Association; canavaninosuccinic acid; carbonyl salicylamide; cell surface antigen; chemical shift anisotropy; chondroitin sulfate A; chorionic somatomammotropin A; colony-stimulating activity; compressed spectral assay; computerized spectral analysis; Controlled Substances Act; cross section area; cyclosporine A

CsA cyclosporine A

CSAA Child Study Association of America

CSAD corporate services administration department

CSAT center for substance abuse treatment

CSAVP cerebral subarachnoid venous pressure

CSB contaminated small bowel; craniosynostosis, Boston type

csb chromosome break

CSBF coronary sinus blood flow

CSBS contaminated small bowel syndrome

CSC blow on blow (administration of small amounts of drugs at short intervals) [Fr. *coup sur coup*]; collagen sponge contraceptive; corticostriatocerebellar; cryogenic storage container

CSCC cutaneous squamous cell carcinoma

CSCD Center for Sickle Cell Disease

CSCI corticosterone side-chain isomerase

CSCR Central Society for Clinical Research

CSCV critical serum chemistry value

CSD carotid sinus denervation; cat scratch disease; combined system disease; conditionally streptomycin dependent; conduction system disease; cortical spreading depression; craniospinal defect; critical stimulus duration

CSDB cat scratch disease bacillus

CSDMS Canadian Society of Diagnostic Medical Sonographers

CSE clinical-symptom/self-evaluation [questionnaire]; cone-shaped epiphysis; conventional spin-echo; cross-sectional echocardiography

C sect, C-section cesarean section

CSEP cortical somatosensory evoked potential

CSER cortical somatosensory evoked response

CSF cancer family syndrome; cerebrospinal fluid; cold stability factor; colony-stimulating factor; coronary sinus flow

CS-F colony-stimulating factor

CSFH cerebrospinal fluid hypotension

CSFP cerebrospinal fluid pressure

CSFR colony-stimulating factor receptor

CSFV cerebrospinal fluid volume

CSF-WR cerebrospinal fluid-Wassermann reaction

CSG cholecystography, cholecystogram

csg chromosome gap

CSGBI Cardiac Society of Great Britain and Ireland

CSGBM collagenase soluble glomerular basement membrane

CSH carotid sinus hypersensitivity; chronic subdural hematoma; combat support [army] hospital; cortical stromal hyperplasia

CSHE California Society for Hospital Engineering

CSHH congenital self-healing histiocytosis

CSI calculus surface index; cancer serum index; cavernous sinus infiltration; cervical spine injury; chemical shift imaging; cholesterol saturation index; computerized severity of illness [index]; coronary sinus intervention

CSICU cardiac surgical intensive care unit

CSIF cytokine synthesis inhibitory factor

CSII continuous subcutaneous insulin infusion

CSIIP continuous subcutaneous insulin infusion pump

CSIN Chemical Substances Information Network

CSIS clinical supplies and inventory system

CSL cardiolipin synthetic lecithin; corticosteroid liposome

CSLM confocal scanning microscopy

CSLU chronic stasis leg ulcer

CSM cardiosynchronous myostimulator; carotid sinus massage; cerebrospinal meningitis; circulation, sensation, motion; Committee on Safety of Medicines; Consolidated Standards Manual; corn-soy milk

CSMA chronic spinal muscular atrophy

CSMAP celiac-superior mesenteric artery portography

CSMB Center for the Study of Multiple Births

CSMMG Chartered Society of Massage and Medical Gymnastics

CSMP chloramphenicol-sensitive microsomal protein

CSMT chorionic somatomammotropin

CSN cardiac sympathetic nerve; carotid sinus nerve

CSNA congenital sensory neuropathy with anhidrosis [syndrome]

CSNB congenital stationary night blindness

CS(NCA) Clinical Laboratory Scientist Certified by the National Certification Agency for Medical Laboratory Personnel

CSNK casein kinase

CSNRT, cSNRT corrected sinus node recovery time

CSNS carotid sinus nerve stimulation

CSNU cystinuria

CSO claims services only; common source outbreak; craniostenosis; craniosynostosis; ostium of coronary sinus

CSOM chronic suppurative otitis media

CSOP coronary sinus occlusion pressure

CSP carotid sinus pressure; cavum septi pellucidi; cell surface protein; cerebrospinal protein; Chartered Society of Physiotherapy; chemistry screening panel; chondroitin sulfate protein; Co-operative Statistical Program; criminal sexual psychopath; cyclosporin

CSPG chondroitin sulfate proteoglycan

Csp, C-spine cervical spine

CSPINE corticosteroid use, seropositive RA, peripheral joint destruction, involvement of cervical nerves, nodules (rheumatoid), established disease [cervical spine disease risk factors]

CSPS continual skin peeling syndrome

CSpT corticospinal tract

CSQ Coping Strategies Questionnaire

CSR central supply room; chart-stimulated recall [test]; Cheyne-Stokes respiration; continued stay review; corrected sedimentation rate; corrected survival rate; cortisol secretion rate; cumulative survival rate

CSRP cysteine-rich protein

CSRT corrected sinus recovery time

CSS Cancer Surveillance System; carotid sinus stimulation; carotid sinus syndrome; cavernous sinus syndrome; central sterile section; central sterile supply; chewing, sucking, swallowing; chronic subclinical scurvy; Churg-Strauss syndrome; client satisfaction scale; cranial sector scan

CSSAE Communication Skills Self-Assessment Exam

CSSD central sterile supply department

CSSU central sterile supply unit

CST cardiac stress test; cavernous sinus thrombosis; certified surgical technologist; chemostatin; Christ-Siemens Touraine [syndrome]; compliance, static; computer scatter tomography; contraction stress test; convulsive shock therapy; corticospinal tract; cosyntropin stimulation test; cystatin

C_{st} static compliance

cSt centistoke

C_{stat} static compliance

CSTI Clearinghouse for Scientific and Technical Information

CSTM cervical prevertebral soft tissue measurement

CSTP Committee for Scientific and Technological Policy

CSTT cold-stimulation time test

CSU casualty staging unit; catheter specimen of urine; central statistical unit; clinical specialty unit

CSUF continuous slow ultrafiltration

CSV chick syncytial virus

CSW Certified Social Worker; current sleep walker

CT calcitonin; calf testis; cardiac tamponade; cardiothoracic [ratio]; carotid tracing; carpal tunnel; cell therapy; cerebral thrombosis; cerebral tumor; cervical traction; cervicothoracic; chemotherapy; chest tube; chicken tumor; *Chlamydia trachomatis*; chlorothiazide; cholera toxin; cholesterol, total; chordae tendineae; chronic thyroiditis; chymotrypsin; circulation time; classic technique; closed thoracotomy; clotting time; coagulation time; coated tablet; cobra toxin; cognitive therapy; coil test; collecting tubule; colon, transverse; combined tumor; compressed tablet; computed tomography; connective tissue; continue treatment; continuous-flow tub; contraceptive technique; contraction time; controlled temperature; Coombs test; corneal transplant; coronary thrombosis; corrected transposition; corrective therapy; cortical thickness; cough threshold; crest time; cystine-tellurite; cytotechnologist; cytotoxic therapy; unit of attenuation [number]

C/T compression/traction [ratio]

C&T color and temperature

Ct carboxyl terminal

ct carat; chromatid; count

C_{T-1824} T-1824 (Evans blue) clearance

CTA Canadian Tuberculosis Association; chemotactic activity; chromotropic acid; Committee on Thrombolytic Agents; congenital trigeminal anesthesia; cyanotrimethyl-androsterone; cystine trypticase agar; cytoplasmic tubular aggregate; cytotoxic assay

CTAB cetyltrimethyl-ammonium bromide

CTAC Cancer Treatment Advisory Committee

cTAL cortical thick ascending limb

CTAP computed tomography in arterial portography; connective tissue activating peptide

CTAT computerized transaxial tomography

CTB ceased to breathe

ctb chromated break

CTC chlortetracycline; Clinical Trial Certificate; computed tomographic colography; computer-aided tomographic cisternography; cultured T cells

CTCL cutaneous T-cell lymphoma

ctCO$_2$ carbon dioxide concentration

CTD carpal tunnel decompression; chest tube drainage; congenital thymic dysplasia; connective tissue disease; cumulative trauma disorder

CT&DB cough, turn, and deep breathe

ctDNA chloroplast deoxyribonucleic acid

CTE calf thymus extract; cultured thymic epithelium

CTEM conventional transmission electron microscopy

CTF cancer therapy facility; certificate; Colorado tick fever; cytotoxic factor

ctf certificate

CTFE chlorotrifluoroethylene

CTFS complete testicular feminization syndrome

CTG cardiotocography; cervicothoracic ganglion; chymotrypsinogen

C/TG cholesterol-triglyceride [ratio]

ctg chromated gap

CTGA complete transposition of great arteries

CTH ceramide trihexoside; chronic tension headache; cystathionase

CTh carrier-specific T-helper [cell]

CTHD chlorthalidone

CTI coffee table injury

CTL cervico-thoraco-lumbar; control; cytolytic C lymphocyte; cytotoxic T-lymphocyte

CTLL cytotoxic lymphoid line

CTLSO cervicothoracolumbosacral orthosis

CTM cardiotachometer; Chlortrimeton; cricothyroid muscle; computed tomographic myelography

CTMC connective tissue mast cell

CTMM computed tomographic metrizamide myelography

CTMM-SF California Test of Mental Maturity–Short Form

CTN calcitonin; clinical trials notification; computer tomography number; continuous noise

cTn-I cardiac troponin I

cTNM TNM (*q.v.*) staging of tumors as determined by clinical noninvasive examination

CTO cervicothoracic orthosis

CTP California Test of Personality; citrate transport protein; clinical terms project; comprehensive treatment plan; cytidine triphosphate; cytosine triphosphate

C-TPN cyclic total parenteral nutrition

CTPP cerebral tissue perfusion pressure

CTPVO chronic thrombotic pulmonary vascular obstruction

CTR cardiothoracic ratio; carpal tunnel release; central tumor registry

ctr central; center; centric

CTRB chymotrypsinogen B

CTRL chymotrypsin-like [protease]

CTRS certified therapeutic recreation specialist

CTRX ceftriaxone

CTS carpal tunnel syndrome; clinical trials support [program]; composite treatment score; computed tomographic scan; contralateral threshold shift; corticosteroid

CTSB cathepsin B

CTSD cathepsin D

CTSE cathepsin E

CTSG cathepsin G

CTSH cathepsin H

CTSL cathepsin L

CTSNFR corrected time of sinoatrial node function recovery

CTSS cathepsin S; closed tracheal suction system

CTT cefotetan; central tegmental tract; central transmission time; compressed tablet triturate; computerized transaxial tomography; critical tracking time

CTTAC clinical trials and treatment advisory committee

CTU cardiac-thoracic unit; centigrade thermal unit; constitutive transcription unit

CTV cervical and thoracic vertebrae; clinical target volume

CTVDR conformal treatment verification, delivery and recording [system]

CTW central terminal of Wilson; combined testicular weight

CTX cefotaxime; cerebrotendinous xanthomatosis; chemotaxis; clinical trials exemption scheme; costotendinous xanthomatosis; cytoxan

CTx cardiac transplantation; conotoxin

CTZ chemoreceptor trigger zone; chlorothiazide

CU cardiac unit; casein unit; cause unknown or undetermined; chymotrypsin unit; clinical unit; color unit; contact urticaria; convalescent unit

Cu copper [Lat. *cuprum*]

C$_u$ urea clearance

cu cubic

CUA cost-utility analysis [ratio]

CuB copper band

CUC chronic ulcerative colitis

cu cm cubic centimeter

CUD cause undetermined; congenital urinary deformity

CuD copper deficiency

CUE cumulative urinary excretion

CUG cystidine, uridine, and guanidine; cystourethrogram, cystourethrography

CUI Cox-Uphoff International [tissue expander]

cu in cubic inch

cult culture

cum cumulative

cu m cubic meter

CUMITECH Cumulative Techniques and Procedures in Clinical Microbiology

cu mm cubic millimeter

CUP carcinoma unknown primary

CUR cystourethrorectal

cur cure, curative; current

CURN Conduct and Utilization of Research in Nursing

CUS carotid ultrasound examination; catheterized urine specimen; contact urticaria syndrome

CuS copper supplement

CUSA Cavitron ultrasonic aspirator

CuTS cubital tunnel syndrome

CV cardiac volume; cardiovascular; carotenoid vesicle; cell volume; central venous; cephalic vein; cerebrovascular; cervical vertebra; Chikungunya virus; closing volume; coefficient of variation; color vision; concentrated volume; conducting vein; conduction velocity; conjugata vera; contrast ventriculography; conventional ventilation; corpuscular volume; costovertebral; cresyl violet; crystal violet; cutaneous vasculitis; cyclic voltometry or voltamogram

C/V coulomb per volt

Cv specific heat at constant volume

C$_v$ constant volume

cv cultivar

CVA cardiovascular accident; cerebrovascular accident; chronic villous arthritis; common variable agammaglobulinemia; costovertebral angle; cyclophosphamide, vincristine, and Adriamycin

CVAH congenital virilizing adrenal hyperplasia

CVAP cerebrovascular amyloid peptide

CVAT costovertebral angle tenderness

CVB chorionic villi biopsy

CVC central venous catheter

CV cath central venous catheter

CVCT cardiovascular computed tomography

CVD cardiovascular disease; cerebrovascular disease; collagen vascular disease; color-vision-deviant

CVF cardiovascular failure; central visual field; cervicovaginal fluid; cobra venom factor

CVFn cardiovascular function

CVG contrast ventriculography; coronary venous graft; cutis verticis gyrata

CVG/MR cutis verticis gyrata/mental retardation [syndrome]

CVH cerebroventricular hemorrhage; cervicovaginal hood; combined ventricular hypertrophy; common variable hypogammaglobulinemia

CVHD chronic valvular heart disease

CVI cardiovascular incident; cardiovascular insufficiency; cerebrovascular incident; cerebrovascular insufficiency; chronic venous insufficiency; common variable immunodeficiency

CVID common variable immunodeficiency

CVLT California Verbal Learning Test; clinical vascular laboratory

CVM cardiovascular monitor; cerebral venous malformation; cyclophosphamide, vincristine, and methotrexate

CVMP Committee on Veterans Medical Problems

CVO central vein occlusion; central venous oxygen; Chief Veterinary Officer; credentialing verification organization

CVOD cerebrovascular obstructive disease

CVP cardioventricular pacing; cell volume profile; central venous pressure; cyclophosphamide, vincristine, and prednisone

cvPO₂, cvP_{O_2} cerebral venous partial pressure of oxygen

CVR cardiovascular-renal; cardiovascular-respiratory; cephalic vasomotor response; cerebrovascular resistance

CVRD cardiovascular-renal disease

CVRR cardiovascular recovery room

CVS cardiovascular surgery; cardiovascular system; challenge virus strain; chorionic villi sampling; clean voided specimen; coronavirus susceptibility; current vital signs

CVT cardiovascular technologist; central venous temperature; congenital vertical talus

CVTR charcoal viral transport medium

CVVH continuous veno-venous hemofiltration

CVVHD continuous veno-venous hemodialysis

CW cardiac work; case work; cell wall; chemical warfare; chemical weapon; chest wall; children's ward; clockwise; continuous wave; crutch walking

Cw crutch walking

C/W compare with; consistent with

CWBTS capillary whole blood true sugar

CWC chest wall compliance

CWD cell wall defect; continuous-wave Doppler

CWDF cell wall-deficient form [bacteria]

CWEQ conditions of work effectiveness scale

CWF Cornell Word Form

CWH cardiomyopathy and wooly haircoat [syndrome]

CWHB citrated whole human blood

CWI cardiac work index

CWL cutaneous water loss

CWMS color, warmth, movement sensation

CWOP childbirth without pain

CWP childbirth without pain; coal worker's pneumoconiosis

CWPEA Childbirth Without Pain Education Association

CWS cell wall skeleton; chest wall stimulation; child welfare service; cold water-soluble; cotton wool spots

CWT cold water treatment

Cwt, cwt hundredweight

CWW clinic without walls

CWXSP Coal Workers' X-ray Surveillance Program

CX cervix; chest x-ray; connexin; critical experiment

Cx cervix; circumflex; clearance; complaint; complex; convex

cx cervix; complex; cylinder axis

CXB3S Coxsackie B3 virus susceptibility

CxCor circumflex coronary [artery]

CXMD canine X-linked muscular dystrophy
CXR, CxR chest x-ray
CY casein-yest autolysate [medium]; cyclophosphamide
Cy cyanogen; cyclophosphamide; cyst; cytarabine
cy, cyan cyanosis
CyA cyclosporine A
CYC cyclophosphamide; cytochrome C
cyc cyclazocine; cycle; cyclotron
CYCLO, Cyclo cyclophosphamide; cyclopropane
Cyclo C cyclocytidine hydrochloride
CYCLOPS cyclically ordered phase sequence
Cyd cytidine
CYE charcoal yeast extract [agar]
CYH chymase, heart
CYL casein yeast lactate
cyl cylinder; cylindrical lens
CYM chymase, mast cell
CYMP chymosin, pseudogene
CYN cyanide

CYP cyclophilin; cyproheptadine
CYPA cyclophilin A
CYPC cyclophilin C
CYPH cyclophilin
CYS cystoscopy
Cys cyclosporine; cysteine
Cys-Cys cystine
CysLT1 cysteinyl leukotriene 1
CYSTO cystogram
cysto cystoscopy
CYT cytochrome
Cyt cytoplasm; cytosine
cyt cytochrome; cytology, cytological; cytoplasm, cytoplasm
Cyto cytotechnologist
cytol cytology, cytological
CY-VA-DIC cyclophosphamide, vincristine, Adriamycin, and dacarbazine
CZ cefazolin
Cz central midline placement of electrodes in electroencephalography
CZI crystalline zine insulin
C_{zn} zinc clearance
CZP clonazepam

D absorbed dose aspartic acid; cholecalciferol; coefficient of diffusion; dacryon; dalton; date; daughter; day; dead; dead air space; debye; deceased; deciduous; decimal reduction time; degree; density; dental; dermatology, dermatologist, dermatologic; deuterium; deuteron; development; deviation; dextro; dextrose; diagnosis; diagonal; diameter; diaphorase; diarrhea; diastole; diathermy; died; difference; diffusion, diffusing; dihydrouridine; dilution [rate]; diopter; diplomate; disease; dispense; displacement [loop]; distal; distance [focus-object]; diuresis; diurnal; divergence; diversity; diverticulum; divorced; doctor; dog; donor; dorsal; drive; drug; dual; duct; duodenum, duodenal; duration; dwarf; electric displacement; mean dose; right [Lat. *dexter*]; unit of vitamin D potency

D̄ mean dose

D₁ diagonal one; first dorsal vertebra

1-D one-dimensional

D₂ diagonal two; second dorsal vertebra

2-D two-dimensional

2,4-D 2,4-dichlorophenoxyacetic acid

D/3 distal third

3-D three-dimensional

D₃₋₁₂ third to twelfth dorsal vertebrae

D4 fourth digit

D₁₀ decimal reduction time

d atomic orbital with angular momentum quantum number 2; day [Lat. *dies*]; dead; deceased; deci-; decrease, decreased; degree; density; deoxy; deoxyribose; dextro-; dextrorotatory; diameter; diastasis; died; diopter; distal; distance [between radiographic grids or between

subject and film or casette]; diurnal; dorsal; dose; doubtful; duration; dyne; right [Lat. *dexter*]

Δ see *delta*

δ see *delta*

1/d once a day

2/d twice a day

DA dark adaptation; dark agouti [rat]; daunomycin; degenerative arthritis; delayed action; Dental Assistant; deoxyadenosine; descending aorta; developmental age; dextroamphetamine; diabetic acidosis; differential analyzer; differentiation antigen; digital angiography; digital to analogue [converter]; diphenylchlorarsine; Diploma in Anesthetics; direct agglutination; disability assistance; disaggregated; dopamine; drug addict, drug addiction; drug administration; ductus arteriosus

D/A date of accident; date of admission; digital-to-analog [converter]; discharge and advise

D-A donor-acceptor

D&A dilatation and aspiration; drugs and allergy

Da dalton

da daughter; day; deca-

DAA decompensated autonomous adenoma; dementia associated with alcoholism; dialysis-associated amyloidosis; diaminoanisole

DAAO diaminoacid oxidase

DAB days after birth; 3,3'-diaminobenzidine; dysrhythmic aggressive behavior

DABA 2,4-diaminobutyric acid

DABP D site albumin promoter binding protein

DAC derived air concentration; digital-to-analog converter; disaster assistance center; Division of Ambulatory Care

dac dacryon

DACL Depression Adjective Check List

DACM N-(7-diethylamino-4-methyl-3-coumarinyl) maleimide

DACMD deputy associate chief medical director

DACS data acquisition and control system

DACT dactinomycin

DAD delayed afterdepolarization; diffuse alveolar damage; dispense as directed

DADA dichloroacetic acid diisopropylammonium salt

DADDS diacetyldiaminodiphenylsulfone

DADS Director Army Dental Service

DAE diphenylanthracene endoperoxide; diving air embolism; dysbaric air embolism

DAF decay-accelerating factor; delayed auditory feedback; drug-adulterated food

DAG diacylglycerol; dianhydrogalactitol; dystrophin-associated glycoprotein

DAGK diacylglycerol kinase

DAGT direct antiglobulin test

DAH disordered action of the heart

DAHEA Department of Allied Health Education and Accreditation

DAHM Division of Allied Health Manpower

DAI diffuse axonal injury

Dal, dal dalton

DALA delta-aminolevulinic acid

DALE Drug Abuse Law Enforcement

DAM data-associated message; degraded amyloid; diacetyl monoxime; diacetylmorphine

dam decameter

DAMA discharged against medical advice

dAMP deoxyadenosine monophosphate; deoxyadenylate adenosine monophosphate

D and C dilatation and curettage

DANS 1-dimethylaminonaphthalene-5-sulfonyl chloride

DANTE delays altered with nutation for tailored excitation

DAO diamine oxidase

DAo descending aorta

DAP data acquisition processor; depolarizing afterpotential; diabetes-associated peptide; diaminopimelic acid; diastolic aortic pressure; dihydroxyacetone phosphate; dipeptidylaminopeptidase; direct latex agglutination pregnancy [test]; dose area product; Draw-a-Person [test]

DAP&E Diploma of Applied Parasitology and Entomology

DAPRE daily adjustable progressive resistive exercise

DAPRU Drug Abuse Prevention Resource Unit

DAPT diaminophenylthiazole; direct agglutination pregnancy test

DAQ Diagnostic Assessment Questionnaire

DAR death after resuscitation; diacereine; differential absorption ratio

DARP drug abuse rehabilitation program

DART developmental and reproductive toxicology

DARTS Drug and Alcohol Rehabilitation Testing System

DAS dead air space; Death Anxiety Scale; delayed anovulatory syndrome; dextroamphetamine sulfate; digital angiography segmentation

DASD direct access storage device

DASH Distress Alarm for the Severely Handicapped

DASI Duke activity specific index

DAST drug abuse screening test; drug and alcohol screening test

DAT delayed-action tablet; dementia Alzheimer's type; dental aptitude test; diacetylthiamine; diet as tolerated; differential agglutination titer; Differential Aptitude Test; diphtheria antitoxin; direct agglutination test; direct antiglobulin test; Disaster Action Team

DATE dental auxiliary teacher education

DATP deoxyadenosine triphosphate

DATTA diagnostic and therapeutic technology assessment

DAU 3-deazauridine; Dental Auxiliary Utilization

dau daughter

DAUs drug abuse testing and urines

DAV data valid; Disabled American Veterans; duck adenovirus

DAVF dural arteriovenous fistula

DAVIT Danish Verapamil Infarction Trial

DAVM dural arteriovenous malformation

DAvMED Diploma in Aviation Medicine

DAVP deamino-arginine vasopressin

DAW dispense as written

DAWN Drug Abuse Warning Network

DB data base; date of birth; deep breath; dense body; dextran blue; diabetes, diabetic; diagonal band; diet beverage; direct bilirubin; disability; distobuccal; double-blind [study]; Dutch belted [rabbit]; duodenal bulb

Db diabetes, diabetic

dB, db decibel

db date of birth; diabetes, diabetic

DBA Diamond-Blackfan anemia; dibenzanthracene; *Dolichos biflorus* agglutinin

DBAE dihydroxyborylaminoethyl

DBC dibencozide; distal balloon catheter; dye-binding capacity

DB&C deep breathing and coughing

DBCL dilute blood clot lysis [method]

DBD definite brain damage; dibromodulcitol

DBDG distobuccal developmental groove

dB/dt change of magnetic flux with time

DBE deep breathing exercise; dibromoethane

DBED penicillin G benzathine

DBH dopamine beta-hydroxylase

DBI development at birth index; phenformin hydrochloride

DBIOC data base input/output control

DBIR Directory of Biotechnology Information Resources

dBk decibels above 1 kilowatt

DBM data base management; dibromomannitol; dobutamine

dBm decibels above 1 milliwatt

DBMS data base management systems

DBO distobucco-occlusal

db/ob diabetic obese [mouse]

DBP diastolic blood pressure; dibutylphthalate; distobuccopulpal; Döhle body panmyelopathy; vitamin D-binding protein

DBR distorted breathing rate

DBRI dysfunctional behavior rating instrument

DBS deep brain stimulation; Denis Browne splint; despeciated bovine serum; Diamond-Blackfan syndrome; dibromosalicil; diminished breath sounds; direct bonding system; Division of Biological Standards; double blind study; double-burst stimulus

DBT dry bulb temperature

DBW desirable body weight

dBW decibels above 1 watt

DC daily census; data communication; data conversion; decrease; deep compartment; Dental Corps; deoxycholate; descending colon; dextran charcoal; diagonal conjugate; diagnostic center; diagnostic cluster; diagnostic code; differentiated cell; diffusion capacity; digit copying; digital computer; dilatation and curettage; dilation catheter; diphenylcyanoarsine; direct Coombs' [test]; direct current; discharge, discharged; discontinue, discontinued; distal colon; distocervical; Doctor of Chiropractic; donor cells; dorsal column; dressing change; duodenal cap; Dupuytren contracture; duty cycle; dyskeratosis congenita; electric defibrillator using DC discharge

Dc critical dilution rate

D/C discontinue

D/c discontinue; discharge

DC65 Darvon compound 65

D&C dilatation and curettage; drugs and cosmetics

dC deoxycytidine

dc decrease; direct current; discharge; discontinue

DCA deoxycholate-citrate agar; deoxycholic acid; desoxycorticosterone acetate; dichloroacetate

DCABG double coronary artery bypass graft

DCB dichlorobenzidine

DCBE double contrast barium enema

DCBF dyamic cardiac blood flow

DCbN deep cerebellar nucleus

DCC day care center; detected in colon cancer; dextran-coated charcoal; diameter of cylindrical collimator; N,N'-dicyclohexylcarbodiimide; digital compact casette; disaster control center; dorsal cell column; double concave

DCCMP daunomycin, cyclocytidine, 6-mercaptopurine, and prednisolone

DC$_{CO2}$ diffusing capacity for carbon dioxide

DCCT diabetes control and complications trial

DCCV direct current cardioversion

DCD Diploma in Chest Diseases

D/c'd, dc'd discontinued

DCE desmosterol-to-cholesterol enzyme

DCET dicarboxyethoxythiamine

DCF 2'-deoxycoformycin; dichlorofluorescin; direct centrifugal flotation; dopachrome conversion factor

DCFDA 2',7'-dichlorofluorescin diacetate

DCG dacryocystography; deoxycorticosterone glucoside; diagnosis related group; disodium cromoglycate; dynamic electrocardiography

DCH delayed cutaneous hypersensitivity; Diploma in Child Health

DCh Doctor of Surgery [Lat. *Doctor Chirurgiae*]

DCHA docosahexaenoic acid

DCHEB dichlorohexafluorobutane

DCHN dicyclohexylamine nitrite

DChO Doctor of Ophthalmic Surgery

DCI dichloroisoprenaline; dichloroisoproterenol; duplicate coverage inquiry

DCIP dichlorophenolindophenol

DCIS ductal carcinoma in situ

DCK deoxycytidine kinase

DCL dicloxacillin; diffuse or disseminated cutaneous leishmaniasis

DCLHb diaspirin cross-linked hemoglobin

DCLS deoxycholate citrate lactose saccharose

DCM dichloromethane; dichloromethotrexate; dilated cardiomyopathy; Doctor of Comparative Medicine; dyssynergia cerebellaris myoclonica

DCML dorsal column medial lemniscus

DCMP daunomycin, cytosine arabinoside, 6-mercaptopurine, and prednisolone

dCMP deoxycytidine monophosphate

DCMT Doctor of Clinical Medicine of the Tropics

DCMX 2,4-dichloro-m-xylenol

DCN data collection network; deep cerebral nucleus; delayed conditioned necrosis; depressed, cognitively normal; dorsal cochlear nucleus; dorsal column nucleus; dorsal cutaneous nerve

DCNU chlorozotocin

DCO Diploma of the College of Optics

D$_{CO}$ diffusing capacity for carbon monoxide

DCOG Diploma of the College of Obstetricians and Gynaecologists

DCP dicalcium phosphate; Diploma in Clinical Pathology; Diploma in Clinical Psychology; District Community Physician; dynamic compression plate

DCR dacryocystorhinostomy; data conversion receiver; direct cortical response

3-DCRT three-dimensional conformal radiation therapy

DCS decompression sickness; dense canalicular system; diffuse cortical sclerosis; dorsal column stimulation, dorsal column stimulator; dynamic condylar screw; dynamic contrast-enhanced subtraction; dynamic contrast-enhanced tomography; dyskinetic cilia syndrome

DCT direct Coombs' test; discrete cosine transform; distal convoluted tubule; diurnal cortisol test; dynamic computed tomography

3DCT three-dimensional computed tomography

DCTMA desoxycorticosterone trimethylacetate

dCTP deoxycytidine triphosphate

DCTPA desoxycorticosterone triphenylacetate

DCTS dynamic carpal tunnel syndrome

DCV distribution of conduction velocities

DCX double charge exchange

DCx double convex

DD dangerous drug; data definition; day of delivery; degenerated disc; degenerative disease; delusional disorder; depth dose [x-ray]; detrusor dyssynergia; developmental disability; diastrophic dysplasia; died of the disease; differential diagnosis; digestive disorder; Di Guglielmo disease; disc diameter; discharge diagnosis; discharged dead; dog dander; double diffusion; drug dependence; dry dressing; Duchenne dystrophy; Dupuytren disease

D6D delta-6-desaturase

dd dideoxy

DDA Dangerous Drugs Act; dideoxyadenosine; digital differential analysis

ddA 2',3'-dideoxyadenosine

DDase deoxyuridine diphosphatase

DDAVP, dDAVP 1-deamino-8-D-arginine vasopressin; 1-deamino-8-N-arginine vasopressin

DDC dangerous drug cabinet; dideoxycytidine; diethyl-dithiocarbamate; direct display console; diverticular disease of the colon

DDc double concave

ddC dideoxycytidine

DDD AV universal [pacemaker]; defined daily dose; degenerative disc disease; dehydroxydinaphthyl disulfide; dense deposit disease; Denver dialysis disease; dichlorodiphenyl-dichloroethane; dihydroxydinaphthyl disulfide; dorsal dural deficiency; Dowling-Degos disease

DDD CT double-dose-delay computed tomography

DDE dichlorodiphenyldichloroethylene

DDG deoxy-D-glucose

DDH developmental dysplasia of the hip; Diploma in Dental Health; dissociated double hypertropia

DDI, ddI dideoxyinosine

DDIB Disease Detection Information Bureau

DDKase deoxynucleoside diphosphate kinase

DDM Diploma in Dermatological Medicine; Doctor in Dental Medicine; Dyke-Davidoff-Masson [syndrome]

dDNA denatured deoxyribonucleic acid

DDNTP dideoxynucleoside triphosphate

DDO Diploma in Dental Orthopaedics

DDP cisplatin; density-dependent phosphoprotein; difficult denture patient; digital data processing; distributed data processing

DDPA Delta Dental Plans Association

DDR diastolic descent rate; Diploma in Diagnostic Radiology

DDRB Doctors' and Dentists' Review Body

DDRT diseases, disorders and related topics

DDS damaged disc syndrome; dendro-dendritic synaptosome; dental distress syndrome; depressed DNA synthesis; dialysis disequilibrium syndrome; diaminodiphenylsulfone; directional Doppler sonography; Director of Dental Services; disability determination service; Disease-Disability Scale; Doctor of Dental Surgery; dodecyl sulfate; double decidual sac; dystrophy-dystocia syndrome

DDSc Doctor of Dental Science

DDSI digital damage severity index

DDSO diaminodiphenylsulfoxide

DDST Denver Developmental Screening Test

DDT dichlorodiphenyltrichloroethane; ductus deferens tumor

DDTC diethyldithiocarbamate

DDTN dideoxy-didehydrothymidine

ddTTP dideoxythymidine triphosphate

DDU dermo-distortive urticaria; duplex Doppler ultrasound

dDVH differential dose-volume histogram

D/DW dextrose in distilled water

D 5% DW 5% dextrose in distilled water

DDx differential diagnosis

DE deprived eye; diagnostic error; dialysis encephalopathy; digestive energy; dose equivalent; dream elements; drug evaluation; duration of ejection

D&E diet and elimination; dilation and evacuation [partial birth abortion]

2DE two-dimensional echocardiography

D=E dates equal to examination

DEA dehydroepiandrosterone; diethanolamine; Drug Enforcement Agency

DEAE diethylaminoethyl [cellulose]

DEAE-D diethylaminoethyl dextran

DEAFF detection of early antigen fluorescent foci

DEALE declining exponential approximation of life expectancy [method]

DEB diepoxybutane; diethylbutanediol; Division of Environmental Biology; dystrophic epidermolysis bullosa

deb debridement

DEBA diethylbarbituric acid

debil debilitation

DEBRA Dystrophic Epidermolysis Bulosa Research Association

DEBS dominant epidermolysis bullosa simplex

DEC decrease; deoxycholate citrate; diagnostic episode cluster; diethylcarbamazine; dynamic environmental conditioning

Dec, dec decant

dec deceased; deciduous; decimal; decompose, decomposition; decrease, decreased

decd deceased

decoct decoction

decomp decompensation; decomposition, decompose

decr decrease, decreased

decub lying down [Lat. *decubitus*]

DED date of expected delivery; defined exposure dose; delayed erythema dose

DEEG depth electroencephalogram, depth electroencephalography

DEF decayed primary teeth requiring filling, decayed primary teeth requiring extraction, and primary teeth successfully filled; dose-effect factor

def defecation; deficiency, deficient; deferred

DEFIANT Doppler Flow and Echocardiography in Functional Cardiac Insufficiency Assessment of Nisoldipine Therapy [trial]

defib defibrillation

defic deficiency, deficient

DEFN Danubian endemic familial nephropathy

DEF$_{NT}$ dose-effect factor for normal tissue

deform deformed, deformity

DEFT direct epifluorescent filter technique

DEF$_T$ dose-effect factor for tumor

DEG diethylene glycol

Deg, deg degeneration, degenerative; degree

degen degeneration, degenerative

DEH dysplasia epiphysealis hemimelica

DEHP di(2-ethylhexyl)phthalate

DEHS Division of Emergency Health Services

DEHT developmental hand function test

dehyd dehydration, dehydrated

DEJ, dej dentino-enamel junction; dermo-epidermal junction

del deletion; delivery; delusion

DELFIA dissociated enhanced lantanide fluoroimmunoassay

deliq deliquescence, deliquescent

DELIRIUM drugs–electrolytes–low temperature and lunacy–intoxication and intracranial processes–retention of urine or feces–infection–unfamiliar surroundings–myocardial infarction [causes of delirium]

Delt deltoid

Δ Greek capital letter *delta*

δ Greek lower case letter *delta*; immunoglobulin D

DEM demerol; diethylmaleate

Dem Demerol

DEN denervation; dengue; dermatitis exfoliativa neonatorum; Device Experience Network [of the CDRH]; diethylnitrosamine

denat denatured

DENT Dental Exposure Normalization Technique

Dent, dent dentistry, dentist, dental, dentition

DENTALPROJ Dental Research Projects

DEP diethylpropanediol; dilution end point

dep dependent; deposit

DEPA diethylene phosphoramide

DEPC diethyl pyrocarbonate

depr depression, depressed

DEPS distal effective potassium secretion

DEP ST SEG depressed ST segment

DEPT distortionless enhancement by polarization transfer

dept department

DEQ Depression Experiences Questionnaire

DER disulfiram-ethanol reaction; dual energy radiography

DeR degeneration reaction

der derivative chromosome

deriv derivative, derived

Derm, derm dermatitis, dermatology, dermatologist, dermatological; dermatome

DES dementia rating scale; dermal-epidermal separation; dialysis encephalopathy syndrome; diethylstilbestrol; diffuse esophageal spasm; disequilibrium syndrome; doctor's emergency service

desat desaturated

desc descendant; descending

Desc Ao descending aorta

DESI drug efficacy study implementation

desq desquamation

DEST Denver Eye Screening Test; dichotic environmental sounds test

DET diethyltryptamine; dipyridamole echocardiography test

DETC diethyldithiocarbamate

Det-6 detroid-6 [human sternal marrow cells]

determ determination, determined

detn detention

detox detoxification

DEUV direct electronic urethrocystometry

DEV deviant, deviation; duck embryo vaccine or virus

dev development; deviation

devel development

DevPd developmental pediatrics

DEX dexamethasone

Dex dextrose

dex dexterity; dextrorotatory; right [Lat. *dexter*]

DEXA dual-energy x-ray absorptiometry

DF decapacitation factor; decontamination factor; deferoxamine; deficiency factor; defined flora [animal]; degree of freedom; diabetic father; dietary fibers; digital fluoroscopy; discriminant function; disseminated foci; distribution factor, dorsiflexion; dysgonic fermenter

Df *Dermatophagoides farinae*

df degrees of freedom

DF-2 dysgonic fermenter 2

DFA direct fluorescent antibody; discriminant function analysis; dorsiflexion assistance

DFB dinitrofluorobenzene; dysfunctional bleeding

DFC developmental field complex; dry-filled capsule

DFD defined formula diets; developmental field defect; diisopropyl phosphorofluoridate

DFDT difluoro-diphenyl-trichloroethane

DFE diffuse fasciitis with eosinophilia; distal femoral epiphysis

DFECT dense fibroelastic connective tissue

3DFEM three-dimensional finite element method

DFG direct forward gaze; German Research Federation [Deutsche Forshungsgemeinschaft]

DFHom Diploma of the Faculty of Homeopathy

DFI disease-free interval

DFL digital film library

DFM decreased fetal movement

DFMC daily fetal movement count

DFMO difluoromethylornithine

DFMR daily fetal movement record

DFO, DFOM deferoxamine

DFP diastolic filling period; diisopropyl-fluorophosphate

DF^{32}P radiolabeled diisopropylfluorophosphate

DFPP double filtration plasmapheresis

DFR diabetic floor routine; digital fluororadiography

DFS disease-free survival

DFSP dermatofibrosarcoma protuberans

DFT diagnostic function test; defibrillation threshold

DFT$_3$ dialyzable fraction of triiodothyronine

DFT$_4$ dialyzable fraction of thryoxine

2DFT two-dimensional Fourier transform

3DFT three-dimensional Fourier transform

DFU dead fetus in utero; dideoxyfluorouridine

DFV diarrhea with fever and vomiting

DG dentate gyrus; deoxyglucose; desmoglein; diacylglycerol; diagnosis; diastolic gallop; DiGeorge [anomaly or syndrome] diglyceride; distogingival

2DG 2-deoxy-*D*-glucose

dg decigram; diagnosis

DGA DiGeorge anomaly

DGAVP desglycinamide-9-[Arg-8]-vasopressin

DGBG dimethylglyoxal bisguanyl-hydrazone

DGCR DiGeorge syndrome chromosome region

DGE delayed gastric emptying

dge drainage

DGF duct growth factor

DGGE denaturing gradient gel electrophoresis

DGI dentinogenesis imperfecta; disseminated gonococcal infection

DGIM Division of General Internal Medicine

DGLA dihomogamma-linolenic acid

dGMP deoxyguanosine monophosphate

DGMS Division of General Medical Sciences

DGN diffuse glomerulonephritis

DGO Diploma in Gynaecology and Obstetrics

DGP 2,3-diglycerophosphate

DGPG diffuse proliferative glomerulonephritis

DGS decompression sickness; developmental Gerstmann syndrome; diabetic glomerulosclerosis; Di George sequence;

Di George syndrome; dysplasia-gigantism syndrome

DGSX X-linked dysplasia gigantism syndrome

dGTP deoxyguanosine triphosphate

DGU uracil deoxyribonucleic acid glycosylase

DGV dextrose-gelatin-Veronal [buffer]

DH daily habits; day hospital; dehydrocholate; dehydrogenase; delayed hypersensitivity; dermatitis herpetiformis; developmental history; diaphragmatic hernia; disseminated histoplasmosis; dominant hand; dorsal horn; drug history; ductal hyperplasia; Dunkin-Hartley [guinea pig]

D/H deuterium/hydrogen [ratio]

DHA dehydroacetic acid; dehydroascorbic acid; dehydroepiandrosterone; dihydroacetic acid; dihydroxyacetone; district health authority

DHAD mitoxantrone hydrochloride

DHAP dihydroxyacetone phosphate

DHAP-AT dihydroxyacetone phosphate acyltransferase

DHAS dehydroandrostenedione

DHB duck hepatitis B

DHBE dihydroxybutyl ether

DHBG dihydroxybutyl guanine

DHBS dihydrobiopterin synthetase

DHBV duck hepatitis B virus

DHC dehydrocholesterol; dehydrocholate

DHCA deep hypothermia and circulatory arrest

DHCC dehydroxycholecalciferol

DHCP decentralized hospital computer program

DHD district health department

DHE dihematoporphirin ether; dihydroergocryptine; dihydroergotamine

DHEA dehydroepiandrosterone

DHEAS dehydroepiandrosterone sulfate

DHEC dihydroergocryptine

DHES Division of Health Examination Statistics

DHESN dihydroergosine

DHEW Department of Health, Education, and Welfare

DHF dengue hemorrhagic fever; dihydrofolate; dorsihyperflexion

DHF/DSS dengue hemorrhagic fever/dengue shock syndrome

DHFR dihydrofolate reductase

DHFRase dihydrofolate reductase

DHFRP dihydrofolate reductase pseudogene

DHg Doctor of Hygiene

DHGG deaggregated human gamma-globulin

DHHS Department of Health and Human Services

DHI Dental Health International; dihydroxyindole

DHIA dehydroisoandrosterol

DHIC dihydroisocodeine

DHL diffuse histiocytic lymphoma

DHLD dihydrolipoamide dehydrogenase

DHM dihydromorphine

DHMA 3,4-dihydroxymandelic acid

DHMO dental health maintenance organization

DHP dehydrogenated polymer; dihydroprogesterone; 1,4-dihydropyridine

DHPA dihydroxypropyl adenine

DHPCCB dihydropyridine calcium channel blocker

DHPG dihydroxyphenylglycol; dihydroxyproproxymethylguanine

DHPR dihydropteridine reductase

DHR delayed hypersensitivity reaction; Department of Human Resources

DHS delayed hypersensitivity; diabetic hyperosmolar state; duration of hospital stay; dynamic hip screw

D-5-HS 5% dextrose in Harman's solution

DHSM dihydrostreptomycin

DHSS Department of Health and Social Security; dihydrostreptomycin sulfate

DHT dehydrotestosterone; dihydroergotoxine; dihydrotachysterol; dihydrotestosterone; dihydrothymine; dihydroxytryptamine

5,7-DHT 5,7-dihydroxytryptamine

DHTP dihydrotestosterone propionate

DHTR dihydrotestosterone receptor

DHy, DHyg Doctor of Hygiene

DHZ dihydralazine

DI date of injury; defective interfering [particle]; dentinogenesis imperfecta; deoxyribonucleic acid index; deterioration index; detrusor instability; diabetes insipidus; diagnostic imaging; dialyzed iron; disability insurance; disto-incisal; dorsoiliac; double indemnity; drug information; drug interactions; dyskaryosis index

DIA depolarization-induced automaticity; diabetes; diaphorase; diazepam; Drug Information Association

DiA Diego antigen

dia diakinesis; diathermy

diab diabetes, diabetic

Diag diagnosis

diag diagonal; diagnosis; diagram

diam diameter

diaph diaphragm

dias diastole, diastolic

diath diathermy

DIB diagnostic interview for borderlines; difficulty in breathing; disability insurance benefits; dot immunobinding; duodenoileal bypass

diBr-HQ 5,7-dibromo-8-hydroxy-quinidine

DIC dicarbazine; differential interference contrast microscopy; diffuse intravascular coagulation; direct isotope cystography; disseminated intravascular coagulation; drug information center

dic dicentric

DICD dispersion-induced circular dichroism

DICO diffusing capacity of carbon monoxide

DICOM digital imaging and communication in medicine

DID dead of intercurrent disease; double immunodiffusion

DIDD dense intramembranous deposit disease

DIDMOA diabetes insipidus-diabetes mellitus-optic atrophy [syndrome]

DIDMOAD diabetis insipidus, diabetes mellitus, otpic atrophy, deafness [syndrome]

DIDS 4,4'diisothiocyanostilbene-2,2-disulfonate

DIE died in emergency department

diEMG diaphragmatic electromyography

DIF diffuse interstitial fibrosis; direct immunofluorescence; dose increase factor

DIFF, diff difference, differential; diffusion

diff diagn differential diagnosis

DIFP diffuse interstitial fibrosing pneumonitis; diisopropyl fluorophosphonate

dif-PIPE diffuse persistent interstitial pulmonary emphysema

DIG digitalis; digoxin; drug-induced galactorrhea

dig digitalis; digoxin

DIH Diploma in Industrial Health

DIHE drug-induced hepatic encephalopathy

diHETE dihydroxyeicosatetraenoic acid

DIHPPA di-iodohydroxyphenylpyruvic acid

DIL, Dil Dilantin; drug-induced lupus [erythematosus]

dil dilute, dilution, diluted

dilat dilatation

DILD diffuse infiltrative lung disease; diffuse interstitial lung disease

DILE drug-induced lupus erythematosus

DILS diffuse infiltrative lymphocytosis syndrome

DIM divalent ion metabolism; medium infective dose [Lat. *dosis infectionis media*]

dim dimension; diminished

DIMIT 3,5-dimethyl-3'-isopropyl-L-thyronine

DIMOAD diabetes insipidus, diabetes mellitus, optic atrophy, deafness

DIMS disorders of initiating and maintaining sleep

DIMSE DICOM message service element

din damage inducible [gene]

DIP desquamative interstitial pneumonitis; diisopropyl phosphate; diisopropylamine; diphtheria; distal interphalangeal; drip infusion pyelogram; dual-in-line package; dynamic integral proctography

Dip diplomate

dip diploid; diplotene

DIPA diisopropylamine

DipBact Diploma in Bacteriology

DIPC diffuse interstitial pulmonary calcification

DipChem Diploma in Chemistry

DipClinPath Diploma in Clinical Pathology

DIPF diisopropylphosphofluoridate

diph diphtheria

diph-tet diphtheria-tetanus [toxoid]

diph-tox AP alum precipitated diphtheria toxoid

DIPI defective interfering particle induction

DIPJ distal interphalangeal joint

DIR double isomorphous replacement

Dir, dir director; direction, directions

DIRD drug-induced renal disease

DIRLINE Directory of Information Resources On-Line

DIS Diagnostic Interview Schedule; draft international standard

DI-S debris index, simplified

dis disability, disabled; disease; dislocation; distal; distance

DISC Diagnostic Interview Schedule for Children

disc discontinue

disch discharge, discharged

DISH diffuse idiopathic skeletal hyperostosis; disseminated idiopathic skeletal hyperostosis

DISI dorsal intercalated segment instability

disinfect disinfection

disl, disloc dislocation, dislocated

disod disodium

disp dispensary, dispense

diss dissolve, dissolved

dissem disseminated, dissemination

dist distal; distill, distillation, distilled; distance; distribution; disturbance, disturbed

DIT deferoxamine infusion test; diet-induced thermogenesis; diiodotyrosine; drug-induced thrombocytopenia

dit dictyate

dITP deoxyinosine triphosphate

div divergence, divergent; divide, divided, division

DIVBC disseminated intravascular blood coagulation

DIVC disseminated intravascular coagulation

DJD degenerative joint disease

DJOA dominant juvenile optic atrophy

DJS Dubin-Johnson syndrome

DK dark; decay; diabetic ketoacidosis; diet kitchen; diseased kidney; dog kidney [cells]

dk deka

DKA diabetic ketoacidosis

DKB deep knee bends

DKC dyskeratosis congenita

dkg dekagram

DKI dextrose potassium insulin

dkl decaliter

dkm dekameter

DKP dikalium phosphate

DKTC dog kidney tissue culture

DKV deer kidney virus

DL danger list; De Lee [catheter]; deep lobe; developmental level; difference limen; diffusion lung [capacity]; direct laryngoscopy; disabled list; distolingual; equimolecular mixture of the dextrorotatory and levorotatory enantiomorphs; lethal dose [Lar. *dosis lethalis*]

DL, D-L Donath-Landsteiner [antibody]

D_L diffusing capacity of the lungs

dl deciliter

DLa distolabial

DLaI distolabioincisal

DLaP distolabiopulpal

DL&B direct laryngoscopy and bronchoscopy

DLBD diffuse Lewy body disease

DLC Dental Laboratory Conference; differential leukocyte count; dual-lumen catheter

DLCO carbon monoxide diffusion in the lung; single-breath diffusing capacity

DL_{CO2} carbon dioxide diffusion in the lungs

$DL_{CO}{}^{SB}$ single-breath carbon monoxide diffusing capacity of the lungs

$DL_{CO}{}^{SS}$ steady-state carbon monoxide diffusing capacity of the lungs

DLD dihydrolipoamide dehydrogenase

DLE delayed light emission; dialyzable leukocyte extract; discoid lupus erythematosus; disseminated lupus erythematosus

D_1LE diagonal 1 lower extremity

D_2LE diagonal 2 lower extremity

DLF Disabled Living Foundation; dorsolateral funiculus

DLG distolingual groove

DLI distolinguoincisal; double label index

DLIS digoxin-like immunoreactive substance

DLL dihomo-gammalinoleic acid

DLLI dulcitol lysine lactose iron

DLMP date of last menstrual period

DLNMP date of last normal menstrual period

DLO Diploma in Laryngology and Otology; distolinguo-occlusal

D_{LO2} diffusing capacity of the lungs for oxygen

DLP delipidized serum protein; direct linear plotting; dislocation of patella; distolinguopulpal; dysharmonic luteal phase

DLR digital luminescence radiography

D/LR dextrose in lactated Ringer solution

D_5LR dextrose in 5% lactated Ringer solution

DLST dihydrolipoamide S-succinyltransferase

DLT dihydroepiandrosterone loading test; double lung transplantation; double-lumen endotracheal tube

DLTS digoxin-like immunoreactive substance

DLV defective leukemia virus

DLW dry lung weight

DM defined medium; dermatomyositis; Descemet's membrane; dextromaltose; dextromethorphan; diabetes mellitus; diabetic mother; diastolic murmur; distal metastases; dopamine; dorsomedial; double minute [chromosome]; duodenal mucosa; dry matter; dystrophia myotonica

D_M membrane component of diffusion

dm decimeter; diabetes mellitus; dorsomedial

dm^2 square decimeter

dm^3 cubic decimeter

DMA department of medical assistance; dimethylamine; dimethylaniline; dimethylarginine; direct memory access; director of medical affairs

DMAB dimethylaminobenzaldehyde

DMAC N,N-dimethylacetamide

DMAD dimethylaminodiphosphate

DMAE dimethylaminoethanol

DMAEM N,N'-dimethylaminoethyl methacrylate

DMAPN dimethylaminopropionitrile

DMARD disease-modifying anti-rheumatic drug

D_{max} maximum denaturation; maximum diameter

DMBA 7,12-dimethylbenz[a]anthracene

DMC demeclocycline; di(p-chlorophenyl)methylcarbinol; direct microscopic count; duration of muscle contraction; Dyggve-Melchior-Clausen [syndrome]

DMCC direct microscopic clump count

DMCL dimethylclomipramine

DMCT, DMCTC dimethylchlortetracycline

DMD disease-modifying drug; Doctor of Dental Medicine; Duchenne muscular dystrophy; dystonia musculorum deformans

DMDC dimethyldithiocarbamate

DMDT dimethoxydiphenyl trichloroethane

DMDZ desmethyldiazepam

DME degenerative myoclonus epilepsy; dimethyl diester; dimethyl ether; diphasic meningoencephalitis; direct medical education; director of medical education; Division of Medical Education [AAMC]; dropping mercury electrode; drug-metabolizing enzyme; Dulbecco modified Eagle [medium]; durable medical equipment

DMEM Dulbecco modified Eagle medium

DMF decayed, missing, and filled [teeth]; N,N-dimethylformamide; diphasic milk fever

DMG dimethylglycine

DMGBL dimethyl-gammabutyrolactone

DMGT deoxyribonucleic acid-mediated gene transfer

DMH diffuse mesangial hypercellularity

DMI Defense Mechanism Inventory; Diagnostic Medical Instruments; diaphragmatic myocardial infarction; direct migration inhibition

D_{min} minimum diameter

dmin double minute

DMJ Diploma in Medical Jurisprudence

DMKA diabetes mellitus ketoacidosis

DMKase deoxynucleoside monophosphate kinase

DML data manipulation language; distal motor latency

DMM dimethylmyleran; disproportionate micromelia

DMN dimethylnitrosamine; dorsal motor nucleus; dysplastic melanocytic nevus

DMNA dimethylnitrosamine

DMNL dorsomedial hypothalamic nucleus lesion

DMO 5,5-dimethyl-2,4-oxazolidinedione (dimethadione)

D_{mo2} membrane diffusing capacity for oxygen

DMOA diabetes mellitus–optic atrophy [syndrome]

DMOOC diabetes mellitus out of control

DMP diffuse mesangial proliferation; dimercaprol; dimethylphthalate

DMPA depot medroxyprogesterone acetate

DMPE, DMPEA 3,4-dimethoxyphenylethylamine

DMPP dimethylphenylpiperazinium

DMPS dysmyelopoietic syndrome

DMR depolarizing muscle relaxant; Diploma in Medical Radiology

DM-R decayed plus missing teeth, minus replaced teeth

DMRD Diploma in Medical Radio-Diagnosis

DMRE Diploma in Medical Radiology and Electrology

DMRF dorsal medullary reticular formation

DMRT Diploma in Medical Radio-Therapy

DMS delayed match-to-sample; delayed microembolism syndrome; demarcation membrane system; department of medicine and surgery; dermatomyositis; diagnostic medical sonographer; diffuse mesangial sclerosis; dimethylsulfate; dimethylsulfoxide; District Management Team; Doctor of Medical Science; dysmyelopoietic syndrome

DMSA dimercaptosuccinic acid; disodium monomethanearsonate

DMSO dimethyl sulfoxide

DMT dermatophytosis; N,N-dimethyltryptamine; Doctor of Medical Technology

DMTU dimethylthiourea

DMU dimethanolurea

DMV diurnal mood variations; Doctor of Veterinary Medicine

DMWP distal mean wave pressure

DN Deiter's nucleus; dextrose-nitrogen; diabetic neuropathy; dibucaine number; dicrotic notch; dinitrocresol; Diploma in Nursing; Diploma in Nutrition; District Nurse; Doctor of Nursing; do not [resuscitate]; duodenum

D/N dextrose/nitrogen [ratio]

D&N distance and near [vision]

Dn dekanem

dn decinem

DNA deoxyribonucleic acid; did not answer

DNAP deoxyribonucleic acid phosphorus

DNAR do not attempt resuscitation

DNASE, DNAse, DNase deoxyribonuclease

DNB dinitrobenzene; Diplomate of the National Board [of Medical Examiners]; dorsal nonadrenergic bundle

DNBP dinitrobutylphenol

DNC did not come; dinitrocarbanilide; dinitrocresol; Disaster Nursing Chairman

DNCB dinitrochlorobenzene

DNCM cytoplasmic membrane-associated deoxyribonucleic acid

DND died a natural death

DNE Director of Nursing Education; Doctor of Nursing Education

DNET dysembryoplastic neuroepithelial tumor

DNFB dinitrofluorobenzene

DNH do-not-hospitalize [order]

DNIC diffuse noxious inhibitory control

DNK did not keep [appointment]

DNKA did not keep appointment

DNLL dorsal nucleus of lateral lemniscus

DNMS Director of Naval Medical Services

DNMT deoxyribonucleic acid methyltransferase

DNO District Nursing Officer

DNOC dinitroorthocresol

DNP deoxyribonucleoprotein; dinitrophenol

DNPH dinitrophenylhydrazine

DNPM dinitrophenol-morphine

DNR daunorubicin; do not resuscitate; dorsal nerve root

DNS deviated nasal septum; diaphragmatic nerve stimulation; did not show [for appointment]; Doctor of Nursing Services; dysplastic nevus syndrome

D/NS dextrose in normal saline [solution]

D5NS 5% dextrose in normal saline [solution]

D_5NSS 5% dextrose in normal saline solution

DNT did not test

DNTM disseminated nontuberculous mycobacterial [infection]

dNTP deoxyribonucleoside triphosphate

DNTT terminal deoxynucleotidyltransferase

DNV dorsal nucleus of vagus nerve; double-normalized value

DO diamine oxidase; digoxin; Diploma in Ophthalmology; Diploma in Osteopathy; dissolved oxygen; disto-occlusal; Doctor of Ophthalmology; Doctor of Optometry; Doctor of Osteopathy; doctor's orders; drugs only

D_O oxygen diffusion

D_{O2} oxygen delivery

DOA date of admission; dead on arrival; Department of Agriculture; depth of anesthesia; differential optical absorption; dominant optic atrophy

DOAC Dubois oleic albumin complex

DOB date of birth; doctor's order book

DObstRCOG Diploma of the Royal College of Obstetricians and Gynaecologists

DOC date of conception; deoxycholate; deoxycorticosterone; died of other causes; disorders of cornification; dissolved organic carbon

doc doctor; document, documentation

DOCA deoxycorticosterone acetate

DOCG deoxycorticosterone glucoside

DOCLINE Documents On-Line

DOCS deoxycorticosteroids

DOcSc Doctor of Ocular Science

DOD date of death; dementia syndrome of depression; depth of discharge; died of disease; dissolved oxygen deficit

DOE date of examination; desoxyephedrine; direct observation evaluation; dyspnea on exertion

DOES disorders of excessive sleepiness

DOFCOSY double-quantum filtered correlated spectroscopy

DOFOS disturbance of function occlusion syndrome

DOG deoxyglucose

DOH department of health

DOHyg Diploma in Occupational Hygiene

DOI date of injury; died of injuries; diffusion of innovations [theory]

Dol dolichol

dol pain [Lat. *dolor*]

DOLLS [Lee] double-loop locking suture

DOLV double outlet left ventricle

DOM deaminated O-methyl metabolite; department of medicine; dimethoxymethylamphetamine; dissolved organic matter; dominance, dominant

dom dominant

DOMA dihydromandelic acid

DOMF 2'7'-dibromo-4'-(hydroxymercuri)fluorescein

DOMS Diploma in Ophthalmic Medicine and Surgery

DON Director of Nursing; diazooxonorleucine

DOOR deafness, onycho-osteodystrophy, mental retardation [syndrome]

DOPA, dopa dihydroxyphenylalanine

DOPAC dihydrophenylacetic acid

DOPAMINE dihydroxyphenylethylamine

dopase dihydroxyphenylalanine oxidase

DOPC determined osteogenic precursor cell

DOph Doctor of Ophthalmology

DOPP dihydroxyphenylpyruvate

DOPS diffuse obstructive pulmonary syndrome; dihydroxyphenylserine

dor dorsal

DORNA desoxyribonucleic acid

Dors dorsal

DOrth Diploma in Orthodontics; Diploma in Orthoptics

DORV double outlet right ventricle

DOS day of surgery; deoxystreptamine; disk operating system; Doctor of Ocular Science; Doctor of Optical Science

dos dosage, dose

DOSC Dubois oleic serum complex

DOSS distal over-shoulder strap; dioctyl sodium sulfosuccinate; docusate sodium

DOT date of transfer; Dictionary of Occupational Titles

DOTC Dameshek's oval target cell

DOTES dosage record and treatment emergent symptoms

DOUBTFUL double quantum transition for finding unresolved lines

Dox doxorubicin

DP data processing; deep pulse; definitive procedure; degradation product; degree of polymerization; dementia praecox; dementia pugillistica; dental prosthodontics;

dental prosthesis; desmoplakin; dexamethasone pretreatment; diastolic pressure; diffuse precipitation; diffusion pressure; diffusion pressure deficit; digestible protein; diphosgene; diphosphate; dipropionate; directional preponderance; disability pension; discrimination power; distal pancreatectomy; distal phalanx; distal pit; distopulpal; docking protein; Doctor of Pharmacy; Doctor of Podiatry; donor's plasma; dorsalis pedis
Dp duplication; dyspnea
D_p pattern difference
DPA D-penicillamine; Department of Public Assistance; diphenylalanine; dipicolinic acid; dipropylacetic acid; direct provider agreement; dual photoabsorptiometry; dynamic physical activity
DPAHC durable power of attorney for health care
DPB days post-burn; diffuse panbronchiolitis
DPBP diphenylbutylpiperidine
DPC delayed primary closure; desaturated phosphatidylcholine; diethylpyrocarbonate; direct patient care; discharge planning coordinator; distal palmar crease
DPCRT double-blind placebo-controlled randomized clinical trial
DPD Department of Public Dispensary; depression pure disease; desoxypyridoxine; diffuse pulmonary disease; diphenamid; Diploma in Public Dentistry
DPDL diffuse poorly differentiated lymphocytic lymphoma
dpdt double-pole double-throw [switch]
dP/dV pressure per unit change in volume
DPE dipiperidinoethane
DPEP dipeptidase
DPF Dental Practitioners' Formulary; dilsopropyl fluorophosphate
DPFC distal flexion palmar crease
DPFR diastolic pressure-flow relationship

DPG 2,3-diphosphoglycerate; displacement placentogram
2,3-DPG 2,3-diphosphoglycerate
2,3-DPGM 2,3-diphosphoglycerate mutase
DPGN diffuse proliferative glomerulonephritis
DPGP diphosphoglycerate phosphatase
DPH Department of Public Health; diphenhydramine; diphenylhexatriene; diphenylhydantoin; Diploma in Public Health; Doctor of Public Health; Doctor of Public Hygiene; dopamine beta-hydrolase
DPhC Doctor of Pharmaceutical Chemistry
DPhc Doctor of Pharmacology
DPHN Doctor of Public Health Nursing
DPhys Diploma in Physiotherapy
DPhysMed Diploma in Physical Medicine
DPI daily permissible intake; days post inoculation; dietary protein intake; diphtheria-pertussis immunization; disposable personal income; drug prescription index; Dynamic Personality Inventory
DPJ dementia paralytica juvenilis
DPKC diagnostic problem-knowledge coupler
DPL diagnostic peritoneal lavage; dipalmitoyl lecithin; distopulpolingual
DPLa distopulpolabial
DPLN diffuse proliferative lupus nephritis
DPM Diploma in Psychological Medicine; discontinue previous medication; Doctor of Physical Medicine; Doctor of Podiatric Medicine; Doctor of Preventive Medicine; Doctor of Psychiatric Medicine; dopamine
dpm disintegrations per minute
DPN dermatosis papulosa nigra; diabetic polyneuropathy; diphosphopyridine nucleotide; disabling pansclerotic morphea
DPNB dorsal penile nerve block

DPNH reduced diphosphopyridine nucleotide

DPO dimethoxyphenyl penicillin

DPP differential pulse polarography; dimethylphenylpenicillin; dipeptidylpeptidase

DPPC dipalmitoylphosphatidylcholine; double-blind placebo-controlled trial

DPR drug price review; dynamic perception resolution

DPS delayed primary suture; descending perineum syndrome; dimethylpolysiloxane; dysesthetic pain syndrome

dps disintegrations per second

dpst double-pole single-throw [switch]

DPT Demerol, Phenergan, and Thorazine; dermatopontin; dichotic pitch discrimination test; diphtheria-pertussis-tetanus [vaccine]; diphtheritic pseudotabes; dipropyltryptamine; dumping provocation test

Dpt house dust mite

DPTA diethylenetriamine penta-acetic acid

DPTI diastolic pressure time index

DPTPM diphtheria-pertussis-tetanus-poliomyelitis-measles [vaccine]

Dptr diopter

DPV disabling positional vertigo

DPVS Denver peritoneovenous shunt

DPW Department of Public Welfare; distal phalangeal width

DQ deterioration quotient; developmental quotient

3DQCT three-dimensional computed tomography

DQE detective quantum efficiency

DR degeneration reaction; delivery room; deoxyribose; diabetic retinopathy; diagnostic radiology; digital radiography; direct repeat; distribution ratio; doctor; dopamine receptor; dorsal raphe; dorsal root; dose ratio; drug receptor

Dr doctor

dr dorsal root; drain; dram; dressing

DRA dextran-reactive antibody

DRACOG Diploma of Royal Australian College of Obstetricians and Gynaecologists

DRACR Diploma of Royal Australasian College of Radiologists

DRAM dynamic random access memory

dr ap dram, apothecary

DRAT differential rheumatoid agglutination test

DRB daunorubicin

DRBC denaturated red blood cell; dog red blood cell; donkey red blood cell

DRC damage risk criterion; dendritic reticulum cell; diagnostic reporting console; digitorenocerebral [syndrome]; dorsal root, cervical; dynamic range compression

DRCOG Diploma of Royal College of Obstetricians and Gynaecologists

DRCPath Diploma of Royal College of Pathologists

DRD dihydroxyphenylalanine-responsive dystonia; dorsal root dilator

DRE digital rectal examination

DREF dose rate effectiveness factor

DRES dynamic random element stimuli

DRESS depth-resolved surface-coil spectroscopy

DREZ dorsal root entry zone

DRF Daily Rating Form; daily replacement factor; Deafness Research Foundation; dose reduction factor

DRG diagnosis-related group; Division of Research Grants [NIH}; dorsal respiratory group; dorsal root ganglion; duodenal-gastric reflux gastropathy

drg drainage

DrHyg Doctor of Hygiene

DRI discharge readiness inventory

dRib deoxyribose

DRID double radial immunodiffusion; double radioisotope derivative

DRIP delirium and drugs-restricted mobility and retention-infection, inflammation and impaction-polyuria [causes of urinary incontinence]

DRL dorsal root, lumbar; drug-related lupus

D5RL 5% dextrose in Ringer lactate [solution]

DRME Division of Research in Medical Education

Dr Med Doctor of Medicine

DRMS drug reaction monitoring system

DrMT Doctor of Mechanotherapy

DRN dorsal raphe nucleus

DRNDP diribonucleoside-3',3'-diphosphate

DRnt diagnostic roentgenology

DRO differential reinforcement of other behavior; Disablement Resettlement Officer

DRP digoxin reduction product; dorsal root potential; dystrophin-related protein

dRp deoxyribose-phosphate

DrPH Doctor of Public Health; Doctor of Public Hygiene

DRQ discomfort relief quotient

DRR digitally reconstructed radiograph; Division of Research Resources [NIH]; dorsal root reflex

DRS descending rectal septum; diagnostic review station; Division of Research Services [NIH]; drowsiness; Duane retraction syndrome; dynamic renal scintigraphy; Dyskinesia Rating Scale

drsg dressing

DRT dorsal root, thoracic

3-DRTP three dimensional radiation treatment planning

DRUJ distal radioulnar joint

dRVVT dilute Russell viper venom time

DS dead air space; dead space; deep sedative; deep sleep; defined substrate; dehydroepiandrosterone sulfate; delayed sensitivity; dendritic spine; density standard; dental surgery; dermatan sulfate; dermatology and syphilology; desynchronized sleep; Devic syndrome; dextran sulfate; dextrose-saline; diaphragm stimulation; diastolic murmur; differential stimulus; diffuse scleroderma; dilute strength; dioptric strength; disaster services; discrimination score; disoriented; disseminated sclerosis; dissolved solids; Doctor of Science; donor's serum; Doppler sonography; double-stranded; double strength; Down syndrome; drug store; dry swallow; dumping syndrome; duplex scan; duration of systole

D/S dextrose/saline

D&S dermatology and syphilology

D-5-S 5% dextrose in saline solution

ds double-stranded

DSA density spectral array; destructive spondyloarthropathy; digital subtraction angiography

DSACT, D-SACT direct sinoatrial conduction time

DSAP disseminated superficial actinic porokeratosis

DSAS discrete subaortic stenosis

DSB double-strand break

Dsb single-breath diffusion capacity

DSBL disabled

DSBT donor-specific blood transfusion

DSC de Sanctis-Cacchione [syndrome]; desmocollin; digital scan converter; disodium chromoglycate; Doctor of Surgical Chiropody; Down syndrome child

DSc Doctor of Science

DSCF Doppler-shifted constant frequency

DSCG disodium chromoglycate

DSCT dorsal spinocerebellar tract

DSD depression spectrum disease; discharge summary dictated; dry sterile dressing

DS-DAT Discomfort Scale for Dementia of the Alzheimer Type

DSDDT double sampling dye dilution technique

dsDNA double-stranded deoxyribonucleic acid

DSE dobutamine stress echoradiography; Doctor of Sanitary Engineering

DSG desmoglein; dry sterile gauze

DSH deliberate self harm; dexamethasone suppressible hyperaldosteronism; disproportionate share hospital

DSHR delayed skin hypersensitivity reaction

DSI deep shock insulin; Depression Status Inventory; disulfide isomerase; Down Syndrome International

DSIM Doctor of Science in Industrial Medicine

DSIP delta sleep-inducing peptide

DSL distal sensory latency

DSL M-U distal sensory latency-m-median-ulnar

dslv dissolve

DSM dextrose solution mixture; Diagnostic and Statistical Manual [of Mental Disorders]; Diploma in Social Medicine; drink skim milk

DSM-III-R Diagnostic and Statistical Manual of Mental Disorders [of APA], third edition, revised

DSM-IV Diagnostic and Statistical Manual of Mental Disorders [of APA], fourth edition

DSNI deep space neck infection

DSO digital storage oscilloscope; distal subungual onychomycosis

DSP decreased sensory perception; delayed sleep phase; desmoplakin; dibasic sodium phosphate; digital signal processor; digital subtraction phlebography

DSPC disaturated phosphatidylcholine

DSPN distal sensory polyneuropathy; distal symmetrical polyneuropathy

DSR distal spleno-renal; double simultaneous recording

dsRNA double-stranded ribonucleic acid

DSRS distal splenorenal shunt

DSS dengue shock syndrome; dioctyl sodium sulfosuccinate; Disability Status Scale; discrete subaortic stenosis; docusate sodium; double simultaneous stimulation

DSSc Diploma in Sanitary Science

DSSEP dermatomal somatosensory evoked potential

DSSI Duke social support index

DSST Digit Symbol Substitution Task

DST desensitization test; dexamethasone suppression test; dihydrostreptomycin; disproportionate septal thickening; donor-specific transfusion

DSUH directed suggestion under hypnosis

DSur Doctor of Surgery

DSVP downstream venous pressure

DSWI deep surgical wound infection

DT defibillation threshold; delirium tremens; dental technician; depression of transmission; dietetic [services]; dietetic technician; digitoxin; diphtheria-tetanus [toxoid]; discharge tomorrow; dispensing tablet; distance test; dorsalis tibialis; double tachycardia; duration of tetany; dye test

D/T date of treatment; total ratio of deaths

d/t due to

dT deoxythymidine

dt due to; dystonic

DTA differential thermal analysis; diphtheria toxin A

DTaP diphtheria-tetanus-pertussis [vaccine]

DTB dedicated time block

DTBC d-tubocurarine

DTBN di-t-butyl nitroxide

DTC day treatment center; differential thyroid carcinoma

dTc d-tubocurarine

DTCD Diploma in Tuberculosis and Chest Diseases

DTCH Diploma in Tropical Child Health

DTD diastrophic dysplasia; document type definition

DTDase deoxyuridine triphosphate diphosphohydrolase

dTDP deoxythymidine diphosphate

DTE desiccated thyroid extract

DTF detector transfer function

DTH delayed-type hypersensitivity; Diploma in Tropical Hygiene

DTI dipyridamole-thallium imaging; Doppler tissue imaging

DTIA Doppler tissue imaging acceleration

DTIC dacarbazine; dimethyltriazenyl imidazole carboxamide

DTICH delayed traumatic intracerebral hemorrhage

DTIE Doppler tissue imaging energy

D time dream time

DTIV Doppler tissue imaging velocity

DTLA Detroit Test of Learning Aptitudes

DTM dermatophyte test medium; Diploma in Tropical Medicine

DTM&H Diplomate of Tropical Medicine and Hygiene

DTMP deoxythymidine monophosphate

DTN diphtheria toxin, normal

DTNB 5,5'-dithiobis-(2-nitrobenzoic) acid

DTO deodorized tincture of opium

DTP diphtheria-tetanus-pertussis [vaccine]; distal tingling on percussion; Tinel's sign

DTPA diethylenetriaminepentaacetic acid

DTPH Diploma in Tropical Public Health

dTPM deoxythymidine monophosphate

DTR deep tendon reflex; dietetic technician registered

DTRTT digital temperature recovery time test

DTS dense tubular system; diphtheria toxin sensitivity; donor transfusion, specific

DT's delirium tremens

DTT diagnostic and therapeutic team; diphtheria tetanus toxoid; direct transverse traction; dithiothreitol

dTTP deoxythymidine triphosphate

DTUS diathermy, traction, and ultrasound

DT-VAC diphtheria-tetanus vaccine

DTVM Diploma in Tropical Veterinary Medicine

DTVMI developmental test of visual motor integration

DTVP developmental test of visual perception

DTX detoxification

DTZ diatrizoate

DU decubitus ulcer; density unknown; deoxyuridine; dermal ulcer; diagnosis undetermined; diazouracil; dog unit; duodenal ulcer; duroxide uptake; Dutch [rabbit]

dU deoxyuridine

du dial unit

DUA dorsal uterine artery

DUB dysfunctional uterine bleeding

dUDP deoxyuridine dephosphate

DUE drug use evaluation

D₁UE diagonal 1 upper extremity

D₂UE diagonal 2 upper extremity

DUF Doppler ultrasonic flowmeter; drug use forecast

DUFSS Duke-University of North Carolina Functional Social Support [questionnaire]

DUHP Duke-University Health Profile

DUI driving under the influence

DUL diffuse undifferentiated lymphoma

dulc sweet [Lat. *dulcis*]

dUMP deoxyuridine monophosphate

duod duodenum, duodenal

dup duplication

DUR drug use review; drug utilization review

dur during

DUS diagnostic ultrasonography; Doppler flow ultrasound

DUSN diffuse unilateral subacute neuroretinitis

DUSOCS Duke social support and stress scale

DUV damaging ultraviolet [radiation]

DV dependent variable; diagnostic variable; difference in volume; digital vibration; dilute volume; distemper virus; domestic violence; domiciliary visit; dorsoventral; double vibration; double vision; ductus venosus

3-DV three dimensional visualization

D&V diarrhea and vomiting

dv double vibrations

DVA developmental venous anomaly; distance visual acuity; duration of voluntary apnea; vindesine

DVB divinylbenzene

DVC divanillylcyclohexane

DVCC Disease Vector Control Center

DVD dissociated vertical deviation

DV&D Diploma in Venereology and Dermatology

dVDAVP 1-deamine-4-valine-D-arginine vasopressin

DVE duck virus enteritis

DVH Diploma in Veterinary Hygiene; Division for the Visually Handicapped; dose volume histogram

DVI deep venous insufficiency; diastolic velocity integral; digital vascular imaging; Doppler velocity index; AV sequential [pacemaker]

DVIS digital vascular imaging system

DVIU direct-vision internal urethrotomy

DVL deep vastus lateralis

DVM digital voltmeter; Doctor of Veterinary Medicine

DVMS Doctor of Veterinary Medicine and Surgery

DVN dorsal vagal nucleus

DVR digital vascular reactivity; Doctor of Veterinary Radiology; double valve replacement; double ventricular response

DVS Doctor of Veterinary Science; Doctor of Veterinary Surgery

DVSc Doctor of Veterinary Science

DVT deep venous thrombosis

DW daily weight; deionized water; dextrose in water; distilled water; doing well; dry weight

D/W dextrose in water

D5W 5% dextrose in water

D$_5$W 5% dextrose in water

D10W 10% aqueous dextrose solution

dw dwarf [mouse]

DWA died from wounds by the action of the enemy

DWD died with disease

DWDL diffuse well-differentiated lymphocytic lymphoma

DWI driving while impaired; driving while intoxicated

DWM Dandy-Walker malformation

DWS Dandy-Walker syndrome; disaster warning system

DWT dichotic word test; discrete wave transform

dwt pennyweight

DX dextran; dicloxacillin

Dx, dx diagnosis

DXA dual-energy x-ray absorptiometry

DXD discontinued

DXM dexamethasone

DXP digital x-ray prototype

DxPLAIN Massachusetts General Hospital's expert diagnostic system

DXPNET Digital X-Ray Prototype Network

DXR deep x-ray

DXRT deep x-ray therapy

DXT deep x-ray therapy; dextrose

dXTP deoxyxanthine triphosphate

DY dense parenchyma

Dy dysprosium

dy dystrophia muscularis [mouse]

dyn dynamic; dynamometer; dyne

DYS dysautonomia

dysp dyspnea

DZ diazepam; dizygotic; dizziness

dZ impedance change

dz disease; dozen

DZM dorsal zone of membranelle

DZP diazepam

E air dose; cortisone [compound E]; each; eating; edema; elastance; electric charge; electric field vector; electrode potential; electromotive force; electron; embryo; emmetropia; encephalitis; endangered [animal]; endogenous; endoplasm; enema; energy; *Entamoeba*; enterococcus; enzyme; eosinophil; epicondyle; epinephrine; error; erythrocyte; erythroid; erythromycin; *Escherichia;* esophagus; ester; estradiol; ethanol; ethyl; examination; exhalation; expectancy [wave]; expected frequency in a cell of a contingency table; experiment, experimenter; expiration; expired air; exposure; extract, extracted, extraction; extraction fraction; extralymphatic; eye; glutamic acid; internal energy; kinetic energy; mathematical expectation; redox potential; stereodescriptor to indicate the configuration at a double bond [Ger. *entgegen* opposite]; unit [Ger. *Einheit*]

E* lesion on the erythrocyte cell membrane at the site of complement fixation

$\bar{E}$ average beta energy

E_0 electric affinity

E_1 estrone

E_2 17β-estradiol

E_3 estriol

E_4 estetrol

4E four-plus edema

E° standard electrode potential

e base of natural logarithms, approximately 2.7182818285; egg transfer; ejection; electric charge; electron; elementary charge; exchange

e^- negative electron

e^+ positron

ε see *epsilon*

η see *eta*

EA early antigen; educational age; egg albumin; electric affinity; electrical activity; electroacupuncture; electroanesthesia; electrophysiological abnormality; embryonic antibody; endocardiographic amplifier; Endometriosis Association; enteral alimentation; enteroanastomosis; enzymatically active; epiandrosterone; erythrocyte antibody; erythrocyte antiserum; esophageal atresia; estivo-autumnal; ethacrynic acid

E/A emergency admission

E&A evaluate and advise

ea each

Eα kinetic energy of alpha particles

EAA electroacupuncture analgesia; Epilepsy Association of America; essential amino acid; excitatory amino acid; extrinsic allergic alveolitis

EAAC excitatory amino acid carrier

EAB elective abortion; Ethics Advisory Board

EABV effective arterial blood volume

EAC Ehrlich ascites carcinoma; electroacupuncture; epithelioma adenoides cysticum; erythema annulare centrifugum; erythrocyte, antibody, complement; external auditory canal

EACA epsilon-aminocaproic acid

EACD eczematous allergic contact dermatitis

EACH essential access community hospital

EAD early afterdepolarization; extracranial arterial disease

EA-D early antigen, diffuse

E-ADD epileptic attentional deficit disorder

EADS early amnion deficit spectrum or syndrome

EAE experimental allergic encephalomyelitis; experimental autoimmune encephalitis

EAEC enteroadherent *Escherichia coli*

EAG electroarteriography

EAHF eczema, asthma, and hay fever

EAHLG equine antihuman lymphoblast globulin

EAHLS equine antihuman lymphoblast serum

EAI Emphysema Anonymous, Inc.; erythrocyte antibody inhibition

EAK ethyl amyl ketone

EAM episodic ataxia with myokymia; external acoustic meatus

EAMG experimental autoimmune myasthenia gravis

EAN experimental allergic neuritis

EAO experimental allergic orchiitis

EAP electric acupuncture; employee assistance program; epiallopregnanolone; Epstein-Barr associated protein; erythrocyte acid phosphatase; evoked action potential

EAQ eudismic affinity quotient

EAR European Association of Radiology

EA-R early antigen, restricted

Ea R reaction of degeneration [Ger. *Entartungs-Reaktion*]

EARR extended aortic root replacement

EASI European applications in surgical interventions

EAST elevated-arm stress test; Emory angioplasty vs. surgery trial; external rotation, abduction stress test

EAT Eating Attitudes Test; Ehrlich ascites tumor; electro-aerosol therapy; epidermolysis acuta toxica; experimental autoimmune thymitis; experimental autoimmune thyroiditis

EATC Ehrlich ascites tumor cell

EAV equine abortion virus

EAVC enhanced atrioventricular conduction

EAVM extramedullary arteriovenous malformation

EAVN enhanced atrioventricular nodal [conduction]

EB elective abortion; electron beam; elementary body; emotional behavior; endometrial biopsy; epidermolysis bullosa; Epstein-Barr [virus]; esophageal body; estradiol benzoate; Evans blue

EBA epidermolysis bullosa acquisita; epidermolysis bullosa atrophicans; orthoethoxybenzoic acid

EBC esophageal balloon catheter

EBCDIC Extended Binary Coded Decimal Interchange Code

EBCT electron-beam computed tomography

EBD epidermolysis bullosa dystrophica

EBDCT Cockayne-Touraine type of epidermolysis bullosa dystrophica

EBDD epidermolysis bullosa dystrophica dominant

EBDR epidermolysis bullosa dystrophica recessiva

EBF erythroblastosis fetalis

EBG electroblepharogram, electroblepharography

EBI emetine bismuth iodide; erythroblastic island; estradiol binding index

EB-IORT intraoperative electron beam boost

EBK embryonic bovine kidney

EBL erythroblastic leukemia; estimated blood loss

eBL endemic Burkitt lymphoma

EBL/S estimated blood loss during surgery

EBM electrophysiologic behavior modification; epidermal basement membrane; evidence-based medicine; expressed breast milk

EBMWG evidence-based medicine working group

EBNA Epstein-Barr virus-associated nuclear antigen

EBO Ebola [disease or virus]

E/BOD electrolyte biochemical oxygen demand

EBO-R Ebola Reston virus

EBP estradiol-binding protein

EBRT electron beam radiotherapy; external beam radiation therapy

EBS elastic back strap; electric brain stimulation; Emergency Bed Service; epidermolysis bullosa simplex

EBSS Earle's balanced salt solution

EBT electron beam tomography; external beam therapy

EBV effective blood volume; Epstein-Barr virus; estimated blood volume

EBv Epstein-Barr virus

EBVS Epstein-Barr virus susceptibility

EBZ epidermal basement zone

EC effective concentration; ejection click; electrochemical; electron capture; embryonal carcinoma; emergency center; endemic cretinism; endocrine cells; endothelial cell; energy charge; enteric coating; entering complaint; enterochromaffin; entorhinal cortex; Enzyme Commission; epidermal cell; epithelial cell; equalization-cancellation; error correction; *Escherichia coli*; esophageal carcinoma; excitation-contraction; experimental control; expiratory center; extended care; external carotid [artery]; external conjugate; extracellular; extracellular concentration; extracorporeal; extracranial; eye care; eyes closed

E-C ether-chloroform [mixture]

E/C endocystoscopy; enteric-coated; estrogen/creatinine ratio

Ec ectoconchion

EC$_{50}$ median effective concentration

ECA electrical control activity; electrocardioanalyzer; endothelial cytotoxic activity; enterobacterial common antigen; epidemiological catchment area; esophageal carcinoma; ethacrynic acid; ethylcarboxylate adenosine; external carotid artery

E-CABG endarterectomy and coronary artery bypass graft

ECAO enteric cytopathogenic avian orphan [virus]

ECAQ elderly cognitive assessment questionnaire

ECBD exploration of common bile duct

ECBO enteric cytopathogenic bovine orphan [virus]

ECBV effective circulating blood volume

ECC electrocorticogram, electrocorticography; electronic claim capture; embryonal cell carcinoma; emergency cardiac care; emergency care center; endocervical cone; endocervical curettage; estimated creatinine clearance; external cardiac compression; extracorporeal circulation

ECCE extracapsular cataract extraction

ECCLS European Committee for Clinical Laboratory Standards

ECCO enteric cytopathogenic cat orphan [virus]

ECCO$_2$R extracorporeal carbon dioxide removal

ECD ectrodactyly; electrochemical detector; electron capture detector; endocardial cushion defect; enzymatic cell dispersion; ethylcysteinate dimer

ECDO enteric cytopathic dog orphan [virus]

ECE equine conjugated estrogen

ECEO enteric cytopathogenic equine orphan [virus]

ECETOC European Centre for Ecotoxicity and Toxicology of Chemicals

ECF effective capillary flow; eosinophilic chemotactic factor; erythroid colony formation; extended care facility; extracellular fluid

ECFA, ECF-A eosinophilic chemotactic factor of anaphylaxis

ECFC eosinophilic chemotactic factor complement

ECFMG Educational Commission on Foreign Medical Graduates; Educational Council for Foreign Medical Graduates

ECFMS Educational Council for Foreign Medical Students

ECFV extracellular fluid volume

ECFVD extracellular fluid volume depletion

ECG electrocardiogram, electrocardiography

ECGF endothelial cell growth factor

ECGS endothelial cell growth supplement

ECH educator contact hour

ECHO echocardiography; enteric cytopathic human orphan [virus]; Etoposide, cyclophosphamide, Adriamycin, and vincristine

EchoCG echocardiography

Echo-Eg echoencephalography

Echo-VM echoventriculometry

ECHSCP Exeter Community Health Services Computer Project

ECI electrocerebral inactivity; eosinophilic cytoplasmic inclusions; extracorporeal irradiation

ECIB extracorporeal irradiation of blood

EC-IC extracranial-intracranial

ECIL extracorporeal irradiation of lymph

ECIS equipment control information system

ECK extracellular potassium

ECL emitter-coupled logic; enterochromaffin-like [type]; euglobin clot lysis

ECLT euglobulin clot lysis time

ECM electronic claims management; embryonic chick muscle; erythema chronicum migrans; experimental cerebral malaria; external cardiac massage; extracellular material; extracellular matrix

ECMO enteric cytopathic monkey orphan [virus]; extracorporeal membrane oxygenation

ECN equipment control number

E co *Escherichia coli*

ECochG electrocochleography

ECOG Eastern Cooperative Oncology Group

ECoG electrocorticogram, electrocorticography

E COLI eight nerve action potential, cochlear nucleus, olivary complex (superior), lateral lemniscus, inferior colliculus [hearing test]

E coli *Escherichia coli*

ECP ectrodactyly-cleft palate [syndrome]; effector cell precursor; endocardial potential; eosinophil cationic protein; erythrocyte coproporphyrin; erythroid committed precursor; *Escherichia coli* polypeptide; estradiol cyclopentane propionate; external cardiac pressure; external counterpulsation; free cytoporphyrin of erythrocytes

ECPO enteric cytopathic porcine orphan [virus]

ECPOG electrochemical potential gradient

ECPR external cardiopulmonary resuscitation

ECR effectiveness-cost ratio; electrocardiographic response; emergency care research; emergency chemical restraint; European Congress of Radiology

ECRB extensor carpi radialis brevis

ECRI Emergency Care Research Institute

ECRL extensor carpi radialis longus

ECRO enteric cytopathogenic rodent orphan [virus]

ECR-SCSI European Committee for Recommendation-Standard on Computer Aspects of Diagnostic Imaging

ECS elective cosmetic surgery; electrocerebral silence; electroconvulsive shock, electroshock; endocervical swab; extracellular space

ECSO enteric cytopathic swine orphan [virus]

ECSP epidermal cell surface protein

ECST European carotid surgery trial

ECT electroconvulsive therapy; emission computed tomography; enteric coated tablet; euglobulin clot test; European compression technique

ect ectopic, ectopy

ECTA esophageal gastric tube airway; Everyman's Contingency Table Analysis

ECU environmental control unit; extended care unit; extensor carpi ulnaris

ECV epithelial cell vacuolization; extracellular volume; extracorporeal volume

ECVAM European Centre for the Validation of Alternative Methods

ECVD extracellular volume of distribution

ECW extracellular water

ED early-decision [applicant]; early differentiation; ectodermal dysplasia; ectopic depolarization; effective dose; Ehlers-Danlos [syndrome]; elbow disarticulation; electrodialysis; electron diffraction; embryonic death; emergency department; emotional disorder, emotionally disturbed; end-diastole; entering diagnosis; Entner-Doudoroff [pathway]; enzyme deficiency; epidural; epileptiform discharge; equine dermis [cells]; erythema dose; ethyl dichlorarsine; ethynodiol; evidence of disease; exertional dyspnea; extensive disease; extensor digitorum; external diameter; extra-low dispersion

E-D ego-defense; Ehlers-Danlos [syndrome]

ED$_{50}$ median effective dose

E$_d$ depth dose

ed edema

EDA electrodermal activity; electrodermal audiometry; electrolyte-deficient agar; electron donor acceptor

EDAM electron-dense amorphous material

EDAX energy dispersive x-ray analysis

EDB early dry breakfast; electron-dense body; extensor digitorum brevis

EDBP erect diastolic blood pressure

EDC emergency decontamination center; end-diastolic count; estimated date of conception; expected date of confinement; expected delivery, cesarean; extensor digitorum communis

ED&C electrodesiccation and curettage

EDCF endothelium-derived contracting factor

EDCI energetic dynamic cardiac insufficiency

EDCS end-diastolic chamber stiffness; end-diastolic circumferential stress

EDD effective drug duration; electron dense deposit; end-diastolic dimension; esophageal detection device; estimated due date; expected date of delivery

EDDA expanded duty dental auxiliary

EDDS electronic development delivery system

EDE effective dose equivalent

edent edentia, edentulous

EDF eosinophil differentiation factor; erythroid differentiation factor; extradural fluid

EDG electrodermography

EDH epidural hematoma

EDI eating disorder inventory; electronic data interchange

EDIM epizootic diarrhea of infant mice

E-diol estradiol

EDL end-diastolic length; end-diastolic load; estimated date of labor; extensor digitorum longus

ED/LD emotionally disturbed and learning disabled

ED LOS emergency department length of stay

EDM early diastolic murmur; extramucosal duodenal myotomy

EDMA ethylene glycol dimethacrylate

EDMD Emery-Dreifuss muscular dystrophy

EDN electrodesiccation; eosinophil-derived neurotoxin

EDNA Emergency Department Nurses Association

EDNF endogenous digitalis-like natriuretic factor

EDOC estimated date of confinement

EDP electron dense particle; electronic data processing; end-diastolic pressure

EDQ extensor digiti quinti

EDR early diastolic relaxation; effective direct radiation; electrodermal response

EDRF endothelium-derived relaxing factor

EDS edema disease of swine; egg drop syndrome; Ehlers-Danlos syndrome; Emery-Dreifus syndrome; energy-dispersive spectrometry; epigastric distress syndrome; excessive daytime sleepiness; extradimensional shift

EDSR electronic document storage and retrieval

EDSS expanded disability status scale

EDT end-diastolic thickness; erythrocyte density test

EDTA ethylenediamine tetraacetic acid

EDTR emergency department-based trauma response

Educ education

EDV end-diastolic volume; epidermodysplasia verruciformis

EDVI end-diastolic volume index

EDVX X-linked epidermodysplasia verruciformis

EDWTH end-diastolic wall thickness

EDX, EDx electrodiagnosis

EDXA energy-dispersive x-ray analysis

EE embryo extract; end-to-end; end expiration; energy expenditure; *Enterobacteriaceae* enrichment [broth]; equine encephalitis; ethinyl estradiol; expressed emotion; external ear; eye and ear

E&E eye and ear

E-E erythema-edema [reaction]

EEA electroencephalic audiometry; end-to-end anastomosis

EEC ectrodactyly–ectodermal dysplasia–clefting [syndrome]; enteropathogenic *Escherichia coli*

EECD endothelial-epithelial corneal dystrophy

EECG electroencephalography

EEE eastern equine encephalitis; eastern equine encephalomyelitis; experimental enterococcal endocarditis; external eye examination

EEEP end-expiratory esophageal pressure

EEEV eastern equine encephalomyelitis virus

EEG electroencephalogram, electroencephalography

EEGA electroencephalographic audiometry

EEG-CSA electroencephalography with computerized spectral analysis

EEGL low-voltage electroencephalography

EEGV1 electroencephalographic variant pattern 1

EELS electron energy loss spectroscopy

EEM ectodermal dysplasia, ectrodactyly, macular dystrophy [syndrome]; erythema exudativum multiforme

EEME, EE3ME ethinylestradiol-3-methyl ether

EEMG evoked electromyogram

EENT eye, ear, nose, and throat

EEP end-expiratory pressure; equivalent effective photon

EEPI extraretinal eye position information

EER electroencephalographic response

EES erythromycin ethylsuccinate; ethyl ethanesulfate

EESG evoked electrospinogram

EF ectopic focus; edema factor; ejection fraction; elastic fibril; electric field; elongation factor; embryo-fetal; embryo fibroblasts; emergency facility; encephalitogenic factor; endothoracic fascia; endurance factor; eosinophilic fasciitis; epithelial focus; equivalent focus; erythroblastosis fetalis; erythrocyte fragmentation; exposure factor; extrafine; extended field [radiotherapy]; extrinsic factor

EFA Epilepsy Foundation of America; essential fatty acid; extrafamily adoptee

EFAD essential fatty acid deficiency

EFAS embryofetal alcohol syndrome

EFC elastin fragment concentration; endogenous fecal calcium; ephemeral fever of cattle

EFD estimated fluid deficit

EFDA expanded function dental assistant

EFE endocardial fibroelastosis

EFF electromagnetic field focusing

eff effect; efferent; efficiency; effusion

effect effective

effer efferent

EFFU epithelial focus-forming unit

EFH explosive follicular hyperplasia

EFL effective focal length

EFM elderly fibromyalgia; electronic fetal monitoring; external fetal monitor

EFP early follicular phase; effective filtration pressure; endoneural fluid pressure

EFR effective filtration rate

EFS electric field stimulation; event-free survival

EFT Embedded Figures Test

EFV extracellular fluid volume

EFVC expiratory flow-volume curve

EFW estimated fetal weight

EG enteroglucagon; eosinophilic granuloma; esophagogastrectomy; ethylene glycol; external genitalia

eg for example [Lat. *exempli gratia*]

EGA estimated gestational age

EGBUS external genitalia, Bartholin, urethral, Skene glands

EGC early gastric cancer; epithelioid-globoid cell

EGD esophagogastroduodenoscopy

EGDF embryonic growth and development factor

EGF epidermal growth factor

EGFR, EGF-R epidermal growth factor receptor

EGF-URO epidermal growth factor, urogastrone

EGG electrogastrogram

EGH equine growth hormone

EGL eosinophilic granuloma of the lung

EGLT euglobin lysis time

EGM electrogram; extracellular granular material

EGME ethylene glycol monomethyl ether

EGN experimental glomerulonephritis

EGOT erythrocytic glutamic oxaloacetic transaminase

EGR early growth response; erythema gyratum repens

E-GR erythrocyte glutathione reductase

EGRA equilibrium-gated radionuclide angiography

EGRAC erythrocyte glutathione reductase activity coefficient

EGS electrogalvanic stimulation; electron gamma-shower; external guide sequence

EGT ethanol gelation test

EGTA esophageal gastric tube airway; ethyleneglycol-bis-(β-aminoethylether)-N,N,N',N'-tetraacetic acid

EH enlarged heart; external hyperalimentation; epidermolytic hyperkeratosis; epoxide hydratase; essential hypertension

E/H environment and heredity

E&H environment and heredity

E$_h$ redox potential

eh enlarged heart

EHA Emotional Health Anonymous; Environmental Health Agency

EHAA epidemic hepatitis-associated antigen

EHB elevate head of bed

EHBA extrahepatic biliary atresia

EHBD extrahepatic bile duct

EHBF estimated hepatic blood flow; exercise hyperemia blood flow; extrahepatic blood flow

EHC enterohepatic circulation; enterohepatic clearance; essential hypercholesterolemia; ethylhydrocupreine hydrochloride; extended health care; extrahepatic cholestasis

EHD electrohemodynamics; epizootic hemorrhagic disease

EHDP ethane-1-hydroxy-1,1-diphosphate

EHDV epizootic hemorrhagic disease virus

EHEC enterohemorrhagic *Escherichia coli*

EHF epidemic hemorrhagic fever; exophthalmos-hyperthyroid factor; extreme high frequency

EHG electrohysterogram, electrohysterography

EHH esophageal hiatal hernia

EHI employer's health insurance

EHK epidermolytic hyperkeratosis

EHL effective half-life; electrohydraulic lipotripsy; endogenous hyperlipidemia; Environmental Health Laboratory; essential hyperlipemia; extensor hallucis longus

EHME employee health maintenance examination

EHMS electrohemodynamic ionization mass spectometry

EHNA 9-erythro-2-(hydroxy-3-nonyl) adenine

EHO extrahepatic obstruction

EHP di-(20-ethylhexyl) hydrogen phosphate; Environmental Health Perspectives; excessive heat production; extrahigh potency

EHPAC Emergency Health Preparedness Advisory Committee

EHPH extrahepatic portal hypertension

EHPT Eddy hot plate test

EHQ Eating Habits Questionnaire

EHSDS experimental health services delivery system

EHT electrohydrothermoelectrode; essential hypertension

EHV electric heart vector; equine herpes virus

EI Edmonton injector; electrolyte imbalance; electron impact; electron ionization; emotionally impaired; energy index; enzyme inhibitor; eosinophilic index; Evans index; excretory index

E/I expiration/inspiration [ratio]

EIA electroimmunoassay; enzyme immunoassay; enzyme-linked immunosorbent assay; equine infectious anemia; erythroimmunoassay; exercise-induced asthma; an interface between a computer and a system for transmitting digital information

EIAB extracranial-intracranial arterial bypass

EIAV equine infectious anemia virus

EIB electrophoretic immunoblotting; exercise-induced bronchospasm

EIC elastase inhibition capacity; enzyme inhibition complex

EID egg infectious dose; electroimmunodiffusion; emergency infusion device

EIEC enteroinvasive *Escherichia coli*

EIEE early infantile epileptic encephalopathy

EIF erythrocyte initiation factor; eukaryotic initiation factor

eIF erythrocyte initiation factor

EIM excitability-inducing material

EIMS electron ionization mass spectrometry

EINECS European Inventory of Existing Commercial Chemical Substances

EIP end-expiratory pause; extensor indicis proprius

EIPS endogenous inhibitor of prostaglandin synthase

eIPV enhanced inactivated polio vaccine

EIRnv extra incidence rate of non-vaccinated groups

EIRP effective isotropic radiated power

EIRv extra incidence in vaccinated groups

EIS Environmental Impact Statement; Epidemic Intelligence Service

EIT electrical impedance tomography; erythroid iron turnover

EIV external iliac vein

EIVA equine infectious anemia virus

EJ elbow jerk; external jugular

EJB ectopic junctional beat

EJP excitation junction potential
EJV external jugular vein
EK enterokinase; erythrokinase
EKC epidemic keratoconjunctivitis
EKG electrocardiogram, electrocardiography
EKS epidemic Kaposi sarcoma
EKV erythrokeratodermia variabilis
EKY electrokymogram, electrokymography
EL early latent; elbow; electroluminescence; erythroleukemia; exercise limit; external lamina
El elastase
el elixir
ELA elastase; elastomer-lubricating agent; endotoxin-like activity
ELAM endothelial leukocyte adhesion molecule
ELAS extended lymphadenopathy syndrome
ELB early light breakfast; elbow
elb elbow
ELBW extremely low birth weight
ELD egg lethal dose
elec electricity, electric
elect elective; electuary
ELECTZ electrosurgical loop excision of the cervical transformation zone
ELEM equine leukoencephalomalacia
elem elementary
elev elevation, elevated, elevator
ELF elective low forceps; extremely low frequency
ELH egg-laying hormone
ELI exercise lability index
ELIA enzyme-linked immunoassay
ELICT enzyme-linked immunocytochemical technique
ELIEDA enzyme-linked immunoelectron diffusion assay
ELIRA enzyme-linked immunoreceptor assay
ELISA enzyme-linked immunosorbent assay

elix elixir
ELM external limiting membrane; extravascular lung mass
ELN elastin; electronic noise
ELND elective lymph node dissection
ELOP estimated length of program
ELOS estimated length of stay
ELP elastase-like protein; endogenous limbic potential
ELS Eaton-Lambert syndrome; electron loss spectroscopy; extended least square; extracorporeal life support; extralobar sequestration
ELSI ethical, legal, and social issues
ELSO Extracorporeal Life Support Organization
ELSS emergency life support system
ELT endless loop tachycardia; euglobulin lysis time
ELV erythroid leukemia virus
elx elixir
EM early memory; ejection murmur; electromagnetic; electron micrograph; electron microscopy, electron microscope; electrophoretic mobility; Embden-Meyerhof [pathway]; emergency medicine; emmetropia; emotional disorder, emotionally disturbed; ergonovine maleate; erythema migrans; erythema multiforme; erythrocyte mass; erythromycin; esophageal manometry; esophageal motility; extracellular matrix
E/M electron microscope, electron microscopy; evaluation and management
E&M endocrine and metabolic
Em emmetropia
E_m mid-point redox potential
EMA electronic microanalyzer; emergency medical assistance, emergency medical assistant; endothelial monocyte antigen; epithelial membrane antigen
EMAB endothelial monocyte antigen B
EMAP evoked muscle action potential
EMB embryology; endomyocardial biopsy; engineering in medicine and biology;

eosin-methylene blue; ethambutol; explosive mental behavior

emb embolism; embryo; embryology

EMBASE Excerpta Medica Database

EMBL European Molecular Biology Laboratory

EMBO European Molecular Biology Organization

embryol embryology

EMC electromagnetic compatibility; electron microscopy; emergency medical care; emergency medical coordinator; encephalomyocarditis; essential mixed cryoglobulinemia

EMC&R emergency medical care and rescue

EMCRO Experimental Medical Care Review Organization

EMCV encephalomyocarditis virus

EMD electromechanical dissociation; emergency medical dispacher; emergency medical doctor; Emery-Dreifuss muscular dystrophy; esophageal mobility disorder

EMEM Eagle minimal essential medium

EMER electromagnetic molecular electron resonance

emer emergency

EMF electromagnetic flowmeter; electromotive force; Emergency Medicine Foundation; endomyocardial fibrosis; erythrocyte maturation factor; evaporated milk formula

emf electromotive force

EMG electromyogram, electromyography; eye movement gauge; exomphalos-macroglossia-gigantism [syndrome]

EMGN extramembranous glomerulonephritis

EMG/NCV electromyography/nerve conduction velocity [test]

EMI electromagnetic interference; emergency medical information

EMIC emergency maternal and infant care; Environmental Mutagen Information Center

EMICBACK Environmental Mutagen Information Center Backfile

EMIT enzyme multiplied immunoassay technique

EMJH Ellinghausen-McCullough-Johnson-Harris [medium]

EML erythema nodosum leprosum

EMLA eutectic mixture of local anesthetics

EMM erythema multiforme major

EMMA eye movement measuring apparatus

EMO Epstein-Macintosh-Oxford [inhaler]; exophthalmos, myxedema circumscriptum praetibiale, and osteoarthropathia hypertrophicans [syndrome]

emot emotion, emotional

EMP electric membrane property; electromagnetic pulse; Embden-Meyerhof pathway; external membrane potential or protein; extramedullary plasmacytoma; malignant proliferation of eosinophils

EMPS exertional muscle pain syndrome

EMR educable mentally retarded; electromagnetic radiation; electronic medical record; emergency mechanical restraint; emergency medicine resident; essential metabolism ratio; eye movement record

EMRA Emergency Medicine Residents Association

EMRC European Medical Research Council

EMRD emergency medicine residency director

EMRS electronic medical record system

EMS early morning specimen; early morning stiffness; electrical muscle stimulation; Electronic Medical Service; emergency medical services; endometriosis; eosinophilia myalagia syndrome; ethyl methane-sulfonate

EMSA electrophoretic mobility shift assay

EMSS emergency medical services system

EMT emergency medical tag; emergency medical team; emergency medical technician; emergency medical treatment; endocardial mapping technique

EMTA endomethylene tetrahydrophthalic acid

EMT-A emergency medical technician-ambulance; emergency medical technician providing basic life support or cardiopulmonary resuscitation

EMTALA Emergency Medical Treatment and Active Labor Act

EMT-B basic emergency medical technician

EMT-D emergency medical technician providing basic life support or defibrillation

EMT-I emergency medical technician-intermediate

EMT-M or **EMT-MAST** emergency medical technician–military antishock trousers

EMT-P emergency medical technician-paramedic

EMT-W emergency medical technician-wilderness

EMU early morning urine; energy-mode ultrasound

emu electromagnetic unit

emul emulsion

EMV eye, motor, voice [Glasgow coma scale]

EMVC early mitral valve closure

EN endoscopy; enrolled nurse; enteral nutrition; epidemic nephritis; erythema nodosum

En, en enema

ENA epithelial neutrophil-activating [protein]; extractable nuclear antigen

ENC environmental control

END early neonatal death; endocrinology; endorphin; endothelin

end endoreduplication

Endo endocardial, endocardium; endocrine, endocrinology; endodontics; endotracheal

endo endoscopy

ENDOR electron nuclear double resonance

ENDR endothelin receptor

ENDRB endothelin receptor B

ENE ethylnorepinephrine

ENeG electroneurography

enem enema

ENG electronystagmogram, electronystagmography

Eng English

ENI elective neck irradiation

ENK enkephalin

ENL erythema nodosum leproticum

ENO, Eno enolase

ENOG, ENoG electroneuronography

ENP electromagnetic pulse; ethyl-p-nitrophenylthiobenzene phosphate; excellence for nursing practice; extractable nucleoprotein

ENR eosinophilic nonallergic rhinitis; extrathyroid neck radioactivity

ENS enteral nutritional support; ethylnorsuprarenin

ENT ear, nose, and throat; enzootic nasal tumor; extranodular tissue

ent enterotoxin

ent A enterotoxin A

Entom entomology

ENU N-ethyl–nitrosourea

env, environ environment, environmental

ENX endonexin

enz enzyme, enzymatic

EO eosinophil; ethylene oxide; eyes open

E_o skin dose

EOA effective orifice area; erosive osteoarthritis; esophageal obturator airway; examination, opinion, and advice

EOB emergency observation bed; explanation of benefits

EOCA early onset cerebellar ataxia

EOD entry on duty; every other day
EOF end of file
E of M error of measurement
EOG electro-oculogram, electro-oculography; electro-olfactogram, electro-olfactography
EOGBS early onset group B streptococcal [infection]
EOJ extrahepatic obstructive jaundice
EOL end of life
EOM end of message; equal ocular movement; external otitis media; extraocular movement; extraocular muscle
EOMA emergency oxygen mask assembly
EOMB explanation of Medicare benefits
EOMI extraocular muscles intact
EOM NL extraocular eye movements normal
EOP efficiency of plating; emergency outpatient
EOR European Organization for Research; exclusive operating room
EORTC European Organization for Research and Treatment of Cancer
EOS end of study; eosinophil; European Orthodontic Society
eos, eosin eosinophil
Eosm effective osmolarity
EOT effective oxygen transport
EOU epidemic observation unit
EP echo planar; ectopic pregnancy; edible portion; electrophoresis; electrophysiologic; electroprecipitin; emergency physician; emergency procedure; endogenous pyrogen; endoperoxide; endorphin; end point; enteropeptidase; environmental protection; enzyme product; eosinophilic pneumonia; epicardial electrogram; epirubicin; epithelium, epithelial; epoxide; erythrocyte protoporphyrin; erythrophagocytosis; erythropoietic porphyria; erythropoietin; esophageal pressure; evoked potential; extramustine phosphate; extreme pressure

EPA eicosapentaenoic acid; empiric phrase association; Environmental Protection Agency; erect posterior-anterior; erythroid potentiating activity; extrinsic plasminogen activator
EPAP expiratory positive airway pressure
EPAQ Extended Personal Attitudes Questionnaire
EPA/RCRA Environmental Protection Agency Resource Conservation and Recovery Act
EPB extensor pollicis brevis
EPC end-plate current; epilepsia partialis continua; external pneumatic compression
EPCA external pressure circulatory assistance
EPCG endoscopic pancreatocholangiography
EPCS emergency portocaval shunt
EPDML epidemiology, epidemiologic
EPE erythropoietin-producing enzyme
EPEC enteropathogenic *Escherichia coli*
EPEG etoposide
EPF early pregnancy factor; endocarditis parietalis fibroplastica; endothelial proliferating factor; established program financing; estrogenic positive feedback; exophthalmos-producing factor
EPG eggs per gram [count]; electropneumography, electropneumogram; ethanolamine phosphoglyceride
EPH edema-proteinuria-hypertension; episodic paroxysmal hemicrania; extensor proprius hallucis
EPI echo planar imaging; electronic portal imaging; Emotion Profile Index; epilepsy; epinephrine; epithelium, epithelial; Estes Park Institute; evoked potential index; Expanded Programme of Immunization (WHO); extrapyramidal involvement; extrinsic pathway inhibitor
EPID electronic portal imaging device
epid epidemic
epil epilepsy, epileptic

epineph epinephrine

epis episiotomy

EPI/STAR echo planar imaging with signal targeting and alternating radiofrequency

epith epithelium

EPL effective patient's life; equivalent path length; essential phospholipid; extensor pollicis longus; extracorporeal piezoelectric lithotriptor

EPM electron probe microanalysis; electrophoretic mobility; energy-protein malnutrition

EPN O-ethyl O-p-nitrophenylphosphonothionate

EPO eosinophil peroxidase; erythropoiesis; erythropoietin; evening primrose-oil; exclusive provider organization; expiratory port occlusion

EPOB employee per occupied bed

EPOR erythropoietin receptor

EPP end-plate potential; equal pressure point; erythropoietic protoporphyria

epp end-plate potential

EPPB end positive-pressure breathing

EPPS Edwards Personal Preference Schedule

EPQ Eysenck Personality Questionnaire

EPR early progressive resistance; electron paramagnetic resonance; electronic patient record; electrophrenic respiration; emergency physical restraint; estradiol production rate; extraparenchymal resistance

EPROM erasable programmable read-only memory

EPS ear-patella-short stature [syndrome]; elastosis perforans serpiginosa; electrophysiologic study; enzyme pancreatic secretion; exophthalmos-producing substance; extracellular polysaccharide; extrapyramidal symptom, extrapyramidal syndrome

ep's epithelial cells

EPSC excitatory postsynaptic current

EPSDT early and periodic screening diagnosis and treatment program

EPSE extrapyramidal side effects

EPSEM equal probability of selection method

EPSI echo planar spectroscopic imaging

ε Greek letter *epsilon*; heavy chain of IgE; permittivity; specific absorptivity

EPSP excitatory postsynaptic potential

EPSS E-point septal separation

EPT early pregnancy test

EPTE existed prior to enlistment

EPTFE expanded polytetrafluoroethylene

EPTS existed prior to service

EPV encephaloclastic proliferative vasculopathy; entomopoxvirus

EPXMA electron probe x-ray microanalyzer

EQ educational quotient; encephalization quotient; energy quotient; equal to

Eq, eq equation; equivalent

EQA external quality assessment

EQAM Ervin quality assessment measure

equip equipment

equiv equivalency, equivalent

ER efficiency ratio; epigastric region; ejection rate; electroresection; emergency room; endoplasmic reticulum; enhanced reactivation; enhancement ratio; environmental resistance; equine rhinopneumonia; equivalent roentgen [unit]; erythrocyte receptor; estradiol receptor; estrogen receptor; etretinate; evoked response; expiratory reserve; extended release; extended resistance; external resistance; external rotation

ER⁻ decreased estrogen receptor

ER⁺ increased estrogen receptor

Er erbium; erythrocyte

er endoplasmic reticulum

ERA electrical response activity; electroencephalic response audiometry; Electroshock Research Association; estrogen receptor assay; estradiol receptor assay; evoked response audiometry

ERAS electronic residency application service

ERBF effective renal blood flow

ERC endoscopic retrograde cholangiography; enteric cytopathic human orphan-rhino-coryza [virus]; erythropoietin-responsive cell

Erc erythrocyte

ERCP endoscopic retrograde cholangiopancreatography

ERD evoked response detector

ERDA Energy Research and Development Administration

ERE external rotation in extension

eRF eukaryotic release factor

ERF Education and Research Foundation; external rotation in flexion; Eye Research Foundation

E-RFC E-rosette forming cell

ERFS electrophysiological ring finger splinting

ERG electron radiography; electro-retinography, electroretinogram

ERHD exposure-related hypothermic death

ERI E-rosette inhibitor

ERIA electroradioimmunoassay

ERIC Educational Resource Information Center; Educational Resource Information Clearinghouse

ERISA Employee Retirement Income Security Act

ERK extracellular signal-regulated kinase

ERM electrochemical relaxation method; extended radical mastectomy

ERMSa embryonal rhabdomyosarcoma

ERNST European Resuscitation Nimodipine Study

ERP early receptor potential; effective refractory period; elodoisin-related peptide; endoscopic retrograde pancreatography; enzyme-releasing peptide; equine

rhinopneumonitis; estrogen receptor protein; event-related potential

ERPC evacuation of retained products of conception

ERPF effective renal plasma flow

ERPLV effective refractory period of left ventricle

ERS enamel-renal syndrome; endoscopic retrograde sphincterectomy

ERSP event-related slow potential

ERT esophageal radionuclide transit; estrogen replacement therapy; examination room terminal; external radiation therapy

ERTAS extended reticulo-thalamic activating system

ERU endorectal ultrasound

ERV equine rhinopneumonitis virus; expiratory reserve volume

ERY erysipelas

Ery *Erysipelothrix*

ES ejection sound; elastic stocking; electrical stimulus, electrical stimulation; electroshock; emergency service; emission spectrometry; endometritis-salpingitis; endoscopic sphincterotomy; end-systole; end-to-side; enzyme substrate; epileptic syndrome; esophageal, esophagus; esophageal scintigraphy; esterase; Ewing sarcoma; exfoliation syndrome; Expectation Score; experimental study; exterior surface; extrasystole

Es einsteinium; estrid

ESA Electrolysis Society of America; endocardial surface area; epidermal surface antigen; esterase; esterase A

ESAT esterase activator

ESB electrical stimulation of the brain; enhanced skill building [program]; esterase B

ESC electromechanical slope computer; endosystolic count; erythropoietin-sensitive stem cell; esterase C

ESCA electron spectroscopy for chemical analysis

ESCC epidural spinal cord compression

Esch *Escherichia*
ESCN electrolyte and steroid cardiopathy with necrosis
ESD electronic summation device; electrostatic discharge; emission spectrometric device; end-systolic dimension; esterase-D; exoskeletal device
ESE electrostatic unit [Ger. *electrostatische Einheit*]
ESF electron scatter function; electrosurgical filter; erythropoietic stimulating factor
ESFL end-systolic force-length relationship
ESG electrospinogram; estrogen; exfoliation syndrome glaucoma
ESHEL Association for Planning and Development of Services for the Aged in Israel
ESI elastase-specific inhibitor; enzyme substrate inhibitor; epidural steroid injection
ESIMV expiratory synchronized intermittent mandatory ventilation
ESL end-systolic length; extracorporeal shockwave lithotripsy
ESLD end-stage liver disease
ESLF end-stage liver failure
ESM ejection systolic murmur; endoscopic specular microscope; ethosuximide
ESMIS Emergency Medical Services Management Information System
ESN educationally subnormal; estrogen-stimulated neurophysin
ESN(M) educationally subnormal-moderate
ESN(S) educationally subnormal-severe
ESO electrospinal orthosis
eso esophagoscopy; esophagus
ESP early systolic paradox; echo spacing; effective sensory projection; effective systolic pressure; endometritis-salpingitis-peritonitis; end-systolic pressure; eosinophil stimulation promoter;

epidermal soluble protein; especially; evoked synaptic potential; extrasensory perception
ESPA electrical stimulation–produced analgesia
ESPVR end-systolic pressure-volume relationship
ESQ early signs questionnaire
ESR Einstein stoke radius; electric skin resistance; electron spin resonance; equipment service report; erythrocyte sedimentation rate; estrogen receptor
ESRD end-stage renal disease
ESRF end-stage renal failure
ESS empty sella syndrome; endostreptosin; erythrocyte-sensitizing substance; euthyroid sick syndrome; evolutionary stable energy; excited skin syndrome; squamous self-healing epithelioma
ess essential
EST electric shock threshold; electroshock therapy; endometrial sinus tumor; endoscopic sphincterectomy; esterase; exercise stress test; expressed sequence tags
est ester; estimation, estimated
esth esthetics, esthetic
ESU electrosurgical unit; electrostatic unit
E-sub excitor substance
ESV end-systolic volume; esophageal valve
ESVI end-systolic volume index
ESVS epiurethral suprapubic vaginal suspension
ESWL extracorporeal shock wave lithotripsy
ESWS end-systolic wall stress
ET educational therapy; effective temperature; ejection time; embryo transfer; endothelin; endotoxin; endotracheal; endotracheal tube; end-tidal; endurance time; enterotoxin; epidermolytic toxin; epithelial tumor; esotropia; essential thrombocythemia; essential tremor; ethanol;

etiocholanolone test; etiology; eustachian tube; examination terminal; exchange transfusion; exercise test; exercise treadmill; exfoliative toxin; expiration time

ET_3 erythrocyte triiodothyronine

ET_4 effective thyroxine [test]

Et ethyl; etiology

et and [Lat. *et*]

ETA electron transfer agent; endotracheal airways; ethionamide

η Greek letter *eta*; absolute viscosity

ETAB extrathoracic assisted breathing

et al and others [Lat. *et alii*]

ETAR equivalent tissue air ratio

ETC electron transport chain; esophageal tracheal combitude; estimated time of conception

ET_c corrected ejection time

$ETCO_2$ end-tidal carbon dioxide [concentration]

ETD eustachian tube dysfunction

ETEC enterotoxin of *Escherichia coli*, enterotoxic *Escherichia coli*

ETF electron-transferring flavoprotein; eustachian tube function

ETFB electron transfer flavoprotein, beta polypeptide

ETH elixir terpin hydrate; ethanol; ethmoid

eth ether

ETHC elixir terpin hydrate with codeine

ETI endotracheal intubation

ETIBACK Environmental Teratology Information Center Backfile

ETICBACK Environmental Toxicology Information Center Backfile

ETIO etiocholanolone

etiol etiology

ETK erythrocyte transketolase

ETKTM every test known to man

ETL echo train length; expiratory threshold load

ETM erythromycin

EtNU ethyl nitrosourea

ETO estimated time of ovulation

Eto ethylene oxide

ETOH, EtOH ethyl alcohol

ETOX ethylene oxide

ETP electron transport particle; entire treatment period; ephedrine, theophylline, phenobarbital; eustachian tube pressure

$ETPCO_2$ end-tidal partial carbon dioxide [concentration]

ETR effective thyroxine ratio; endothelin receptor

ETS educational testing service; electrical transcranial stimulation

ETT endotracheal tube; epinephrine tolerance test; exercise tolerance test; exercise treadmill test; extrathyroidal thyroxine

ETU emergency and trauma unit; emergency treatment unit

ETV extravascular thermal volume

EU Ehrlich unit; elementary unit; emergency unit; endotoxin unit; entropy unit; enzyme unit; esterase unit; etiology unknown

Eu europium; euryon

EUA examination under anesthesia

EUL expected upper limit

EUM external urethral meatus

EUP extrauterine pregnancy

EURONET European On-Line Network

EuroQol European quality of life [scale]

EUROTOX European Committee on Chronic Toxicity Hazards

EUS endoscopic ultrasound; external urethral sphincter

Eust eustachian

EUV extreme ultraviolet laser

EV electronic vehicle; emergency vehicle; enterovirus; epidermodysplasia verruciformis; estradiol valerate; eustachian valve; evoked potential [response]; excessive ventilation; expected utility; expected value; extravascular

Ev, ev eversion

eV, ev electron volt

EVA ethyl violet azide; ethylene vinyl acetate

evac evacuate, evacuated, evacuation
eval evaluate, evaluated, evaluation
evap evaporation, evaporated
EVB electronic view box; esophageal variceal bleeding
EVC Ellis-van Creveld [syndrome]
EVCI expected value of clinical information
EVD external ventricular drainage; extravascular [lung] density
ever eversion, everted
EVF ethanol volume fraction
EVFMG exchange visitor foreign medical graduate
EVG electroventriculography
EVLW extravascular lung water
EVM electronic voltmeter; extravascular mass
EVP episcleral venous pressure; evoked visual potential
EVR evoked visual response; exudative vitreoretinopathy
EVRS early ventricular repolarization syndrome
EVS eligibility verification system; endovaginal sonography
EVTV extravascular thermal volume
EVXX exudative vitreoretinopathy, X-linked
EW emergency ward; estrogen withdrawal
E-W Edinger-Westphal [nucleus]
EWB estrogen withdrawal bleeding
EWHO elbow-wrist-hand orthosis
EWL egg-white lysozyme; evaporation water loss
EWS Ewing sarcoma
EWSR Ewing sarcoma breakpoint region
EX exfoliation; exsmoker
E(X) expected value of the random variable X
ex exacerbation; examination, examined, examiner; example; excision; exercise; exophthalmos; exposure; extraction

EXA electronic X-ray archives
exac exacerbation
EXAFS extended x-ray absorption fine structure
exam examination, examine, examined
EXBF exercise hyperemia blood flow
exc excision
exch exchange
excr excretion
ExEF ejection fraction during exercise
EXELFS extended electron-loss line fine structure
exer exercise
EXO exonuclease; exophoria
exog exogenous
exoph exophthalmia
exos exostosis
exp expansion; expectorant; experiment, experimental; expiration, expired; exponential function; exposure
exp lap exploratory laparotomy
expect expectorant
exper experiment, experimental
ExPGN extracapillary proliferative glomerulonephritis
expir expiration, expiratory, expired
expl exploratory
Expl Lap exploratory laparotomy
exptl experimental
EXREM external radiation-emission man [dose]
EXS external support
EXT exercise testing
Ext extraction, extract
ext extension; extensive; extensor; exterior; external; extract; extreme, extremity
extr extract
extrav extravasation
ext rot external rotation
extub extubation
EXU excretory urogram
exud exudate, exudation
EY egg yolk; epidemiological year
EYA egg yolk agar
Ez eczema

F bioavailability; a cell that donates F factor in bacterial conjugation; a conjugative plasmid in F$^+$ bacterial cells; degree of fineness of abrasive particles; facies; factor; Fahrenheit; failure; false; family; farad; Faraday constant; fascia; fasting; fat; father; feces; fellow; female; fermentation; fertility; fetal; fiat; fibroblast; fibrous; field of vision; filament; *Filaria*; fine; finger; flexion; flow; fluorine; flux; focal [spot]; focus; foil; fontanel; foramen; force; form, forma; formula; fornix; fossa; fraction, fractional; fracture; fragment; free; French [catheter]; frequency; frontal; frontal electrode placement in electroencephalography; function; fundus; *Fusiformis*; *Fusobacterium*; gilbert; Helmholz free energy; hydrocortisone [compound F]; inbreeding coefficient; left foot electrode in vectorcardiography; phenylalanine; variance ratio

F$_0$, F$_1$ coupling factor

F$_1$, F$_2$ etc. first, second, etc., filial generation

FI, FII, etc. factors I, II, etc.

F344 Fischer 344 [rat]

°F degree on the Fahrenheit scale

F' a hybrid F plasmid

F$^-$ a bacterial cell lacking an F plasmid

F$^+$ a bacterial cell having an F plasmid

f atomic orbital with angular momentum quantum number 3; farad; father; female; femto; fiber, fibrous; fingerbreadth; fission; flexion; fluid; focal; foot; form, forma; formula; fostered [experimental animal]; fraction; fracture; fragment; frequency; frontal; function; fundus; numerical expression of the relative aperture of a camera lens

FA false aneurysm; Families Anonymous; Fanconi anemia; far advanced; fatty acid; febrile antigen; femoral artery; fibrinolytic activity; fibroadenoma; fibrosing alveolitis; field ambulance; field assessment; filterable agent; filtered air; first aid; flip angle; fluorescent antibody; fluorescent assay; fluoroalanine; folic acid; follicular area; food allergy; forearm; fortified aqueous [solution]; free acid; Freund adjuvant; Friedreich ataxia; functional activity; functional administration

F/A fetus active

fa fatty [rat]

FAA folic acid antagonist; formaldehyde, acetic acid, alcohol

FAAN Fellow of the American Academy of Nursing

FAB fast atom bombardment; formalin ammonium bromide; fragment, antigen-binding [of immunoglobulins]; French-American-British [carcinoma staging]; functional arm brace

Fab fragment, antigen-binding [of immunoglobulins]

F(ab')$_2$ fragment, antigen-binding [of immunoglobulins]

Fabc fragment, antigen and complement binding [of immunoglobulins]

FABER flexion in abduction and external rotation

FABF femoral artery blood flow

FABP fatty acid-binding protein; folate-binding protein

FAC familial adenomatosis coli; femoral arterial cannulation; ferric ammonium citrate; 5-fluorouracil, Adriamycin, and cyclophosphamide; foamy alveolar cast; fractional area changes; free available chlorine

Fac factor

fac facility; to make [Lat. *facere*]

FACA Fanconi anemia complementation group A; Fellow of the American College of Anesthetists; Fellow of the American College of Angiology; Fellow of the American College of Apothecaries

FACAI Fellow of the American College of Allergy and Immunology

FACB Fanconi anemia complementation group B

Facb fragment, antigen, and complement binding

FACC Fanconi anemia complementation group C; Fellow of the American College of Cardiologists

FACCP Fellow of the American College of Chest Physicians

FACD Fanconi anemia complementation group D; Fellow of the American College of Dentists

FACEP Fellow of the American College of Emergency Physicians

FACES unique facies, anorexia, cachexia, and eye and skin lesions [syndrome]

FACFS Fellow of the American College of Foot Surgeons

FACG Fellow of the American College of Gastroenterology

FACH forceps to after-coming head

FACHA Fellow of the American College of Health Administrators; Fellow of the American College of Hospital Administrators

FACHE Fellow of the American College of Healthcare Executives

FACIT fibril-associated collagen with interrupted triple helices

FACL fatty acid coenzyme ligase

FACMTA Federal Advisory Council on Medical Training Aids

FACNHA Foundation of American College of Nursing Home Administrators

FACO Fellow of the American College of Otolaryngology

FACOG Fellow of the American College of Obstetricians and Gynecologists

FACOSH Federal Advisory Committee on Occupational Safety and Health

FACP Fellow of the American College of Physicians

FACPE Fellow of the American College of Physician Executives

FACPM Fellow of the American College of Preventive Medicine

FACS Fellow of the American College of Surgeons; fluorescence-activated cell sorter

FACSM Fellow of the American College of Sports Medicine

FACT Flannagan Aptitude Classification Test

FACWA familial amyotrophic chorea with acanthocytosis

FAD familial Alzheimer dementia; familial autonomic dysfunction; fetal activity-acceleration determination; flavin adenine dinucleotide

FADF fluorescent antibody dark field

FADH$_2$ reduced form of flavin adenine dinucleotide

FADIR flexion in adduction and internal rotation

FADN flavin adenine dinucleotide

FADS fetal akinesia deformation sequence

FAE fetal alcohol effect

FAEES fatty acid ethyl ester synthase

FAF fatty acid free; fibroblast-activating factor

FAH Federation of American Hospitals

Fahr Fahrenheit

FAI first aid instruction; free androgen index; functional aerobic impairment; functional assessment inventory

FAJ fused apophyseal joint

FALG fowl antimouse lymphocyte globulin

FALP fluoro-assisted lumbar puncture

FAM 5-fluorouracil, Adriamycin, and mitomycin C

Fam, fam family, familial

FAMA Fellow of the American Medical Association; fluorescent antibody to membrane antigen

FAME fatty acid methyl ester

fam hist family history

FAMMM familial atypical multiple mole–melanoma [syndrome]

FAN fuchsin, amido black, and naphthol yellow

FANA fluorescent antinuclear antibody

F and R force and rhythm [of pulse]

FANEL Federation for Accessible Nursing Education and Licensure

FANPT Freeman Anxiety Neurosis and Psychosomatic Test

FAOF family assessment of occupational functioning

FAP familial adenomatous polyposis; familial amyloid polyneuropathy; fatty acid polyunsaturated; fatty acid poor; femoral artery pressure; fibrillating action potential; fixed action potential; frozen animal procedure

FAPA Fellow of the American Psychiatric Association; Fellow of the American Psychoanalytical Association

FAPHA Fellow of the American Public Health Association

FAQ frequently asked question; functional asessment questionnaire

FAR Federal acquisitions regulation; fractional albumin rate; fresh bone marrow

far faradic

FARE Federation of Alcoholic Rehabilitation Establishments

FARS fatal accident reporting system

FAS fatty acid synthetase; Federation of American Scientists; fetal alcohol syndrome

FASB Financial Accounting Standards Board

FASC free-standing ambulatory surgical center

fasc fasciculus, fascicular

FASEB Federation of American Societies for Experimental Biology

FASHP Federation of Associations of Schools of the Health Professions

FAST flow-assisted, short-term [balloon catheter]; fluorescent antibody staining technique; fluoro-allergosorbent test; Fourier acquired steady state; Frenchay Aphasia Screening Test; functional assessment stages

FAT family attitudes test; fluorescent antibody technique; fluorescent antibody test

FATS face and thigh squeeze [position for bag mask ventilation]

FAV facio-auriculovertebral [sequence]; feline ataxia virus; floppy aortic valve; fowl adenovirus

FAX, fax facsimile

FAZ Fanconi-Albertini-Zellweger [syndrome]; foveal avascular zone; fragmented atrial activity zone

FB fasting blood [sugar]; feedback; fiberoptic bronchoscopy; fingerbreadth; foreign body; *Fusobacterium*

FBA fecal bile acid

FBAO foreign-body airway obstruction

FBC full blood count

FBCOD foreign body of the cornea, oculus dexter (right eye)

FBCOS foreign body of the cornea, oculus sinister (left eye)

FBCP familial benign chronic pemphigus

FBD functional bowel disorder

FbDP fibrin degradation products

FBE full blood examination

FBEC fetal bovine endothelial cell

FBF forearm blood flow

FBG fasting blood glucose; fibrinogen; foreign body granulomatosis

fbg fibrinogen

FBH familial benign hypercalcemia

FBHH familial benign hypocalciuric hypercalcemia

FBI flossing, brushing, and irrigation

FBL follicular basal lamina
FBLN fibulin
FBM fetal breathing movements
FBN Federal Bureau of Narcotics; fibribillin
FBP femoral blood pressure; fibrin breakdown product; folate-binding protein; fructose-1, 6-biphosphatase
FBPsS Fellow of the British Psychological Society
FBS fasting blood sugar; feedback system; fetal bovine serum
FBSS failed back surgery syndrome
FC fasciculus cuneatus; fast component [of a neuron]; febrile convulsions; feline conjunctivitis; ferric citrate; fibrocyte; finger clubbing; finger counting; flow compensation; fluorocarbon; fluorocytosine; Foley catheter; foster care; fowl cholera; free cholesterol; frontal cortex; functional castration
5-FC 5-fluorocytosine
Fc centroid frequency; fraction/centrifuge; fragment, crystallizable [of immunoglobulin]
Fc' a fragment of an immunoglobulin molecule produced by papain digestion
fc foot candles
F + C flare ;pl cells
FCA ferritin-conjugated antibodies; Freund's complete adjuvant; functional capacity assessment
FCAH familial cytomegaly adrenocortical hypoplasia [syndrome]
FCAP Fellow of the College of American Pathologists
F cath Foley catheter
FCC follicular center cells
fcc face-centered-cubic
f/cc fibers per cubic centimeter of air
FCCL follicular center cell lymphoma
FCCSET Federal Coordinating Committee for Science, Engineering and Technology
FCD feces collection device; fibrocystic disease; fibrocystic dysplasia; focal cytoplasmic degradation
FCE fibrocartilaginous embolism
FCF fetal cardiac frequency; fibroblast chemotactic factor
FCFC fibroblast colony-forming cell
FCH faculty contact hour; family case home; fetal cystic hygroma
FCHL familial combined hyperlipidemia
FChS Fellow of the Society of Chiropodists
FCI fixed-cell immunofluorescence; food chemical intolerance
FCIM Federated Council for Internal Medicine
FCL fibroblast cell line
fcly face lying
FCM flow cytometry
FCMC familial chronic mucocutaneous candidiasis; family centered maternity care
FCMD Fukuyama congenital muscular dystrophy
FCMS Fellow of the College of Medicine and Surgery; Foix-Chavany-Marie syndrome
FCMW Foundation for Child Mental Welfare
FCO Fellow of the College of Osteopathy
FCP F-cell production; final common pathway; Functional Communication Profile
FCPS Fellow of the College of Physicians and Surgeons
FCR flexor carpi radialis; fractional catabolic rate
FcR Fc receptor
FCRA fecal collection receptacle assembly; Fellow of the College of Radiologists of Australasia
FCRC Frederick Cancer Research Center
FCS faciocutaneoskeletal syndrome; fecal containment system; feedback control system; fetal calf serum; foot compartment syndrome

FCSP Fellow of the Chartered Society of Physiotherapy

FCST Fellow of the College of Speech Therapists

FCT food composition table; fucosyl transferase

FCU flexor carpi ulnaris

FCx frontal cortex

FCXM flow cytometric cross-matching

FD familial dysautonomia; family doctor; fan douche; fatal dose; fetal danger; fibrin derivative; fibrous dysplasia; focal distance; Folin-Denis [assay]; follicular diameter; foot drop; forceps delivery; freeze drying

Fd the amino-terminal portion of the heavy chain of an immunoglobulin molecule; ferredoxin

fd fundus

FD$_{50}$ median fatal dose

FDA fluorescein diacetate; Food and Drug Administration; right frontoanterior [position of the fetus]

FDAW film digitizer acquisition workstation

FDBL fecal daily blood loss

FDC factor-dependent cell [line]; follicular dendritic cell

FD&C Food, Drug and Cosmetic Act; food, drugs, and cosmetics

FDCPA Food, Drug, and Consumer Product Agency

FDD Food and Drugs Directorate

FDDC ferric dimethyldithiocarbonate

FDDI film distribution data interface

FDDS Family Drawing Depression Scale

FDE female day-equivalent; final drug evaluation

FDF fast death factor

FDFQ Food/Drink Frequency Questionnaire

FDFT farnesyldiphosphate farnesyltransferase

FDG F-deoxyglucose; fluorodeoxyglucose

fdg feeding

FDGF fibroblast-derived growth factor

FDH familial dysalbuminemic hyperthyroxinemia; focal dermal hypoplasia; formaldehyde dehydrogenase

FDI first dorsal interosseous [muscle]; International Dental Federation [Fédération Dentaire Internationale]

FDIU fetal death in utero

FDL flexor digitorum longus

FDLMP first day of last menstrual period

FDLV fer de lance virus

FDM fetus of diabetic mother; fibrous dysplasia of the mandible

FDMP fluid depth at Morison's pouch

FDNB fluorodinitrobenzene

FDO Fleet Dental Officer

FDP fibrin degradation product; fibrinogen degradation product; flexor digitorum profundus; frontodextra posterior [position of fetus]; fructose-1,6-diphosphate

FDPase fructose-1,6-diphosphatase

FDPS farnesyl diphosphate synthetase

FDPSL farnesyl diphosphate synthetase-like

FDQB flexor digiti quinti brevis

FDR fractional disappearance rate

FDS Fellow in Dental Surgery; fiber duodenoscope; flexor digitorum superficialis

FDSRCSEng Fellow in Dental Surgery of the Royal College of Surgeons of England

FDT frontodextra transversa [position of fetus]

FDTD finite difference time domain [method]

FDV Friend disease virus

FDZ fetal danger zone

FE fatty ester; fecal emesis; fetal erythroblastosis; fetal erythrocyte; fluid extract; fluorescent erythrocyte; forced expiration; formaldehyde-ethanol; frequency-encoded; frozen embryo

Fe female; ferret; iron [Lat. *ferrum*]

fe female
feb fever [Lat. *febris*]
FEBP fetal estrogen-binding protein
FEBS Federation of European Biochemical Societies
FEC forced expiratory capacity; free erythrocyte coproporphyrin; freestanding emergency center; Friend erythroleukemia cell
FECH ferrochelatase
FECG fetal electrocardiogram
F_{ECO2} fractional concentration of carbon dioxide in expired gas
FECP free erythrocyte coproporphyrin
FECT fibroelastic connective tissue
FECU factor [VIII] correctional unit
FECV feline enteric coronavirus
FECVC functional extracellular fluid volume
FED fish eye disease
FeD iron deficiency
Fed federal
FEDRIP Federal Research in Progress [database]
FEE forced equilibrating expiration
FEEG fetal electroencephalography
FEER field echo with even echo rephasing
FEF forced expiratory flow
FEF_{50} forced expiratory flow at 50% of forced vital capacity
FEF_{50}/FIF_{50} ratio of expiratory flow to inspiratory flow at 50% of forced vital capacity
FEFV forced expiratory flow volume
FEGO International Federation of Gynecology and Obstetrics
FEH focal epithelial hyperplasia
FEHBARS Federal Employee Health Benefit Acquisition Regulations
FEHBP Federal Employee Health Benefits Program
$Fe+^2Hgb$ ferromethemoglobin
$Fe+^3Hgb$ ferrimethemoglobin
FEKG fetal electrocardiogram

FEL familial erythrophagocytic lymphohistiocytosis
FELC Friend erythroleukemia
FeLV feline leukemia virus
FEM female; femur, femoral; finite element method
fem female; femur, femoral
fem intern at inner side of the thighs [Lat. *femoribus internus*]
FENa, FE_{Na} fractional excretion of sodium
FEO familial expansile osteolysis
FE_{O2}, F_{EO2} fractional concentration of oxygen in expired gas
FEP fluorinated ethylene-propylene; free erythrocyte protoporphyrin; front-end processing; front-end processor
FEPB functional electronic peroneal brace
FEPP free erythrocyte protoporphyrin
FER flexion, extension, rotation; fractional esterification rate
fert fertility, fertilized
FES family environment scale; fat embolism syndrome; flame emission spectroscopy; forced expiratory spirogram; functional electrical stimulation
Fe/S iron/sulfur [protein]
FESS functional endoscopic sinus surgery
FeSV feline sarcoma virus
FET field-effect transistor; forced expiratory time
FETE Far Eastern tick-borne encephalitis
FETs forced expiratory time in seconds
FEUO for external use only
FEV familial exudative vitreoretinopathy; forced expiratory volume
fev fever
FEV1, FEV_1 forced expiratory volume in one second
$FEV_{1\%}$ ratio of FEV_1 to FVC
FEVB frequency ectopic ventricular beat

FEVR familial exudative vitreoretinopathy

FF degree of fineness of abrasive particles; fat-free; father factor; fecal frequency; fertility factor; field of Forel; filtration fraction; fine fiber; fine focus; finger flexion; finger-to-finger; fixation fluid; flat feet; flip-flop; fluorescent focus; follicular fluid; force fluids; forearm flow; forward flexion; foster father; free fraction; fresh frozen; fundus firm

F2F face-to-face

ff⁺ fertility inhibition positive

ff⁻ fertility inhibition negative

FFA Fellow of the Faculty of Anaesthetists; free fatty acid

FFAP free fatty acid phase

FFARCS Fellow of the Faculty of Anaesthetists of the Royal College of Surgeons

FFB flexible fiberoptic bronchoscopy

FFC fixed flexion contracture; fluorescence flow cytometry; free from chlorine

FFCM Fellow of the Faculty of Community Medicine

FFD Fellow in the Faculty of Dentistry; focus-film distance

FFDCA Federal Food, Drug, and Cosmetic Act

FFDD focal facial dermal dysplasia

FFDSRCS Fellow of the Faculty of Dental Surgery of the Royal College of Surgeons

FFDW fat-free dry weight

FFE fast field echo; fecal fat excretion

FFF degree of fineness of abrasive particles; field-flow fractionation; flicker fusion frequency

FFG free fat graft

FFHC federally funded health center

FFHom Fellow of the Faculty of Homeopathy

FFI family function index; free from infection; fundamental frequency indicator

FFIT fluorescent focus inhibition test

FFM fat-free mass; fundus flavimaculatus

FFOM Fellow of the Faculty of Occupational Medicine

FFP freedom from progression; fresh frozen plasma

FFR Fellow of the Faculty of Radiologists

FFROM full and free range of motion

FFS fat-free solids; fee for services

FFT fast Fourier transform; flicker fusion test or threshold

FFU femur-fibula-ulna [syndrome]; focal forming unit

FFW fat-free weight

FFWC fractional free water clearance

FFWW fat-free wet weight

FG fasciculus gracilis; fast-glycolytic [fiber]; Feeley-Gorman [agar]; fibrinogen; Flemish giant [rabbit]

fg femtogram

FGA fibrinogen alpha

FGB fibrinogen beta

FGC fibrinogen gel chromatography

FGD fatal granulomatous disease

FgDP fibrinogen degradation products

FGDS fibrogastroduodenoscopy

FGDY faciogenital dysplasia

FGF father's grandfather; fibroblast growth factor; fresh gas flow

FGFA fibroblast growth factor, acidic

FGFB fibroblast growth factor, basic

FGFR fibroblast growth factor receptor

FGG fibrinogen gamma; focal global glomerulosclerosis; fowl gamma-globulin

FGH formylglutathione hydrolase

FGL fasting gastrin level

FGM father's grandmother

FGN fibrinogen; focal glomerulonephritis

FGP fundic gland polyp

FGS fibrogastroscopy; focal glomerular sclerosis

FGT fluorescent gonorrhea test

FH facial hemihyperplasia; familial hypercholesterolemia; family history; fasting hyperbilirubinemia; favorable histology; femoral hernia; femoral hypoplasia; fetal head; fetal heart; fibromuscular hyperplasia; follicular hyperplasia; Frankfort horizontal [plane]; fumarate hydratase

FH$^+$ family history positive

FH$^-$ family history negative

FH$_4$ tetrahydrofolic acid

fh fostered by hand [experimental animal]

FHA familial hypoplastic anemia; Fellow of the Institute of Hospital Administrators; filamentous hemagglutinin

FH/BC frontal horn/bicaudate [ratio]

FHC familial hypercholesterolemia; family health center; Ficoll-Hypaque centrifugation; Fuchs heterochromic cyclitis

FHD familial histiocytic dermatoarthritis; family history of diabetes

FHF fetal heart frequency; fulminant hepatic failure

fHg free hemoglobin

FHH familial hypocalciuric hypercalcemia; fetal heart heard

FHI Fuchs' heterochromic iridocyclitis

FHIP family health insurance plan

FHIT fragile histidine triad [gene]

FHL flexor hallucis longus; functional hearing loss

FHM familial hemiplegic migraine; fathead minnow [cells]

FHN family history negative

FHNH fetal heart not heard

FHP family history positive

FHR familial hypophosphatemic rickets; fetal heart rate

FHRNST fetal heart rate nonstress test

FHS fetal heart sound; fetal hydantoin syndrome; Floating Harbor syndrome

FHT fast Hartley transform; fetal heart; fetal heart tone

FHTG familial hypertriglyceridemia

FH-UFS femoral hypoplasia-unusual facies syndrome

FHV falcon herpesvirus

FHVP free hepatic vein pressure

FHx family history

FI fasciculus intrafascicularis; fever caused by infection; fibrinogen; fixed interval; flame ionization; follicular involution; food intolerance; forced inspiration; frontoiliac

FIA fistula in ano; fluorescent immunoassay; focal immunoassay; Freund incomplete adjuvant

FIAC 2'-fluoro-5-iodo-aracytosine

FIB Fellow of the Institute of Biology; fibrin; fibrinogen; fibrositis; fibula

fib fiber; fibrillation; fibrin; fibrinogen; fibula

FIC Fogarty International Center; fractional inhibitory concentration

FICA Federal Insurance Contributions Act

FICD Fellow of the Institute of Canadian Dentists; Fellow of the International College of Dentists

FiCO$_2$, FI$_{CO_2}$ fractional concentration of carbon dioxide in inspired gas

FICS Fellow of the International College of Surgeons

FICU fetal intensive care unit

FID flame ionization detector; free induction decay; fungal immunodiffusion

FIDD fetal iodine deficiency disorder

FIF feedback inhibition factor; fibroblast interferon; forced inspiratory flow; formaldehyde-induced fluorescence

FIF$_{50}$ forced inspiratory flow at 50% of forced vital capacity

FIFO first in, first out

FIFR fasting intestinal flow rate

FIGD familial idiopathic gonadotropin deficiency

FIGE field inversion gel electrophoresis

FIGLU, FIGlu formiminoglutamate, formiminoglutamic acid

FIGLU-uria formiminoglutaminaciduria
FIGO International Federation of Gynecology and Obstetrics
FIH familial isolated hypoparathyroidism; fat-induced hyperglycemia
fil filament; filial
filt filter, filtration
FIM field ion microscopy; functional independence measure
FIMG familial infantile myasthenia gravis
FIMLT Fellow of the Institute of Medical Laboratory Technology
FIN fine intestinal needle
FINCC familial idiopathic nonarteriosclerotic cerebral calcification
FI$_{O2}$ forced inspiratory oxygen; fractional concentration of oxygen in inspired gas
FiO$_2$ fractional concentration of oxygen in inspired gas
FIP feline infectious peritonitis
FIPA familial intestinal polyatresia [syndrome]
FIPV feline infectious peritonitis virus
FIQ full-scale intelligence quotient
FIR far infrared; fold increase in resistance
FIRDA frontal, intermittent delta activity
FIS forced inspiratory spirogram; free induction signal
fis fission
FISH fluorescence in situ hybridization
FISP fast imaging with steady state precession
fist fistula
FIT fluorescein isothiocyanate; fusion inferred threshold
FITC fluorescein isothiocyanate
FIUO for internal use only
FIV feline immunodeficiency; forced inspiratory volume
FIV$_1$ forced inspiratory volume in one second
FIVC forced inspiratory vital capacity
FJN familial juvenile nephrophthisis

FJRM full joint range of movement
FJS finger joint size
FK feline kidney
FKBP FK 506 [macrolide] binding protein
FL fatty liver; feline leukemia; femur length; fibers of Luschka; fibroblast-like; filtration leukapheresis; focal length; follicular lymphoma; Friend leukemia; frontal lobe; full liquid [diet]; functional length
FL-2 feline lung [cells]
Fl fluid; fluorescence
fl femtoliter; filtered load; flexion, flexible; fluorescent; flow; fluid; flutter; foot lambert
FLA fluorescent-labeled antibody; left frontoanterior [position of the fetus] [Lat. *fronto-laeva anterior*]
flac flaccidity, flaccid
FLAIR fluid attenuated inversion recovery
FLAP 5-lipoxygenase activating protein
FLASH fast low angle shot; fluorescence in situ hybridization
FLC family life cycle; fatty liver cell; fetal liver cell; Friend leukemia cell
FLD fibrotic lung disease
fld fluid
fl dr fluid dram
FLEX Federation Licensing Examination
flex flexor, flexion
FLG filaggrin
FLIC functional living index-cancer
FLICC Federal Library and Information Center Committee
FLK funny looking kid
FLKS fatty liver and kidney syndrome
FLM fasciculus longitudinalis medialis
floc flocculation
fl oz fluid ounce
FLP left frontoposterior [position of the fetus] [Lat. *fronto-laeva posterior*]; functional limitations profile
FLR funny looking rash

FLS fatty liver syndrome; Fellow of the Linnean Society; fibrous long-spacing [collagen]; flow-limiting segment

FLSP fluorescein-labeled serum protein

FLT left frontotransverse [position of the fetus] [Lat. *fronto-laeva transversa*]

FLU 5-fluorouracil; flunitrazepam; fluphenazine; flutamide

flu influenza

fluor fluorescence; fluorescent; fluorometry; fluoroscopy

fluoro fluoroscope, fluoroscopy

FLV feline leukemia virus; Friend leukemia virus

FM face mask; facilities management; family medicine; feedback mechanism; fetal movement; fibromuscular; filtered mass; flavin mononucleotide; flowmeter; foramen magnum; forensic medicine; foster mother; frequency modulation; functional movement

Fm fermium

f-M free metanephrine

fm femtometer

FMA Frankfort mandibular plane angle

FMAT fetal movement acceleration test

FMC family medicine center; flight medicine clinic; focal macular choroidopathy; foundation for medical care

FMCG fetal magnetocardiography

FMD facility medical director; family medical doctor; fibromuscular dysplasia; foot and mouth disease; frontometaphyseal dysplasia

FMDV foot and mouth disease virus

FME full mouth extraction

Fmed median frequency

FMEG fetal magnetoencephalography

FMEL Friend murine erythroleukemia

FMEN familial multiple endocrine neoplasia

F-met, fMet formyl methionine

FMF familial Mediterranean fever; fetal movement felt; flow microfluorometry; forced midexpiratory flow

FMFD V familial multiple coagulation factor deficiency V

FMG five-mesh gauze; foreign medical graduate

FMGEMS Foreign Medical Graduate Examination in Medical Sciences

FMH family medical history; fat-mobilizing hormone; feto-maternal hemorrhage; fibromuscular hyperplasia

FMI Foods and Moods Inventory

FML flail mitral leaflet; fluorometholone

FMLP N-formyl-methionyl-leucyl-phenylalanine; formylpeptide

f-MLP N-formyl-methyonyl-leucyl-phenylalanine

FMN first malignant neoplasm; flavin mononucleotide; frontomaxillonasal [suture]

FMNH, FMNH$_2$ reduced form of flavin mononucleotide

FMO falvin-containing monooxygenase; Fleet Medical Officer; Flight Medical Officer

fmol femtomole

FMP faculty mentorship program; first menstrual period; fructose monophosphate

FMR fragile site mental retardation [syndrome]; Friend-Moloney-Rauscher [antigen]

fMRI functional magnetic resonance imaging

FMS fat-mobilizing substance; Fellow of the Medical Society; fibromyalgia syndrome; full mouth series

FMTC familial medullary thyroid cancer

FMU first morning urine

F-MuLV Friend murine leukemia virus

FMX full mouth x-ray

FN false negative; fibronectin; fluoride number

F-N finger to nose

fn function

FNA fine-needle aspiration

FNAB fine-needle aspiration biopsy
FNAC fine-needle aspiration cytology
FNC fatty nutritional cirrhosis
FNCJ fine needle catheter jejunostomy
FND febrile neutrophilic dermatosis; frontonasal dysplasia
f-NE free norepinephrine
Fneg false negative
FNF false-negative fraction; femoral neck fracture
FNFMG foreign national foreign medical school graduate
FNH focal nodular hyperplasia
FNL fibronectin-like
f-NM free normetanephrine
FNP family nurse practitioner
FNR fibronectin receptor
FNRA fibronectin receptor alpha
FNRB fibronectin receptor beta
FNRBL fibronectin receptor beta-like
FNS frontier nursing service; functional neuromuscular stimulation
FNT false neurochemical transmitter; farnesyltransferase
FNTA farnesyltransferase alpha
FNTB farnesyltransferase beta
FO fiberoptic; fish oil; foot arthrosis; foramen ovale; forced oscillation; fronto-occipital
Fo fomentation, fomenting
FOA Federation of Orthodontic Associations
FOAR facio-oculo-acoustico-renal [syndrome]
FOAVF failure of all vital forces
FOB fecal occult blood; feet out of bed; fiberoptic bronchoscopy; foot of bed; functional observational battery
FOBT fecal occult blood test
FOC fronto-occipital circumference
FOCAL formula calculation
FOD focus-to-object distance; free of disease
FOG fast oxidative glycolytic [fiber]
FOL folate

FOLR folate receptor
FOM figure-of-merit
FOMi 5-fluorouracil, vincristine, and mitomycin C
FOOB fell out of bed
FOOSH fell onto [his or her] outstretched hand
FOP fibrodysplasia ossificans progressiva; forensic pathology
FOPR full outpatient rate
For foramen; forensic
for foreign; formula
FORIMG foreign national international medical school graduate
form formula
FORTRAN formula translation
FOS fiberoptic sigmoidoscopy; fractional osteoid surface
FOV field of view
FP false positive; family physician; family planning; family practice; family practitioner; Fanconi pancytopenia; femoropopliteal; fetoprotein; fibrinopeptide; filling pressure; filter paper; fixation protein; flash point; flavin phosphate; flavoprotein; flexor profundus; fluid pressure; fluorescence polarization; food poisoning; forearm pronated; freezing point; frontoparietal; frozen plasma; full period; fusion point
F1P, F-1-P fructose-1-phosphate
F6P, F-6-P fructose-6-phosphate
Fp frontal polar electrode placement in electroencephalography
fp flexor pollicis; foot-pound; forearm pronated; freezing point
FPA Family Planning Association; fibrinopeptide A; filter paper activity; fluorophenylalanine
FPB femoral popliteal bypass; fibrinopeptide B; flexor pollicis brevis
FPC familial polyposis coli; family planning clinic; fish protein concentrate
FPCA family practice comfort assessment

FpCA 1-fluoromethyl-2-p-chlorophenyl-ethylamine

FPD feto-pelvic disproportion; flame photometric detector

FPDM fibrocalculous pancreatic diabetes mellitus

FPE fatal pulmonary embolism; field placement error; final prediction error

FPF false positive fraction; fibroblast pneumocyte factor

FPG fasting plasma glucose; fluorescence plus Giemsa; focal proliferative glomerulonephritis

FPGS folylpolyglutamate synthetase

FPH$_2$ reduced form of flavin phosphate

FPHE formaldehyde-treated pyruvaldehyde-stabilized human erythrocytes

FPI femoral pulsatility index; fluid percussion injury; formula protein intolerance; Freiburg Personality Identification Questionnaire

FPIA fluorescence polarization immunoassay

FPK fructose phosphokinase

FPL fasting plasma lipids; flexor pollicis longus

FPLC fast protein liquid chromatography

FPM filter paper microscopic [test]; full passive movements

fpm feet per minute

FPN ferric chloride, perchloric acid, and nitric acid [solution]

FPO faciopalatooseous [syndrome]; Federation of Prosthodontic Organizations; freezing point osmometer

FPP faculty practice plan; free portal pressure

FPPH familial primary pulmonary hypertension

FPR false-positive rate; finger peripheral resistance; fluorescence photobleaching recovery; N-formylpeptide receptor; fractional proximal resorption

FPRA first pass radionuclide angiogram

FPRH N-formylpeptide homolog

FPS farnesylpyrophosphate synthetase; Fellow of the Pathological Society; Fellow of the Pharmaceutical Society; fetal PCB (polychlorinated biphenyl) syndrome; footpad swelling

fps feet per second; frames per second

FPSL farnesylpyrophosphate synthetase-like

FPSTS false-positive serologic test for syphilis

FPV feline pseudoleukopenia virus; fowl plague virus

FPVB femoral popliteal vein bypass

FQHC federally qualified health center

FR failure rate; film-screen radiograph; fasciculus retroflexus; febrile reaction; feedback regulation; Fischer-Race [notation]; fixed ratio; flocculation reaction; flow rate; fluid restriction; fluid resuscitation; fluid retention; free radical; frequency of respiration; frequent relapses

F2R [blood coagulation] factor II receptor

F&R force and rhythm [pulse]

Fr fracture; francium; franklin [unit charge]; French; frequency or frequent

Fr1 first fraction

F( )R:Ag factor ( ) related antigen

F( )R:C factor ( ) related cofactor activity

FRA fibrinogen-related antigen; fluorescent rabies antibody

fra fragil [site]

FRAC Food Research and Action Center

frac fracture

fract fracture

FRAME Fund for the Replacement of Animals in Medical Experiments

FRAP fluorescence recovery after photo-bleaching

FRAT free radical assay technique

FRAX fragile [chromosome] X

fra(X) fragile X chromosome, fragile X syndrome

FRAXA fragile X syndrome

FRAXE X-linked mental retardation-fragile site [syndrome]

FRAX-MR fragile X-mental retardation [syndrome]

Fr BB fracture of both bones

FRC Federal Radiation Council; frozen red cells; functional reserve capacity; functional residual capacity

FRCD Fellow of the Royal College of Dentists; fixed ratio combination drug

FRCGP Fellow of the Royal College of General Practitioners

FRCOG Fellow of the Royal College of Obstetricians and Gynaecologists

FRCP Fellow of the Royal College of Physicians

FRCPA Fellow of the Royal College of Pathologists of Australia

FRCPath Fellow of the Royal College of Pathologists

FRCP(C) Fellow of the Royal College of Physicians of Canada

FRCPE Fellow of the Royal College of Physicians of Edinburgh

FRCPI Fellow of the Royal College of Physicians of Ireland

FRCPsych Fellow of the Royal College of Psychiatrists

FRCS Fellow of the Royal College of Surgeons

FRCS(C) Fellow of the Royal College of Surgeons of Canada

FRCSEd Fellow of the Royal College of Surgeons of Edinburgh

FRCSEng Fellow of the Royal College of Surgeons of England

FRCSI Fellow of the Royal College of Surgeons of Ireland

FRCVS Fellow of the Royal College of Veterinary Surgeons

FRDA Friedreich ataxia

FRE Fischer rat embryo; flow-related enhancement

FREIR Federal Research on Biological and Health Effects of Ionizing Radiation

frem fremitus

freq frequency

FRES Fellow of the Royal Entomological Society

FRF Fertility Research Foundation; follicle-stimulating hormone-releasing factor

FRFC functional renal failure of cirrhosis

FRH follicle-stimulating hormone-releasing hormone

FRh fetal rhesus monkey kidney [cell]

FRHS fast-repeating high sequence

frict friction

FRIPHH Fellow of the Royal Institute of Public Health and Hygiene

FRJM full range joint movement

FRMedSoc Fellow of the Royal Medical Society

FRMS Fellow of the Royal Microscopical Society

FRO floor reaction orthosis

FROM full range of movements

FRP follicle-stimulating hormone releasing protein; functional refractory period

FRS Fellow of the Royal Society; ferredoxin-reducing substance; first rank symptom; furosemide

FRSH Fellow of the Royal Society of Health

FRT Family Relations Test; full recovery time

Fru fructose

FRV full-length retroviral [sequence]; functional residual volume

Frx fracture

FS factor of safety; Fanconi syndrome; Felty syndrome; fibromyalgia syndrome; field stimulation; Fisher syndrome; food service; forearm supination; fractional shortening; fracture site; fragile site; Friesinger score; frozen section; full scale [IQ]; full soft [diet]; full strength; function study; human foreskin [cells]; simple fracture

F/S female, spayed [animal]; frozen section

FSA flexible spending account

FSB fetal scalp blood

FSBA fluorosulfonylbenzoyladenosine

FSBP finger systolic blood pressure

FSBT Fowler single breath test

FSC Food Standards Committee

FSD focus-skin distance

FSE fast spin echo; filtered smoke exposure

FSF fibrin stabilizing factor; front surface fluorescence

FSG fasting serum glucose; focal segmental sclerosis

FSGHS focal segmental glomerular hyalinosis and sclerosis

FSGN focal sclerosing glomerulonephritis

FSGS focal segmental glomerulosclerosis

FSH fascioscapulohumeral; focal and segmental hyalinosis; follicle-stimulating hormone

FSHB follicle-stimulating hormone, beta chain

FSHD facioscapulohumeral dystrophy

FSH/LR-RH follicle-stimulating hormone and luteinizing hormone releasing hormone

FSHR follicle-stimulating hormone receptor

FSH-RF follicle-stimulating hormone-releasing factor

FSH-RH follicle-stimulating hormone-releasing hormone

FSHSMA facioscapulohumeral spinal muscular atrophy

FSI foam stability index; Food Sanitation Institute; functional status index; function status index

FSIQ full-scale intelligence quotient

FSL fasting serum level

FSMB Federation of State Medical Boards

FSN functional stimulation, neuromuscular

FSOP free-standing surgical outpatient facility

FSP familial spastic paraplegia; fibrin split products; fibrinogen split products; fine suspended particles

F-SP special form [Lat. *forma specialis*]

FSQ Functional Status Questionnaire

FSR Fellow of the Society of Radiographers; film screen radiography; force sensing resistor; fragmented sarcoplasmic reticulum; fusiform skin revision

FSRS functional status rating system

FSS focal segmental sclerosis; Freeman-Sheldon syndrome; French steel sound

FST foam stability test

FSU family service unit; functional spine unit

FSV feline fibrosarcoma virus; forward stroke volume; functional subunit

FSW field service worker

FT Fallot tetralogy; false transmitter; family therapy; fast twitch; fatigue trial; fibrous tissue; fingertip; follow through; Fourier transform; free testosterone; free thyroxine; full term; function test

FT$_3$ free triiodothyronine

FT$_4$ free thyroxine

Ft ferritin

fT free testosterone

ft foot, feet

FTA fluorescent titer antibody; fluorescent treponemal antibody

FTA-ABS, FTA-Abs fluorescent treponemal antibody, absorbed [test]

FTAG, F-TAG fast-binding target-attaching globulin

FTAS familial testicular agenesis syndrome

FTAT fluorescent treponemal antibody test

FTBD fit to be detained; full-term born dead

FTBE focal tick-borne encephalitis

FTBI fractionated total body irradiation

FTBS Family Therapist Behavioral Scale

FTC Federal Trade Commission; follicular thyroid carcinoma; frequency threshold curve; frequency tuning curve

ftc foot candle

FTD femoral total density

FDTS familial testicular dysgenesis syndrome

FTE full-time equivalent

FTEE full-time employe equivalent

FTF finger to finger

FTFT fast time frequency transform

FTG full-thickness graft

FTH ferritin heavy chain; fracture threshold

FTI free thyroxine index

FT$_3$I free triiodothyronine index

FT$_4$I free thyroxine index

FTIR Fourier-transformed infrared; functional terminal innervation ratio

FTKA failed to keep appointment

FTL ferritin light chain

ftL foot lambert

FTLB full-term live birth

ft lb foot pound

FTLV feline T-lymphotropic lentivirus

FTM fluid thioglycolate medium; fractional test meal

FTN finger to nose

FTNB full-term newborn

FTND full-term normal delivery

FTO fructose-terminated oligosaccharide

FTP file transfer protocol

FTR fractional tubular reabsorption

FTS family tracking system; feminizing testis syndrome; fetal tobacco syndrome; fissured tongue syndrome; flexortenosynovitis; thymulin [Fr. *facteur thymique sérique*]

FTSG full thickness skin graft

FTT failure to thrive; fat tolerance test

FTU fluorescence thiourea

FTVD full term vaginal delivery

FU fecal urobilinogen; fetal urobilinogen; fluorouracil; follow-up; flux unit [ion]; fractional urinalysis; fundus

Fu Finsen unit

F/U follow-up, fundus of umbilicus

F&U flanks and upper quadrants

5-FU 5-fluorouracil

FUB functional uterine bleeding

FUC fucosidase

Fuc fucose

FUCA fucosidase alpha

FUDR, FUdR fluorodeoxyuridine

FUFA free volatile fatty acid

FUM 5-fluorouracil and methotrexate; fumarate; fumigation

FUMIR 5-fluorouracil, mitomycin C, radiation

FUMP fluorouridine monophosphate

FUN follow-up note

funct function, functional

FUO fever of unknown origin

FUOV follow-up office visit

FUR 5-fluorouracil and radiation; fluorouracil riboside; fluorouridine; follow-up report; furin membrane-associated receptor

FUS feline urologic syndrome; first-use syndrome

FUT fibrinogen uptake test; fucosyl transferase

FUTP fluoridine triphosphate

FV femoral vein; fluid volume; Friend virus

FVA Friend virus anemia

FVC false vocal cord; forced vital capacity

FVE forced volume expiration

FVIC forced inspiratory vital capacity

FVL femoral vein ligation; flow volume loop; force, velocity, length

FVOP finger venous opening pressure

FVP Friend virus polycythemia

FVR feline viral rhinotracheitis; forearm vascular resistance

FVS fetal valproate syndrome

FVT follicular-variant-translocation

FW Felix-Weil [reaction]; Folin-Wu [reaction]; fragment wound

Fw F wave

fw fresh water

FWA Family Welfare Association

FWB full weight bearing

FWHM full width at half maximum

FWPCA Federal Water Pollution Control Administration

FWR Felix-Weil reaction; Folin-Wu reaction

FWTM full width tenth maximum

FX fluoroscopy; fornix; fracture frozen section

Fx fracture

fx fracture; friction

Fx-dis fracture-dislocation

FXN function

FXS fragile X syndrome

FY fiscal year

FYI for your information

FYMS fourth-year medical student

FZ focal zone; furazolidone

Fz frontal midline placement of electrodes in electroencephalography

FZS Fellow of the Zoological Society

G acceleration [force]; conductance; free energy; gallop; ganglion; gap; gas; gastrin; gauge; gauss; geometric efficiency; giga; gingiva, gingival; glabella; globular; globulin; glucose; glycine; glycogen; goat; gold inlay; gonidial; good; goose; grade; Grafenberg spot; gram; gravida; gravitation constant; Greek; green; guanidine; guanine; guanosine; gynecology; unit of force of acceleration

G_0 quiescent phase of cells leaving the mitotic cycle

G_1 presynthetic gap [phase of cells prior to DNA synthesis]

G_2 postsynthetic gap [phase of cells following DNA synthesis]

GI primigravida

GII secundigravida

GIII tertigravida

G° standard free energy

g force [pull of gravity]; gap; gender; grain; gram; gravity; group; ratio of magnetic moment of a particle to the Bohr magneton; standard acceleration due to gravity, 9.80665 m/s^2

^{g} relative centrifugal force

γ see *gamma*

GA Gamblers Anonymous; gastric analysis; gastric antrum; general anesthesia; general angiography; general appearance; gentisic acid; germ-cell antigen; gestational age; gibberellic acid; gingivoaxial; glucoamylase; glucose; glucose/acetone; glucuronic acid; Golgi apparatus; gramicidin A; granulocyte adherence; granuloma annulare; guessed average; gut-associated; gyrate atrophy

G/A globulin/albumin [ratio]

Ga gallium; granulocyte agglutination

ga gauge

GAA gossypol acetic acid

GAAS Goldberg Anorectic Attitude Scale

GABA, gaba gamma-aminobutyric acid

GABAT, GABA-T gamma-aminobutyric acid transaminase

GABHS group A beta-hemolytic streptococcus

GABOA gamma-amino-beta-hydroxybutyric acid

GABRA gamma-aminobutyric acid alpha receptor

GAD generalized anxiety disorder; glutamic acid decarboxylase

GADH gastric alcohol dehydrogenase

GADS gonococcal arthritis/dermatitis syndrome

GAF global assessment of functioning [scale]

GAFG goal attainment follow-up guide

GAG glycosaminoglycan; group-specific antigen gene

GAHS galactorrhea-amenorrhea hyperprolactinemia syndrome

GaIN Georgia Interactive Network for Medical Information

GAIPAS General Audit Inpatient Psychiatric Assessment Scale

GAL galactose; galactosyl; glucuronic acid lactone

Gal galactose

gal galactose; gallon

GALBP galactose-binding protein

GalC galactocerebroside

GALE galactose epimerase

GALK galactokinase

GalN galactosamine

Gal-1-P galactose-1-phosphate

GALT galactose-1-p-uridyltransferase; gut-associated lymphoid tissue

GALV gibbon ape leukemia virus

Galv, galv galvanic

γ Greek letter *gamma*; a carbon separated from the carboxyl group by two other carbon atoms; a constituent of the gamma protein plasma fraction; heavy chain of immunogammaglobulin; a monomer in fetal hemoglobin; photon

γG immunoglobulin G

GAME immunoglobulins G, A, M, and E

GAN giant axon neuropathy

G and D growth and development

gang, gangl ganglion, ganglionic

GANS granulomatous angiitis of the nervous system

GAO general accounting office

GAP D-glyceraldehyde-3-phosphate; growth associated protein; guanosine triphosphatase-activating protein

GAPD glyceraldehyde-3-phosphate dehydrogenase

GAPDH glyceraldehyde-3-phosphate dehydrogenase

GAPDP glyceraldehyde-3-phosphate dehydrogenase pseudogene

GAPO growth retardation, alopecia, pseudo-anodontia, and optic atrophy [syndrome]

GARS glycine amide phosphoribosyl synthetase

GAS galactorrhea-amenorrhea syndrome; gastric acid secretion; gastrin; gastroenterology; general adaptation syndrome; generalized arteriosclerosis; global anxiety score; global assessment scale; goal attainment scale; growth arrest-specific [gene]

GASA growth-adjusted sonographic age

gastroc gastrocnemius [muscle]

GAT gelatin agglutination test; geriatric assessment team; Gerontological Apperception Test; group adjustment therapy

GAWTS genomic amplification with transcript sequencing

GB gallbladder; glial bundle; goof balls; Guillain-Barré [syndrome]

Gb gilbert

GBA ganglionic blocking agent; gingivobuccoaxial

GBAP glucocerebrosidase pseudogene

GBD gallbladder disease; gender behavior disorder; glass blower's disease; granulomatous bowel disease

GBG glycine-rich beta-glycoprotein; gonadal steroid-binding globulin

GBH gamma-benzene hexachloride; graphite benzalkonium-heparin

GBHA glyoxal-bis-(2-hydroxyanil)

GBI globulin-binding insulin

GBIA Guthrie bacterial inhibition assay

GBL glomerular basal lamina

GBM glomerular basement membrane

GBP galactose-binding protein; gastric bypass; gated blood pool

Gbq gigabequerel

GBS gallbladder series; gastric bypass surgery; group B *Streptococcus*; general biopsychosocial screening; Guillain-Barré syndrome; glycerine-buffered saline [solution]

GBSS Gey's balanced saline solution; Guillain-Barré-Strohl syndrome

GC ganglion cell; gas chromatography; general circulation; general closure; general condition; generalizability coefficient; geriatric care; germinal center; glucocorticoid; goblet cell; Golgi cell; gonococcus; gonorrhea; granular casts; granulomatous colitis; granulosa cell; group-specific component; guanine cytosine; guanylcyclase

Gc gigacycle; gonococcus; group-specific component

GCA gastric cancer area; giant cell arteritis

g-cal gram calorie

GCAP germ-cell alkaline phosphatase

GCB gonococcal base

GCBM glomerular capillary basement membrane

GCD graft coronary disease

GCF growth-rate-controlling factor

GCFT gonococcal/gonorrhea complement fixation test

GCG glucagon

GCGR glucagon receptor; glucocorticoid receptor

GCI General Cognitive Index

GCIIS glucose controlled insulin infusion system

GCK glomerulocystic kidney; glucokinase

GCL globoid cell leukodystrophy

GCLO gastric *Campylobacter*-like organism

GCM Gorlin-Chaudhry-Moss [syndrome]

g-cm gram-centimeter

GC-MS gas chromatography-mass spectrometry

GCN geometric constraint network; giant cerebral neuron

g-coef generalizability coefficient

GCP geriatric cancer population; granulocyte chemotactic protein

GCPS Greig cephalopolysyndactyly syndrome

GCR glucocorticoid receptor; Group Conformity Rating

GCRC General Clinical Research Center [of NIH]

GCRS gynecological chylous reflux syndrome

GCS general clinical services; Gianotti-Crosti syndrome; Glasgow Coma Scale; glucocorticosteroid; glutamylcysteine synthetase; glycine cleavage system

GCSA Gross cell surface antigen

G-CSF granulocyte colony-stimulating factor

GCSFR granulocyte colony-stimulating factor receptor

GCSP glycine cleavage system protein

GCT general care and treatment; germ-cell tumor; giant cell thyroiditis; giant cell tumor

GC(T)A giant cell (temporal) arteritis

GCU gonococcal urethritis

GCV great cardiac vein

GCVF great cardiac vein flow

GCW glomerular capillary wall

GCWM General Conference on Weights and Measures

GCY gastroscopy

GD gastroduodenal; Gaucher disease; general diagnostics; general dispensary; gestational day; Gianotti disease; gonadal dysgenesis; Graves disease; growth and development; growth delay

Gd gadolinium

G&D growth and development

GDA gastroduodenal artery; germine diacetate; Graves disease autoantigen

GDB gas density balance; guide dogs for the blind

GDC giant dopamine-containing cell; General Dental Council

Gd-CDTA gadolinium-cyclohexane-diamine-tetraacetic acid

Gd-DOTA gadolinium-tetra-azacyclo-dodecatetraacetic acid

Gd-DTPA gadolinium-diethylene-triamine-pentaacetic acid

Gd-EDTA gadolinium diethylene-triamine-pentaacetic acid

GDF gel diffusion precipitin

GDH glucose dehydrogenase; glutamate dehydrogenase; glycerophosphate dehydrogenase; glycol dehydrogenase; gonadotropin hormone; growth and differentiation hormone

GDID genetically determined immunodeficiency disease

g/dl grams per deciliter

GDM gestational diabetes mellitus

GDMO General Duties Medical Officer

gDNA genomic deoxyribonucleic acid

GDNF giant cell line-derived neutrophilic factor

GDP gel diffusion precipitin; gross domestic product; guanosine diphosphate

GDS geriatric depression scale; Global Deterioration Scale; Gordon Diagnostic System [for attention disorders]; gradual dosage schedule; guanosine diphosphate dissociation stimulator

GDT geometrically deformable template

GDU gastroduodenal ulcer

GDW glass-distilled water

GDXY XY gonadal dysgenesis

GE gastric emptying; gastroemotional; gastroenteritis; gastroenterology; gastroenterostomy; gastroesophageal; gastrointestinal endoscopy; gel electrophoresis; generalized epilepsy; generator of excitation; gentamicin; glandular epithelium; gradient echo

Ge germanium

Ge⁻ Gerbich negative

G/E granulocyte/erythroid [ratio]

GEA gastric electrical activity

GEC galactose elimination capacity; glomerular epithelial cell

GECC Government Employees' Clinic Centre

GEE generalized estimating equation

GEF gastroesophageal fundoplication; glossoepiglottic fold; gonadotropin enhancing factor

GEH glycerol ester hydrolase

gel gelatin

GEMISCH Generalized Medical Information System for Community Health

GEMSS glaucoma-lens ecopia-microspherophakia-stiffness-shortness syndrome

GEN gender; generation

Gen genetics, genetic; genus

gen general; genital

genet genetic, genetics

GENETOX Genetic Toxicology [data base]

genit genitalia, genital

GENOVA generalized analysis of variance

GENPS genital neoplasm-papilloma syndrome

GENT gentamicin

GEP gastroenteropancreatic; gustatory evoked potential

GEPG gastroesophageal pressure gradient

GER gastroesophageal reflux; geriatrics; granular endoplasmic reticulum

Ger geriatric(s); German

GERD gastroesophageal reflux disease

geriat geriatrics, geriatric

GeriROS geriatric review of systems

GERL Golgi-associated endoplasmic reticulum lysosome

Geront gerontology, gerontologist, gerontologic

GERRI geriatric evaluation by relative rating instrument

GES gastroesophageal sphincter; glucose-electrolyte solution

GESICA Argentinian Study Group for the Prevention of Cardiac Insufficiency [Grupo de Estudio de la Sobrevida en la Insuficiencia Cardiaca en Argentina]

GEST, gest gestation; gestational

GET gastric emptying time; general endotracheal [anesthesia]; graded treadmill exercise test

GEU geriatric evaluation unit

Gev giga electron volt

GEWS Gianturco expandable wire stent

GEX gas exchange

GF gastric fistula; gastric fluid; germ-free; glass factor; glomerular filtration; gluten-free; grandfather; growth factor; growth failure

gf gram-force

GFA glial fibrillary acidic [protein]

GF-AAS graphite furnace atomic absorption spectroscopy

GFAP glial fibrillary acidic protein

GFAT glutamine:fructose-6-phosphate amidotransferase

GFCI ground-fault circuit-interrupter

GFD gingival fibromatosis-progressive deafness [syndrome]; gluten-free diet
GFFS glycogen and fat-free solid
GFH glucose-free Hanks [solution]
GFI glucagon-free insulin; goodness-of-fit index; ground-fault interrupter
GFL giant follicular lymphoma
GFP gamma-fetoprotein; gel-filtered platelet; glomerular filtered phosphate
GFR glomerular filtration rate
GFRP growth factor response protein
GFS global focal sclerosis; guafenesin
GG gamma globulin; genioglossus; glycylglycine
GGA general gonadotropic activity
GGC gamma-glutamyl carboxylase
GGCS gamma-glutamyl cysteine synthetase
GGE generalized glandular enlargement; gradient gel electrophoresis
GGFC gamma-globulin-free calf [serum]
GGG glycine-rich gamma-glycoprotein
GGM glucose-galactose malabsorption
GG or S glands, goiter, or stiffness [of neck]
GGPNA gamma-glutamyl-p-nitroanilide
GGT gamma-glutamyl transferase; gamma-glutamyl transpeptidase; geranylgeranyltransferase
GGTB glycoprotein 4-beta-galactosyl transferase
GGTP gamma-glutamyl transpeptidase
GGVB gelatin, glucose, and veronal buffer
GH general health; general hospital; genetic hypertension; genetically hypertensive [rat]; geniohyoid; growth hormone
GHA Group Health Association
GHAA Group Health Association of America
GHB gamma hydroxybutyrate
GHb glycated hemoglobin
GHBA gamma-hydroxybutyric acid
GHBP growth hormone binding protein

GHC group health cooperative
GHD growth hormone deficiency
GHDD ghosal hematodiaphyseal dysplasia
GHF growth hormone factor
GHL growth hormone-like
GHPM general health policy model
GHPQ General Health Perception Questionnaire
GHQ General Health Questionnaire
GHR granulomatous hypersensitivity reaction
GHRF growth hormone-releasing factor
GHRFR growth hormone-releasing releasing factor
GH-RH growth hormone-releasing hormone
GHRHR growth hormone-releasing hormone receptor
GHRI general health rating index
GH-RIF growth hormone-release inhibiting factor
GH-RIH growth hormone-release inhibiting hormone
GHV goose hepatitis virus; growth hormone variant
GHz gigahertz
GI gastrointestinal; gelatin infusion [medium]; gingival index; globin insulin; glomerular index; glucose intolerance; granuloma inguinale; growth inhibition
gi gill
GIA gastrointestinal anastomosis
GIB gastrointestinal bleeding
GIBF gastrointestinal bacterial flora
GICA gastrointestinal cancer
GID gender identity disorder
GIF gastric intrinsic factor; growth hormone-inhibiting factor
GIFB growth hormone inhibitory factor, brain
GIFT gamete intrafallopian transfer; granulocyte immunofluorescence test
GIGO garbage in, garbage out

GIH gastrointestinal hemorrhage; growth-inhibiting hormone
GII gastrointestinal infection
GIK glucose-insulin-potassium [solution]
GIM general internal medicine; gonadotropin-inhibiting material
Ging, ging gingiva, gingival
g-ion gram-ion
GIP gastric inhibitory polypeptide; giant cell interstitial pneumonia; glucose-dependent insulinotropic peptide; gonorrheal invasive peritonitis
GIPR gastric inhibitory polypeptide receptor
GIR global improvement rating
GIS gas in stomach; gastrointestinal series; geographic information system; guaranteed income supplement
GISSI Italian Study Group for the Prevention of Myocardial Infarction [Gruppo Italiano per lo Studio della Sopravivenza nell'Infarto Miocardico]
GIT gastrointestinal tract
GITS gastrointestinal therapeutic system
GITSG gastrointestinal tumor study group
GITT gastrointestinal transit time; glucose insulin tolerance test
GJ gap junction; gastric juice; gastrojejunostomy
GJA-S gastric juice aspiration syndrome
GK galactokinase; glomerulocystic kidney; glycerol kinase
GKD glycerol kinase deficiency
GKI glucose potassium insulin
GL gland; glomerular layer; glycolipid; glycosphingolipid; glycyrrhizin; greatest length; gustatory lacrimation
Gl beryllium [Lat. *glucinium*]; glabella
gl gill; gland, glandular
g/l grams per liter
GL-4 glycophospholipid
GLA galactosidase A; gamma-linolenic acid; gingivolinguoaxial
glac glacial
GLAD gold-labelled antigen detection

gland glandular
GLAT galactose + activator
GLB galactosidase beta
GLC gas-liquid chromatography
Glc glucose
glc glaucoma
GlcA gluconic acid
GLC-MS gas-liquid chromatography-mass spectrometry
GlcN glucosamine
GlcUA D-glucuronic acid
GLD globoid leukodystrophy; glutamate dehydrogenase
GLDH glutamic dehydrogenase
GLH germinal layer hemorrhage; giant lymph node hyperplasia
GLI glicentin; glucagon-like immunoreactivity
GLIM generalized linear interactive model
GLM general linear model
GLN glutamine
Gln glucagon; glutamine
GLNH giant lymph node hyperplasia
GLNN galanin
GLO glyoxylase
GLO1 glyoxylase 1
glob globular; globulin
GLP glucagon-like peptide; glucose-L-phosphate; glycolipoprotein; good laboratory practice; group living program
GLPR glucagon-like peptide receptor
GLR graphic level recorder
GLRA glycine receptor alpha
GLRB glycine receptor beta
GLS generalized lymphadenopathy syndrome
GLTN glomerulotubulonephritis
GLTT glucose-lactate tolerance test
GLU glucose; glucuronidase; glutamate; glutamic acid
Glu glucuronidase; glutamic acid; glutamine
glu glucose; glutamate
GLU-5 five-hour glucose tolerance test

GLUC glucosidase

gluc glucose

GLUD glutamate dehydrogenase

GLUDP glutamate dehydrogenase pseudogene

GLUL glutamate (ammonia) ligase

GLUR glutamate receptor

GLUT glucose transporter

GLV gibbon ape leukemia virus; Gross leukemia virus

GLVR gibbon ape leukemia virus receptor

Glx glucose; glutamic acid

GLY, gly glycine

glyc glyceride

GM gastric mucosa; Geiger-Müller [counter]; general medicine; genetic manipulation; geometric mean; giant melanosome; gram; grand mal [epilepsy]; grandmother; grand multiparity; granulocyte-macrophage; gray matter; growth medium

GM⁺ gram-positive

GM⁻ gram-negative

G-M Geiger-Müller [counter]

G/M granulocyte/macrophage

Gm an allotype marker on the heavy chains of immunoglobins

gm gram

g-m gram-meter

GMA glyceral methacrylate

GMB gastric mucosal barrier; granulomembranous body

GMBF gastric mucosa blood flow

GMC general medical clinic; general medical council; giant migratory contraction; grivet monkey cell

gm cal gram calorie

gm/cc grams per cubic centimeter

GMCD grand mal convulsive disorder

GM-CFU granulocyte-macrophage colony forming unit

GM-CSA granulocyte-macrophage colony-stimulating activity

GM-CSF granulocyte-macrophage colony-stimulating factor

GMD geometric mean diameter; glycopeptide moiety modified derivative

GME graduate medical education

GMENAC Graduate Medical Education National Advisory Committee

GMH germinal matrix hemorrhage

GMK green monkey kidney [cells]

GML gut mucosa lymphocyte

g/ml grams per milliliter

gm/l grams per liter

gm-m gram-meter

GMN gradient moment nulling

g-mol gram-molecule

GMP glucose monophosphate; good manufacturing practice; granule membrane protein; guanosine monophosphate

3':5'-GMP guanosine 3':5'-cyclic phosphate

GMPR guanine monophosphate reductase

GMR gallops, murmurs, rubs; gradient motion rephasing

GMRH germinal matrix related hemorrhage

GMRI gated magnetic resonance imaging

GMS General Medical Service; geriatric mental state; Gilbert-Meulengracht syndrome; Gomori methenamine silver [stain]; goniodysgenesis-mental retardation-short stature [syndrome]; glyceryl monostearate

GM&S general medicine and surgery

GMSC General Medical Services Committee

GMT geometric mean titer; gingival margin trimmer

GMV gram molecular volume

GMW gram molecular weight

GN gaze nystagmus; glomerulonephritis; glucose nitrogen [ratio]; gnotobiote; graduate nurse; gram-negative; guanine nucleotide

G/N glucose/nitrogen ratio

Gn gnathion; gonadotropin

GNA general nursing assistance

GNAT guanine nucleotide-binding protein, alpha-transducing

GNAZ guanosine nucleotide-binding alpha Z polypeptide

GNB ganglioneuroblastoma; gram-negative bacillus; guanine nucleotide-binding [protein]

GNBM gram-negative bacillary meningitis

GNBT guanine nucleotide-binding protein, beta transducing

GNC general nursing care; General Nursing Council; geriatric nurse clinician

GND Gram-negative diplococci

GNID gram-negative intracellular diplococci

GNP geriatric nurse practitioner; gerontologic nurse practitioner

GNR gram-negative rods

GnRF gonadotropin-releasing factor

GnRH gonadotropin-releasing hormone

GnRHR gonadotropin-releasing hormone receptor

G/NS glucose in normal saline [solution]

GNTP Graduate Nurse Transition Program

GO gastro-[o]esophageal; geroderma osteodysplastica; gonorrhea; glucose oxidase

G&O gas and oxygen

Go gonion

GOA generalized osteoarthritis

GOAT Galveston Orientation and Amnesia Test

GOBAB gamma-hydroxy-beta-aminobutyric acid

GOE gas, oxygen, and ether

GOG Gynecologic Oncology Group

GOH geroderma osteodysplastica hereditaria

GΩ gigaohm [one billion ohms]

GON gonococcal ophthalmia neonatorum

GOND glaucomatous optic nerve damage

GOQ glucose oxidation quotient

GOR gastroesophageal reflux; general operating room

GOS Glasgow outcome score

GOT aspartate aminotransferase; glucose oxidase test; glutamate oxaloacetate transaminase; goal of treatment

GOTM glutamic-oxaloacetic transaminase, mitochondrial

GP gangliocytic paraganglioma; gastroplasty; general paralysis, general paresis; general practice, general practitioner; genetic prediabetes; geometric progression; globus pallidus; glucose phosphate; glutathione peroxidase; glycerophosphate; glycopeptide; glycophorin; glycoprotein; Goodpasture syndrome; grampositive; guinea pig; gutta percha

G/P gravida/para

G-1-P glucose-1-phosphate

G3P, G-3-P glyceraldehyde-3-phosphate; glycerol-3-phosphate

G6P, G-6-P glucose-6-phosphate

Gp glycoprotein

gp gene product; glycoprotein; group

GPA Goodpasture antigen; grade point average; Group Practice Association; guinea pig albumin

GPAIS guinea pig anti-insulin serum

G6Pase, G-6-Pase glucose-6-phosphatase

GPB glossopharyngeal breathing; glycophorin B

GPC gastric parietal cell; gel permeation chromatography; giant papillary conjunctivitis; glycophorin C; granular progenitor cell; guinea pig complement

GPCI geographic practice cost index

GPD glucose-6-phosphate dehydrogenase; glycerol-phosphate dehydrogenase

G3PD glucose-3-phosphate dehydrogenase

G6PD, G-6-PD glucose-6-phosphate dehydrogenase

G-6-PDA glucose-6-phosphate dehydrogenase enzyme variant A

G6PDH, G-6-PDH glucose-6-phosphate dehydrogenase reduced

G6PDL glucose-6-phosphate dehydrogenase-like

GPE guinea pig embryo; granulocyte colony-stimulating factor promoter element

GPEBP granulocyte colony-stimulating factor promoter element binding protein

GPEP General Professional Education of the Physician

GPET graphic plan evaluation tool

GPF glomerular plasma flow; granulocytosis-promoting factor

GPGG guinea pig gamma-globulin

GPh Graduate in Pharmacy

GPHN giant pigmented hairy nevus

GPHV guinea pig herpes virus

GPI general paralysis of the insane; glucose phosphate isomerase; glycoprotein I; glycosylphosphatidylinositol; guinea pig ileum

GpIb glycoprotein Ib

GPIMH guinea pig intestinal mucosal homogenate

GPIPID guinea pig intraperitoneal infectious dose

GPK guinea pig kidney [antigen]

GPKA guinea pig kidney absorption [test]

GPLV guinea pig leukemia virus

Gply gingivoplasty

GPM general preventive medicine; giant pigmented melanosome

GPMAL gravida, para, multiple births, abortions, and live births

GPN graduate practical nurse

GPOA primary open angle glaucoma

GPP generalist physician program; gross primary production

GPPQ General Purpose Psychiatric Questionnaire

GPRBC guinea pig red blood cell

GPS Goodpasture syndrome; gray platelet syndrome; guinea pig serum; guinea pig spleen

GPT glutamate-pyruvate transaminase; glutamic-pyruvic transaminase

GpTh group therapy

GPU guinea pig unit

GPUT galactose phosphate uridyl transferase

GPWW group practice without wall

GPX glutathione peroxidase

GPx glutathione peroxidase

GQAP general question-asking program

GR gamma-rays; gastric resection; general research; generalized rash; glucocorticoid receptor; glutathione reductase

gr grade; graft; grain; gram; gravity; gray; gross

gr⁻ gram-negative

gr⁺ gram-positive

GRA gated radionuclide angiography; glucocorticoid-remedial aldosteronism; gonadotropin-releasing agent

GRABS group A beta-hemolytic streptococcal pharyngitis

grad gradient; gradually; graduate

GRAE generally regarded as effective

gran granule, granulated

GRANDDAD growth delay-aged facies-normal development-deficiency of subcutaneous fat [syndrome]

GRAS generally recognized as safe

GRASS gradient recalled acquisition in a steady state

grav gravid

grav I pregnancy one, primigravida

grav II pregnancy two, secundagravida

GRB growth factor receptor-binding protein

GRD gastroesophageal reflux disease; gender role definition

grd ground

GRE glucocorticoid response element; gradient-recalled echo; Graduate Record Examination

GRECC Geriatric Research and Education Clinical Center

GREPCO Rome Group for the Epidemiology and Prevention of Cholelithiasis

GRF gastrin-releasing factor; genetically related macrophage factor; gonadotropin-releasing factor; growth hormone-releasing factor

GRG glycine-rich glycoprotein

GRH growth hormone-releasing hormone

GRHR gonadotropic-releasing hormone receptor

GRIA glutamate receptor, ionotropic, ampa

GRID gay-related immunodeficiency [syndrome]

GRIF growth hormone release-inhibiting factor

GRIK glutamate receptor, ionotropic, kainate

GRINA glutamate receptor, ionotropic, N-methyl-D-aspartate A

GRINB glutamate receptor, ionotropic, N-methyl-D-aspartate B

GRMP granulocyte membrane protein

GRN granules; granulin

GrN gram-negative

Grn green

GRO growth-related [protein]

GROB growth-related protein beta

GROG growth-related protein gamma

GRP gastrin-releasing peptide; glucose-regulated protein

GrP gram-positive

Gr$_1$P$_0$AB$_1$ one pregnancy, no births, one abortion

GRPR gastrin-releasing peptide receptor

GRPS glucose-Ringer-phosphate solution

GRS Golabi-Rosen syndrome

GRV ground reaction vector

GRW giant ragweed [test]

gr wt gross weight

GS gallstone; Gardner syndrome; gastric shield; general surgery; gestational score; Gilbert syndrome; glomerular sclerosis; glutamine synthetase; goat serum; Goldenhar syndrome; Goodpasture syndrome; graft survival; granulocytic sarcoma; grip strength; group section; group-specific

G6S glucosamine-6-sulfatase

gs group specific

G/S glucose and saline

g/s gallons per second

GSA general somatic afferent; group-specific antigen; Gross virus antigen; guanidinosuccinic acid

GSBG gonadal steroid-binding globulin

GSC gas-solid chromatography; gravity settling culture

GSCN giant serotonin-containing neuron

GSD genetically significant dose; Gerstmann-Sträussler disease; glutathione synthetase deficiency; glycogen storage disease

GSD-0 glycogen storage disease-zero

GSE general somatic efferent; gluten-sensitive enteropathy

GSF galactosemic fibroblast; genital skin fibroblast

GSFR granulocyte colony-stimulating factor receptor

GSH glomerulus-stimulating hormone; golden Syrian hamster; reduced glutathione; L-alpha-glutamyl-L-cysteinyl-glycine

GSH-Px glutathione peroxidase

GSI global severity index

GSN gelsonin; giant serotonin-containing neuron

GSoA Gerontological Society of America

GSP galvanic skin potential

GSR galvanic skin response; generalized Shwartzman reaction; glutathione reductase

GSS gamete-shedding substance; General Social Survey; Gerstmann-Sträussler-Scheinker [disease]

GSSD Gerstmann-Sträussler-Scheinker disease
GSSG oxidized glutathione
GSSG-R glutathione reductase
GSSR generalized Sanarelli-Shwartzman reaction
GST glutathione-S-transferase; gold salt therapy; gold sodium thiomalate; graphic stress telethermometry; group striction
GSTA glutathione-S-transferase, alpha
GST1L glutathione-S-transferase-1-like
GSTM glutathione-S-transferase, mu
GSV gestational sac volume
GSW gunshot wound
GSWA gunshot wound, abdominal
GT gait training; galactosyl transferase; gastrostomy; generation time; genetic therapy; gingiva treatment; Glanzmann thrombasthenia; glucose therapy; glucose tolerance; glucose transport; glucuronyl transferase; glutamyl transpeptidase; glycityrosine; granulation tissue; great toe; greater trochanter; group tensions; group therapy
GT1-GT10 glycogen storage disease, types 1 to 10
gt drop [Lat. *gutta*]
g/t granulation time; granulation tissue
G&T gowns and towels
GTA gene transfer agent; Glanzmann thrombasthenia; glycerol teichoic acid
GTB gastrointestinal tract bleeding
GTD gestational trophoblastic disease
GTEM gigahertz transverse electromagnetic [cell]
GTF glucose tolerance factor; glucosyltransferase
GTH gonadotropic hormone
GTHR generalized thyroid hormone resistance
GTI grid tiler
GTM generalized tendomyopathy
GTN gestational trophoblastic neoplasia; glomerulotubulonephritis; glyceryl trinitrate

GTO Golgi tendon organ
GTP glutamyl transpeptidase; guanosine triphosphate
GTPase guanosine triphosphatase
GTR galvanic tetanus ratio; granulocyte turnover rate
GTS Gilles de la Tourette syndrome; glucose transport system
GTT gelatin-tellurite-taurocholate [agar]; glucose tolerance test
GTV gross tumor volume
GU gastric ulcer; genitourinary; glucose uptake; glycogenic unit; gonococcal urethritis; gravitational ulcer; guanethidine
GUA group of units of analysis
Gua guanine
GUCA guanylate cyclase activator
GUD genitourinary dysplasia
GUI graphic user interface
GUK guanylate kinase
GULHEMP general physique, upper extremity, lower extremity, hearing, eyesight, mentality, and personality
Guo guanosine
GUS genitourinary sphincter; genitourinary system
GUSTO Global Utilization of Streptokinase and Tissue Plasminogen Activator for Occluded Coronary Arteries [trial]
GV gastric volume; gas ventilation; gentian violet; germinal vesicle; granulosis virus; griseoviridan; Gross virus
GVA general visceral afferent [nerve]
GVB gelatin-Veronal buffer
GVBD germinal vesicle breakdown
GVE general visceral efferent [nerve]
GVF good visual fields
GVG gamma-vinyl-gamma-aminobutyric acid
GVH, GvH graft-versus-host
GVHD, GvHD graft-versus-host disease
GVHR, GvHR graft-versus-host reaction
GVL graft versus leukemia

G vs HD graft versus host disease
GVTY gingivectomy
GW germ warfare; gigawatt; glycerin in water; gradual withdrawal; group work
G/W glucose in water
GWB general well-being [schedule]
GWE glycerol and water enema
GWG generalized Wegener granulomatosis

GWUHP George Washington University Health Plan
GX glycinexylidide
GXT graded exercise test
Gy gray
GY-1 graduate year one
GYN, Gyn, gyn gynecologic, gynecologist, gynecology
GZ Guilford-Zimmerman [test]

H bacterial antigen in serologic classification of bacteria [Ger. *Hauch*, film]; deflection in the His bundle in electrogram [spike]; dose equivalent; draft [Lat. *haustus*]; electrically induced spinal reflex; enthalpy; fucosal transferase-producing gene; heart; heavy [strand]; height; hemagglutination; hemisphere; hemolysis; *Hemophilus;* henry; heparin; heroin; high; histidine; *Histoplasma;* histoplasmosis; Holzknecht unit; homosexual; horizontal; hormone; horse; hospital; Hounsfield unit; hour; human; hydrogen; hydrolysis; hygiene; hyoscine; hypermetropia; hyperopia; hypodermic; hypothalamus; magnetic field strength; magnetization; mustard gas; oersted; the region of a sarcomere containing only myosin filaments [Ger. *heller,* lighter] [band]

H⁺ hydrogen ion

[H⁺] hydrogen ion concentration

H_0 null hypothesis

H1, ¹H, H¹ protium

H_1 alternative hypothesis

H2, ²H, H² deuterium

H₂ blockers histamine blockers

H3, ³H, H³ tritium

h hand-rearing [of experimental animals]; heat transfer coefficient; hecto; height; henry; hour [Lat. *hora*]; human; hundred; hypodermic; negatively staining region of a chromosome; Planck constant; secondary constriction; specific enthalpy

H1/2 half-value layer

HA H antigen; Hakim-Adams [syndrome]; halothane anesthesia; Hartley [guinea pig]; headache; health alliance; hearing aid; height age; hemadsorption; hemagglutinating antibody; hemagglutination; hemagglutinin; hemolytic anemia; hemophiliac with adenopathy; hepatic adenoma; hepatic artery; hepatitis A; hepatitis-associated; heterophil antibody; Heyden antibiotic; high anxiety; hippuric acid; histamine; histocompatibility antigen; Horton arteritis; hospital administration; hospital admission; hospital apprentice; Hounsfield unit; human albumin; hyaluronic acid; hydroxyapatite; hyperalimentation; hyperandrogenism; hypersensitivity alveolitis; hypothalamic amenorrhea

H/A head to abdomen; headache

HA2 hemadsorption virus 2

Ha absolution hypermetropia; hafnium; hamster; Hartmann number

ha hectare

HAA hearing aid amplifier; hemolytic anemia antigen; hepatitis-associated antigen; hospital activity analysis

HA Ag hepatitis A antigen

HAB histoacryl blue

HABA 2(4'-hydroxyazobenzene) benzoic acid

HABF hepatic artery blood flow

HACEK *Haemophilus, Actinobacillus, Cardiobacterium, Eikinella, Kingella*

HAChT high affinity choline transport

HACR hereditary adenomatosis of the colon and rectum

hACSP human adenylate cyclase-stimulating protein

HACS hyperactive child syndrome

HAD health care alternatives development; hemadsorption; hospital administration, hospital administrator

HAd hemadsorption; hospital administrator

HADH hydroxyacyl CoA dehydrogenase

HAd-I hemadsorption-inhibition

HADS hospital anxiety and depression scale
HAE health appraisal examination; hearing aid evaluation; hepatic artery embolism; hereditary angioneurotic edema
HAF hyperalimentation fluid
HaF Hageman factor
HAFP human alpha-fetoprotein
HAG heat-aggregated globulin
HAGG hyperimmune antivariola gammaglobulin
HAGH hydroxyacyl-glutathione hydrolase
HAHTG horse antihuman thymus globulin
HAI hemagglutination inhibition; hepatic arterial infusion
H&A Ins health and accident insurance
HAIR-AN hyperandrogenism, insulin resistance, and acanthosis nigricans [syndrome]
HaK hamster kidney
HAL hepatic artery ligation; hypoplastic acute leukemia
hal halogen; halothane
HALC high affinity-low capacity
HALFD hypertonic albumin-containing fluid demand
halluc hallucinations
HALO Halotestin
HALP hyperalphalipoproteinemia
HaLV hamster leukemia virus
HAM hearing aid microphone; helical axis in motion; human albumin microsphere; human alveolar macrophage; hypoparathyroidism, Addison disease, and mucocutaneous candidiasis [syndrome]
HAm human amnion
HAMA Hamilton anxiety [scale]; human anti-murine antibody
HAMD Hamilton depression [scale]
Ha-MSV Harvey murine sarcoma virus
HAN heroin-associated nephropathy; hyperplastic alveolar nodule
HANA hemagglutinin neuraminidase

H and E hematoxylin and eosin [stain]
Handicp handicapped
HANE hereditary angioneurotic edema
HANES Health and Nutrition Examination Survey
hANF human atrial natriuretic factor
h-ANP human atrial natriuretic polypeptide
HAP Handicapped Aid Program; Hazardous Air Pollutants [List]; hazardous air pollution; health alliance plan; heredopathia atactica polyneuritiformis; high-altitude peristalsis; histamine acid phosphate; hospital admissions program; humoral antibody production; hydrolyzed animal protein; hydroxyapatite
HAp hydroxyapatite
HAPA hemagglutinating anti-penicillin antibody
HAPC high-amplitude peristaltic contraction; hospital-acquired penetration contact
HAPE high-altitude pulmonary edema
HAPPHY Heart Attack Primary Prevention in Hypertension
HAPS hepatic arterial perfusion scintigraphy
HAPVC hemi-anomalous pulmonary venous connection
HAPVD hemi-anomalous pulmonary venous drainage
HAPVR hemi-anomalous pulmonary venous return
HAQ health assessment questionnaire
HAR high-altitude retinopathy
HARD hydrocephalus-agyria-retinal dysplasia [syndrome]
HARD +/– E hydrocephalus-agyria-retinal dysplasia plus or minus encephalocele [syndrome]
HAREM heparin assay rapid easy method
HARH high-altitude retinal hemorrhage
HARM heparin assay rapid method
HARP homeless and at-risk population

HARS histidyl-RNA synthetase

HART Heparin-Aspirin Reinfarction Trial

HAS Hamilton Anxiety Scale; health advisory service; highest asymptomatic [dose]; hospital administrative service; hospital advisory service; human albumin solution; hyperalimentation solution; hypertensive arteriosclerotic

HASCVD hypertensive arteriosclerotic cardiovascular disease

HASHD hypertensive arteriosclerotic heart disease

HASP Hospital Admissions and Surveillance Program

HASS highest anxiety subscale score

HAT Halsted Aphasia Test; head, arm, trunk; heparin-associated thrombocytopenia; heterophil antibody titer; hospital arrival time; hypoxanthine, aminopterin, and thymidine; hypoxanthine, azaserine, and thymidine

HATG horse antihuman thymocyte globulin

HATH Heterosexual Attitudes Toward Homosexuality [scale]

HATT heparin-associated thrombocytopenia and thrombosis

HATTS hemagglutination treponemal test for syphilis

HAU hemagglutinating unit

HAV hemadsorption virus; hepatitis A virus

HAWIC Hamburg-Wechsler Intelligence Test for Children

HAZ MAT hazardous material

HAZWOPER Hazardous Waste Operation and Emergency Response [of OSHA]

HB health board; heart block; heel to buttock; held back; hemoglobin; hepatitis B; His bundle; hold breakfast; housebound; hybridoma bank; hyoid body

Hb hemoglobin

HbA hemoglobin A, adult hemoglobin

HBA$_1$ glycosylated hemoglobin

HBAb hepatitis B antibody

HBABA hydroxybenzeneazobenzoic acid

HBAg hepatitis B antigen

HB$_s$AG hepatitis B surface virus

HBB hemoglobin beta-chain; hospital blood bank; hydroxybenzyl benzimidazole

HbBC hemoglobin binding capacity

HBBW hold breakfast blood work

HBC hereditary breast cancer

HB$_c$, HBC, HBc hepatitis B core [antigen]

HbC hemoglobin C

HB$_c$Ag, HBcAg, HBCAG hepatitis B core antigen

HBCG heat-aggregated Calmette-Guérin bacillus

HbCO carboxyhemoglobin

Hb CS hemoglobin Constant Spring

HbCV *Haemophilus influenzae* conjugate vaccine

HBD has been drinking; hydroxybutyric dehydrogenase; hypophosphatemic bone disease

HbD hemoglobin D

HBDH hydroxybutyrate dehydrogenase

HBDT human basophil degranulation test

HBE His bundle electrogram

HbE hemoglobin E

HB$_e$Ag, HBeAg, HBEAG hepatitis B early [antigen]

HBF hand blood flow; hemispheric blood flow; hemoglobinuric bilious fever; hepatic blood flow; hypothalamic blood flow

HbF fetal hemoglobin, hemoglobin F

Hbg hemoglobin

HBGF heparin-binding growth factor

HBGM home blood glucose monitoring

HBGR hemoglobin-gamma regulator

HbH hemoglobin H

Hb-Hp hemoglobin-haptoglobin [complex]

HBI high serum-bound iron
HBIG, HBIg hepatitis B immunoglobulin
HBL hepatoblastoma
HBLA human B-cell lymphocyte antigen
HBLV human B-cell lymphotropic virus
HBM health belief model; hypertonic buffered medium
HbM hemoglobin Milwaukee
HbMet methemoglobin
HBO hyperbaric oxygenation, hyperbaric oxygen
HbO oxyhemoglobin
HbO$_2$ oxyhemoglobin
HBOC hereditary breast-ovarian cancer
HBOT hyperbaric oxygen therapy
HBP heartbeat period; hepatic binding protein; high blood pressure; hospital-based practice
HbP primitive hemoglobin
HBr hydrobromic acid
HbR reduced hemoglobin
HBS hepatitis B surface [antigen]; hyperkinetic behavior syndrome
HB$_s$ hepatitis B surface [antigen]
HbS hemoglobin S, sickle-cell hemoglobin
HBSAg IgG antibody to HBsAg
HB$_s$Ag, HBsAg, HBSAG hepatitis B surface antigen
HBsAg/adr hepatitis B surface antigen manifesting group-specific determinant *a* and subtype-specific determinants *d* and *r*
HBSC hematopoietic blood stem cell
HBSS Hank's balanced salt solution
HbSS hemoglobin SS
HBT human brain thromboplastin; human breast tumor
Hb$_{tot}$ total hemoglobin
HBV hepatitis B vaccine; hepatitis B virus
HBV-MN membranous nephropathy associated with hepatitis B virus
HBVS hepatitis B virus integration site

HBW high birth weight
HbZ hemoglobin Z, hemoglobin Zürich
HC hair cell; hairy cell; handicapped; head circumference; head compression; health care; healthy control; heat conservation; heavy chain; hemoglobin concentration; hemorrhagic colitis; heparin cofactor; hepatic catalase; hepatocellular; hereditary coproporphyria; hippocampus; histamine challenge; histochemistry; home care; Hospital Corps; house call; Huntington chorea; hyaline casts; hydraulic concussion; hydrocarbon; hydrocortisone; hydroxycorticoid; hyoid cornu; hypercholesterolemia; hypertrophic cardiomyopathy
H&C hot and cold
Hc hydrocolloid
HCA heart cell aggregate; hepatocellular adenoma; home care aide; Hospital Corporation of America; hydrocortisone acetate
HCAP handicapped
HCA/W home care aide or worker
HCB hexachlorobenzene
HCC hepatitis contagiosa canis; hepatocellular carcinoma; history of chief complaint; hydroxycholecalciferol
25-HCC 25-hydroxycholecalciferol
HCD health care delivery; heavy-chain disease; high-calorie diet; high-carbohydrate diet; homologous canine distemper
HCE hypoglossal carotid entrapment
HCF [fetal] head-to-cervix force; heparin cofactor; hereditary capillary fragility; highest common factor; hypocaloric carbohydrate feeding
HCFA Health Care Financing Administration (pronounced Hickfa)
hCFSH human chorionic follicle-stimulating hormone
HCG, hCG human chorionic gonadotropin
HCH Health Care for the Homeless; hexachlorocyclohexane; hemochromatosis

HCHP Harvard Community Health Plan
HCHWA hereditary cerebral hemorrhage with amyloidosis
HCI Health Commons Institute; human collagenase inhibitor
HcImp hydrocolloid impression
HCIS Health Care Information System
HCK hematopoietic cell kinase
HCL hairy-cell leukemia; human cultured lymphoblasts
HCl hydrogen chloride
HCLF high carbohydrate, low fiber [diet]
HCM health care management; hypertrophic cardiomyopathy
HCMM hereditary cutaneous malignant melanoma
HCMV human cytomegalovirus
HCN hereditary chronic nephritis
HCO health care organization
HCO$_3^-$ bicarbonate
HCOP health center opportunity program
HCP handicapped; hepatocatalase peroxidase; hereditary coproporphyria; hexachlorophene; high cell passage
H&CP hospital and community psychiatry
HCPCS Health Care Financing Administration common procedural collecting system; Health Care Financing Administrators Common Procedure Coding System
HCPH hematopoietic cell phosphatase
HCPOTP health care professionals other than physicians
HCPP health care prepayment plan
HCQI health care quality improvement (pronounced Hicky)
HCQIA Health Care Quality Improvement Act
HCQIP Health Care Quality Improvement Program [of HCFA]
HCR heme-controlled repressor; host-cell reactivation; hysterical conversion reaction

HCRE Homeopathic Council for Research and Education
hCRH human corticotropin-releasing hormone
Hcrit hematocrit
HCS Hajdu-Cheney syndrome; Hazard Communication Standard; health care support; hourglass contraction of the stomach; human chorionic somatotropin; human cord serum
17-HCS 17-hydroxycorticosteroid
hCS human chorionic somatomammotropin
HCSD Health Care Studies Division
hCSM human chorionic somatomammotropin
HCSS hypersensitive carotid sinus syndrome
HCT health check test; hematocrit; historic control trial; homocytotrophic; human calcitonin; hydrochlorothiazide; hydroxycortisone
Hct hematocrit
hCT human calcitonin; human chorionic thyrotropin
HCTA health care technology assessment
HCTC Health Care Technology Center
HCTD hepatic computed tomography density
HCTS high cholesterol and tocopherol supplement
HCTU home cervical traction unit
HCTZ hydrochlorothiazide
HCU homocystinuria; hyperplasia cystica uteri
HCV hepatitis C virus; hog cholera virus
HCVD hypertensive cardiovascular disease
HCVS human coronavirus sensitivity
HCW health care worker
Hcy homocysteine
HD Haab-Dimmer [syndrome]; Hajna-Damon [broth]; Hansen disease; hearing distance; heart disease; helix destabilizing

[protein]; hemidiaphragm; hemodialysis; hemolytic disease; hemolyzing dose; herniated disc; high density; high dose; hip disarticulation; Hirschsprung disease; histopathologic damage; Hodgkin disease; hormone-dependent; house dust; human diploid [cells]; Huntington disease; hydatid disease; hydroxydopamine

H&D Hunter and Driffield [curve]

HD$_{50}$ 50% hemolyzing dose of complement

HDA heteroduplex analysis; Huntington Disease Association; hydroxydopamine

HDAg hepatitis delta antigen

HDARAC high dose cytarabine (ARA C)

HDBH hydroxybutyric dehydrogenase

HDC histidine decarboxylase; human diploid cell; hypodermoclysis

HDCS human diploid cell strain

HDCV human diploid cell rabies vaccine

HDD high-dosage depth; Higher Dental Diploma

HDF host defense factor; human diploid fibroblast

HDFP Hypertension Detection and Follow-up Program

³H-DFP tritiated diisopropyl-fluoro-phosphonate

HDG high-dose group

HDH heart disease history

3H-DHE tritiated dihydroergocriptine

HDI hemorrhagic disease of infants; hexamethylene diisocyanate; hospital discharge index

HDL high-density lipoprotein

HDLBP high-density lipoprotein binding protein

HDL-C high-density lipoprotein-cholesterol

HDL-c high-density lipoprotein-cell surface

HDLP high-density lipoprotein

HDLS hereditary diffuse leukoencephalopathy with spheroids

HDLW distance from which a watch ticking is heard by left ear

HDMP high-dose methylprednisolone

HDMTX high-dose methotrexate

HDMTX-CF high-dose methotrexate citrovorum factor

HDMTX-LV high-dose methotrexate leucovorin

HDN hemolytic disease of the newborn

hDNA hybrid deoxyribonucleic acid

HDP hexose diphosphate; high-density polyethylene; hydrogen diphosphonate; hydroxydimethylpyrimidine

HDPAA heparin-dependent platelet-associated antibody

HDR high dose rate

HDRBC head-damaged red blood cells

HDRF Heart Disease Research Foundation

HDRS Hamilton Depression Rating Scale

HDRV human diploid rabies vaccine

HDRW distance from which a watch ticking is heard by right ear

HDS Hamilton Depression Scale; Health Data Services; health delivery system; Healthcare Data Systems; herniated disc syndrome; Hospital Discharge Survey

HDU hemodialysis unit; high dependency unit

HDV hepatitis D virus; hepatitis delta virus

HDZ hydralazine

HE half-scan with extrapolation; hard exudate; hektoen enteric [agar]; hemagglutinating encephalomyelitis; hematoxylin-eosin [stain]; hemoglobin electrophoresis; hepatic encephalopathy; hereditary eliptocytosis; high exposure; hollow enzyme; human enteric; hydroxyethyl [cellulose]; hyperextension; hypertensive encephalopathy; hypogonadotropic eunuchoidism

H&E hematoxylin and eosin [stain]; hemorrhage and exudate; heredity and environment

He heart; helium

HEA hexone-extracted acetone; human erythrocyte antigen

HEAL health education assistance loan

HealSB Health Standards Board

HEAT human erythrocyte agglutination test

HEB hemato-encephalic barrier

HEC hamster embryo cell; Health Education Council; human endothelial cell; hydroxyergocalciferol; hydroxyethyl cellulose

HED hereditary ectodermal dysplasia; hydrotropic electron-donor; hypohidrotic ectodermal dysplasia; unit skin dose [of x-rays] [Ger. *Haut-Einheits-Dosis*]

HEDH hypohidrotic ectodermal dysplasia-hypothyroidism [syndrome]

HEDIS Health Plan Employer Data and Information Set; health employer data and information set

HEENT head, ears, eyes, nose, and throat

HEEP health effects of environmental pollutants

HEF hamster embryo fibroblast; human embryo fibroblast

HEG hemorrhagic erosive gastritis

HEHR highest equivalent heart rate

HEI Health Effects Institute; high-energy intermediate; homogenous enzyme immunoassay; human embryonic intestine [cells]

HEIR health effects of ionizing radiation; high-energy ionizing radiation

HEIS high-energy ion scattering

HEK human embryo kinase; human embryonic kidney

HEL hen egg white lysozyme; human embryonic lung; human erythroleukemia

HeLa Helen Lake [human cervical carcinoma cells]

HELF human embryo lung fibroblast

HELLIS Health, Literature, Library and Information Services

HELLP hemolysis, elevated liver enzymes, and low platelet count [syndrome]

HELP Hawaii early learning profile; Health Education Library Program; Health Emergency Loan Program; Health Evaluation and Learning Program; heat escape lessening posture; Heroin Emergency Life Project; Hospital Equipment Loan Project

HEM hematology, hematologist; hematuric; hemophilia; hemorrhage; hemorrhoids

HEMA Health Education Media Association; 2-hydroxyethyl methacrylate

hemat hematology, hematologist

HEMB hemophilia B

hemi hemiparesis, hemiparalysis; hemiplegia

HEMPAS hereditary erythrocytic multinuclearity with positive acidified serum

HEMRI hereditary multifocal relapsing inflammation

HEMS hospital engineering management system

HEN home enteral nutrition

HeNe helium neon [laser]

HEP hemolysis end point; hepatoerythropoietic porphyria; high egg passage [virus]; high-energy phosphate; human epithelial cell

Hep hepatic; hepatitis

hEP human endorphin

HEp-1 human cervical carcinoma cells

HEp-2 human laryngeal tumor cells

HEPA high-efficiency particulate air [filter]

HEP A hepatitis A

HEP B hepatitis B

HEPBsAg hepatitis B surface antigen

HEP C hepatitis C

HEP D hepatitis D

HEPES N-2-hydroxyethylpiperazine-N-2-ethanesulfonic [acid]

HEPM human embryonic palatal mesenchymal [cell]

HEPOD hereditary expansile polyostotic dysplasia

HER hemorrhagic encephalopathy of rats; hernia

hered heredity, hereditary

hern hernia, herniated

HERS Health Evaluation and Referral Service; hemorrhagic fever with renal syndrome

HES health examination survey; hematoxylin-eosin stain; human embryonic skin; human embryonic spleen; hydroxyethyl starch; hypereosinophilic syndrome; hyperprostaglandin E syndrome

HESCA Health Sciences Communications Association

HET Health Education Telecommunications; helium equilibration time

Het heterophil

het heterozygous

HETE hydroxy-eicosatetraenoic [acid]

HETP height equivalent to a theoretical plate; hexaethyltetraphosphate

HEV health and environment; hemagglutinating encephalomyelitis virus; hepatitis E virus; hepato-encephalomyelitis virus; high endothelial venule; human enteric virus

HeV hepatitis virus

HEW [Department of] Health, Education, and Welfare

HEX hexaminidase; hexosaminidase

Hex hexamethylmelamine

HEX A, hex A hexosaminidase A

HEX B, hex B hexosaminidase B

HEX C, hex C hexosaminidase C

HF Hageman factor; haplotype frequency; hard filled [capsule]; hay fever; head of fetus; head forward; heart failure; helper factor; hemofiltration; hemorrhagic factor; hemorrhagic fever; Hertz frequency; high fat [diet]; high flow; high frequency; human fibroblast; hydrogen fluoride; hyperflexion

Hf hafnium

hf half; high frequency

HFAK hollow-fiber artificial kidney

HFC hard filled capsule; high-frequency current; histamine-forming capacity

HFD hemorrhagic fever of deer; high-fiber diet; high forceps delivery; hospital field director; human factors design

HFDA high film density area

HFDK human fetal diploid kidney

HFDL human fetal diploid lung

HFE, HFe hemochromatosis

HFEC human foreskin epithelial cell

HFF human foreskin fibroblast

HFG hand-foot-genital [syndrome]

HFH hemifacial hyperplasia

HFHV high frequency, high volume

HFI hereditary fructose intolerance; human fibroblast interferon

HFIF human fibroblast interferon

HFJV high-frequency jet ventilation

HFL human fetal lung

HFM hemifacial microsomia

HFMA Healthcare Financial Management Association

HFO high-frequency oscillator; high-frequency oscillatory [ventilation]

HFO-A high-frequency oscillatory [ventilation]-active [expiratory phase]

HFOV high-frequency oscillatory ventilation

HFP hexafluoropropylene; high-frequency pulsation; hypofibrinogenic plasma

HFPPV high-frequency positive pressure ventilation

HFR high-frequency recombination

Hfr heart frequency; high frequency

HFRS hemorrhagic fever with renal syndrome

HFS hemifacial spasm; Hospital Financial Support

hfs hyperfine structure

hFSH, HFSH human follicle-stimulating hormone

HFSP Hanukah factor serine protease

HFST hearing for speech test

HFT high-frequency transduction; high-frequency transfer

Hft high-frequency transfer

HFU hand-foot-uterus [syndrome]

HFV high-frequency ventilation

HG hand grip; herpes gestationis; Heschl's gyrus; high glucose; human gonadotropin; human growth; hypoglycemia

Hg mercury [Lat. *hydrargyrum*]

hg hectogram; hemoglobin

HGA homogentisic acid

Hgb hemoglobin

Hge hemorrhage

HGF hepatocyte growth factor; hyperglycemic-glucogenolytic factor

Hg-F fetal hemoglobin

HGFL hepatocyte growth factor-like [protein]

HGG herpetic geniculate ganglionitis; human gammaglobulin; hypogammaglobulinemia

HGH, hGH human gamma globulin; human growth hormone

HGHRF human growth hormone releasing factor

HGL heregulin

HGM hog gastric mucosa; human gene mapping; human glucose monitoring

HGMCR human genetic mutant cell repository

HGO hepatic glucose output; human glucose output

HGP hepatic glucose production; hyperglobulinemic purpura

HGPRT hypoxanthine guanine phosphoribosyl transferase

HGPS hereditary giant platelet syndrome; Hutchinson-Gilford progeria syndrome

hGR human glucocorticoid receptor

hGRH human growth hormone-releasing hormone

HH halothane hepatitis; hard-of-hearing; healthy hemophiliac; healthy human; hiatal hernia; holistic health; home help; hydroxyhexamide; hypergastrinemic hyperchlorhydria; hyperhidrosis; hypogonadotropic hypogonadism; hyporeninemic hypoaldosteronism

H&H hematocrit and hemoglobin

HHA health hazard appraisal; hereditary hemolytic anemia; home health agency; home health aid; hypothalamo-hypophyseo-adrenal [system]

HHb hypohemoglobinemia; un-ionized hemoglobin

HHC home health care; hypocalciuric hypercalcemia

HHCC home health care classification

HHCS high-altitude hypertrophic cardiomyopathy syndrome

HHD high heparin dose; home dialysis; hypertensive heart disease

HHE health hazard evaluation; hemiconvulsion-hemiplegia-epilepsy [syndrome]

HHG hypertrophic hypersecretory gastropathy

HHH hyperornithinemia, hyperammonemia, homocitrillinuria [syndrome]

HHHH hereditary hemihypotrophy-hemiparesis-hemiathetosis [syndrome]

HHHO hypotonia, hypomentia, hypogonadism, obesity [syndrome]

HHIE Hearing Handicap Inventory for the Elderly

HHIE-S Hearing Handicap Inventory for the Elderly-Screening Version

HHM humoral hypercalcemia of malignancy

H + Hm compound hypermetropic astigmatism

HHMI Howard Hughes Medical Institutes

HHNC hyperosmolar nonketotic diabetic coma

HHNK hyperglycemic hyperosmoler nonketotic [coma]

HHNS hyperosmolar hyperglycemic nonketotic syndrome

HHR hydralazine, hydrochlorothiazide, and reserpine

HHRH hereditary hypophosphatemic rickets with hypercalciuria; hypothalamic hypophysiotropic releasing hormone

HHS [Department of] Health and Human Services; Hearing Handicap Scale; hereditary hemolytic syndrome; human hypopituitary serum; hyperglycemic hyperosmolar syndrome; hyperkinetic heart syndrome

HHSSA Home Health Services and Staffing Association

HHT head halter traction; hereditary hemorrhagic telangiectasia; heterotopic heart transplantation; homoharringtonine; hydroxyheptadecatrienoic acid

HHV human herpes virus

HI half-scan with interpolation; head injury; health insurance; hearing impaired; heart infusion; hemagglutination inhibition; hepatobiliary imaging; high impulsiveness; histidine; hormone-independent; hormone insensitivity; hospital insurance; humoral immunity; hydroxyindole; hyperglycemic index; hypomelanosis of Ito; hypothermic ischemia

H-I hemagglutination-inhibition

Hi histamine; histidine

HIA Hearing Industries Association; heat infusion agar; hemagglutination inhibition antibody or assay

HIAA Health Insurance Association of America

5-HIAA 5-hydroxyindoleacetic acid

HIB heart infusion broth; hemolytic immune body; *Hemophilus influenzae* type B [vaccine]

HIBAC Health Insurance Benefits Advisory Council

HIC handling-induced convulsions; health insurance claim; Heart Information Center

HICA hydroxyisocaproic acid

HIC-CPR high-impulse compression cardiopulmonary resuscitation

HICH hypertensive intracranial hemorrhage

HiCn cyanomethemoglobin

HI-CPR high impulse cardiopulmonary resuscitation

HID headache, insomnia, depression [syndrome]; herniated intervertebral disc; human infectious dose; hyperkinetic impulse disorder

HIDA Health Industry Distributors Association; hepato-iminodiacetic acid (lidofenin) [nuclear medicine scan]; 12-hydroxy-heptadecatrienoic acid

HIE human intestinal epithelium; hyper-IgE [syndrome]; hypoxic-ischemic encephalopathy

HIES hyper-IgE syndrome

HIF higher integrative functions

HIFBS heat-inactivated fetal bovine serum

HIFC hog instrinsic factor concentrate

HIFCS heat-inactivated fetal calf serum

HIG, hIG human immunoglobulin

HIg hyperimmunoglobulin

HIH hypertensive intracerebral hemorrhage

HIHA high impulsiveness, high anxiety

HiHb hemiglobin (methemoglobin)

HII Health Industries Institute; Health Insurance Institute; hemagglutination inhibitor immunoassay

HILA high impulsiveness, low anxiety

HILDA human interleukin in DA [cells]

HIM hepatitis-infectious mononucleosis; hexosephosphate isomerase

HIMA Health Industry Manufacturers Association

HIMC hepatic intramitochondrial crystalloid

HIMP high-dose intravenous methylprednisolone

HIMSS Healthcare Information and Management Systems Society

HIMT hemagglutination inhibition morphine test

HINT hierarchical interpolation; Holland Interuniversity Nifedipine/Metoprolol Trial

Hint Hinton [test]

HIO health insuring organization; hypoiodism

HIOMT hydroxyindole-O-methyl transferase

HIOS high index of suspicion

HIP health illness profile; health insurance plan or program; homograft incus prosthesis; hospital insurance program; hydrostatic indifference point

HIPA heparin-induced platelet activation

HIPC health insurance purchasing collective; health insurance purchasing cooperative

HIPDM N-trimethyl-n-(2-hydroxyl-3-methyl-5-iodobenzyl)-1,3-propendiamine

HIPE Hospital Inpatient Enquiry

HiPIP high potential iron protein

HIPO hemihypertrophy, intestinal web, preauricular skin tag, and congenital corneal opacity [syndrome]; Hospital Indicator for Physicians Orders

HiPRF high pulse repetition frequency

HIR head injury routine

HIS health information system; Health Interview Survey; histatin; histidine; hospital information system; hyperimmune serum

His histidine

HISB Health Insurance Standards Board

HISKEW Health Information Skeletonized Eligibility Write-off [file, Medicare]

HISSG Hospital Information Systems Sharing Group

HIST hospital in-service training

hist histamine, history

HISTLINE History of Medicine On-Line [NLM database]

Histo histoplasmin skin test

histol histological, histologist, histology

HIT hemagglutination inhibition test; heparin-induced thrombocytopenia; histamine inhalation test; hypertrophic infiltrative tendonitis

HITB, HiTB *Hemophilus influenzae* type B

HITF Health Insurance Trust Fund

HITT heparin-induced thrombocytopenia and thrombosis

HITTS heparin-induced thrombosis-thrombocytopenia syndrome

HIU hyperplasia interstitialis uteri

HIV human immunodeficiency virus

HIV1 human immunodeficiency virus type 1

HIV Ag human immunodeficiency virus antigen

HIVAN human immunodeficiency virus-associated nephropathy

HIV-G human immunodeficiency virus-associated gingivitis

HJ Howell-Jolly [bodies]

HJR hepatojugular reflex

HK hand to knee; heat-killed; heel-to-knee; hexokinase; human kidney

H-K hand to knee

HKAFO hip, knee, ankle, and foot orthosis

HKAO hip-knee-ankle orthosis

HKC human kidney cell

HKLM heat-killed *Listeria monocytogenes*

HKS hyperkinesis syndrome

HL hairline; hairy leukoplakia; half life; hearing level; hearing loss; heparin lock; histiocytic lymphoma; histocompatibility locus; Hodgkin lymphoma; human leukocyte; hyperlipidemia; hypermetropia, latent; hypertrichosis lanuginosa

H&L heart and lung [machine]

H/L hydrophil/lipophil [ratio]

Hl hypermetropia, latent

hl hectoliter

HL7 health level 7

HLA histocompatibility leukocyte antigen; histocompatibility locus antigen; homologous leukocyte antibody; human leukocyte antigen; human lymphocyte antigen

HL-A human leukocyte antigen

HLAA human leukocyte antigen A

HLAB human leukocyte antigen B

HLAC human leukocyte antigen C

HLAD human leukocyte antigen D

HLA-LD human lymphocyte antigen-lymphocyte defined

HLA-SD human lymphocyte antigen-serologically defined

HLB hydrophilic-lipophilic balance; hypotonic lysis buffer

HLBI human lymphoblastoid interferon

HLC heat loss center

HLCL human lymphoblastoid cell line

HLD hepatolenticular degeneration; herniated lumbar disk; Hippel-Lindau disease; hypersensitivity lung disease

HLDH heat-stable lactic dehydrogenase

HLEG hydrolysate lactalbumin Earle glucose

HLF heat-labile factor; hepatic leukemia factor

HLH helix-loop-helix; hemophagocytic lymphohistiocytosis

hLH human luteinizing hormone

HLHS hypoplastic left heart syndrome

HLI human leukocyte interferon

H-L-K heart, liver, and kidneys

HLL hypoplastic left lung

HLN hilar lymph node; hyperplastic liver nodules

HLP hepatic lipoperoxidation; hind leg paralysis; holoprosencephaly; hyperkeratosis lenticularis perstans; hyperlipoproteinemia

HLQ high-level question

HLR heart-lung resuscitation

HLS Health Learning System; Hippel-Lindau syndrome

HLT heart-lung transplantation; human lipotropin; human lymphocyte transformation

HLTx heart-lung transplant

HLV hamster leukemia virus; herpes-like virus; hypoplastic left ventricle

HLVS hypoplastic left ventricle syndrome

HM hand movements; health maintenance; heart murmur; hemifacial microsomia; Holter monitoring; home management; homosexual male; hospital management; human milk; hydatidiform mole; hyperbaric medicine; hyperimmune mouse

Hm manifest hypermetropia

hm hectometer

HMA health care management alternatives; human monocyte antigen; hydroxymethionine analog

HMAB human monocyte antigen B

HMAC Health Manpower Advisory Council

HMAS hyperimmune mouse ascites

HMB homatropine methobromide

HMBA hexamethylene bisacetamide

HMBS hydroxymethylbilane synthetase

HMC hand-mirror cell; health maintenance cooperative; heroin, morphine, and cocaine; histocompatibility complex, major; hospital management committee; hypertelorism-microtia-clefting [syndrome]

HMCCMP human mammary carcinoma cell membrane proteinase

HMD hyaline membrane disease

HMDC health maintenance and diagnostic center

HMDP hydroxymethylenediphosphonate

HME Health Media Education; heat and moisture exchanger; heat, massage, and exercise

HMF hydroxymethylfurfural

HMG high-mobility group; human menopausal gonadotropin; 3-hydroxy-3-methyl-glutaryl

hMG human menopausal gonadotropin

HMG CoA 3-hydroxy-3-methylglutaryl coenzyme A

HMI healed myocardial infarct; hypomelanosis of Ito

HMIS hazardous materials identification system; hospital medical information system

HML human milk lysosome

HMM heavy meromyosin; hexamethylmelamine

HMMA 4-hydroxy-3-methoxymandelic acid

HMN hereditary motor neuropathy

H-MNPM [Department of] Health Education and Welfare-Medicus Nursing Process Methodology

HMO health maintenance organization; heart minute output

HMOX heme oxygenase

HMP hexose monophosphate pathway; hot moist packs

HMPA hexamethylphosphoramide

HMPAO hexamethyl-propyleneamine oxine

HM-PAO hexamethyl-propyleneamineoxime

HMPG hydroxymethoxyphenylglycol

HMPS hexose monophosphate shunt

HMPT hexamethylphosphorotriamide

HMQC heteronuclear multiple-quantum correlation

HMR histiocytic medullary reticulosis

HMRI Hospital Medical Record Institute

H-mRNA H-chain messenger ribonucleic acid

HMRTE human milk reverse transcriptase enzyme

HMS hexose monophosphate shunt; hypermobility syndrome

HMSA health manpower shortage area

HMSAS hypertrophic muscular subaortic stenosis

HMSN hereditary motor and sensory neuropathy

HMSS Hospital Management Systems Society

HMT hematocrit; histamine-N-methyltransferase; hospital management team

HMTA hexamethylenetetramine

HMW high-molecular-weight

HMWC high-molecular-weight component

HMWGP high-molecular-weight glycoprotein

HMWK high-molecular-weight kininogen

HMX heat, massage, and exercise

HN head and neck; head nurse; hemagglutinin neuraminidase; hematemesis neonatorum; hemorrhage of newborn; hereditary nephritis; high necrosis; hilar node; histamine-containing neuron; home nursing; human nutrition; hypertrophic neuropathy

H&N head and neck

HNA heparin neutralizing activity

HNB human neuroblastoma

HNC hypernephroma cell; hyperosmolar nonketotic coma; hypothalamoneurohypophyseal complex

HNF hepatocyte nuclear factor

HNF1A hepatocyte nuclear factor-1-alpha

HNKC hyperosmolar nonketotic coma

HNKDS hyperosmolar nonketotic diabetic state

HNL histiocytic necrotizing lymphadenitis

HNP hereditary nephritic protein; herniated nucleus pulposus; human neurophysin

HNPCC hereditary nonpolyposis colorectal cancer

HNPP hereditary neuropathy with liability to pressure palsies

hnRNA heterogeneous nuclear ribonucleic acid

hnRNP heterogeneous nuclear ribonucleoprotein

HNRP heterogenous nuclear ribonucleoprotein

HNRPG heterogenous nuclear ribonucleoprotein peptide G

HNS head and neck surgery; home nursing supervisor

HNSHA hereditary nonspherocytic hemolytic anemia

HNTD highest nontoxic dose

HNV has not voided

HO hand orthosis; heterotopic ossification; high oxygen; hip orthosis; history of; Holt-Oram [syndrome]; house officer; hyperbaric oxygen

H/O, h/o history of

Ho holmium; horse

HOA hip osteoarthritis; hypertrophic osteoarthropathy

HoaRhLG horse anti-rhesus lymphocyte globulin

HoaTTG horse anti-tetanus toxoid globulin

HOB head of bed

HOC human ovarian cancer; hydroxycorticoid

HOCM high-osmolar contrast medium; hypertrophic obstructive cardiomyopathy

HOD hyperbaric oxygen drenching

HOF hepatic outflow

HofF height of fundus

HOGA hyperornithinemia with gyrate atrophy

HOH hard of hearing

HOI hospital onset of infection

HoIg horse immunoglobulin

HOKPP hypokalemic periodic paralysis

HOME Home Observation for Measurement of the Environment

Homeop homeopathy

HOMO highest occupied molecular orbital; homosexual

homo homosexual

HONC hyperosmolar nonketotic coma

HONK hyperosmolar nonketosis

HOOD hereditary onycho-osteodysplasia

HOODS hereditary onycho-osteodysplasia syndrome

HOOE heredopathia ophthalmo-oto-encephalica

HOP high oxygen pressure

HOPE Healthcare Options Plan Entitlement; health-oriented physical education; holistic orthogonal parameter estimation

HOPI history of present illness

HOPP hepatic occluded portal pressure

hor horizontal

HOS health opinion survey; Holt-Oram syndrome; human osteosarcoma; hypo-osmotic swelling [test]

HoS horse serum

Hosp, hosp hospital

HOST hypo-osmotic shock treatment

HOT health-oriented telecommunication; human old tuberculin; hyperbaric oxygen therapy; Hypertension Optimal Treatment [study]

HOTS hypercalcemia-osteolysis-T-cell syndrome

HP halogen phosphorus; handicapped person; haptoglobin; hard palate; Harvard pump; health profession(al); heat production; heel to patella; hemiparkinsonism; hemipelvectomy; hemiplegia; hemoperfusion; *Hemophilus pleuropneumoniae*; heparin; hepatic porphyria; high potency; high power; high pressure; high protein; highly purified; horizontal plane; horsepower; hospital participation; hot pack; house physician; human pituitary; hydrophilic petrolatum; hydrostatic pressure; hydroxypyruvate; hyperparahyroidism; hypersensitivity pneumonitis; hypophoria

H&P history and physical examination

Hp haptoglobin; hematoporphyrin; hemiplegia

HPA Health Care Practice Act; Health Policy Agenda for the American People; health promotion advocates; *Helix pomatia* agglutinin; hemagglutinating penicillin antibody; *Histoplasma capsulatum* polysaccharide antigen; humeroscapular periarthritis; hypertrophic pulmonary arthropathy; hypothalamo-pituitary-adrenocortical [system]

HPAA hydroperoxyarachidonic acid; hydroxyphenlacetic acid; hypothalamo-pituitary-adrenal axis

HPAC high-performance anion-exchange chromatography; hypothalamo-pituitary-adreno-cortical

HPAFT hereditary persistence of alfa-fetoprotein

H-PAGE horizontal polyacrylamide gel

HPB hepatobiliary

HPBC hyperpolarizing bipolar cell

HPBF hepatotrophic portal blood factor

HPBL human peripheral blood leukocyte

HPC hemangiopericytoma; hippocampal pyramidal cell; history of present complaint; holoprosencephaly; hydroxypropylcellulose

HPCA human progenitor cell antigen

HPCC health plan purchasing cooperative; high performance computing and communication

HPCHA high red-cell phosphatidylcholine hemolylic anemia

HPD hearing protective device; high-protein diet; home peritoneal dialysis

HPDR hypophosphatemic D-resistant rickets

HPE hepatic portoenterostomy; high-permeability edema; history and physical examination; holoprosencephaly; hydrostatic permeability edema

HPES holoprosencephaly

HPETE hydroxyperoxy-eicosotetranoic [acid]

HPF heparin-precipitable fraction; hepatic plasma flow; high-pass filter; high-power field [microscope]; hypocaloric protein feeding

HPFH hereditary persistence of fetal hemoglobin

hPFSH, HPFSH human pituitary follicle-stimulating hormone

hPG, HPG human pituitary gonadotropin

HpGe hyperpure germanium

HPH *Helix pomatia* hemocyanin

HPI hepatic perfusion index; history of present illness

HPL human parotid lysozyme; human peripheral lymphocyte; human placental lactogen

hPL human placental lactogen; human platelet lactogen

HPLA hydroxyphenyl lactic acid

HPLAC high-pressure liquid-affinity chromatography

HPLC high-performance liquid chromatography; high-power liquid chromatography; high-pressure liquid chromatography

HPLE hereditary polymorphic light eruption

HPM high-performance membrane

HPMC human peripheral mononuclear cell

HPN hepsin; home parenteral nutrition; hypertension

hpn hypertension

HPNS high pressure neurological syndrome

HPO high-presure oxygen; hydroperoxide; hydrophilic ointment; hypertrophic pulmonary osteoarthropathy

HPOA hypertrophic pulmonary osteoarthropathy

HPP hereditary pyropoikilocytosis; history of presenting problems

HPP, hPP hydroxyphenylpyruvate; hydroxypyrozolopyrimidine; human pancreatic polypeptide

HPPA hydroxyphenylpyruvic acid

HPPD hours per patient day

HPPH 5-(4-hydroxyphenyl)-5-phenyl-hydantoin

HPPO high partial pressure of oxygen; hydroxyphenyl pyruvate oxidase

HPQ Health Perceptions Questionnaire

HPR haptoglobin-related gene; health practices research

HPr human prolactin

hPRL human prolactin

HPRP human platelet-rich plasma

HPRT hypoxanthine-guanine phosphoribosyltransferase

HPS Hantavirus pulmonary syndrome; hematoxylin, phloxin, and saffron; Hermansky-Pudlak syndrome; high-protein supplement; His-Purkinje system; human platelet suspension; hypertrophic pyloric stenosis; hypothalamic pubertal syndrome

HPSA health professional shortage area

HPSL health professions student loan

HPT histamine provocation test; human placental thyrotropin; hyperparathyroidism; hypothalamo-pituitary-thyroid [system]

1°HPT primary hyperparathyroidism

2°HPT secondary hyperparathyroidism

HPTH hyperparathyroid hormone

HPTIN human pancreatic trypsin inhibitor

HPU heater probe unit

HPV *Hemophilus pertussis* vaccine; hepatic portal vein; human papillomavirus; human parvovirus; hypoxic pulmonary vasoconstriction

HPVD hypertensive pulmonary vascular disease

HPV-DE high-passage virus-duck embryo

HPV-DK high-passage virus-dog kidney

HPVG hepatic portal venous gas

HPW hypergammaglobulinemic purpura of Waldenström

HP/W health promotion/wellness [program]

HPX high peroxidase [content]; hypophysectomized

HPZ high pressure zone

[3H]QNB (-)[3H]quinuclidinyl benzilate

HR heart rate; hemorrhagic retinopathy; high resolution; higher rate; histamine receptor; hormonal response; hospital record; hospital report; hyperimmune reaction; hypophosphatemic rickets

hr hairless [mouse]; host-range [mutant]; hour

H&R hysterectomy and radiation

HRA health record analyst; health risk appraisal; heart rate audiometry; hereditary renal adysplasia; histamine release activity; Human Resources Administration

HRAE high right atrium electrogram

HRBC horse red blood cell

HRC hereditary renal cancer; high-resolution chromatography; horse red cell; human rights committee

HRCT, HR-CT high-resolution computed tomography

HRE hepatic reticuloendothelial [cell]; high-resolution electrocardiography; hormone receptor enzyme

HREH high-renin essential hypertension

HREM high-resolution electron microscopy

HRF heart rate fluctuations

HRG histidine-rich glycoprotein

HRGP histidine-rich glycoprotein

HRH2 histamine receptor H2

HRIG, HRIg human rabies immunoglobulin

HRL head rotation to the left

HRLA human reovirus-like agent

hRNA heterogeneous ribonucleic acid

HRNB Halstead-Reitan Neuropsychological Battery

HRP high-risk patient; high-risk pregnancy; histidine-rich protein; horseradish peroxidase

HRPD Hamburg Rating Scale for Psychiatric Disorders

HRPT hyperparathyroidism

HRQOL health-related quality of life

HRR head rotation to the right; heart rate range

HRRI heart rate retardation index

HRS Hamilton Rating Scale; Hamman-Rich syndrome; health and rehabilitative services; hepatorenal syndrome; high rate of stimulation; hormone receptor site; humeroradial synostosis

HRSA Health Resources and Services Administration

HRS-D Hamilton Rating Scale for Depression; Hirschsprung disease

HRSP high-resolution storage phosphor

HRSUB submaximal heart rate

HRT heart rate; hormone replacement therapy

HRTE human reverse transcriptase enzyme

HRTEM high-resolution transmission electron microscopy

HRV heart rate variability; human reovirus; human rotavirus

HS Haber syndrome; half strength; hamstring; hand surgery; Hartmann solution; head sling; healthy subject; heart sounds; heat-stable; heavy smoker; Hegglin syndrome; heme synthetase; Henoch-Schönlein [purpura]; heparan sulfate; hereditary spherocytosis; herpes simplex; hidradenitis suppurativa; home surgeon; homologous serum; horizontally selective; Horner syndrome; horse serum; hospital ship; hospital staff; hospital stay; hours of sleep; house surgeon; human serum; Hurler syndrome; hypereosinophilic syndrome; hypersensitivity; hypertonic saline

hs history; hospitalization

H/S helper-suppressor [ratio]

H&S hemorrhage and shock; hysterectomy and sterilization

HSA Hazardous Substances Act; Health Services Administration; health systems agency; hereditary sideroblastic anemia; horse serum albumin; human serum albumin; hypersomnia-sleep apnea

HSAG N-2-hydroxyethylpiperazine-N-2-ethanesulfonate-saline-albumin-gelatin

HSAN hereditary sensory and autonomic neuropathy

HSAP heat-stable alkaline phosphatase

HSAS hydrocephalus due to stenosis of aqueduct of Sylvius; hypertrophic subaortic stenosis

HSC Hand-Schüller-Christian [syndrome]; Health and Safety Commission; health sciences center; health screening center; hematopoietic stem cell; human skin collagenase

HSCD Hand-Schüller-Christian disease

HSCL Hopkins Symptom Check List

HS-CoA reduced coenzyme A

HSCS health state classification system

HSD Hallervorden-Spatz disease; honestly significant difference; hydroxysteroid dehydrogenase; hypertonic saline and dextran

H(SD) Holtzman Sprague-Dawley [rat]

HSDB hazardous substances data bank

HSDO health services delivery organization

HSE herpes simplex encephalitis; hemorrhagic shock and encephalopathy

HSEES Hazardous Substances Emergency Events Surveillance [system]

HSEP heart synchronized evoked potential

HSES hemorrhagic shock-encephalopathy syndrome

HSF heat shock factor; hepatocyte stimulatory factor; histamine sensitizing factor; human serum esterase; hypothalamic secretory factor

HSG herpex simplex genitalis; hystero-salpingogram, hysterosalpingography
hSGF human skeletal growth factor
HSGP human sialoglycoprotein
HSH hypomagnesemia with secondary hypocalcemia
HSHC hydrocortisone hemisuccinate
HSI heat stress index; human seminal plasma inhibitor
HSIL high-grade squamous intraepithelial lesion
HSK herpes simplex keratitis
HSL herpes simplex labialis; hormone-sensitive lipase
HSLC high-speed liquid chromatography
HSM hepatosplenomegaly; holosystolic murmur
HSMHA Health Services and Mental Health Administration
HSN hereditary sensory neuropathy; hospital satellite network
hSOD human superoxide dismutase
HSP Health Systems Plan; heat shock protein; hemostatic screening profile; Henoch-Schönlein purpura; hereditary spastic paraparesis; Hospital Service Plan; human serum prealbumin; human serum protein
hsp heat shock protein [gene]
HS PACS high-speed picture archive and communication system
HS-PG heparan sulfate-proteoglycan
HSPM hippocampal synaptic plasma membrane
HSPN Henoch-Schönlein purpura nephritis
HSQB Health Standards and Quality Bureau
HSQC heteronuclear single-quantum correlation
HSR Harleco synthetic resin; heated serum reagin; homogeneously staining region
HSRC Health Services Research Center; Human Subjects Review Committee

HSRD hypertension secondary to renal disease
HSR&D health services research and development
HSRI Health Systems Research Institute
HSRS Health-Sickness Rating Scale
HSRV human spuma retrovirus
HSS Hallermann-Streiff syndrome; Hallervorden-Spatz syndrome; Henoch-Schönlein syndrome; high-speed supernatant; hyperstimulation syndrome; hypertrophic subaortic stenosis
HSSCC hereditary site-specific colon cancer
HSSD hospital sterile supply department
HSSU hospital sterile supply unit
HSTAR health services and technology assessment research
HSTAT health services/technology assessment text
HSTF heat shock transcription factor; human serum thymus factor
HSV herpes simplex virus; high selective vagotomy; hop stunt viroid; hyperviscosity syndrome
HSV-1 herpes simplex virus type 1
HSV-2 herpes simplex virus type 2
HSVE herpes simplex virus encephalitis
HSVtk herpes simplex virus thymidine kinase
HSyn heme synthase
HT Hashimoto thyroiditis; hearing test; hearing threshold; heart; heart transplantation, heart transplant; hemagglutination titer; hereditary tyrosinemia; high-frequency transduction; high temperature; high tension; histologic technician; home treatment; hospital treatment; Hubbard tank; human thrombin; hydrocortisone test; hydrotherapy; hydroxytryptamine; hypermetropia, total; hypertension; hyperthyroidism; hypertransfusion; hypodermic tablet; hypothalamus; hypothyroidism
H&T hospitalization and treatment

³HT tritiated thymidine

5-HT 5-hydroxytryptamine [serotonin]

Ht height of heart; heterozygote; hyperopia, total; hypothalamus

H_t dose equivalent to individual tissues

ht heart; heart tones; height; high tension

HTA heterophil transplantation antigen; human thymocyte antigen; hydroxytryptamine; hypophysiotropic area

HTACS human thyroid adenyl-cyclase stimulator

ht aer heated aerosol

HT(ASCP) Histologic Technician certified by the American Society of Clinical Pathologists

HTB house tube feeding; human tumor bank

HTC hepatoma cell; hepatoma tissue culture; homozygous typing cell

HTCVD hypertensive cardiovascular disease

HTD human therapeutic dose

HTDW heterosexual development of women

HTF heterothyrotropic factor; house tube feeding; HpaII tiny fragment

HTG hypertriglyceridemia

HTGL hepatic triglyceride lipase

HTH homeostatic thymus hormone; hypothalamus

Hth hypothermic

HTHD hypertensive heart disease

HTI hemispheric thrombotic infarction

HTIG human tetanus immune globulin

HTK heel to knee

HTL hamster tumor line; hearing threshold level; high-L-leucine transport; histotechnologist; human T-cell leukemia; human thymic leukemia

HTLA high-titer, low acidity; human T-lymphocyte antigen

HTL(ASCP) Histotechnologist certified by the American Society of Clinical Pathologists

HTLF human T-cell leukemia virus enhancer factor

HTLV human T-cell leukemia/lymphoma virus; human T-lymphotropic virus

HTLV-MA cell membrane antigen associated with the human T-cell leukemia virus

HTLV-I-MA human T-cell leukemia virus-I-associated membrane antigen

HTLVR human T-cell leukemia virus receptor

HTML hypertext markup language

HTN Hantaan-[like virus]; histatin; hypertension; hypertensive nephropathy

HTO hospital transfer order

HTOR 5-hydroxytryptamine oxygenase regulator

HTP House-Tree-Person [test]; hydroxytryptophan; hypothromboplastinemia

5-HTP 5-hydroxy-L-tryptophan

HtPA hexahydrophthalic anhydride

HTPN home total parenteral nutrition

HTR histidine transport regulator; 5-hydroxytryptamine receptor

HTS head traumatic syndrome; HeLa tumor suppression; human thyroid-stimulating hormone, human thyroid stimulator

HTSAB human thyroid-stimulating antibody

HTSH, hTSH human thyroid-stimulating hormone

HTST high temperature, short time

HTT 5-hydroxytryptamine transformer

HTTP hypertext transfer protocol

HTV herpes-type virus

HTVD hypertensive vascular disease

HTX heterotaxy, X-linked; histrionicotoxin

HU heat unit; hemagglutinating unit; hemolytic unit; Hounsfield unit; human urine, human urinary; hydroxyurea; hyperemia unit

Hu human

HUAA home uterine activity assessment

HUC hypouricemia

HuEPO human erythropoietin

HU-FSH human urinary follicle-stimulating hormone

HUI headache unit index

HUIFM human leukocyte interferon meloy

HuIFN human interferon

HUK human urinary kallikrein

Hum humerus

HUP Hospital Utilization Project

HUR hydroxyurea

HURA health in underserved rural areas

HURT hospital utilization review team

HUS hemolytic uremic syndrome; hyaluronidase unit for semen

HuSA human serum albumin

hut histidine utilization [gene]

HUTHAS human thymus antiserum

HUV human umbilical vein

HUVEC human umbilical vein endothelial cell

HV hallux valgus; Hantaan virus; heart volume; hepatic vein; herpesvirus; high voltage; high volume; hospital visit; hyperventilation

hv hypervariable region

H&V hemigastrectomy and vagotomy

HVA homovanillic acid

HVAC heating, ventilating, and air conditioning

HVC Health Visitor's Certificate

HVD hypertensive vascular disease

HVDRR hypocalcemic vitamin D-resistant rickets

HVE hepatic venous effluence; high-voltage electrophoresis

HVG host versus graft [disease]

HVGS high-voltage galvanic stimulation

HVH *Herpesvirus hominis*

HVJ hemagglutinating virus of Japan

HVL, hvl half-value layer

HVLP high volume, low pressure

HVM high-velocity missile

HVPC high-voltage pulsed current

HVPE high-voltage paper electrophoresis

HVPG hepatic venous pressure gradient

HVR hypervariable region; hypoxic ventilation response

HVS herpesvirus of Saimiri; herpesvirus sensitivity; high vaginal swab; high-volt stiumulation; hyperventilation syndrome; hyperviscosity syndrome

HVSD hydrogen-detected ventricular septal defect

HVT half-value thickness; herpesvirus of turkeys

HVTEM high-voltage transmission electron microscopy

HVUS hypocomplementemic vasculitis urticaria syndrome

HVWP hepatic vein wedge pressure

HW healing well

HWB hot water bottle

HWC Health and Welfare, Canada

HWCD Hans-Weber-Christian disease

HWD heartworm disease

HWE healthy worker effect; hot water extract

HWP hepatic wedge pressure; hot wet pack

HWS hot water-soluble

HX histiocytosis X; hydrogen exchange; hypophysectomized

Hx history; hypoxanthine

hx hospitalization

HXB hexabrachion

HXIS hard x-ray imaging spectrometry

HXM hexamethylmelamine

HXR hypoxanthine riboside

Hy hypermetropia; hyperopia; hypophysis; hypothenar; hysteria

HYD hydralazine; hydration, hydrated; hydrocortisone; hydroxyurea

hydr hydraulic

hydro hydrotherapy

HYE healthy years equivalent

hyg hygiene, hygienic, hygienist

HYL, Hyl hydroxylysine
HYP hydroxyproline; hypnosis
Hyp hydroxyproline; hyperresonance; hypertrophy; hypothalamus
hyp hypophysis, hypophysectomy
hyper-IgE hyperimmunoglobulinemia E
hypn hypertension
hypno hypnosis
Hypo hypodermic, hypodermic injection
hypox hypophysectomized

HYPP hyperkalemic periodic paralysis
HypRF hypothalamic releasing factor
Hypro hydroxyproline
hys, hyst hysterectomy; hysteria, hysterical
HZ herpes zoster
Hz hertz
Hz/G hertz/gauss
HZO herpes zoster ophthalmicus
HZV herpes zoster virus

I electric current; impression; incisor [permanent]; independent; index; indicated; induction; inertia; inhalation; inhibition, inhibitor; inosine; insoluble; inspiration, inspired; insulin; intake; intensity; intermittent; internal medicine; intestine; iodine; ionic strength; isoleucine; isotope; nuclear spin quantum number; region of a sarcomere that contains only actin filaments; Roman numeral one

I-131 iodine-131

i electric current; incisor [deciduous]; insoluble; isochromosome; optically inactive

ι see *iota*

IA ibotenic acid; immune adherence; immunoadsorbent; immunobiologic activity; impedance angle; indolaminergic accumulation; indolic acid; indulin agar; infantile autism; infected area; inferior angle; inhibitory antigen; internal auditory; intra-alveolar; intra-amniotic; intra-aortic; intra-arterial; intra-articular; intra-atrial; intra-auricular; intrinsic activity; irradiation area

I&A irrigation and aspiration

Ia immune response gene-associated antigen

IAA imidazoleacetic acid; indoleacetic acid; infectious agent, arthritis; insulin autoantibody; International Antituberculosis Association; interruption of the aortic arch; iodoacetic acid

IAAA inflammatory abdominal aortic aneurysm

IAAR imidazoleacetic acid ribonucleotide

IAB Industrial Accident Board; intra-abdominal; intra-aortic balloon

IABA intra-aortic balloon assistance

IABC, IABCP intra-aortic balloon counter-pulsation

IABM idiopathic aplastic bone marrow

IABP intra-aortic balloon pump

AIBS International Association for Biological Standards

IAC image analysis cytometry; ineffective airway clearance; internal auditory canal; interposed abdominal compression; intra-arterial catheter; intra-arterial chemotherapy

IAC CPR interposed abdominal compression cardiopulmonary resuscitation

IACD implantable automatic cardioverter-defibrillator; intra-arterial conduction defect

IACI idiopathic arterial calcification of infancy

IACP intra-aortic counterpulsation

IACS International Academy of Cosmetic Surgery

IACV International Association of Cancer Victims and Friends

IAD inactivating dose; instructional advance directive; internal absorbed dose

IADH inappropriate antidiuretic hormone

IADHS inappropriate antidiuretic hormone syndrome

IADL instrumental or intermediate activities of daily living

IADR International Association for Dental Research

IADSA intra-arterial digital subtraction angiography

IAds immunoadsorption

IAEA International Atomic Energy Agency

IAET International Association for Enterostomal Therapy

IAF idiopathic alveolar fibrosis

IAFI infantile amaurotic familial idiocy

IAG International Association of Gerontology; International Academy of Gnathology

IAGP International Association of Geographic Pathology

IAGUS International Association of Genito-Urinary Surgeons

IAH idiopathic adrenal hyperplasia; implantable artificial heart

IAHA idiopathic autoimmune hemolytic anemia; immune adherence hemagglutination

IAHD idiopathic acquired hemolytic disorder

IAHS infection-associated hemophagocytic syndrome; International Association of Hospital Security

IAI intra-abdominal infection

IAIMS integrated advanced information management system

IAIS insulin autoimmune syndrome

IAM Institute of Applied Microbiology [Japan]; Institute of Aviation Medicine; internal auditory meatus

i am intra-amniotic

IAMM International Association of Medical Museums

IAMS International Association of Microbiological Societies

IAN idiopathic aseptic necrosis; indole acetonitrile

iANP immunoreactive atrial natriuretic peptide

IAO immediately after onset; intermittent aortic occlusion; International Association of Orthodontists

IAOM International Association of Oral Myology

IAP immunosuppressive acidic protein; inosinic acid pyrophosphorylase; Institute of Animal Physiology; intermittent acute porphyria; International Academy of Pathology; International Academy of Proctology; intra-abdominal pressure; intracellular action potential; intracisternal A-type particle; islet-activating protein

IAPB International Association for Prevention of Blindness

IAPG interatrial pressure gradient

IAPM International Academy of Preventive Medicine

IAPP International Association for Preventive Pediatrics; islet amyloid polypeptide

IAPSRS International Association of Psychosocial Rehabilitation Services

IAPV intermittent abdominal pressure ventilation

IAR immediate asthma reaction; inhibitory anal reflex; iodine-azide reaction

IARC International Agency for Research on Cancer

IARF ischemic acute renal failure

IARS image archival and retrieval system

IARSA idiopathic acquired refractory sideroblastic anemia

IAS immunosuppressive acidic substance; infant apnea syndrome; insulin autoimmune syndrome; interatrial septum; interatrial shunting; internal anal sphincter; International Acquired Immune Deficiency Syndrome Society; intra-amniotic saline

IASA interatrial septal aneurysm

IASD interatrial septal defect; inter-auricular septal defect

IASH isolated asymmetric septal hypertrophy

IASHS Institute for Advanced Study in Human Sexuality

IASL International Association for Study of the Liver

IASP International Association for Study of Pain

IAT instillation abortion time; iodine azide test; invasive activity test

IATI inter-alpha-trypsin inhibitor

IATIL inter-alpha-trypsin inhibitor, light chain

IAV intermittent assisted ventilation; intra-arterial vasopressin

IAVM intramedullary arteriovenous malformation

IB idiopathic blepharospasm; immune body; inclusion body; index of body build; infectious bronchitis; Institute of Biology; interface bus

ib in the same place [Lat. *ibidem*]

IBAT intravascular bronchoalveolar tumor

IBB intestinal brush border

IBBBB incomplete bilateral bundle branch block

IBC Institutional Biosafety Committee; iodine-binding capacity; iron-binding capacity; isobutyl cyanoacrylate

IBCA isobutyl-2-cyanoacrylate

IBD inflammatory bowel disease; irritable bowel disease

IBE International Bureau for Epilepsy

IBED Inter-African Bureau for Epizootic Diseases

iB-EP immunoreactive beta-endomorphin

IBF immature brown fat; immunoglobulin-binding factor; Insall-Burstein-Freeman [total knee instrumentation]

IBG insoluble bone gelatin

IBI intermittent bladder irrigation; ischemic brain infarction

ibid in the same place [Lat. *ibidem*]

IBIDS ichthyosis-brittle hair-impaired intelligence-decreased fertility-short stature [syndrome]

IBK infectious bovine keratoconjunctivitis

IBM inclusion body myositis

IBMP International Board of Medicine and Psychology

IBMX 3-isobutyl-1-methylxanthine

IBNR incurred but not reported

IBP insulin-like growth factor binding protein; International Biological Program; intra-aortic balloon pumping; iron-binding protein

IBPMS indirect blood pressure measuring system

IBQ Illness Behavior Questionnaire

IBR infectious bovine rhinotracheitis

IBRO International Brain Research Organization

IBRV infectious bovine rhinotracheitis virus

IBS imidazole buffered saline; immunoblastic sarcoma; irritable bowel syndrome; isobaric solution

IBSA iodinated bovine serum albumin

IBSN infantile bilateral striated necrosis

IBSP integrin-binding sialoprotein

IBT ink blot test

IBU ibuprofen; international benzoate unit

i-Bu isobutyl

IBV infectious bronchitis vaccine; infectious bronchitis virus

IBW ideal body weight

IC icteric, icterus; immune complex; immunoconjugate; immunocytochemistry; immunocytotoxicity; impedance cardiogram; indirect calorimetry; individual counseling; infection control; inferior colliculus; inner canthal [distance]; inorganic carbon; inspiratory capacity; inspiratory center; institutional care; integrated circuit; integrated concentration; intensive care; intercostal; intermediate care; intermittent catheterization; intermittent claudication; internal capsule; internal carotid; internal conjugate; interstitial cell; intracapsular; intracardiac; intracarotid; intracavitary; intracellular; intracerebral; intracisternal; intracranial; intracutaneous; irritable colon; islet cells; isovolumic contraction

IC 1/2/3 intermediate care 1/2/3

IC$_{50}$ inhibitory concentration of 50%

ic between meals [Lat. *inter cibos*]

ICA Institute of Clinical Analysis; internal carotid artery; intracranial aneurysm; islet cell antibody

ICAA International Council on Alcohol and Addictions; Invalid Children's Aid Association

ICAAC Interscience Conference on Antimicrobial Agents and Chemotherapy

ICAb islet cell antibody

ICAM intercellular adhesion molecule

ICAMI International Committee Against Mental Illness

ICAO internal carotid artery occlusion

ICASO International Committee of Acquired Immunodeficiency Syndrome Service Organisations

ICBF inner cortical blood flow

ICBG idiopathic calcification of basal ganglia

ICBP intracellular binding protein

ICBR increased chromosomal breakage rate

ICC immunocompetent cells; immunocytochemistry; Indian childhood cirrhosis; intensive coronary care; intercanthal distance; interchromosomal crossing over; interclass correlation coefficient; internal conversion coefficient; International Certification Commission; interventional cardiac center; intracervical device; intraclass correlation coefficient

ICCE intracapsular cataract extraction

ICCS International Classification of Clinical Services

ICDS International Cardiac Doppler Society

ICG impedance cardiogram; impedance cardiography

iCCK immunoreactive cholecystokinin

ICCM idiopathic congestive cardiomyopathy

ICCR International Committee for Contraceptive Research

ICCU intensive coronary care unit; intermediate coronary care unit

ICD I-cell disease; immune complex disease; implantable cardioverter defibrillator; impulse-control disorder; induced circular dichroism; Institute for Crippled and Disabled; International Center for the Disabled; International Classification of Diseases, Injuries, and Causes of Death; International Statistical Classification of Diseases and Health-related Problems; intrauterine contraceptive device; ischemic coronary disease; isocitrate dehydrogenase; isolated conduction defect

ICDA International Classification of Diseases, Adapted

ICDC implantable cardioverter-defibrillator catheter

ICD-9-CM International Classification of Diseases-ninth revision-Clinical Modification

ICD-10 International Statistical Classification of Diseases and Health-related Problems, 10th revision

ICDH isocitrate dehydrogenase

ICD-O International Classification of Diseases-Oncology

ICDRC International Contact Dermatitis Research Center

ICDS Integrated Child Development Scheme

ICE ice, compression, elevation; ichthyosis-cheek-eyebrow [syndrome]; immunochemical evaluation; interleukin converting enzyme; iridocorneal endothelial [syndrome]

ICES information collection and evaluation system

ICF immunodeficiency-centromeric instability-facial anomalies [syndrome]; indirect centrifugal flotation; intensive care facility; intercellular fluorescence; interciliary fluid; intermediate-care facility; International Cardiology Foundation; intracellular fluid; intravascular co-agulation and fibrinolysis

ICFA incomplete Freund adjuvant; induced complement-fixing antigen

ICF(M)A International Cystic Fibrosis (Mucoviscidosis) Association

ICF-MR intermediate-care facility for the mentally retarded

ICF/MR intensive care facilities for mental retardation

ICG indocyanine green; isotope cisternography

ICGC indocyanine-green clearance

ICGN immune-complex glomerulo-nephritis

ICH idiopathic cortical hyperostosis; infectious canine hepatitis; intracerebral hematoma; intracranial hemorrhage; intracranial hypertension

ICHD Inter-Society Commission for Heart Disease Resources

ICHPPC International Classification of Health Problems in Primary Care

ICI intracardiac infection

ICi intracisternal

ICIDH International Classification of Impairments, Disabilities, and Handicaps

ICL idiopathic CD4 T-cell lymphocytopenia; iris-clip lens; isocitrate lyase

ICLA International Committee on Laboratory Animals

ICLH Imperial College, London Hospital

ICM inner cell mass; integrated conditional model; intercostal margin; International Confederation of Midwives; intracytoplasmic membrane; introduction to clinical medicine; ion conductance modulator; isolated cardiovascular malformation

ICMI Inventory of Childhood Memories and Imaginings

ICMSF International Commission on Microbiological Specifications for Foods

ICN intensive care nursery; International Council of Nurses

ICNa intracellular concentration of sodium

ICNB International Committee on Nomenclature of Bacteria

ICNC intracerebral nuclear cell

ICNND Interdepartmental Committee on Nutrition in National Defense

ICNP International Classification of Nursing Practice

ICNV International Committee on Nomenclature of Viruses

ICO idiopathic cyclic oedema; impedance cardiac output

ICP incubation period; indwelling catheter program; infantile cerebral palsy; infection-control practitioner; infectious cell protein; inflammatory cloacogenic polyp; interdisciplinary care plan; intermittent catheterization protocol; intracranial pressure; intracytoplasmic; intrahepatic cholestasis of pregnancy

ICPA International Commission for the Prevention of Alcoholism

ICPB International Collection of Phytopathogenic Bacteria

ICPEMC International Commission for Protection against Environmental Mutagens and Carcinogens

ICPI Intersociety Committee on Pathology Information

ICP-MS inductively coupled plasma mass spectrometry [or spectrometer]

ICR [distance between] iliac crests; Institute for Cancer Research; Institute for Cancer Research [mouse]; intermittent catheter routine; International Congress of Radiology; intracardiac catheter recording; intracavitary radium; intracranial reinforcement; ion cyclotron resonance

ICRC infant care review committee; International Committee of the Red Cross

ICRD Index of Codes for Research Drugs

ICRE International Commission on Radiological Education

ICRETT International Cancer Research Technology Transfer

ICREW International Cancer Research Workshop

ICRF Imperial Cancer Research Fund [UK]

I-CRF immunoreactive corticotropin-releasing factor

ICRF-159 razoxane

ICRP International Commission on Radiological Protection

ICRS Index Chemicus Registry System

ICRU International Commission on Radiation Units and Measurements

ICS ileocecal sphincter; immotile cilia syndrome; impulse-conducting system; integrated case study; intensive care, surgical; intercellular space; intercostal space; International College of Surgeons; intracranial stimulation; irritable colon syndrome

ICSA islet cell surface antibody

ICSB International Committee on Systematic Bacteriology

ICSC idiopathic central serous choroidopathy

ICSH International Committee for Standardization in Hematology; interstitial cell-stimulating hormone

ICSI Institute for Clinical Systems Integration

ICSK intracoronary streptokinase

ICSO intermittent coronary sinus occlusion

ICSP International Council of Societies of Pathology

ICSS intracranial self-stimulation

ICSTI International Council for Scientific and Technical Information

ICSU International Council of Scientific Unions

ICT icteric, icterus; indirect Coombs test; inflammation of connective tissue; insulin coma therapy; intensive conventional therapy; intermittent cervical traction; interstitial cell tumor; intracardiac thrombus; intracranial tumor; isovolumic contraction time

Ict icterus

iCT immunoreactive calcitonin

ICTMM International Congress on Tropical Medicine and Malaria

ICTS idiopathic carpal tunnel syndrome

ICTV International Committee for the Taxonomy of Viruses

ICTX intermittent cervical traction

ICU infant care unit; immunologic contact urticaria; intensive care unit; intermediate care unit

ICV intracellular volume; intracerebroventricular

ICVS International Cardiovascular Society

ICW intensive care ward; intracellular water

ICx immune complex

ID identification; iditol dehydrogenase; immunodeficiency; immunodiffusion; immunoglobulin deficiency; inappropriate disability; inclusion disease; index of discrimination; individual dose; infant death; infectious disease; infective dose; inhibitory dose; initial diagnosis; initial dose; initial dyskinesia; injected dose; inside diameter; interdigitating; interhemispheric disconnection; interstitial disease; intradermal; intraduodenal

I-D intensity-duration

I&D incision and drainage

ID$_{50}$ median infective dose

Id infradentale; interdentale

id the same [Lat. *idem*]

IDA idamycin; image display and analysis; iminodiacetic acid; insulin-degrading activity; iron deficiency anemia

IDAV immunodeficiency-associated virus

IDB image data baser

IDBS infantile diffuse brain sclerosis

IDC idiopathic dilated cardiomyopathy; interdigitating cell

IDCI intradiplochromatid interchange

IDD insulin-dependent diabetes; intraluminal duodenal diverticulum; Inventory to Diagnose Depression

IDDF investigational drug data form

IDDM insulin-dependent diabetes mellitus

IDDM-MED insulin-dependent diabetes mellitus-multiple epiphyseal dysplasia [syndrome]

IDDT immune double diffusion test

IDE insulin-degrading enzyme; investigational device exemption

IDEA Individuals with Disabilities Education Act

IDF inverse document frequency

IDG intermediate dose group

IDI immunologically detectable insulin; induction-delivery interval; inter-dentale inferius

IDIC Internal Dose Information Center

idic isodicentric

IDISA intraoperative digital subtraction angiography

IDK internal derangement of knee

IDL Index to Dental Literature; interface definition language; intermediate density lipoprotein; intermediate differentiation of lymphocytic lymphoma

IDLH immediate danger to life and health

IDM idiopathic disease of myocardium; immune defense mechanism; indirect method; infant of diabetic mother; intermediate-dose methotrexate

ID-MS isotope dilution-mass spectrometry

iDNA intercalary deoxyribonucleic acid

IDP immunodiffusion procedure; inflammatory demyelinating neuropathy; initial dose period; inosine diphosphate

IDPH idiopathic pulmonary hemosiderosis

IDPN iminodipropionitrile

IDQ Individualized Dementia Questionnaire

IDR intradermal reaction

IDS iduronate sulfatase; immune deficiency state; inhibitor of DNA synthesis; integrated delivery system; intraduodenal stimulation; Inventory for Depressive Symptomatology; investigational drug service

IdS interdentale superius

IDSA Infectious Disease Society of America

IDSAN International Drug Safety Advisory Network

IDS-SR Inventory for Depressive Symptomatology-Systems Review

IDT immune diffusion test; instillation delivery time; intradermal typhoid [vaccine]

IDU idoxuridine; injection or intravenous drug user; iododeoxyuridine

IdUA iduronic acid

IDUR idoxuridine

IdUrd idoxuridine

IDV intermittent demand ventilation

IDVC indwelling venous catheter

Idx cross-reactive idiotype

IE imaging equipment; immunizing unit [Ger. *Immunitäts Einheit*]; immunoelectrophoresis; infectious endocarditis; inner ear; intake energy; internal elastica; intraepithelial

ie that is [Lat. *id est*]

I/E inspiratory/expiratory [ratio]; internal/external

I:E inspiratory/expiratory [ratio]

IEA immediate early antigen; immunoelectroadsorption; immunoelectrophoretic analysis; infectious equine anemia; inferior epigastric artery; International Epidemiological Association; intravascular erythrocyte aggregation

IEC injection electrode catheter; International Electrotechnical Commission; intraepithelial carcinoma; ion-exchange chromatography

IECa intraepithelial carcinoma

IED inherited epidermal dysplasia; intermittent explosive disorder

IEE inner enamel epithelium

IEEE Institute of Electrical and Electronics Engineers

IEF International Eye Foundation; isoelectric focusing

IEG immediate early gene

IEI isoelectric interval

IEL internal elastic lamina; intraepithelial lymphocyte

IEM immuno-electron microscopy; inborn error of metabolism

IEMA immunoenzymatic assay

IEMCT individualized epidural morphine conversion tool

IEMG integrated electromyogram; integrated electromyography

IEOP immunoelectro-osmophoresis

IEP immunoelectrophoresis; individualized education program; isoelectric point

IESS Intergroup Ewing Sarcoma Study

IET intrauterine exchange transfusion

IF idiopathic fibroplasia; idiopathic flushing; immersion foot; immunofluorescence; indirect fluorescence; infrared; inhibiting factor; initiation factor; instantaneous flow; interferon; interior facet; intermediate filament; intermediate frequency; internal fixation; interstitial fluid;interventional fluoroscopy; intrinsic factor; involved field [radiotherapy]

IF1, IF2, IF3 interferon 1, 2, 3

IFA idiopathic fibrosing alveolitis; immunofluorescence assay; immunofluorescent antibody; incomplete Freund's adjuvant; indirect fluorescent antibody; indirect fluorescent assay; International Fertility Association; International Filariasis Association

IFAP ichthyosis follicularis-atrichia-photophobia [syndrome]

IFAT indirect fluorescent antibody test

IFC intermittent flow centrifugation; intrinsic factor concentrate

IFCC International Federation of Clinical Chemistry

IFCR International Foundation for Cancer Research

IFCS inactivated fetal calf serum

IFDS isolated follicle-stimulating hormone deficiency syndrome

IFE immunofixation electrophoresis; interfollicular epidermis

IFF inner fracture face

IFFH International Foundation for Family Health

IFG inferior frontal gyrus; interferon gamma

IFGO International Federation of Gynecology and Obstetrics

IFGS interstitial fluid and ground substance

IFHP International Federation of Health Professionals

IFHPMSM International Federation for Hygiene, Preventive Medicine, and Social Medicine

IFI immune interferon

IFL immunofluorescence

IFLrA recombinant human leukocyte interferon A

IFM internal fetal monitor

IFMBE International Federation for Medical and Biological Engineering

IFME International Federation for Medical Electronics

IFMP International Federation for Medical Psychotherapy

IFMSA International Federation of Medical Student Associations

IFMSS International Federation of Multiple Sclerosis Societies

IFN interferon

IFNA interferon alpha

If nec if necessary

IFNG interferon gamma

IFNGT interferon gamma transducer

IFP inflammatory fibroid polyp; insulin, compound F [hydrocortisone], prolactin; intermediate filament protein; intrapatellar fat pad

IFPM International Federation of Physical Medicine

IFR infrared; inspiratory flow rate

IFRA indirect fluorescent rabies antibody [test]

IFRP International Fertility Research Program

IFRT involved field radiotherapy

IFS interstitial fluid space

IFSM International Federation of Sports Medicine

IFSP individualized family service plan

IFSSH International Federation of Societies for Surgery of the Hand

IFT immunofluorescence test

IFU interferon unit

IFV interstitial fluid volume; intracellular fluid volume

IG immature granule; immunoglobulin; insulin and glucose; intragastric; irritable gut

Ig immunoglobulin

IGA infantile genetic agranulocytosis

IgA immunoglobulin A

IgA1, IgA2 subclasses of immunoglobulin A

IgAGN immunoglobulin A glomerulonephritis

IgAN immunoglobulin A nephropathy

IGC immature germ cell; intragastric cannula

IGD idiopathic growth hormone deficiency; interglobal distance; isolated gonadotropin deficiency

IgD immunoglobulin D

IgD1, IgD2 subclasses of immunoglobulin D

IGDM infant of mother with gestational diabetes mellitus

IGE impaired gas exchange

IgE immunoglobulin E

IgE1 subclass of immunoglobulin E

IGF insulin-like growth factor

IGFPB insulin-like growth factor binding protein

IGFBP-3 IGF-binding protein 3

IGFET insulated gate field effect transistor

IGFL integral green fluorescence

IGFR insulin-like growth factor receptor

IgG immunoglobulin G

IgG1, IgG2, IgG3, IgG4 subclasses of immunoglobulin G

IGH immunoreactive growth hormone

IGHD immunoglobin delta heavy chain; isolated growth hormone deficiency

IGHE immunoglobulin epsilon heavy chain

IGHV immunoglobulin heavy chain variable region

IGIV immune globulin intravenous

IGKDEL immunoglobulin kappa deleting element

IGL immunoglobulin lambda

IGLJ immunoglobulin lambda light chain J

IGLL immunoglobulin lambda-like

IgM immunoglobulin M

IgM1 subclass of immunoglobulin M

IgMN immunoglobulin M nephropathy

IGO1 immunoglobulin kappa orphan 1

IGP intestinal glycoprotein

IGR immediate generalized reaction; integrated gastrin response

IGS image-guided surgery; inappropriate gonadotropin secretion; internal guide sequence

Igs immunoglobulins

IgSC immunoglobulin-secreting cell

IGT impaired glucose tolerance

IGTT intravenous glucose tolerance test

IGV intrathoracic gas volume

IH idiopathic hirsutism; idiopathic hypercalciuria; immediate hypersensitivity; incompletely healed; indirect hemagglutination; industrial hygiene; infantile hydrocephalus; infectious hepatitis; inguinal hernia; inhibiting hormone; in hospital; inner half; inpatient hospital; intermittent heparinization; intracranial hematoma; iron hematoxylin

IHA idiopathic hyperaldosteronism; indirect hemagglutination; indirect hemagglutination antibody

IHAC Industrial Health and Advisory Committee

IHBT incompatible hemolytic blood transfusion

IHC idiopathic hemochromatosis; idiopathic hypercalciuria; immunohistochemistry; inner hair cell; intrahepatic cholestasis

IHCA individual health care account; isocapnic hyperventilation with cold air

IHCP Institute of Hospital and Community Psychiatry

IHCM ichthyosis hystrix, Curth-Macklin [type]

IHD in-center hemodialysis; ischemic heart disease

IHES idiopathic hypereosinophilic syndrome

IHF Industrial Health Foundation; integration host factor; International Hospital Foundation

IHGD isolateral human growth deficiency

IHH idiopathic hypogonadotropic hypogonadism; idiopathic hypothalamic hypogonadism; infectious human hepatitis

IHHS idiopathic hyperkinetic heart syndrome

IHI Institute for Healthcare Improvement

IHIS integrated hospital information system

IHL International Homeopathic League

IHO idiopathic hypertrophic osteoarthropathy

IHP idiopathic hypoparathyroidism; idiopathic hypopituitarism; individualized health plan; inositol hexaphosphate; interhospitalization period; inverted hand position

IHPC intrahepatic cholestasis

IHPH intrahepatic portal hypertension

IHPP Intergovernmental Health Project Policy

IHQL index of health-related quality of life

IHR intrahepatic resistance; intrinsic heart rate

IHRA isocapnic hyperventilation with room air

IHRB Industrial Health Research Board

IHS idiopathic hypereosinophilic syndrome; inactivated horse serum; Indian Health Service; integrated health system; International Headache Society; International Health Society

IHSA iodinated human serum albumin

IHSC immunoreactive human skin collagenase

IHSS idiopathic hypertrophic subaortic stenosis

IHT insulin hypoglycemia test; intravenous histamine test; ipsilateral head turning

I5HT intraplatelet serotonin

Ii incision inferius

II icterus index; image intensification or intensifier; Roman numeral two

I&I illness and injuries

IICP increased intracranial pressure

II-para secundipara

IID insulin-independent diabetes

IIDM insulin-independent diabetes mellitus

IIE idiopathic ineffective erythropoiesis

IIF immune interferon; indirect immunofluorescence

IIFT itraoperative intraarterial fibrinolytic therapy

IIG interactive image-guided [surgery]

IIGR ipsilateral instinctive grasp reaction

III Roman numeral three

III-para tertipara

IIME Institute of International Medical Education

IIMS Interest in Internal Medicine Scale

IIP idiopathic interstitial pneumonia; idiopathic intestinal pseudo-obstruction; increased intracranial pressure

IIS intensive immunosuppression; International Institute of Stress

IIT ineffective iron turnover

IJ ileojejunal; internal jugular; intrajejunal; intrajugular

IJCAI International Joint Conference on Artificial Intelligence

IJD inflammatory joint disease

IJP inhibitory junction potential; internal jugular pressure

IJV internal jugular vein

IK immobilized knee; immune body [Ger. *Immunekörper*]; *Infusoria* killing [unit]; interstitial keratitis

IKE ion kinetic energy

IKU *Infusoria* killing unit

IL ileum; incisolingual; independent laboratory; iliolumbar; independent laboratory; inspiratory load; intensity load; interleukin; intralumbar

Il promethium [*illinium*]

IL-1 interleukin 1

IL-2 interleukin 2

IL-3 interleukin 3

ILA insulin-like activity; International Leprosy Association

ILa incisolabial

ILAR Institute of Laboratory Animal Research

ILB infant, low birth [weight]; initial lung burden

ILBBB incomplete left bundle branch block

ILBW infant, low birth weight

ILC ichthyosis linearis circumflex; incipient lethal concentration

ILD interstitial lung disease; intraoperative localization device; ischemic leg disease; ischemic limb disease; isolated lactase deficiency

ILDBP interleukin-dependent deoxyribonucleic acid-binding protein

ILE, ILe, Ileu isoleucine

ILGF insulin-like growth factor

ILH immunoreactive luteinizing hormone

ILL intermediate lymphocytic lymphoma

ILM insulin-like material; internal limiting membrane

ILNR intralobar nephrogenic rest

ILo iodine lotion

ILP inadequate luteal phase; insufficiency of luteal phase; interstitial laser photocoagulation; interstitial lymphocytic pneumonia

ILR interleukin receptor; irreversible loss rate

ILRA interleukin receptor alpha

ILRB interleukin receptor beta

ILS idiopathic leucine sensitivity; idiopathic lymphadenopathy syndrome; increase in life span; infrared liver scanner; intermittent light stimulation; intralobal sequestration

ILSI International Life Sciences Institute

ILSS integrated life support system; intraluminal somatostatin

ILT iliotibial tract

ILTV infectious laryngotracheitis virus

ILV independent lung ventilation

IM idiopathic myelofibrosis; immunosuppressive method; implementation monitoring; Index Medicus; indomethacin; industrial medicine; infection medium; infectious mononucleosis; inner membrane; innocent murmur; inspiratory muscles; intermediate; intermediate megaloblast; internal malleolus; internal mammary [artery]; internal medicine; intramedullary; intramuscular; invasive mole

im intramuscular

IMA Industrial Medical Association; inferior mesenteric artery; Interchurch Medical Assistance; internal mammary artery; Irish Medical Association

IMAA iodinated macroaggregated albumin

IMAB internal mammary artery bypass

IMAC information management, archiving, and communication

IMACS image archiving and communication system

IMAGE International Multicenter Angina Exercise [study]

IMAI internal mammary artery implant

IMB intermenstrual bleeding

IMBC indirect maximum breathing capacity

IMBI Institute of Medical and Biological Illustrators

IMC indigent medical care; information-memory-concentration [test]; interdigestive migrating contractions; International Medical Corps; intestinal mast cell

IMCT Information-Memory-Concentration Test

IMCU intermediate medical care unit

IMD immunodeficiency; immunologically mediated disease; institution for mentally disabled

ImD$_{50}$ immunizing dose sufficient to protect 50% of the animals in a test group

IMDC intramedullary metatarsal decompression

IMDD idiopathic midline destructive disease

IMDG International Maritime Dangerous Goods [code]

IMDP imidocarb diproprionate

IME independent medical examination; indirect medical education

IMEG innovations in medical education grant

IMEM improved minimum essential medium

IMET isometric endurance test

IMF idiopathic myelofibrosis; immunofluorescence; intermaxillary fixation; intermediate filament

IMG inferior mesenteric ganglion; internal medicine group [practice]; international medical graduate

IMGG intramuscular gammaglobulin

IMH idiopathic myocardial hypertrophy; indirect microhemagglutination [test]

IMHP 1-iodomercuri-2-hydroxypropane

IMHT indirect microhemagglutination test

IMI immunologically measurable insulin; impending myocardial infarction; Imperial Mycological Institute [UK]; inferior myocardial infarction; intermeal interval; intramuscular injection

Imi imipramine

IMIA International Medical Informatics Association

IMIC International Medical Information Center

IMLA intramural left anterior [artery]

IMLAD intramural left anterior descending [artery]

IMLNS idiopathic minimal lesion nephrotic syndrome

ImLy immune lysis

IMM inhibitor-containing minimal medium; internal medial malleolus

immat immaturity, immature

IMMC interdigestive migrating motor complex

IMO idiopathic multicentric osteolysis

immobil immobilization, immobilize

immun immune, immunity, immunization

IMN internal mammary node

IMP idiopathic myeloid proliferation; impression; incomplete male pseudohermaphroditism; individual Medicaid practitioner; inosine 5'-monophosphate; intramembranous particle; intramuscular compartment pressure; N-isopropyl-p-iodoamphetamine

Imp impression

imp impacted, impaction

IMPA incisal mandibular plane angle

IMPAC Information for Management, Planning, Analysis and Coordination

IMPATH interactive microcomputer patient assessment tool for health

IMPC International Myopia Prevention Center

IMPD inosine-5'-monophosphate dehydrogenase

IMPDH inosine-5'-monophosphate dehydrogenase

IMPDHL inosine-5'-monophosphate dehydrogenase-like

IMPS Inpatient Multidimensional Psychiatric Scale; intact months of patient survival

Impx impacted

IMR individual medical record; infant mortality rate; infant mortality risk; Institute for Medical Research; institution for mentally retarded

IMS incurred in military service; Indian Medical Service; industrial methylated spirit; information management system; integrated medical services; international metric system

IMSS in-flight medical support system

IMT indomethacin; induced muscular tension; inspiratory muscle training

IMU Index of Medical Underservice

IMV inferior mesenteric vein; intermittent mandatory ventilation; intermittent mechanical ventilation; isophosphamide, methotrexate, and vincristine

IMViC, imvic indole, methyl red, Voges-Proskauer, citrate [test]

IMVP idiopathic mitral valve prolapse

IMVS Institute of Medical and Veterinary Science

IN icterus neonatorum; impetigo neonatorum; incidence; incompatibility number; infundibular nucleus; insulin; interneuron; interstitial nephritis; intranasal; irritation of nociceptors

In index; indium; inion; insulin; inulin

in inch

in² square inch

in³ cubic inch

INA infectious nucleic acid; inferior nasal artery; International Neurological Association

INAA instrumental neutron activation analysis

INAD infantile neuroaxonal dystrophy

INAH isonicotinic acid hydrazide

INB internuclear bridging; ischemic necrosis of bone

inbr inbreeding

INC internodular cortex; inside needle catheter

inc incision; inclusion; incompatibility; incontinent; increase; increased; increment; incurred

INCB International Narcotics Control Board

IncB inclusion body

INCD infantile nuclear cerebral degeneration

incl inclusion or include

incr increase, increased; increment

incur incurable

IND indomethacin; industrial medicine; investigational new drug

ind indirect; induction

indic indication, indicated

indig indigestion

indiv individual

INDM infant of nondiabetic mother

INDO indoleamine-2,3-dioxygenase; indomethacin

INDOR internuclear double resonance

indust industrial

INE infantile necrotizing encephalomyelopathy

INEPT insensitive nuclei enhanced by polarization transfer

INET image network
INF infant, infantile; infection, infective, infected; inferior; infirmary; infundibulum; infusion; interferon
inf infant, infantile; inferior
infect infection, infected, infective
Inflamm inflammation, inflammatory
inf mono infectious mononucleosis
ING isotope nephrogram
ing inguinal
InGP indolglycerophosphate
INH inhalation; isoniazid; isonicotinic acid hydrazide
INHA inhibin alpha
inhal inhalation
INHB inhibin beta
inhib inhibition, inhibiting
INI intranuclear inclusion
inj injection; injury, injured, injurious
inject injection
INK injury not known
INLSD ichthyosis and neutral lipid storage disease
INN International Nonproprietary Names
innerv innervation, innervated
innom innominate
INO internuclear ophthalmoplegia; inosine
Ino inosine
INOC isonicotinoyloxycarbonyl
inoc inoculation, inoculated
inorg inorganic
iNOS inducible macrophage-type nitric oxide synthase
Inox inosine, oxidized
INP idiopathic neutropenia
INPAV intermittent negative pressure assisted ventilation
INPEA isopropyl nitrophenylethanolamine
INPH iproniazid phosphate
INPP1 inositol polyphosphate 1-phosphatase
INPV intermittent negative-pressure ventilation

INQ interior nasal quadrant
InQ inquiry mode questionnaire
InQ(R) inquiry mode questionnaire, reliability assessment
INR international normalized ratio
INREM internal roentgen-equivalent, man
INRIA National Institute for Research in Computers and Automation [France] [Institut National de la Recherche Informatique et Automatique]
INS idiopathic nephrotic syndrome; insulin; insurance
Ins insulin; insurance, insured
ins insertion; insulin; insurance, insured
insem insemination
INSIGHT International Nifedipine Study Intervention as a Goal in Hypertension Treatment
insol insoluble
Insp inspiration
INSR insulin receptor
INSRR insulin receptor-related receptor
INSS international neuroblastoma staging system
Inst institute
instab instability
instill instillation
insuf insufflation
insuff insufficient, insufficiency; insufflation
INT intermediate; intermittent; intern, internship; internal; interval; intestinal; intima; p-iodonitrotetrazolium
Int international; intestinal
int internal
INTACT International Nifedipine Trial on Antiatherosclerotic Therapy
INTEG integument
intern internal
Internat international
intes intestine
Intest intestine, intestinal
Int/Ext internal/external
INTH intrathecal

Intmd intermediate
Int Med internal medicine
INTOX, Intox intoxication
INTR intermittent
Int Rot internal rotation
INTRP Inventory of Negative Thoughts in Response to Pain
Int trx intermittent traction
intub intubation
INV inferior nasal vein
Inv, inv inversion; involuntary
Inv/Ev inversion/eversion
invest investigation
inv ins inverted insertion
invol involuntary
involv involvement, involved
inv(p+q-) pericentric inversion
inv(p-q+) pericentric inversion
IO incisal opening; inferior oblique; inferior olive; internal os; interorbital; intestinal obstruction; intraocular; intraoperative
I&O in and out; intake and output
I/O input/output; intake/output
Io ionium
IOA inner optic anlage; International Osteopathic Association
IOC International Organizing Committee on Medical Librarianship; intern on call
IOCG intraoperative cholangiogram
IOD injured on duty; integrated optical density; interorbital distance
IOFB intraocular foreign body
IOH idiopathic orthostatic hypotension
IOL induction of labor; intraocular lens
IOM Institute of Medicine
IOMP International Organization for Medical Physics
ION ischemic optic neuropathy
IOP improving organizational performance; intraocular pressure
IOR index of response
IORT intraoperative radiotherapy
IOS infant observation scale; International Organization for Standardization

IOT intraocular tension; intraocular transfer; ipsilateral optic tectum
IOTA information overload testing aid
ι Greek letter *iota*
IOU intensive care observation unit; international opacity unit
IOUS intraoperative ultrasound [examination]
IOV inside-out vesicle
IP icterus praecox; imaging plate; immune precipitate; immunoblastic plasma; immunoperoxidase technique; inactivated pepsin; incisoproximal; incisopulpal; incontinentia pigmenti; incubation period; induced potential; induction period; infection prevention; infundibular process; infusion pump; inhibition period; inorganic phosphate; inosine phosphorylase; inpatient; instantaneous pressure; L'Institut Pasteur; International Pharmacopoeia; Internet protocol; interpeduncular; interphalangeal; interpupillary; intestinal pseudo-obstruction; intramuscular pressure; intraperitoneal; intraphalangeal; intrapulmonary; ionization potential; isoelectric point; isoproterenol
ip intraperitoneal
i/p inpatient
IP$_1$ inositol-1-phosphate
IP$_3$ inositol-1,4,5-triphosphate
IPA immunoperoxidase assay; incontinentia pigmenti achromians; independent physician or practice association; individual practice association; infantile papular acrodermatitis; International Pediatric Association; International Pharmaceutical Association; International Psychoanalytical Association; intrapleural analgesia; isopropyl alcohol
I$_{pa}$ pulse average intensity
IPAA International Psychoanalytical Association
IPAP inspiratory positive airway pressure
I-para primipara

IPAT Institute of Personality and Ability Testing; Iowa Pressure Articulation Test

IPB injury-prone behavior; integrated problem-based curriculum

IPC intermittent pneumatic compression; International Poliomyelitis Congress; ion pair chromatography; isopropyl carbamate; isopropyl chlorophenyl

IPCD infantile polycystic disease

IPCP interdisciplinary patient care plan

IPCS intrauterine progesterone contraception system

IPD idiopathic Parkinson disease; idiopathic protracted diarrhea; immediate pigment darkening; increase in pupillary diameter; incurable problem drinker; inflammatory pelvic disease; intermittent peritoneal dialysis; intermittent pigment darkening; interocular phase difference; interpupillary distance; Inventory of Psychosocial Development

IPE infectious porcine encephalomyelitis; interstitial pulmonary emphysema

IPEH intravascular papillary endothelial hyperplasia

IPF idiopathic pulmonary fibrosis; infection-potentiating factor; interstitial pulmonary fibrosis

IPFM integral pulse frequency modulation

IPG impedance plethysmography; inspiration-phase gas

iPGE immunoreactive prostaglandin E

IPH idiopathic portal hypertension; idiopathic pulmonary hemosiderosis; idiopathic pulmonary hypertension; inflammatory papillary hyperplasia; interphalangeal; intraparenchymal hemorrhage

IPHR inverted polypoid hamartoma of the rectum

IPI interpulse interval

IPIA immunoperoxidase infectivity assay

IPITA International Pancreas and Islet Transplant Association

IPJ interphalangeal joint

IPK intractable plantar keratosis

IPKD infantile polycystic kidney disease

IPL inner plexiform layer; intrapleural

IPM impulses per minute; inches per minute

IPMS inhibited power motive syndrome

IPN infantile polyarteritis nodosa; infectious pancreatic necrosis [of trout]; intern progress note; interpeduncular nucleus; interstitial pneumonitis

IPNA isopropyl noradrenalin

IPO improved pregnancy outcome

IPOF immediate postoperative fitting

IPOP immediate postoperative prosthesis

IPP independent practice plan; individual patient profile; inflatable penile prosthesis; inorganic pyrophosphate; intermittent positive pressure; intracisternal A particle-promoted polypeptide; intrahepatic partial pressure; intrapericardial pressure

Ipp interpulse potential

IPPA inspection, palpation, percussion, and auscultation

IPPB intermittent positive-pressure breathing

IPPB-I intermittent positive-pressure breathing-inspiration

IPPI interruption of pregnancy for psychiatric indication

IPPO intermittent positive-pressure inflation with oxygen

IPPR integrated pancreatic polypeptide response; intermittent positive-pressure respiration

IPPV intermittent positive-pressure ventilation

IPQ intimacy potential quotient

IPR insulin production rate; intraparenchymal resistance; ipratropium

i-Pr isopropyl

IPRL isolated perfused rat liver or lung

IPRT interpersonal reaction test

IPS idiopathic pain syndrome; idiopathic postprandial syndrome; inches per second; infundibular pulmonary stenosis; initial prognostic score; intrapartum stillbirth; intraperitoneal shock; ischiopubic synchondrosis

ips inches per second

IPSC inhibitory postsynaptic current

IPSC-E Inventory of Psychic and Somatic Complaints in the Elderly

IPSF immediate postsurgical fitting

IPSID immunoproliferative small intestine disease

IPSP inhibitory postsynaptic potential

IPT immunoperoxidase technique; immunoprecipitation; interpersonal psychotherapy; isoproterenol

IPTG isopropyl thiogalactose

iPTH immunoassay for parathyroid hormone; immunoreactive parathyroid hormone

IPTX intermittent pelvic traction

IPU inpatient unit

IPV inactivated poliomyelitis vaccine or virus; infectious pustular vaginitis; infectious pustular vulvovaginitis; intrapulmonary vein

IPW interphalangeal width

IPZ insulin protamine zinc

IQ institute of quality; intelligence quotient

IQAS internal quality assurance system

IQB individual quick blanch

IQCODE information questionnaire on cognitive decline in the elderly

IQR interquartile range

IQ&S iron, quinine, and strychnine

IR drop of voltage across a resistor produced by a current; ileal resection; immune response; immunization rate; immunoreactive; immunoreagent; index of response; impedance rheography; individual reaction; inferior rectus [muscle]; inflow resistance; information retrieval; infrared; infrarenal; inside radius; insoluble residue; inspiratory reserve; inspiratory resistance; insulin resistance; internal resistance; internal rotation; interventional radiology; intrarectal; intrarenal; inversion recovery; inverted repeat; irritant reaction; isovolumic relaxation

I-R Ito-Reenstierna [reaction]

I/R ischemia/reperfusion

Ir immune response [gene]; iridium

ir immunoreactive; intrarectal; intrarenal

IRA immunoradioassay; immunoregulatory alpha-globulin; inactive renin activity

IR-ACTH immunoreactive adrenocorticotropic hormone

IrANP immunoreactive atrial natriuretic peptide

IR APAP immediate release acetaminophen

IR-AVP immunoreactive arginine-vasopressin

IRB Institutional Review Board

IRBBB incomplete right bundle branch block

IRBC immature or infected red blood cell

IRBP intestinal retinol-binding protein

IRC inspiratory reserve capacity; instantaneous resonance curve; International Red Cross; International Research Communications System

IRCA intravascular red cell aggregation

IRCC International Red Cross Committee

IRCU intensive respiratory care unit

IRD infantile Refsum syndrome; isorhythmic dissociation

IRDP insulin-related DNA polymorphism

IRDS idiopathic respiratory distress syndrome; infant respiratory distress syndrome

IRE internal rotation in extension; iron-responsive element; isolated rabbit eye

IREBP iron-responsive element binding protein

IRED infrared light-emitting diode

IRF idiopathic retroperitoneal fibrosis; impulse response function; interferon regulatory factor; internal rotation in flexion

IRFL integral red fluorescence

IRG immunoreactive gastrin; immunoreactive glucagon

IRGH immunoreactive growth hormone

IRGl immunoreactive glucagon

IRH Institute for Research in Hypnosis; Institute of Religion and Health; intrarenal hemorrhage

IRHCS immunoradioassayable human chorionic somatomammotropin

IRhGH immunoreactive human growth hormone

IRhPL immunoreactive human growth hormone

IRI immunoreactive insulin; insulin resistance index

IRIA indirect radioimmunoassay

IRIg insulin-reactive immunoglobulin

IRIS integrated risk information system; interleukin regulation of immune system; International Research Information Service

IR-LED infrared light emitting diode

IRM innate releasing mechanism; Institute of Rehabilitation Medicine

IRMA immunoradiometric assay; intraretinal microvascular abnormalities

iRNA immune ribonucleic acid; informational ribonucleic acid

IROS ipsilateral routing of signal

IRP immunoreactive plasma; immunoreactive proinsulin; incus replacement prosthesis; insulin-releasing polypeptide; interstitial radiation pneumonitis

IRR insulin receptor-related receptor; intrarenal reflux

Irr irradiation; irritation

IRRD Institute for Research in Rheumatic Diseases

irreg irregularity, irregular

irrig irrigation, irrigate

IRS immunoreactive secretion; infrared spectrophotometry; insulin receptor species; insulin receptor substrate; intergroup rhabdomyosarcoma study; internal resolution site; International Rhinologic Society

IRS-1 insulin receptor substrate 1

IRS-2 insulin receptor substrate 2

IRSA idiopathic refractory sideroblastic anemia; iodinated rat serum albumin

IRT immunoreactive trypsin; interresponse time; interstitial radiotherapy

IRTIS Integrated Radiation Therapy Information System

IRTO immunoreactive trypsin output

IRTU integrating regulatory transcription unit

IRU industrial rehabilitation unit; interferon reference unit

IRV inferior radicular vein; inspiratory reserve volume; inverse ratio ventilation

IS ileal segment; immediate sensitivity; immune serum; immunosuppression; impingement syndrome; incentive spirometer; index of sexuality; infant size; infantile spasms; information system; insertion sequence; in situ; insulin secretion; intercellular space; intercostal space; interictal spike; interstitial space; intracardial shunt; intraspinal; intrasplenic; intrastriatal; intraventricular septum; invalided from service; inversion sequence; ischemic score; isoproterenol

Is incision superius

is in situ; island; islet; isolated

ISA Instrument Society of America; intracarotid sodium amytal; intrinsic simulating activity; intrinsic sympathomimetic activity; iodinated serum albumin; irregular spiking activity

I$_{sa}$ spatial average intensity [pulse]

ISADH inappropriate secretion of antidiuretic hormone

I$_{sapa}$ spatial average pulse average

I$_{sapt}$ spatial peak, temporal average intensity [pulse]

I$_{sata}$ spatial average, temporal average intensity [pulse]

ISB incentive spirometry breathing

ISBI International Society for Burn Injuries

ISBP International Society for Biochemical Pharmacology

ISBT International Society for Blood Transfusion

ISC immunoglobulin-secreting cells; insoluble collagen; International Society of Cardiology; International Society of Chemotherapy; intensive supportive care; intershift coordination; interstitial cell; irreversibly sickled cell

ISCF interstitial cell fluid

ISCLT International Society for Clinical Laboratory Technology

ISCM International Society of Cybernetic Medicine

ISCN International System for Human Cytogenetic Nomenclature

ISCO immunostimulating complex [vaccine]

ISCP infection surveillance and control program; International Society of Comparative Pathology

ISCW immunosuppression of streptococcal wall [antigen]

ISD immunosuppressive drug; Information Services Division; inhibited sexual desire; interstimulus distance; interventricular septal defect; isosorbide dinitrate

ISDN integrated services digital network; isosorbide dinitrate

ISE inhibited sexual excitement; International Society of Endocrinology; International Society of Endoscopy; inversion spin-echo pulse sequence; ion-selective electrode

ISEK International Society of Electromyographic Kinesiology

ISEM immunosorbent electron microscopy

ISF interstitial fluid

ISFC International Society and Federation of Cardiology

ISFV interstitial fluid volume

ISG immune serum globulin

ISGE International Society of Gastroenterology

ISH icteric serum hepatitis; in situ hybridization; internal self helper; International Society of Hematology; isolated septal hypertrophy

ISI infarct size index; initial slope index; injury severity index; Institute for Scientific Information; insulin sensitivity index; International Sensitivity Index; International Standardized Index; interstimulus interval

ISIH interspike interval histogram

ISIS image selected in vivo spectroscopy; imaging science and information system; information system-imaging system; interactive system for image selection; International Study of Infarct Survival

ISKDC International Study of Kidney Diseases in Childhood

ISL inner scapular line; interspinous ligament; isoleucine

ISM information sources map [of UMLS]; International Society of Microbiologists; intersegmental muscle

ISMED International Society on Metabolic Eye Disorders

ISMH International Society of Medical Hydrology

ISMHC International Society of Medical Hydrology and Climatology

ISMN isosorbide mononitrate

ISN integrated service network; International Society of Nephrology; International Society of Neurochemistry

ISO International Standards Organization

iso isoproterenol; isotropic

isol isolation, isolated

isom isometric

ISO-OSI International Standards Organization-Open Systems Interconnection

ISP distance between iliac spines; interspace; intraspinal; isoproterenol

I$_{sp}$ spatial peak intensity [pulse]

ISPO International Society for Prosthetics and Orthotics

I$_{sppa}$ spatial peak pulse average intensity

ISPT interspecies ovum penetration test

isq unchanged [Lat. *in status quo*]

ISR information storage and retrieval; Institute for Sex Research; Institute of Surgical Research; insulin secretion rate

ISRM International Society of Reproductive Medicine

ISS idiopathic short stature; injury severity score; International Society of Surgery; ion-scattering spectroscopy; ion surface scattering

ISSI interview schedule for social interaction; Israeli Study of Surgical Infections

ISSN International Standard Serial Number

IST inappropriate sinus tachycardia; insulin sensitivity test; insulin shock therapy; International Society on Toxicology; isometric systolic tension

ISTD International Society of Tropical Dermatology

ISTU isometric strength testing unit

ISU International Society of Urology

I-sub inhibitor substance

ISW interstitial water

ISWI incisional surgical wound infection

ISY intrasynovial

IT immunological test; immunotherapy; implantation test; individual therapy; information technology; inhalation test; inhalation therapy; injection time; insulin therapy; intensive therapy; intentional tremor; intermittent traction; interstitial tissue; intradermal test; intratesticular; intrathecal; intrathoracic; intratracheal; intratracheal tube; intratuberous; intratumoral; ischial tuberosity; isolation transformer; isomeric transition

I/T intensity/time

I&T intolerance and toxicity

ITA inferior temporal artery; internal thoracic artery; International Tuberculosis Association

I$_{ta}$ temporal average intensity [pulse]

ITB iliotibial band

ITC imidazolyl-thioguanine chemotherapy; Interagency Testing Committee; in the canal [hearing aid]

ITc International Table calorie

ITCP idiopathic thrombocytopenic purpura

ITCVD ischemic thrombotic cerebrovascular disease

ITD idiopathic torsion dystonia; intensely transfused dialysis; iodothyronine deiodinase

ITE insufficient therapeutic effect; in the ear [hearing aid]; in-training examination; intrapulmonary interstitial emphysema

ITET isotonic endurance test

ITF interferon

ITFS iliotibial tract friction syndrome; incomplete testicular feminization syndrome

ITG integrin

ITGA integrin alpha

ITGB integrin beta

ITH interstitial hyperthermia

ITh, ith intrathecal

IThP intrathyroidal parathyroid

ITI inter-alpha-trypsin inhibitor; intertrial interval

ITIH2 inter-alpha-trypsin inhibitor, heavy chain 2

ITIL inter-alpha-trypsin inhibitor, light chain

ITIM immunoreceptor tyrosine-based inhibition motif

ITLC instant thin-layer chromatography

ITM improved Thayer-Martin [medium]; intrathecal methotrexate; Israel turkey meningoencephalitis

ITMTX intrathecal methotrexate

ITO indium tin oxide

ITOU intensive therapy observation unit

ITP idiopathic thrombocytopenic purpura; immune thrombocytopenia; immunogenic thrombocytopenic purpura; individualized treatment plan; inosine triphosphate; inositol 1,4,5-triphosphate; islet-cell tumor of the pancreas; isotachophoresis

I$_{tp}$ temporal peak intensity [pulse]

ITPA Illinois Test of Psycholinguistic Abilities; inosine triphosphatase

ITPK inositol 1,4,5-triphosphate-3-kinase

ITPKA inositol 1,4,5-triphosphate-3-kinase A

ITPKB inositol 1,4,5-triphosphate-3-kinase B

ITPR inositol 1,4,5-triphosphate receptor

ITQ inferior temporal quadrant

ITR intraocular tension recorder; intratracheal

ITS infective toxic shock

ITSHD isolated thyroid-stimulating hormone deficiency

ITT insulin tolerance test; internal tibial torsion

ITU intensive therapy unit

ITV inferior temporal vein

IU immunizing unit; international unit; intrauterine; in utero; 5-iodouracil

iu infectious unit

IUA intrauterine adhesions

IUB International Union of Biochemistry

IUBS International Union of Biological Sciences

IUC idiopathic ulcerative colitis

IUCD intrauterine contraceptive device

IUD intrauterine death; intrauterine device

IUDR, IUdR iodeoxyuridine

IUF isolated ultrafiltration

IUFB intrauterine foreign body

IUG infusion urogram; intrauterine growth

IUGR intrauterine growth rate; intrauterine growth retardation

IUI intrauterine insemination

IU/l international units per liter

IUM internal urethral meatus; intrauterine [fetus] malnourished; intrauterine membrane

IU/min international units per minute

IUP intrauterine pregnancy; intrauterine pressure

IUPAC International Union of Pure and Applied Chemistry

IUPAP International Union of Pure and Applied Physics

IUPAT intrauterine pregnancy at term

IUPD intrauterine pregnancy delivered

IUPHAR International Union of Pharmacology

IUPS International Union of Physiological Sciences

IUPTB intrauterine pregnancy, term birth

IURES International Union of Reticuloendothelial Societies

IUT intrauterine transfusion

IUVDT International Union against Venereal Diseases and the Treponematoses

IV ichthyosis vulgaris; initial visit; interventricular; intervertebral; intravaginal; intravascular; intravenous; intraventricular; intravertebral; invasive; in vivo; in vitro; iodine value; Roman numeral four; symbol for class 4 controlled substances

iv intravascular; intravenous

IVA intraoperative vascular angiography; isovaleric acid

IVAP in-vivo adhesive platelet

IVB intraventricular block; intravitrial blood

IVBAT intravascular bronchioalveolar tumor

IVBC intravascular blood coagulation

IVC inferior vena cava; inspiratory vital capacity; integrated vector control; intravascular coagulation; intravenous cholangiogram, intravenous cholangiography; intraventricular catheter

IVCC intravascular consumption coagulopathy

IVCD intraventricular conduction defect

IVCH intravenous cholangiography

IVCP inferior vena cava pressure

IVCR inferior vena cava reconstruction

IVCT inferior vena cava thrombosis; intravenously enhanced computed tomography

IVCV inferior venocavography

IVD intervertebral disc

IVDA/IVDU intravenous drug abuse/abuser; intravenous drug use/user

IVDSA intravenous digital subtraction angiography

IVET in vivo expression technology

IVF interventricular foramen; intervertebral foramen; intravascular fluid; intravenous fluid; in vitro fertiliztion

IVF-ET in vitro fertilization-embryo transfer

IVGG intravenous gammaglobulin

IVGTT intravenous glucose tolerance test

IVH intravenous hyperalimentation; intraventricular hemorrhage; in vitro hyperploidy

IVI intravenous infusion

IVIG intravenous immunoglobulin

IVJC intervertebral joint complex

IVL involucrin

IVM intravascular mass

IVMP intravenous methylprednisolone

IVN intravenous nutrition

IVOTTS Irvine viable organ-tissue transport system

IVOX intravascular oxygenator

IVP intravenous push; intravenous pyelogram, intravenous pyelography; intraventricular pressure

IVPB intravenous piggyback

IVPF isovolume pressure flow curve

IVR idioventricular rhythm; intravaginal ring; isolated volume responder

IVRT isovolumic relaxation time

IVS inappropriate vasopressin secretion; intervening sequence; interventricular septum; intervillous space

IVSA International Veterinary Students Association

IVSCT in vitro skin corrosivity test

IVSD interventricular septal defect

IVT index of vertical transmission; interventional video tomography; intrasound vibration test; intravenous transfusion; intraventricular; in vitro tetraploidy; isovolumetric time

IVTT in vitro transcription and translation

IVTTT intravenous tolbutamide tolerance test

IVU intravenous urography

IVUS intravascular ultrasound

IVV influenza virus vaccine; intravenous vasopressin

IW inner wall; inpatient ward

IWB indeterminate [HIV-1] Western blot; index of well being

IWGMT International Working Group on Mycobacterial Taxonomy

IWI inferior wall infarction; interwave interval

IWL insensible water loss

IWMI inferior wall myocardial infarct

IWRP Individualized Written Rehabilitation Program

IWS Index of Work Satisfaction

IZ infar

J dynamic movement of inertia; electric current density; flux density; joint; joule; journal; juvenile; juxtapulmonary-capillary receptor; magnetic polarization; a polypeptide chain in polymeric immunoglobulins; a reference point following the QRS complex, at the beginning of the ST segment, in electrocardiography; sound intensity

J flux [density]

j jaundice [rat]

JA judgment analysis; juvenile atrophy; juxta-articular

JAI juvenile amaurotic idiocy

JAMA Journal of the American Medical Association

JAMG juvenile autoimmune myasthenia gravis

JAMIA Journal of the American Medical Informatics Association

JAN Japanese accepted name

JAS Jenkins Activity Survey; juvenile ankylosing spondylitis

jaund jaundice

JBE Japanese B encephalitis

JBS Johanson-Blizzard syndrome

JC Jakob-Creutzfeldt; joint contracture

J/C joules per coulomb

jc juice

JCA juvenile chronic arthritis

JCAE Joint Committee on Atomic Energy

JCAH Joint Commission on Accreditation of Hospitals

JCAHO Joint Commission on Accreditation of Healthcare Organizations

JCAI Joint Council of Allergy and Immunology

JCC Joint Committee on Contraception

JCD Jakob-Creutzfeldt disease

JCF juvenile calcaneal fracture

JCM Japanese Collection of Microorganisms

JCML juvenile chronic myelogenous leukemia

JCN Jefferson Cancer Network

JCP juvenile chronic polyarthritis

jct junction

JCV Jamestown Canyon virus

JD jejunal diverticulitis; juvenile delinquent; juvenile diabetes

JDF Juvenile Diabetes Foundation

JDM juvenile diabetes mellitus

JDMS juvenile dermatomyositis

JE Japanese encephalitis; junctional escape

JEBL junctional epidermolysis bullosa letalis

JEE Japanese equine encephalitis

Jej, jej jejunum

JEMBEC agar plates for transporting cultures of gonococci

JER junctional escape rhythm

JEV Japanese encephalitis virus

JF joint fluid; jugular foramen; junctional fold

JFET junction field effect transistor

JFS jugular foramen syndrome

JG, jg juxtaglomerular

JGA juxtaglomerular apparatus

JGC juxtaglomerular cell

JGCT juvenile granulosa cell tumor; juxtaglomerular cell tumor

JGI jejunogastric intussusception; juxtaglomerular granulation index

JGP juvenile general paresis

JH juvenile hormone

J_H heat transfer factor

JHA juvenile hormone analog

JHMO Junior Hospital Medical Officer

JHR Jarisch-Herxheimer reaction

JI jejunoileal; jejunoileitis; jejunoileostomy

JIB jejunoileal bypass
JIH joint interval histogram
JIS Japanese industrial standard; juvenile idiopathic scoliosis
JJ jaw jerk; jejunojejunostomy
J/kg joules per kilogram
JLP juvenile laryngeal papilloma
JMD juvenile macular degeneration
JME juvenile myoclonus epilepsy
JMS junior medical student
JN Jamaican neuropathy
Jn junction
JNA Jena Nomina Anatomica
JNC Joint National Committee
JND just noticeable difference
jnt joint
JOD juvenile-onset diabetes
JODM juvenile-onset diabetes mellitus
jour journal
JP Jackson-Pratt [drain]; joining peptide; juvenile periodontitis
JPA juvenile pilocytic astrocytoma
JPB junctional premature beat
JPC junctional premature contraction
JPD juvenile plantar dermatosis
JPEG Joint Photographic Experts Group
JPI Jackson Personality Inventory
JPS joint position sense
JR Jolly reaction; junctional rhythm
JRA juvenile rheumatoid arthritis
JRC CVT Joint Review Committee on Education in Cardiovascular Technology

JRC DMS Joint Review Committee on Diagnostic Medical Sonography
JROM joint range of motion
JRT junctional recovery time
JS jejunal segment; Job syndrome; junctional slowing
J/s joules per second
JSAIR Japanese Society of Angiography and Interventional Radiology
JSATO$_2$ jugular vein oxygen saturation
JSV Jerry-Slough virus
JT jejunostomy tube
J/T joules per tesla
jt joint
JTPS juvenile tropical pancreatitis syndrome
Ju jugale
JUA joint underwriting association
jug jugular
junct junction
juv juvenile
JV jugular vein; Junin virus
JVC jugular venous catheter
JVD jugular venous distention
JVP jugular vein pulse; jugular venous pressure
JVPT jugular venous pulse tracing
juxt near [Lat. *juxta*]
JWS Jackson-Weiss syndrome
Jx junction
JXG juvenile xanthogranuloma

K absolute zero; capsular antigen [Ger. *Kapsel*, capsule]; carrying capacity; cathode; coefficient of heat transfer; constant improvement factor [in imaging]; in electroencephalography, a burst of diphasic slow waves in response to stimuli during sleep; electron capture; electrostatic capacity; equilibrium constant; ionization constant; kallikrein inhibiting unit; kanamycin; Kell factor; kelvin; kerma; kidney; killer [cell]; kilo-; kinetic energy; *Klebsiella;* knee; lysine; modulus of compression; the number 1024 in computer core memory; potassium [Lat. *kalium*]; vitamin K

°K degree on the Kelvin scale

K_1 phylloquinone

17-K 17-ketosteroid

k Boltzmann constant; constant; kilo; kilohm

κ see *kappa*

KA alkaline phosphatase; kainic acid; keratoacanthoma; keto acid; ketoacidosis; King-Armstrong [unit]

K/A ketogenic/antiketogenic ratio

Ka cathode

K_a acid ionization constant

kA kiloampere

ka cathode

KAAD kerosene, alcohol, acetic acid, and dioxane

KAAS Keele assessment of auditory style

KABC Kaufman Assessment Battery for Children

KAF conglutinogen-activating factor; killer-assisting factor; kinase activating factor

KAFO knee-ankle-foot orthosis

KAL Kallmann [syndrome]

Kal potassium [Lat. *kalium*]

KAO knee-ankle orthosis

KAP knowledge, aptitude, and practice

κ Greek letter *kappa*; magnetic susceptibility

kappa a light chain of human immunoglobulins [chain]

KAS Katz Adjustment Scales; Kennedy-Alter-Sung [syndrome]

KAT kanamycin acetyltransferase

kat katal

kat/l katals per liter

KAU King-Armstrong unit

KB human oral epidermoid carcinoma cells; Kashin-Bek [disease]; ketone body; kilobyte; Kleihauer-Betke [test]; knee brace; knowledge [data] base

K_b base ionization constant

kb kilobase; kilobyte

KBG syndrome of multiple abnormalities designated with the original patient's initials

kbp kilobase pair

kBq kilobecquerel

KBS Klüver-Bucy syndrome

KC cathodal closing; keratoconus; keratoconjunctivitis; knee-to-chest; Kupffer cell

kC kilocoulomb

kc kilocycle

K Cal, Kcal, kcal kilocalorie

KCC cathodal closing contraction; Kulchitzky cell carcinoma

KCCT kaolin-cephalin clotting time

K cell killer cell

KCF key clinical finding

KCG kinetocardiogram

kCi kilocurie

KCO transfer coefficient

kcps kilocycles per second

KCS keratoconjunctivitis sicca

kc/s kilocycles per second

KCT, KCTe cathodal closing tetanus

KD cathodal duration; Kawasaki disease; Kennedy disease; killed

K_d dissociation constant; distribution coefficient; partition coefficient

kd, kDa kilodalton

KDA known drug allergies

KDB kinase insert domain; knowledge database

KDC kidney disease treatment center

KDNA kinetoblast deoxyribonucleic acid

KDO ketodeoxyoctonate

KDS Kaufman Developmental Scale; King-Denborough syndrome; Kocher-Debré-Semelaigne [syndrome]; Kupfer-Detre system

KDT cathodal duration tetanus

kdyn kilodyne

KE Kendall compound E; kinetic energy

K_e exchangeable body potassium

KED Kendrick extrication device

Kera keratitis

KERMA kinetic energy released per unit mass

KERV Kentucky equine respiratory virus

keV kiloelectron volt

KF Kenner-fecal medium; kidney function; Klippel-Feil [syndrome]

KF, K-F Kayser-Fleischer [rings]

kf flocculation rate in antigen-antibody reaction

KFAB kidney-fixing antibody

KFAO knee-foot-ankle orthosis

K_{fc} filtration coefficient

KFD Kyasanur forest disease

KFR Kayser-Fleischer ring

KFS Klippel-Feil syndrome

KFSD keratosis follicularis spinulosa decalvans

KG ketoglutarate

kG kilogauss

kg kilogram

KG-1 Koeffler Golde-1 [cell line]

kg-cal kilocalorie

kg/cm² kilogram per square centimeter

KGD ketoglutarate dehydrogenase

KGF keratocyte growth factor

kgf kilogram-force

KGFR keratocyte growth factor receptor

kg/l kilograms per liter

KGM keratinocyte growth medium

kg-m kilogram-meter

kg/m kilograms per meter

kg-m/s² kilogram-meter per second squared

Kgn kininogen

kgps kilograms per second

KGS ketogenic steroid

17-KGS 17-ketogenic steroid

KH Krebs-Henseleit [buffer]

K24H potassium, urinary 24-hour

KHB Krebs-Henseleit buffer

KHb potassium hemoglobinate

KHC kinetic hemolysis curve

KHD kinky hair disease

KHF Korean hemorrhagic fever

KHM keratoderma hereditaria mutilans

KHN Knoop hardness number

KHP King's Honorary Physician

KHS King's Honorary Surgeon; kinky hair syndrome; Krebs-Henseleit solution

kHz kilohertz

KI karyopyknotic index; Krönig's isthmus

KIA Kligler iron agar

KIC ketoisocaproate; keto isocaproic acid

KICB killed intracellular bacteria

KID keratitis, ichthyosis, and deafness [syndrome]

kilo kilogram

KIMSA Kirsten murine sarcoma

KIMSV, Ki-MSV Kirsten murine sarcoma virus

KIP key intermediary protein

KiP kilopascal

KIPS key indicators, probes, and scoring method [for evaluating compliance with requirements for accreditation]

KISS key integrative social system; saturated solution of potassium iodide

KIT Kahn Intelligence Test
KIU kallikrein inactivation unit
KIVA keto isovaleric acid
KJ, kj knee jerk
kJ kilojoule
KK knee kick
kkat kilokatal
KKS kallikrein-kinin system
KL kidney lobe; Klebs-Loeffler [bacillus]; Kleine-Levin [syndrome]
kl kiloliter
Klebs *Klebsiella*
KLH keyhole limpet hemocyanin
KLK kallikrein
KLKR kallikrein
KLS kidneys, liver, and spleen; Kreuzbein lipomatous syndrome
KM kanamycin
km kilometer
km² square kilometer
K$_m$ Michaelis-Menten constant
kMc kilomegacycle
K-MCM potassium-containing minimum capacitation medium
kMc/s kilomegacycles per second
KMEF keratin, myosin, epidermin, and fibrin
kmps kilometers per second
KMS kabuki make-up syndrome; knowledge management system; kwashiorkor-marasmus syndrome
K-MSV Kirsten murine sarcoma virus
KMV killed measles virus vaccine
Kn knee; Knudsen number
kN kilonewton
kn knee
K nail Küntscher nail
KNG kininogen
KNRK Kirsten sarcoma virus in normal rat kidney
KNS kinesin
KNSL kinesin-like
KO keep on; keep open; killed organism; knee orthosis; knock out
KOC cathodal opening contraction

KOPS thousand of operations per second
kΩ kilohm
KP Kaufmann-Peterson [base]; keratitic precipitate; keratitis punctata; kidney protein; killed parenteral [vaccine]; *Klebsiella pneumoniae*
K-P Kaiser-Permanente [diet]
kPa kilopascal
kPa·s/l kilopascal seconds per liter
KPB ketophenylbutazone; potassium phosphate buffer
KPC keratoconus posticus circumscriptus
KPE Kelman pharmacoemulsification
KPI kallikrein-protease inhibitor; karyopyknotic index
KPR key pulse rate
KPS Karnofsky Performance Status
KPT kidney punch test
KPTI Kunitz pancreatic trypsin inhibitor
KPTT kaolin partial thromboplastin time
KPV key process variable; killed parenteral vaccine
KQC key quality characteristics
KR key-ridge; Kopper Reppart [medium]
Kr krypton
kR kiloroentgen
KRB Krebs-Ringer buffer
KRBG Krebs-Ringer bicarbonate buffer with glucose
KRBS Krebs-Ringer bicarbonate solution
KRP Kolmer test with Reiter protein [antigen]; Krebs-Ringer phosphate
KRR knowledge representation and reasoning
KRRS kinetic resonance Raman spectroscopy
KRT keratin
KS Kallmann syndrome; Kaposi sarcoma; Kartagener syndrome; Kawasaki syndrome; keratan sulfate; ketosteroid; Klinefelter syndrome; Korsakoff syndrome; Kveim-Siltzbach [test]

K-S Kearns-Sayre [syndrome]
17-KS 17-ketosteroid
ks kilosecond
KSC cathodal closing contraction
KS/OI Kaposi sarcoma with opportunistic infection
K_{sp} solubility product
KSP Karolinska Scales of Personality; kidney-specific protein
17-KSR 17-ketosteroid reductase
KSS Kearns-Sayre syndrome; Kearns-Sayre-Shy [syndrome]
KST cathodal closing tetanus; kallistatin
KT kidney transplant, kidney transplantation
KTI kallikrein-trypsin inhibitor
KTS Klippel-Trenaunay syndrome
KTSA Kahn test of symbol arrangement
KTW, KTWS Klippel-Trenaunay-Weber [syndrome]
KTx kidney transplant
KU kallikrein unit; Karmen unit
Ku kurchatovium; Peltz factor
KUB kidneys and upper bladder; [x-ray examination of the] kidneys, ureter, and bladder
KUS, kidney, ureter, spleen

KV kanamycin and vancomycin; killed vaccine
kV, kv kilovolt
kVA kilovolt-ampere
kvar kilovar
KVBA kanamycin-vancomycin blood agar
kVcp, kvcp kilovolt constant potential
KVE Kaposi's varicelliform eruption
KVLBA kanamycin-vancomycin laked blood agar
KVO keep vein open
kVp, kvp kilovolt peak
KW Keith-Wagener [ophthalmoscopic finding]; Kimmelstiel-Wilson [syndrome]; Kugelberg-Welander [syndrome]
Kw weighted kappa
K_w dissociation constant of water
kW, kw kilowatt
KWB Keith-Wagener-Barker [hypertension classification]
KWD Kimmelstiel-Wilson disease
kWh, kW-hr, kw-hr kilowatt-hour
K wire Kirschner wire
KWS Kimmelstiel-Wilson syndrome; Kugelberg-Welander syndrome
K-XRF K x-ray fluorescence
KYN kynurenic acid
KZ ketoconazole

L angular momentum; Avogadro constant; boundary [Lat. *limes*]; coefficient of induction; diffusion length; inductance; *Lactobacillus*; lambda; lambert; latent heat; latex; Latin; leader sequence; left; *Legionella; Leishmania*; length; lente insulin; lethal; leucine; levo-; lidocaine; ligament; light; light sense; lingual; *Listeria;* liter; liver; low; lower; lumbar; luminance; lymph; lymphocyte; outer membrane layer of cell wall of gram-negative bacteria [layer]; pound [Lat. *libra*]; radiance; self-inductance; syphilis [Lat. *lues*]; threshold [Lat. *limen*]

L-variant a defective bacterial variant that can multiply on hypertonic medium

L_0 limes zero [*limes nul*]

L_+ limes tod

L1, L2, L3, L4, L5 first, second, third, fourth, and fifth lumbar vertebrae

LI, LII, LIII first, second, third stage of syphilis

L/3 lower third

l azimuthal quantum number; left; length; lethal; levorotatory; liter; long; longitudinal; specific latent heat

Λ see *lambda*

λ see *lambda*

LA lactic acid; large amount; laser angioplasty; late abortion; late antigen; latex agglutination; left angle; left arm; left atrium; left auricle; leucine aminopeptidase; leukemia antigen; leukoagglutination; leuprolide acetate; levator ani; linguo-axial; linoleic acid; lobuloalveolar; local anesthesia; local anesthetic; long-acting [drug]; long arm; low anxiety; Ludwig angina; lupus anticoagulant; lymphocyte antibody

L&A light and accommodation; living and active

LA50 total body surface area of burn that will kill 50% of patients (lethal area)

La labial; lambda; lambert; lanthanum

LAA left atrial appendage; left atrial area; leukemia-associated antigen; leukocyte ascorbic acid

LAAM L-alpha acetyl methadol

LAAO L-amino acid oxidase

LA/Ao left atrial/aortic [ratio]

LAB, lab laboratory

LABV left atrial ball valve

LAC La Crosse [virus]; lactase; left atrial circumflex [artery]; left atrial contraction; linguoaxiocervical; long-arm cast; low-amplitude contraction; lung adenocarcinoma cells; lupus anticoagulant

LaC labiocervical

lac laceration; lactation

LACN local area communications network

LACI lipoprotein-associated coagulation inhibitor

lacr lacrimal

LACS long chain acyl-coenzyme A synthetase

lact lactate, lactating, lactation; lactic

lact hyd lactalbumin hydrolysate

LAD lactic acid dehydrogenase; left anterior descending [artery]; left axis deviation; leukocyte adhesion deficiency; ligament augmentation device; linoleic acid depression; lipoamide dehydrogenase; lymphocyte-activating determinant

LADA laboratory animal dander allergy; left acromio-dorso-anterior [position]; left anterior descending artery

LADCA left anterior descending coronary artery

LADD lacrimo-auriculo-dento-digital [syndrome]; left anterior descending diagonal [coronary artery]

LADH lactic acid dehydrogenase; liver alcohol dehydrogenase

LAD-MIN left axis deviation, minimal

LADP left acromio-dorso-posterior [position]; left anterior descending arterial pressure

LAE left atrial enlargement

LAEDV left atrial volume in end diastole

LAEI left atrial emptying index

LAESV left atrial volume in end systole

LAF laminar air flow; Latin American female; leukocyte-activating factor; lymphocyte-activating factor

LAFB left anterior fascicular block

LAFR laminar air flow room

LAFU laminar air flow unit

LAG labiogingival; leukocyte antigen group; linguo-axiogingival; lymphangiogram; lymphocyte activation gene

LaG labiogingival

LAH lactalbumin hydrolysate; left anterior hemiblock; left atrial hypertrophy; Licentiate of Apothecaries Hall; lithium, aluminum, hydroxide

LAHB left anterior hemiblock

LAHC low affinity-high capacity

LAHV leukocyte-associated herpesvirus

LAI latex particle agglutination inhibition; leukocyte adherence inhibition

LaI labioincisal

LAIF leukocyte adherence inhibition factor

LAIT latex agglutination inhibition test

LAK lymphokine-activated killer [cells]

LAL left axillary line; *Limulus* amebocyte lysate; low air loss; lysosomal acid lipase

LaL labiolingual

LALB low air-loss bed

LALI lymphocyte antibody-lymphocytolytic interaction

LALL lymphomatous acute lymphoblastic leukemia

LAM laminectomy; laminin; late ambulatory monitoring; Latin American male; left anterior measurement; left atrial myxoma; lymphangioleiomyomatosis; lymphocyte adhesion molecule

lam laminectomy

LAMA laminin A

LAMB laminin B; lentigines, atrial myxoma, mucocutaneous myxomas, blue nevi [syndrome]

λ Greek lower case letter *lambda*; craniometric point; decay constant; an immunoglobulin light chain; mean free path; microliter; thermal conductivity; wavelength

LAMBR laminin B receptor

LAMC laminin C

LAMMA laser microprobe mass analyzer

LAMP lysosome-associated membrane protein

LAN local area network; long-acting neuroleptic [agent]

LANC long-arm navicular cast

LANE lidocaine, atropine, naloxone, epinephrine [drugs that may be administered via endotracheal tube]

LANV left atrial neovascularization

LAO left anterior oblique; left atrial overload; Licentiate of the Art of Obstetrics

LAP laparoscopy; laparotomy; left arterial pressure; left atrial pressure; leucine aminopeptidase; leukemia-associated phosphoprotein; leukocyte alkaline phosphatase; liver-enriched transcriptional activator protein; low atmospheric pressure; lyophilized anterior pituitary

lap laparoscopy; laparotomy

lap & dye laparoscopy and injection of dye

LAPW left atrial posterior wall

LAR laryngology; late asthmatic response; late reaction; left arm recumbent; leukocyte antigen-related

lar larynx; left arm reclining

LARC leukocyte automatic recognition computer

LARD lacrimoauriculoradiodental [syndrome]

LARS leucyl-tRNA synthetase

Laryngol laryngology

LAS laboratory automation system; lateral amyotrophic sclerosis; laxative abuse syndrome; left anterior-superior; leucine acetylsalicylate; linear alkylsulfonate; local adaptation syndrome; long arm splint; lower abdominal surgery; lymphadenopathy syndrome

LASA linear-analogue self assessment

LASA-P linear-analogue self-assessment-Pristman

LASA-S linear-analogue self-assessment-Selby

LASER light amplification by stimulated emission of radiation

LASH left anterior superior hemiblock

L-ASP L-asparaginase

LASS labile aggregation stimulating substance

LAST left anterior small thoracotomy

LAT lateral; latex agglutination test; left atrial thrombus; lysolecithin acyltransferase

Lat Latin

lat latent; lateral

lat bend lateral bending

LATCH literature attached to charts

l·atm liter atmosphere

LATP left atrial transmural pressure

LATPT left atrial transesophageal pacing test

LATS long-acting thyroid stimulator

LATS-P long-acting thyroid stimulator-protector

LATu lobulo-alveolar tumor

LAUP laser-assisted uvulopalatoplasty

LAV leafhopper A virus; lymphadenopathy-associated virus

lav lavoratory

LAVH laparoscopy-assisted vaginal hysterectomy

LAW left atrial wall

LAX, LAx long axis

lax laxative; laxity

LAX-DSS long axis-discrete subaortic stenosis

lax oc laxative of choice

LB lamellar body; large bowel; left breast; left bronchus; left bundle; left buttock; leiomyoblastoma; lipid body; live birth; liver biopsy; loose body; low back [pain]; lung biopsy; Luria-Bertani [medium]

L&B left and below

Lb pound force

lb pound [Lat. *libra*]

LBA left basal artery

LBB left bundle branch; low back bending

LBBB left bundle branch block

LBBsB left bundle branch system block

LBC lidocaine blood concentration; lymphadenosis benigna cutis

LBCD left border of cardiac dullness

LBCF Laboratory Branch complement fixation [test]

LBD large bile duct; left border of dullness

LBF *Lactobacillus bulgaricus* factor; limb blood flow; liver blood flow

lbf pound force

lbf-ft pound force foot

LBH length, breadth, height

LBI low back injury; low serum-bound iron

lb/in² pounds per square inch

LBL labeled lymphoblast; lymphoblastic lymphoma

LBM lean body mass; loose bowel movement; lung basement membrane

L-BMAA L-beta-N-methylamino-L-alanine

LBNP lower body negative pressure

LBO large bowel obstruction

LBP lipopolysaccharide-binding protein; low back pain; low blood pressure; lumbar back pain

LBPF long bone or pelvic fracture

LBPQ Low Back Pain Questionnaire

LBRF louse-borne relapsing fever

LBS low back syndrome; lumbar back strain

LBSA lipid-bound sialic acid

LBT low back tenderness or trouble

LBTI lima bean trypsin inhibitor

lb tr pound troy

LBV left brachial vein; lung blood volume

LBW lean body weight; low birth weight

LBWI low-birth-weight infant

LBWR lung-body weight ratio

LC Laennec cirrhosis; Langerhans cell; late clamped; large chromophobe; lecithin cholesterol acyltransferase; lethal concentration; Library of Congress; life care; light chain; linguocervical; lipid cytosomes; liquid chromatography; liver cirrhosis; living children; locus ceruleus; long chain; low calorie; lung cancer; lung cell

LC$_{50}$ median lethal concentration

LCA left circumflex artery; left coronary artery; leukocyte common antigen; lithocholic acid; lymphocyte chemotactic activity

LCAM liver cell adhesion molecule

LCAO linear combination of atomic orbitals

LCAR late cutaneous anaphylactic reaction

LCAT lecithin cholesterol acyltransferase

LCATA lecithin cholesterol acetyltransferase alpha

LCB Laboratory of Cancer Biology; Leber congenital blindness; left costal border; lymphomatosis cutis benigna

LCBF local cerebral blood flow

LCC lactose coliform count; left circumflex coronary (artery); left common carotid; left coronary cusp; life cycle cost [analysis]; lipid-containing cell; liver cell carcinoma

LCCA late cortical cerebellar atrophy; leukoclastic angiitis

LCCME Liaison Committee on Continuing Medical Education

LCCS lower cervical cesarean section

LCCSCT large-cell calcifying Sertoli cell tumor

LCD coal tar solution [liquor carbonis detergens]; lattice corneal dystrophy; liquid crystal diode; localized collagen dystrophy

LCDD light chain deposition disease

LCF least common factor; lymphocyte culture fluid

LCFA long-chain fatty acid

L-cFA long chain fatty acid

LCFU leukocyte colony-forming unit

LCG Langerhans cell granule

LCGL large-cell granulocytic leukemia

LCGME Liaison Committee on Graduate Medical Education

LCGR lutropin-choriogonadotropin receptor

LCGU local cerebral glucose utilization

LCH Langerhans cell histiocytosis

LCh Licentiate in Surgery

LCI length complexity index

LCIS lobular carcinoma in situ

LCL Levinthal-Coles-Lillie [body]; lower confidence limit; lower control limit; lymphoblastoid cell line; lymphocytic lymphosarcoma; lymphoid cell line

LCM latent cardiomyopathy; left costal margin; leukocyte-conditioned medium; lowest common multiple; lymphatic choriomeningitis; lymphocytic choriomeningitis

LCME Liaison Committee on Medical Education

LCMG long-chain monoglyceride

L/cm H$_2$O liters per centimeter of water

LCMV lymphocytic choriomeningitis virus

LCN lateral cervical nucleus; left caudate nucleus; lipocalin

LCO low cardiac output

LCOS low cardiac output syndrome

LCP long-chain polysaturated [fatty acid]; lymphocyte cytosol polypeptide

LCPD Legg-Calvé-Perthes disease

LCPS Licentiate of the College of Physicians and Surgeons

LCQ Learning Climate Questionnaire

LCR locus control region

LCRB locus control region beta

LCS cerebrospinal fluid [Lat. *liquor cerebrospinalis*]; left coronary sinus; life care service; low constant suction; low continuous suction; lymphocyte culture supernatants

LCSB Liaison Committee for Specialty Boards

LCSS lethal congenital contracture syndrome

LCT liver cell tumor; long-chain triglyceride; lymphocytotoxicity; lymphocytotoxin

LCTA lymphocytotoxic antibody

LCU life change unit

LCV lecithovitellin; leukocytoclastic vasculitis

LCx left circumflex artery

LD labor and delivery; laboratory data; labyrinthine defect; lactate dehydrogenase; laser Doppler; learning disability; learning disorder; left deltoid; Legionnaires' disease; lethal dose; light differentiation; limited disease; linear dichroism; linguodistal; lipodystrophy; liver disease; living donor; loading dose; Lombard-Dowell [agar]; longitudinal diameter; low density; low dose; lymphocyte-defined; lymphocyte depletion

L-D Leishman-Donovan [body]

L/D light/darkness [ratio]

L&D labor and delivery

LD$_1$ isoenzyme of lactate dehydrogenase found in the heart, erythrocytes, and kidneys

LD$_2$ isoenzyme of lactate dehydrogenase found in the lungs

LD$_3$ isoenzyme of lactate dehydrogenase found in the lungs

LD$_4$ isoenzyme of lactate dehydrogenase found in the liver

LD$_5$ isoenzyme of lactate dehydrogenase found in the liver and muscles

LD$_{50}$ median lethal dose

LD$_{50/30}$ a dose that is lethal for 50% of test subjects within 30 days

LD$_{100}$ lethal dose in all exposed subjects

Ld *Leishmania donovani*

LDA laser Doppler anemometry; left dorso-anterior [fetal position]; linear discriminant analysis; lymphocyte-dependent antibody

LDAC low-dose cytosine arabinoside

LDAR latex direct agglutination reaction

LDB lamb dysentery bacillus; Legionnaires' disease bacillus

LDC lymphoid dendritic cell; lysine decarboxylase

LDCC lectin-dependent cellular cytotoxicity

LDCI low-dose continuous infusion

LDCT late distal cortical tubule

LDD late dedifferentiation; light-darkness discrimination

LDER lateral-view dual-energy radiography

LD-EYA Lombard-Dowell egg yolk agar

LDF laser Doppler flux, laser Doppler fluxometry; limit dilution factor

LDG lactic dehydrogenase; lingual developmental groove

LDH lactate dehydrogenase; low-dose heparin

LDHA lactic dehydrogenase A

LDHB lactic dehydrogenase-B

LDHC lactic dehydrogenase-C

LDHK lactic dehydrogenase-K

LDIH left direct inguinal hernia

LDL loudness discomfort level; low density lipoprotein

LDLA low-density lipoprotein apheresis

LDLC low-density lipoprotein cholesterol

LDLP low-density lipoprotein

LDLR, LDL-R low density lipoprotein receptor

LDM lactate dehydrogenase, muscle; limited dorsal myeloschisis

LD-NEYA Lombard-Dowell neomycin egg yolk agar

L-DOPA, L-dopa levodopa, levo-3, 4-dihydroxyphenylalanine

LDP left dorsoposterior [fetal position]

LDR labor, delivery, recovery

LDRPS labor-delivery-recovery-postpartum suite

LDRS labor-delivery-recovery suite

LDS Licentiate in Dental Surgery; locked door seclusion

LDSc Licentiate in Dental Science

LDT left dorsotransverse [fetal position]

LDUB long double upright brace

LDUH low-dose unfractionated heparin

LDV lactic dehydrogenase virus; large dense-cored vesicle; laser Doppler velocimetry; lateral distant view

LE lactate extraction; left ear; left eye; leukocyte elastase; leukoerythrogenic; live embryo; Long Evans [rat]; low exposure; lower extremity; lupus erythematosus [cell]

LEA lower extremity amputation

LEC leukoencephalitis; lower esophageal contractility

LECP low-energy charged particle

LED light-emitting diode; lowest emitting dose; lupus erythematosus disseminatus

LEED low-energy electron diffraction

LEEDS low-energy electron diffraction spectroscopy

LEEP left end-expiratory pressure; loop electrosurgical excision procedure

LEF leukokinesis-enhancing factor; lupus erythematosus factor; lymphoid-enhanced binding factor

leg legislation; legal

LeIF leukocyte interferon

LEIS low-energy ion scattering

LEL lower explosive limit; lowest effect level

LEM lateral eye movement; Leibovitz-Emory medium; leukocyte endogenous mediator; light emission microscopy

LEMO lowest empty molecular orbital

LEMS Lambert-Eaton myasthenic syndrome

lenit lenitive

LEOPARD lentigines, EKG abnormalities, ocular hypertelorism, pulmonary stenosis, abnormalities of genitalia, retardation of growth, and deafness [syndrome]

LEP lethal effective phase; lipoprotein electrophoresis; low egg passage; lower esophagus

lep leptotene

L$_{EPN}$ effective perceived noise level

Leq loudness equivalent

LER lysozomal enzyme release

LERG local electroretinogram

LES Lambert-Eaton syndrome; Lawrence Experimental Station [agar]; local excitatory state; Locke egg serum; low excitatory state; lower esophageal sphincter; lupus erythematosus, systemic

les lesion

LESD Letterer-Siwe disease

LESP lower esophageal sphincter pressure

LESS lateral electrical spine stimulation

LESTR leukocyte-derived seven-transmembrane domain receptor

LET lidocaine, epinephrine, and tetracaine [solution]; linear or low energy transfer

LETD lowest effective toxic dose

LETS large external transformation-sensitive [protein]

LEU leucine; leucovorin; leukocyte equivalent unit

Leu leucine

leuc leukocyte

LEUT leucine transport

LEV Levamisole

LEW Lewis [rat]

l/ext lower extremity

LF labile factor; lactoferrin; laryngofissure; Lassa fever; latex fixation; left foot; left forearm; lethal fctor; leukotactic factor; ligamentum flavum; limit of flocculation; low fat [diet]; low forceps; low frequency

L/F Latin female

Lf limit of flocculation

lf lactoferrin; low frequency

LFA left femoral artery; left frontal craniotomy; left fronto-anterior [fetal position]; leukocyte function associated antigen; leukotactic factor activity; low-friction arthroplasty; lymphocyte function-associated antigen

LFB luxol fast blue [stain]

LFC living female child; low fat and cholesterol [diet]

LFD lactose-free diet; large for date [fetus]; late fetal death; lateral facial dysplasia; least fatal dose; low-fat diet; low-fiber diet; low forceps delivery

LFER linear free-energy relationship

LFH left femoral hernia

LFHL low-frequency hearing loss

LFL left frontolateral; leukocyte feeder layer; lower flammable limit

LFN lactoferrin

L-[form] a defective bacterial variant that can multiply on hypertonic medium

LFP left frontoposterior [fetal position]

LFPPV low-frequency positive pressure ventilation

LFPS Licentiate of the Faculty of Physicians and Surgeons

LFR lymphoid follicular reticulosis

LFS lateral facet syndrome; Li-Fraumeni syndrome; limbic forebrain structure; liver function series

LFT latex fixation test; latex flocculation test; left fronto-transverse [fetal position]; liver function test; low-frequency tetanus; low-frequency transduction; low-frequency transfer; lung function test

LFU lipid fluidity unit

LFV Lassa fever virus; low-frequency ventilation

LFx linear fracture

LG lactoglobulin; lamellar granule; laryngectomy; left gluteal; Lennox-Gastaut [syndrome]; leucylglycine; linguogingival; lipoglycopeptide; liver graft; low glucose; lymphatic gland

lg large; leg

LGA large for gestational age; left gastric artery

LGALS lecithin, galactoside-binding, soluble

LGB Landry-Guillain-Barré [syndrome]; lateral geniculate body

LGBS Landry-Guillain-Barré syndrome

LGD limb girdle dystrophy

LGE Langat encephalitis

LGF lateral giant fiber

LGH lactogenic hormone

LGI large glucagon immunoreactivity; low gastrointestinal

LGL large granular leukocyte; large granular lymphocyte; Lown-Ganong-Levine [syndrome]

LGL-NK large granular lymphocyte-natural killer

LGMD limb-girdle muscular dystrophy

LGN lateral geniculate nucleus; lateral glomerulonephritis

LGS Langer-Giedion syndrome; Lennox-Gastaut syndrome; limb girdle syndrome

LGT late generalized tuberculosis

LGTI lower genital tract infection

LGV large granular vesicle; lymphogranuloma venereum

LGVHD lethal graft-versus-host disease

LgX lymphogranulomatosis X

LH late healing; lateral hypothalamic [syndrome]; left hand; left heart; left hemisphere; left hyperphoria; liver homogenate; lower half; lues hereditaria; lung homogenate; luteinizing hormone

LHA lateral hypothalamic area; left hepatic artery

LHB luteinizing hormone beta chain

LHBV left heart blood volume

LHC Langerhans cell histiocytosis; left heart catheterization; left hypochondrium; light-harvesting complex; Local Health Council

LHCGR luteinizing hormone-choriogonadotropin receptor

LHD lateral head displacement [sperm]

LHEG local healthcare executive group

LHF left heart failure

LHFA lung Hageman factor activator

LHG left hand grip; localized hemolysis in gel

LHI lipid hydrocarbon inclusion

LHL left hepatic lobe

LHM lysuride hydrogen maleate

LHMP Life Health Monitoring Program

LHN lateral hypothalamic nucleus

LHNCBC Lister Hill National Center for Biomedical Communication

LHON Leber hereditary optic neuropathy

LHPZ low high-pressure zone

LHR leukocyte histamine release; lymph node homing receptor

l-hr lumen-hour

LHRF luteinizing hormone-releasing factor

LHRH, LH-RH luteinizing hormone-releasing hormone

LHRHR luteinizing hormone-releasing hormone receptor

LHS left hand side; left heart strain; left heelstrike; lymphatic/hematopoietic system

LHT left hypertropia

LHV left hepatic vein

LI labeling index; lactose intolerance; lacunar infarct; lamellar ichthyosis; Langerhans islet; large intestine; *Leptospira icterohaemorrhagica;* linguoincisal; lithogenic index; low impulsiveness

L&I liver and iron

Li a blood group system; labrale inferius; lithium

LIA Laser Institute of America; leukemia-associated inhibitory activity; lock-in amplifier; lymphocyte-induced angiogenesis; lysine iron agar

LIAFI late infantile amaurotic familial idiocy

lib a pound [Lat. *libra*]

LIBC latent iron-binding capacity

LIC left internal carotid [artery]; limiting isorrheic concentration; local intravascular coagulation

Lic licentiate

LICA left internal carotid artery

LICM left intercostal margin

LicMed Licentiate in Medicine

LICS left intercostal space

LID large intraluminal density; late immunoglobulin deficiency; lymphocytic infiltrative disease

LIF laser-induced fluorescence; left iliac fossa; left index finger; leukemia-inhibiting factor; leukocyte inhibitory factor; leukocytosis-inducing factor

LIFE lung imaging fluorescence endoscope

LIFO last in, first out

LIFR leukemia inhibitory factor receptor

LIFT lymphocyte immunofluorescence test

lig ligament; ligation

LIH left inguinal hernia

LIHA low impulsiveness, high anxiety

LIJ left internal jugular [vein]

LILA low impulsiveness, low anxiety

LIM line isolation monitor

lim limit, limited

LIMA left internal mammary artery

LIMM lethal infantile mitochondrial myopathy

LINAC linear accelerator

LINC laboratory instrumentation computer

Linim, lin liniment

LIO left inferior oblique

LIP lipase; lipocortin; lithium-induced polydipsia; lymphoid interstitial pneumonitis

Lip lipoate

LIPB lipase B

LIPD lipase D

lipoMM lipomyelomeningocele

LIPP laser-induced pressure pulse

LIQ low inner quadrant

liq liquid [Lat. *liquor*]

liq dr liquid dram

liq oz liquid ounce

liq pt liquid pint

liq qt liquid quart

LIR left iliac region; left inferior rectus

LIRBM liver, iron, red bone marrow

LIS laboratory information system; lateral intercellular space; left intercostal space; library information service; lobular *in situ*; locked-in syndrome; low intermittent suction; low ionic strength

LISA Library and Information Science Abstracts

LISP List Processing Language

LISREL linear structural relation

LISS low-ionic-strength saline

LITA left internal thoracic artery

LIV left innominate vein

liv live, living

LIV-BP leucine, isoleucine, and valine-binding protein

LIVC left inferior vena cava

LIVEN linear inflammatory verrucous epidermal nevus

LJI List of Journals Indexed

LJM limited joint mobility; Lowenstein-Jensen medium

LK left kidney; lichenoid keratosis; lymphokine

LKKS liver, kidneys, spleen

LKM liver-kidney microsomal [antibody]

LKP lamellar keratoplasty

LKS Landau-Kleffner syndrome; liver, kidneys, spleen

LKSB liver, kidney, spleen, bladder

LKV laked kanamycin vancomycin [agar]

LL large lymphocyte; lateral leminiscus; left lateral; left leg; left lower; left lung; lepromatous [in Ridley-Jopling Hansen disease classification]; lepromatous leprosy; lipoprotein lipase; loudness level; lower [eye]lid; lower limb; lower lip; lower lobe; lumbar length; lymphocytic lymphoma; lymphoid leukemia; lysolecithin

LLA limulus lysate assay

L lat left lateral

LLB left lateral border; long-leg brace

LLBCD left lower border of cardiac dullness

LLC Lewis lung carcinoma; liquid-liquid chromatography; long-leg cast; lymphocytic leukemia

LLCC long-leg cylinder cast

LLC-MK1 rhesus monkey kidney cells

LLC-MK2 rhesus monkey kidney cells

LLC-MK3 *Cercopithecus* monkey kidney cells

LLC-RK1 rabbit kidney cells

LLD left lateral decubitus [muscle]; leg length discrepancy; long-lasting depolarization

LLE left lower extremity

LLETZ large loop excision of the transformation zone

LLF Laki-Lóránd factor; left lateral femoral; left lateral flexion

LLL left lower [eye]lid; left liver lobe; left lower leg; left lower lobe

LLLE lower lid left eye

LLM localized leukocyte mobilization

LLN lower limit of normal

LLO *Legionella*-like organism

LLP late luteal phase; long-lasting potentiation

LLPV left lower pulmonary vein

LLQ left lower quadrant; low-level question

LLR large local reaction; left lateral rectus [muscle]; left lumbar region

LLRE lower lid right eye

LLS lazy leukocyte syndrome; long-leg splint

LLSB left lower scapular border; left lower sternal border

LLT left lateral thigh; lysolecithin

LLV lymphatic leukemia virus

LLV-F lymphatic leukemia virus, Friend associated

LLVP left lateral ventricular preexcitation

LLWC long-leg walking cast

LLX left lower extremity

LLZ left lower zone

LM lactic acid mineral [medium]; lactose malabsorption; laryngeal mask; laryngeal muscle; lateral malleolus; left median; legal medicine; lemniscus medialis; Licentiate in Medicine; Licentiate in Midwifery; light microscope, light microscopy; light minimum; lincomycin; lingual margin; linguomesial; lipid mobilization; liquid membrane; *Listeria monocytogenes;* localized movement; longitudinal muscle; lower motor [neuron]

L/M Latin male

Lm *Listeria monocytogenes*

lm lower midline; lumen

l/m liters per minute

LMA laryngeal mask airway; left mentoanterior [fetal position]; limbic midbrain area; liver cell membrane autoantibody

LMB left main bronchus; leiomyoblastoma; leukomethylene blue

LMBB Laurence-Moon-Bardet-Biedl [syndrome]

LMBS Laurence-Moon-Biedl syndrome

LMC large motile cell; lateral motor column; left main coronary [artery]; left middle cerebral [artery]; living male child; lymphocyte-mediated cytotoxicity; lymphomyeloid complex

LMCA left main coronary artery; left middle cerebral artery

LMCAD left main coronary artery disease

LMCC Licentiate of the Medical Council of Canada

LMCL left midclavicular line

LMCAO left marginal coronary artery occlusion

LMD lipid-moiety modified derivative; local medical doctor; low molecular weight dextran

LMDX low-molecular-weight dextran

LME left mediolateral episiotomy; leukocyte migration enhancement

LMed&Ch Licentiate in Medicine and Surgery

LMF left middle finger; lymphocyte mitogenic factor

lm/ft² lumens per square foot

LMG lethal midline granuloma

LMH lipid-mobilizing hormone

lmh lumen hour

LMI leukocyte migration inhibition

LMIF leukocyte migration inhibition factor

l/min liters per minute

LML large and medium lymphocytes; left mediolateral; left middle lobe

LMM *Lactobacillus* maintenance medium; lentigo maligna melanoma; light meromyosin

lm/m² lumens per square meter
LMN lower motor neuron
LMNL lower motor neuron lesion
LMO localized molecular orbital
LMP large multifunctional protease; last menstrual period; latent membrane potential; left mentoposterior [fetal position]; lumbar puncture
LMR left medial rectus [muscle]; localized magnetic resonance; lymphocytic meningpolyradiculitis
LMRCP Licentiate in Midwifery of the Royal College of Physicians
LMS lateral medullary syndrome; left main stem [coronary artery]; leiomyosarcoma; Licentiate in Medicine and Surgery
lms lumen-second
LMSSA Licentiate in Medicine and Surgery of the Society of Apothecaries
LMT left mentotransverse [fetal position]; leukocyte migration technique
LMV larva migrans visceralis
LMW low molecular weight
LMWH low molecular weight heparin
LMWP low molecular weight proteinuria
lm/W lumens per watt
LMWD low-molecular-weight dextran
LMZ left midzone
LN Lesch-Nyhan [syndrome]; lipoid nephrosis; Lisch nodule; low necrosis; lupus nephritis; lymph node
LN₂ liquid nitrogen
L/N letter/numerical [system]
ln natural logarithm
LNAA large neutral amino acid
LNBx lymph node biopsy
LNC lymph node cell
LNE lymph node enlargement
LNH large number hypothesis
LNKS low natural killer syndrome
LNL lymph node lymphocyte
LNLS linear-nonlinear least squares
LNMP last normal menstrual period

LNNB Luria-Nebraska Neuropsychological Battery
LNP large neuronal polypeptide
LNPF lymph node permeability factor
LNS lateral nuclear stratum; Lesch-Nyhan syndrome
LO linguo-occlusal
5-LO 5-lipooxygenase
LOA leave of absence; Leber optic atrophy; left occipitoanterior [fetal position]
LOC laxative of choice; level of consciousness; liquid organic compound; locus of control; loss of consciousness
lo cal low calorie
lo calc low calcium
lo CHO low carbohydrate
lo chol low cholesterol
LOCM low molecular contrast medium
LOCS laryngoonychocutaneous syndrome
LOD line of duty
LOF lofexidine
LOG lipoxygenase
log logarithm
LOGIC laryngeal and ocular granulations in children of Indian subcontinent [syndrome]
LOH loop of Henle; loss of heterozygosity
LOI level of incompetence; limit of impurities
LOIH left oblique inguinal hernia
LOINC Laboratory Observation Identifier of Names and Codes [Consortium]
lo k low potassium
LOL left occipitolateral [fetal position]
LOM left otitis media; limitation of motion; loss of motion
LOMSA left otitis media suppurativa acuta
LOMSC, LOMSCh left otitis media suppurativa chronica
lo Na low sodium
long longitudinal

LOP leave on pass; left occipitoposterior [fetal position]

LOPP chlorambucil, vincristine, procarbazine, prednisolone

LOPS length of patient's stay

LOQ lower outer quadrant

LOR long open reading frame; lorazepam; loricrin; loss of righting reflex

Lord lordosis, lordotic

LORF long open reading frame

LOS length of stay; Licentiate in Obstetrical Science; lipo-oligosaccharide; low cardiac output syndrome; lower [o]esophageal sphincter

LOS(P) lower [o]esophageal sphincter (pressure)

LOT lateral olfactory tract; left occipitotransverse [fetal position]

lot lotion

LOV large opaque vesicle

LOWBI low-birth-weight infant

LOX lysyl oxidase

LOXL lysyl oxidase-like

LP labile peptide; labile protein; laboratory procedure; lactic peroxidase; lamina propria; laryngopharyngeal; latent period, latency period; lateral plantar; lateral posterior; lateral pylorus; *Legionella pneumophila;* leukocyte poor; leukocytic pyrogen; lichen planus; light perception; lingua plicata; linguopulpal; lipoprotein; liver plasma [concentration]; loss of privileges; low potency; low power; low pressure; low protein; lumbar puncture; lumboperitoneal; lung parenchyma; lymphoid plasma; lymphomatoid papulosis

L/P lactate/pyruvate [ratio]; liver plasma [concentration]; lymph/plasma [ratio]

Lp lipoprotein; sound pressure level

L$_p$ pathlength

LPA latex particle agglutination; left pulmonary artery; lysophosphatidic acid

LPAM L-phenylalanine mustard

LPB lipoprotein B

LPBP low-profile bioprosthesis

LPC late positive component; lipocortin; longitudinal primary care [program]; lysophosphatidylcholine

LPCM low-placed conus medullaris

LPCT late proximal cortical tubule

LPD low-protein diet; luteal phase defect

LPDF lipoprotein-deficient fraction

LPE lipoprotein electrophoresis; lysophosphatidylethanolamine

LPF leukocytosis-promoting factor; leukopenia factor; lipopolysaccharide factor; localized plaque formation; low-power field; lymphocytosis-promoting factor

lpf low-power field

LPFB left posterior fascicular block

LPFN low-pass filtered noise

LPFS low-pass filtered signal

LPG lipophosphoglycan

LPH lactase-phlorizin hydrolase; left posterior hemiblock; lipotropic pituitary hormone

LPHAS limb/pelvis-hypoplasia/aplasia syndrome

LPI left posterior-inferior; lysinuric protein intolerance

LPIFB left posteroinferior fascicular block

LPIH left posteroinferior hemiblock

LPK liver pyruvate kinase

LPL lichen planus-like lesion; lipoprotein lipase

LPLA lipoprotein lipase activity

LPM lateral pterygoid muscle; liver plasma membrane

lpm lines per minute; liters per minute

lp/mm line pairs per millimeter

LPN Licensed Practical Nurse

LPO lactoperoxidase; left posterior oblique; light perception only; lipid peroxidation

LPP lateral pterygoid plate

LPPH late postpartum hemorrhage

LPR lactate-pyruvate ratio

LPS lateral premotor system; levator palpebrae superioris [muscle]; linear profile scan; lipase; lipopolysaccharide

lps liters per second

LPSR lipopolysaccharide receptor

LPT lipotropin

LPV left portal view; left pulmonary veins

LPVP left posterior ventricular preexcitation

LPW lateral pharyngeal wall

lpw lumens per watt

LPX, Lp-X lipoprotein-X

LQ longevity quotient; lordosis quotient; lower quadrant

LQTS long QT syndrome

LR labeled release; laboratory references; laboratory report; labor room; lactated Ringer [solution]; large reticulocyte; latency reaction; latency relaxation; lateral rectus [muscle]; lateral retinaculum; left rotation; light reaction; light reflex; limb reduction [defect]; limit of reaction; logistic regression; low renin; lymphocyte recruitment

L-R left to right

L/R left-to-right [ratio]

L&R left and right

Lr lawrencium; Limes reacting dose of diphtheria toxin

LRA low right atrium

LRC learning resource center; lower rib cage

LRCP Licentiate of the Royal College of Physicians

LRCS Licentiate of the Royal College of Surgeons

LRCSE Licentiate of the Royal College of Surgeons, Edinburgh

LRD living related donor

LRDT living related donor transplant

LRE lamina rara externa; leukemic reticuloendotheliosis; lymphoreticuloendothelial

LREH low renin essential hypertension

LRES long-range evaluation system

LRF latex and resorcinol formaldehyde; liver residue factor; luteinizing hormone-releasing factor

LRH luteinizing hormone-releasing hormone

LRI lamina rara interna; lower respiratory [tract] illness; lower respiratory [tract] infection; lymphocyte reactivity index

LRM left radical mastectomy

LRMP last regular menstrual period

LRN lateral reticular nucleus

LROP lower radicular obstetrical paralysis

LRP lichen ruber planus; long-range planning

LRQ lower right quadrant

LRR labyrinthine righting reflex; lymph return rate

LRS lactated Ringer solution; lateral recess stenosis; lateral recess syndrome; low rate of stimulation; lumboradicular syndrome

LRSF lactating rat serum factor; liver regenerating serum factor

LRSS late respiratory systemic syndrome

LRT local radiation therapy; long terminal repeat; lower respiratory tract

LRTI lower respiratory tract illness; lower respiratory tract infection

LRV left renal vein

LS lateral suspensor; left sacrum; left septum; left side; legally separated; leiomyosarcoma; length of stay; Leriche syndrome; Licentiate in Surgery; life sciences; light sensitive, light-sensitivity; light sleep; liminal sensation; linear scleroderma; lipid synthesis; liver and spleen; long sleep; longitudinal section; low-sodium [diet]; lower strength; lumbar spine; lumbosacral; lung surfactant; lymphosarcoma

L-S Letterer-Siwe [disease]

L/S lactase/sucrase [ratio]; lecithin/sphingomyelin [ratio]; lipid/saccharide [ratio]; longitudinal section; lumbosacral

L&S liver and spleen

LSA left sacro-anterior [fetal position]; left subclavian artery; leukocyte-specific activity; lichen sclerosus et atrophicus; lymphosarcoma

LS&A lichen sclerosus et atrophicus

LSANA leukocyte-specific antinuclear antibody

LSA/RCS lymphosarcoma-reticulum cell sarcoma

LSB least significant bit; left sternal border; left scapular border; long spike burst

LS-BMD lumbar spine bone mineral density

LSC late systolic click; left side colon cancer; left subclavian; lichen simplex chronicus; liquid scintillation counting; liquid-solid chromatography

LSc local scleroderma

LScA left scapulo-anterior [fetal position]

LSCL lymphosarcoma cell leukemia

LScP left scapulo-posterior [fetal position]

LSCS lower segment cesarean section

LSD laryngeal sound discrimination; least significant difference; least significant digit; low-sodium diet; lysergic acid diethylamide

LSD-25 lysergic acid diethylamide

LSE left sternal edge

LSect longitudinal section

LSEP left somatosensory evoked potential; lumbosacral somatosensory evoked potential

LSF linear spread function; lymphocyte-stimulating factor

LSG labial salivary gland

LSH lutein-stimulating hormone; lymphocyte-stimulating hormone

LSHTM London School of Hygiene and Tropical Medicine

LSI large-scale integration; life satisfaction index; lumbar spine index

LSK liver, spleen, kidneys

LSKM liver-spleen-kidney-megalia

LSL left sacrolateral [fetal position]; left short leg; lymphosarcoma [cell] leukemia

LSM late systolic murmur; lymphocyte separation medium; lysergic acid morpholide

LSN left substantia nigra

LSO lateral superior olive; left salpingo-oophorectomy; left superior oblique; lumbosacral orthosis

LSP left sacroposterior [fetal position]; linguistic string project; liver-specific protein; lymphocyte-specific protein

LS PACS low-speed picture archive and communication system

LSp life span

L-Spar asparaginase (Elspar)

LSSA lipid-soluble secondary antioxidant

LSR lanthanide shift reagent; lecithin/sphingomyelin ratio; left superior rectus [muscle]; liver/spleen ratio

LSRA low septal right atrium

LSS life support station; lumbosacral spine

LST lateral spinothalamic tract; left sacrotransverse [fetal position]; life-sustaining treatment

LSTAT life support for trauma and transport

LSTL laparoscopic tubal ligation

LSU lactose-saccharose-urea [agar]; life support unit

LSV lateral sacral vein; left subclavian vein; longitudinal sound velocity

LSVC left superior vena cava

LSWA large amplitude slow wave activity

LT heat-labile toxin; laminar tomography; left; left thigh; less than; lethal time; leukotriene; Levin tube; levothyroxine;

light; long-term; low temperature; lymphocytotoxin; lymphotoxin; syphilis [lues] test

L-T3 L-triiodothyronine

L-T4 L-thyroxine

lt left; light; low tension

LTA leukotriene A; lipoate transacetylase; lipotechoic acid; local tracheal anesthesia; long-term archives

LTAS lead tetra-acetate Schiff

LTB laryngotracheobronchitis; leukotriene B

LTC large transformed cell; leukotriene C; lidocaine tissue concentration; long-term care

L1TC level 1 trauma center

LTCF long-term care facility

LTCS low transverse cervical section

LTD Laron-type dwarfism; leukotriene D; long-term disability

LTE laryngotracheoesophageal; leukotriene E

LT-ECG long-term electrocardiography

LTF lactotransferrin; lipotropic factor; lymphocyte-transforming factor

LTG low-tension glaucoma

LTH lactogenic hormone; local tumor hyperthermia; low temperature holding; luteotropic hormone

LTI lupus-type inclusions

LTK leukocyte tyrosine kinase

lt lat left lateral

LTM long-term memory

LTN lateral telangiectatic nevus

LTOT long-term oxygen therapy

LTP leukocyte thromboplastin; long-term potentiation; L-tryptophan

LTPP lipothiamide pyrophosphate

LTR location transactivating region; long terminal repeat

LTS long-term survival

LTT lactose tolerance test; leucine tolerance test; limited treadmill test; lymphocyte transformation test

LTV lung thermal volume

LTW Leydig-cell tumor in Wistar rat

LU left upper [limb]; loudness unit; Lupron; lytic unit

Lu lutetium

L&U lower and upper

LUC large unstained cell

LUE left upper extremity

LUF luteinized unruptured follicle

LUFS luteinized unruptured follicle syndrome

LUL left upper eyelid; left upper limb; left upper lobe; left upper lung

lumb lumbar

LUMD lowest usual maintenance dose

LUMO lowest unoccupied molecular orbital

LUO left ureteral orifice

LUOQ left upper outer quadrant

LUP left ureteropelvic

LUPV left upper pulmonary vein

LUQ left upper quadrant

LUSB left upper scapular border; left upper sternal border

LUT look-up table

LUV large unilamellar vesicle

LUZ left upper zone

LV laryngeal vestibule; lateral ventricle; lecithovitellin; left ventricle, left ventricular; leucovorin; leukemia virus; live vaccine; live virus; low volume; lumbar vertebra; lung volume

Lv brightness or luminance

lv leave

LVA left ventricular aneurysm; left vertebral artery

LVAD left ventricular assist device

LVAS left ventricular assist system

LVBP left ventricular bypass pump

LVC low-viscosity cement

LVCS low vertical cesarean section

LVD left ventricular dysfunction

LVDd left ventricular dimension in end-diastole

LVDI left ventricular dimension

LVDP left ventricular developed pressure; left ventricular diastolic pressure

LVDV left ventricular diastolic volume

LVE left ventricular ejection; left ventricular enlargement

LVED left ventricular end-diastole

LVEDC left ventricular end-diastolic circumference

LVEDD left ventricular end-diastolic diameter

LVEDP left ventricular end-diastolic pressure

LVEDV left ventricular end-diastolic volume

LVEF left ventricular ejection fraction

LVEP left ventricular end-diastolic pressure

LVESD left ventricular end-systolic dimension

LVESV left ventricular end-systolic volume

LVET left ventricular ejection time; low volume eye test

LVETI left ventricular ejection time index

LVF left ventricular failure; left ventricular function; left visual field; low-voltage fast; low-voltage foci

LVFP left ventricular filling pressure

LVH large vessel hematocrit; left ventricular hypertrophy

LVI left ventricular insufficiency; left ventricular ischemia

LVID left ventricular internal dimension

LVIV left ventricular infarct volume

LVL left vastus lateralis

LVLG left ventrolateral gluteal

LVM left ventricular mass

LVMF left ventricular minute flow

LVN lateral ventricular nerve; lateral vestibular nucleus; Licensed Visiting Nurse; Licensed Vocational Nurse

LVO left ventricle outflow

LVOH left ventricle outflow [tract] height

LVOT left ventricular outflow tract

LVP large volume parenteral [infusion]; left ventricular pressure; levator veli palatini; lysine-vasopressin

LVPFR left ventricular peak filling rate

LVPW left ventricular posterior wall

LVQ learning vector quantization

LVS left ventricular strain

LVSEMI left ventricular subendocardial ischemia

LVSI left ventricular systolic index

LVSO left ventricular systolic output

LVSP left ventricular systolic pressure

LVST lateral vestibulospinal tract

LVSV left ventricular stroke volume

LVSW left ventricular stroke work

LVSWI left ventricular stroke work index

LVT left ventricular tension; lysine vasotonin

LVV left ventricular volume; Le Veen valve; live varicella vaccine; live varicella virus

LVW left ventricular wall; left ventricular work

LVWI left ventricular work index

LVWM left ventricular wall motion

LVWT left ventricular wall thickness

LW lacerating wound; lateral wall; Lee-White [method]

L&W, L/W living and well

Lw lawrencium

LWBS leaving [hospital] without being seen

LWCT Lee-White clotting time

LWK large white kidney

LWP lateral wall pressure

LWS Lowry-Wood syndrome

LX local irradiation; lower extremity

Lx latex

lx larynx; lower extremity; lux

L-XRF L x-ray fluorescence

LXT left exotopia

LY lactoalbumin and yeastolate [medium]; lymphocyte

Ly a T-cell antigen used for grouping T-lymphocytes into different classes

LYDMA lymphocyte-detected membrane antigen

LYES liver yang exuberance syndrome

LYG lymphomatoid granulomatosis

lym, lymph lymphocyte, lymphocytic

LyNeF lytic nephritic factor

lyo lyophilized

LYP lactose, yeast, and peptone [agar]; lower yield point

LYS, Lys lysine; lysodren; lytes electrolytes

LySLk lymphoma syndrome leukemia

Lyso-PC lysophosphatidyl phosphatidylcholine

LYZ lysozyme

LZM, Lzm lysozyme

M blood factor in the MNS blood group system; chin [Lat. *mentum*]; concentration in moles per liter; death [Lat. *mors*]; dullness [of sound] [Lat. *mutitas*]; macerate; macroglobulin; macroscopic magnetization vector; magnetization; magnification; male; malignant; married; masculine; mass; massage; maternal contribution; matrix; mature; maximum; mean; meatus; median; mediator; medical, medicine; medium; mega; megohm; membrane; memory; mental; mesial; metabolite; metanephrine; metastases; meter; methionine; methotrexate; *Micrococcus*; *Microspora*; minim; minute; mitochondria; mitosis; mix, mixed, mixture; mobility; molar [permanent tooth]; molar [solution]; molarity; mole; molecular; moment of force; monkey; monocyte; month; morgan; morphine; mother; motile; mouse; mucoid [colony]; mucous; multipara; murmur [cardiac]; muscle; muscular response to an electrical stimulation of its motor nerve [wave]; *Mycobacterium*; *Mycoplasma*; myeloma or macroglobulinemia [component]; myopia; strength of pole; thousand [Lat. mille]

M-I first meiotic metaphase

M_1 mitral first [sound]; myeloblast; slight dullness

M-II second meiotic metaphase

M_2 dose per square meter of body surface; marked dullness; promyelocyte

2-M 2-microglobulin

M_3 absolute dullness; myelocyte at the 3rd stage of maturation

3-M [syndrome] initials for Miller,

McKusick, and Malvaux, who first described the syndrome

M/3 middle third

M_4 myelocyte at the 4th stage of maturation

M_5 metamyelocyte

M_6 band form in the 6th stage of myelocyte maturation

M_7 polymorphonuclear neutrophil

M/10 tenth molar solution

M/100 hundredth molar solution

m electron rest mass; electromagnetic moment; magnetic moment; magnetic quantum number; male; mass; median; melting [temperature]; metastable; meter; milli-; minim; minimum; minute; molality; molar [deciduous tooth]

m^2 square meter

m^3 cubic meter

m_8 spin quantum number

μ see mu

MA malignant arrhythmia; management and administration; mandelic acid; masseter; Master of Arts; maternal age; maximum amplitude; mean arterial; medical assistance; medical audit; medical authorization; mega-ampere; megaloblastic anemia; membrane antigen; menstrual age; mental age; mentum anterior [fetal position]; metatarsus adductus; meter-angle; methacrylic acid; microadenoma; microagglutination; microaneurysm; microscopic agglutination; Miller-Abbott [tube]; milliampere; mitochondrial antibody; mitogen activation; mitotic apparatus; mixed agglutination; moderately advanced; monoamine; monoclonal antibody; multiple action; mutagenic activity; myelinated axon

M/A male, altered [animal]; mood and/or affect

MA-104 embryonic rhesus monkey kidney cells

MA-111 embryonic rabbit kidney cells

MA-163 human embryonic thymus cells
MA-184 newborn human foreskin cells
Ma mass of atom
mA, ma milliampere; meter-angle
mÅ milliångström
ma milliampere
MAA macroaggregated albumin; Medical Assistance for the Aged; melanoma-associated antigen; moderate aplastic anemia; monoarticular arthritis
MAAC maximum allowable actual charges
MAACL Multiple Affect Adjective Check List
MAAGB Medical Artists Association of Great Britain
MAB, MAb monoclonal antibody
mAB monoclonal antibody
m-AB m-aminobenzamide
MABP mean arterial blood pressure
Mabs monoclonal antibodies
MAC MacConkey [broth]; major ambulatory category; malignancy-associated changes; maximum allowable concentration; maximum allowable cost; medical alert center; membrane attack complex; midarm circumference; minimum alveolar concentration; minimum antibiotic concentration; mitral anular calcium; modulator of adenylate cyclase; monitored anesthesia care; *Mycobacterium avium* complex
MACDP Metropolitan Atlanta Congenital Defects Program
macer maceration
mAChR muscarinic acetylcholine receptor
MACR mean axillary count rate
macro macrocyte, macrocytic; macroscopic
MACS maximum aortic cusp separation; myristoylated alanine-rich protein kinase C
MACTAR McMaster-Toronto arthritis and rehumatism [questionnaire]

MAD major affective disorder; mandibulo-acral dysplasia; maximum allowable dose; methylandrostenediol; mind-altering drug; minimum average dose; myoadenylate deaminase
mAD, MADA muscle adenylate deaminase; myoadenylate deaminase
MADD Mothers Against Drunk Driving; multiple acyl-CoA dehydrogenase deficiency
MADGE microliter array diagonal gel electrophoresis
MADPA Medicaid Antidiscriminatory Drug Pricing and Patient Benefit Restoration Act
MADRS Montgomery Asberg Depression Rating Scale
MADU methylaminodeoxyuridine
MAE medical air evacuation; moves all extremities
MAF macrophage activation factor; macrophage agglutinating factor; maximum atrial fragmentation; minimum audible field; mouse amniotic fluid
MAFD manic affective disorder
MAFH macroaggregated ferrous hydroxide
MAFI Medic Alert Foundation International
MAG myelin-associated glycoprotein
Mag magnesium
mag, magn large [Lat. *magnus*]; magnification
mag cit magnesium citrate
MAGF male accessory gland fluid
MAggF macrophage agglutination factor
MAGIC microprobe analysis generalized intensity correction; mouth (or mucosal) and genital ulceration with inflamed cartilage [syndrome]
MAGP microfibril-associated glycoprotein
mAH, mA-h milliampere-hours
MAHA microangiopathic hemolytic anemia

MAHH malignancy-associated humoral hypercalcemia

MAI microscopic aggregation index; movement assessment of infants; multilevel assessment instrument; *Mycobacterium avium intracellulare*

MAIDS mouse acquired immunodeficiency syndrome

MAIN medication-induced, autoimmune, infectious, and neoplastic [diseases associated with antiphospholipid antibodies]

MAKA major karyotypic abnormality

MAL midaxillary line

Mal malate; malfunction; malignancy

mal malaise; male; malposition

Mal-BSA maleated bovine serum albumin

MALG Minnesota antilymphoblast globulin

MALiMET Master List of Medical Indexing Terms

MALT male, altered [animal]; mucosa-associated lymphoid tissue; Munich Alcoholism Test

MAM methylazoxymethanol

mam milliampere-minute; myriameter

M+Am compound myopic astigmatism

6-MAM monoacetyl-morphine

MAMA monoclonal anti-malignin antibody

MAM Ac methylazoxymethanol acetate

MAMC mean arm muscle circumference

mA-min, ma-min milliampere-minute

Mammo mammogram, mammography

MAN metropolitan area network

MAN, Man mannose

MAN-6-P mannose-6-phosphate

man manipulate

MANA mannosidase alpha

MANB mannosidase beta

mand mandible, mandibular

manifest manifestation

manip manipulation

MANOVA multivariate analysis of variance

MAO Master of the Art of Obstetrics; maximal acid output; monoamine oxidase

MAOA monoamine oxidase A

MAOB monoamine oxidase B

MAOI monoamine oxidase inhibitor

MAP malignant atrophic papulosis; mandibular angle plane; maturation-activated protein; maximal aerobic power; mean airway pressure; mean aortic pressure; mean arterial pressure; Medical Audit Program; megaloblastic anemia of pregnancy; mercapturic acid pathway; methyl acceptor protein; methylacetoxyprogesterone; methylaminopurine; microtubule-associated protein; minimum audible pressure; mitogen-activated protein; moment angle plotter; monophasic action potential; motor [nerve] action potential; mouse antibody production; muscle action potential

MAPA muscle adenosine phosphoric acid

MAPC migrating action potential complex

MAPF microatomized protein food

MAPI microbial alkaline protease inhibitor; Millon Adolescent Personality Inventory

MAPS Make a Picture Story [test]; Multidimensional Affect and Pain Survey

MAR main admissions room; marasmus; marrow; maximal aggregation ratio; medication administration record; minimal angle resolution; mixed antiglobulin reaction

mar margin; marker [chromosome]

MARC machine-readable cataloging; multifocal and recurrent choroidopathy

MARCKS myristoylated alanine-rich protein C kinase substrate

MARS magnetic anchor retinal stimulation; methionyl-transfer ribonucleic acid synthetase; mouse antirat serum

MARSA methicillin-aminoglycoside-resistant *Staphylococcus aureus*
MART multiplicative algebraic reconstruction technique
mar(X) marker X [chromosome]
MAS magic angle spinning; Manifest Anxiety Scale; maximum average score; McCune-Albright syndrome; meconium aspiration syndrome; medical advisory service; medical audit study; mesoatrial shunt; milk-alkali syndrome; milli-ampere-second; minor axis shortening; mobile arm support; monoclonal antibodies; Morgagni-Adams-Stokes [syndrome]; motion analysis system
mA-s, mas milliampere-second
MASA Medical Association of South Africa; mental retardation-aphasia-shuffling gait-adducted thumbs [syndrome]
masc masculine; mass concentration
MASER microwave amplification by stimulated emission of radiation
MASH mobile Army surgical hospital; multiple automated sample harvester
MASK Medical Anatomy Segmentation Kit
MASS Medicine, Angioplasty, or Surgery Study
mass massage
massc mass concentration
MAST military antishock trousers; Michigan Alcohol Screening Test
mast mastectomy; mastoid
MASU mobile Army surgical unit
MAT manual arts therapist; master of arts in technology; mean absorption time; medical assistance team (emergency medicine); methionine adenosyltransferase; microagglutination test; multifocal atrial tachycardia; multiple agent therapy
Mat, mat maternal [origin]; mature
mat gf maternal grandfather
mat gm maternal grandmother
MATH Modern Approach to Treatment of Hypertension [study]

MATSA Marek-associated tumor-specific antigen
MAU multi-attribute utility [model]
MAUS Mammography Attitudes and Usage Study
MAUT multi-attribute utility theory
MAV mechanical auditory ventricle; minimal alveolar ventilation; minimum apparent viscosity; movement arm vector; myeloblastosis-associated virus
MAVD mixed aortic valve disease
MAVIS mobile artery and vein imaging system
MAVR mitral and aortic valve replacement
max maxilla, maxillary; maximum
MaxEP maximum esophageal pressure
MB Bachelor of Medicine [Lat. *Medicinae Baccalaureus*]; buccal margin; isoenzyme of creatine kinase containing M and B subunits; mammillary body; Marsh-Bender [factor]; maximum breathing; medulloblastoma; megabyte; mesiobuccal; methyl bromide; methylene blue; microbiological assay; muscle balance; myocardial band
Mb megabyte; mouse brain; myoglobin
mb millibar; mix well [Lat. *misce bene*]
MBA methylbenzyl alcohol; methyl bovine albumin
MBAC Member of the British Association of Chemists
MBAR myocardial beta adrenergic receptor
mbar millibar
MBAS methylene blue active substance
MBB modified barbiturate buffer
MBBS British doctoral degree
MBC male breast cancer; maximal bladder capacity; maximal breathing capacity; metastatic breast cancer; methylthymol blue complex; microcrystalline bovine collagen; minimum bactericidal concentration

MB-CK creatine kinase isoenzyme containing M and B subunits

MBCL monocytoid B-cell lymphoma

MbCO carbon monoxide myoglobin

MBD Marchiafava-Bignami disease; Mental Deterioration Battery; methylene blue dye; minimal brain damage; minimal brain dysfunction; Morquio-Brailsford disease

MBDG mesiobuccal developmental groove

MBF medullary blood flow; muscle blood flow; myocardial blood flow

MBFC medial brachial fascial compartment

MBFLB monaural bifrequency loudness balance

MBG Marburg [disease]; mean blood glucose; morphine-benzedrine group [scale]

MBH medial basal hypothalamus

MBH₂ reduced methylene blue

MBHI Millon Behavioral Health Inventory

MBHO managed behavioral healthcare organization

MBI Maslach Burnout Inventory; maximum blink index

MBK methyl butyl ketone

MBL Marine Biological Laboratory; menstrual blood loss; minimum bactericidal level

MBLA methylbenzyl linoleic acid; mouse-specific bone-marrow-derived lymphocyte antigen

MBM mineral basal medium

MBNOA Member of the British Naturopathic and Osteopathic Association

MBO management by objective; mesiobucco-occlusal

MBO₂ oxymyoglobin

MBP major basic protein; maltose-binding protein; management by policy; mannose-binding protein; mean blood pressure; melitensis, bovine, porcine [antigen from *Brucella bovis, B. melitensis,* and *B. suis*]; mesiobuccopulpal; myelin basic protein

MBPS multigated blood pool scanning

Mbps megabits per second; myeloblastic syndrome

MBq megabecquerel

MBR methylene blue, reduced

MBRT methylene blue reduction time

MBS Martin-Bell syndrome

MBSA methylated bovine serum albumin

MBT mercaptobenzothiazole; mixed bacterial toxin; myeloblastin

MBTE meningeal tick-borne encephalitis

MBTH 3-methyl-2-benzothiazoline hydrazone

MBTI Myers-Briggs type indicator

MC mass casualties; mast cell; Master of Surgery [Lat. *Magister Chirurgiae*]; maximum concentration; Medical Corps; medium chain; medullary cavity; medullary cyst; megacoulomb; melanocortin; melanoma cell; menstrual cycle; Merkel cell; mesiocervical; mesocaval; metacarpal; methyl cellulose; microcephaly; microcirculation; microscopic colitis; midcapillary; mineralocorticoid; mini-catheterization; minimal change; mitomycin C; mitotic cycle; mitral commissurotomy; mixed cellularity; mixed cryoglobulinemia; monkey cell; mononuclear cell; mucous cell; myocarditis

M/C male, castrated [animal]

M-C mineralocorticoid

M&C morphine and cocaine

Mc megacurie; megacycle

M_c mitral closure

mC millicoulomb

mc millicurie

MCA major coronary artery; Maternity Center Association; medical care administration; methylcholanthrene; microchannel architecture; middle cerebral artery; monoclonal antibody; multichannel analyzer; multiple congenital anomaly

MCAB monoclonal antibody

MCAD medium chain acyl-CoA dehydrogenase

MCAF monocyte chemotactic and activating factor

MCA/MR multiple congenital anomaly/mental retardation [syndrome]

MCAO middle cerebral artery occlusion

MCAR mixed cell agglutination reaction

MCAS middle cerebral artery syndrome

MCAT medical college admission test; middle cerebral artery thrombosis

MCB membranous cytoplasmic body

McB McBurney [point]

mCBF mean cerebral blood flow

MCBM muscle capillary basement membrane

MCBR minimum concentration of bilirubin

MCC mean corpuscular hemoglobin concentration; medial cell column; Medical Council of Canada; metacerebral cell; metastatic cord compression; microcalcification cluster; microcrystalline collagen; minimum complete-killing concentration; mucocutaneous candidiasis; mutated in colorectal cancer [gene]

MC-C metacarpo-carpal [joint]

MCCA Medicare Catastrophic Care Act; Medicare Catastrophic Coverage Act

MCCD minimum cumulative cardiotoxic dose

MCCI medical care component of the consumer price index; medical cost control initiative

MCCPI medical care component of the consumer price index

MCCU mobile coronary care unit

MCD magnetic circular dichroism; mast-cell degranulation; mean cell diameter; mean of consecutive differences; mean corpuscular diameter; Medicaid competition demonstration; medullary collecting duct; medullary cystic disease; metacarpal cortical density; minimal cerebral dysfunction; minimal change disease; multiple carboxylase deficiency; muscle carnitine deficiency

MCDI Minnesota Child Development Inventory

MCDK multicystic dysplastic kidney

MCDU mercaptolactate-cysteine disulfiduria

MCE medical care evaluation; military clinical engineering; multicystic encephalopathy; multiple cartilaginous exostosis; myocardial contrast echocardiography

MCES medical care evaluation study; multiple cholesterol emboli syndrome

MCF macrophage chemotactic factor; median cleft face; medium corpuscular fragility; microcomplement fixation; mononuclear cell factor; myocardial contraction force

MCFA medium-chain fatty acid; miniature centrifugal fast analyzer

MCFP mean circulating filling pressure

MCG magnetocardiogram; membrane coating granule; monoclonal gammopathy

mcg microgram

MCGC metacerebral giant cell

MCGF mast cell growth factor

MCGN mesangiocapillary glomerulonephritis; minimal change glomerulonephritis; mixed cryoglobulinemia with glomerulonephritis; multiple cutaneous leiomyomata; myeloid cell leukemia

MCGNX mesangiocapillary glumerulonephritis, X-linked

MCH Maternal and Child Health; mean corpuscular hemoglobin; muscle contraction headache

MCh Master of Surgery [Lat. *Magister Chirurgiae*]; methacholine

mc-h, mch millicurie-hour

MCHB maternal and child health bureau

MCHC maternal/child health care; mean corpuscular hemoglobin concentration; mean corpuscular hemoglobin count

MChD Master of Dental Surgery

MCHgb mean corpuscular hemoglobin

MChir Master in Surgery [Lat. *Magister Chirurgiae*]

MChOrth Master of Orthopaedic Surgery

MChOtol Master of Otology

MCHR Medical Committee for Human Rights

mc-hr millicurie-hour

MCHS Maternal and Child Health Service

MCI mean cardiac index; methicillin; mucociliary insufficiency; muscle contraction interference

MCi megacurie

mCi millicurie

MCICU medical coronary intensive care unit

MCID minimum clinically important difference

MCi-hr millicurie-hour

MCINS minimal change idiopathic nephrotic syndrome

MCK multicystic kidney

MCKD multicystic kidney disease

MCL maximum containment laboratory; medial collateral ligament; midclavicular line; midcostal line; minimal change lesion; mixed culture, leukocyte; modified chest lead; most comfortable loudness; multiple cutaneous leiomyomata; myeloid cell leukemia

MCLNS, MCLS mucocutaneous lymph node syndrome

MClSci Master of Clinical Science

MCM methylmalonic coenzyme A mutase; minimum capacitation medium

MCMI Millon Clinical Multiaxial Inventory

MCMV murine cytomegalovirus

MCN maternal child nursing; minimal change nephropathy; mixed cell nodular [lymphoma]

MCNS minimal change nephrotic syndrome

MCO managed care organization; medical care organization; multicystic ovary

MCommH Master of Community Health

mcoul millicoulomb

MCOV modified covariance

MCP maximum closure pressure; maximum contraction pattern; malanocortin receptor; melphalan, cyclophosphamide, and prednisone; membrane cofactor protein; metacarpophalangeal; metoclopramide; mitotic-control protein; monocyte chemotactic protein; mucin clot prevention

MCP-1 monocyte chemotactic protein-1

MCPA Member of the College of Pathologists, Australasia

MCPH metacarpophalangeal

MCPJ metacarpophalangeal joint

MCPP metacarpophalangeal pattern profile; metacarpophalangeal profile; meta-chlorophenylpiperazine

MCPPP metacarpophalangeal pattern profile plot

MCPS Member of the College of Physicians and Surgeons

Mcps megacycles per second

MCQ multiple-choice question

MCR Medical Corps Reserve; melanocortin receptor; message competition ratio; metabolic clearance rate; myotonia congenita, recessive type

MCRA Member of the College of Radiologists, Australasia

MCRE mother-child relationship evaluation

MCRI Multifactorial Cardiac Risk Index

MCS malignant carcinoid syndrome; managed care system; massage of the carotid sinus; mesocaval shunt; methylcholanthrene [induced] sarcoma; microculture and sensitivity; Miles-Carpenter syndrome; moisture-control system; multiple chemical sensitivity; multiple combined sclerosis; myocardial contraction state

MC & S microscopy, culture, and sensitivity

mc/s megacycles per second

MCSA Moloney cell surface antigen

MCSDS Marlowe-Crowne Social Desirability Scale

MCSF macrophage colony-stimulating factor

MCSP Member of the Chartered Society of Physiotherapists

MCSPG melanoma-specific chondroitin sulfate proteoglycan

MCT manual cervical traction; mean cell thickness; mean cell threshold; mean circulation time; mean corpuscular thickness; medial canthal tendon; medium-chain triglyceride; medullary carcinoma of thyroid; medullary collecting tubule; microtoxicity test; multiple compressed tablet

MCTC metrizamide computed tomography cisternography

MCTD mixed connective tissue disease

MCTF mononuclear cell tissue factor

MCU malaria control unit; maximum care unit; micturating cystourethrography; motor cortex unit

MCUG micturating cystogram

MCV mean cell volume; mean clinical value; mean corpuscular volume; median cell volume; motor conduction velocity

MCx main circumflex [artery]

MD Doctor of Medicine [Lat. *Medicinae Doctor*]; magnesium deficiency; main duct; maintenance dose; major depression; malate dehydrogenase; malignant disease; malrotation of duodenum; manic-depressive; Mantoux diameter; Marek disease; maternal deprivation; maximum dose; mean deviation; Meckel diverticulum; mediastinal disease; medical department; Medical Design [brace]; mediodorsal; medium dosage; Ménière disease; mental deficiency; mental depression; mesiodistal; Miller-Dieker [syndrome]; Minamata disease; minimum dose; mitral disease, mixed diet; moderate disability; monocular deprivation; movement disorder; multiple deficiency; muscular dystrophy; myelodysplasia; myocardial damage; myocardial disease; myotonic dystrophy

Md mendelevium

md median

MDA malondialdehyde; manual dilation of anus; methylene dianiline; 3,4-methylenedioxyamphetamine; minimal deviation adenocarcinoma; monodehydroascorbate; motor discriminative acuity; multivariant discriminant analysis; right mentoanterior [fetal position] [Lat. *mento-dextra anterior*]

MDa megadalton

MDAD mineral dust airway disease

MDAP Machover Draw-A-Person [test]

MDB medulloblastoma

MDBDF March of Dimes Birth Defect Foundation

MDBK Madin-Darby bovine kidney [cell]

MDC major diagnostic categories; Metoprolol in Dilated Cardiomyography [trial]; minimum detectable concentration; monocyte-depleted mononuclear cell

MDCK Madin-Darby canine kidney

MDCR Miller-Dieker [syndrome] chromosome region

MDD major depressive disorder; mean daily dose

MDDS medical diagnostic decision support [system]

MDE major depressive episode

MDEBP mean daily erect blood pressure

MDentSc Master of Dental Science

MDF mean dominant frequency; myocardial depressant factor

MDFD map-dot-fingerprint dystrophy

MDG mean diastolic gradient; methyladenine deoxyribonucleic acid glycosylase

MDGF macrophage-derived growth factor

MDH malate dehydrogenase; medullary dorsal horn

MDHR maximum determined heart rate

MDHV Marek disease herpesvirus

MDI manic-depressive illness; metered dose inhaler; multiple daily injection; Multiscore Depression Inventory

MDIA multidimensional interaction analysis

MDIPT Multicenter Diltiazem Postinfarction Trial

MDIS medical diagnostic imaging support; medical diagnostic imaging system

MDIT mean disintegration time

MDK midkine

MDLS Miller-Dieker lissencephaly syndrome

MDM medical decision making; mid-diastolic murmur; minor determinant mix [penicillin]

MDMA methylenedioxymethamphetamine

MD-MPH Doctor of Medicine–Master of Public Health [combined degree in medicine and public health]

MDMU medical devices for military use

mdn median

MDNB mean daily nitrogen balance; metadinitrobenzene

MDOPA, mdopa methyldopa

MDP manic-depressive psychosis; maximum diastolic potential; maximum digital pulse; methylene diphosphate; microsomal dipeptidase; muramyldipeptide; muscular dystrophy, progressive; right mentoposterior [fetal position] [Lat. *mento-dextra posterior*]

MDPD maximum daily permissible dose

MD-PhD combined degree in medicine and science

MDPK myotonic dystrophy protein kinase

MDQ memory deviation quotient; Menstrual Distress Questionnaire; minimum detectable quantity

MDR median duration of response; medical device reporting; minimum daily requirement; multidrug resistance

MDRD Modification of Diet in Renal Disease [study]

MDRS Mattis Dementia Rating Scale

MDR TB multidrug-resistant tuberculosis

MDS Master of Dental Surgery; maternal deprivation syndrome; medical data screening; medical data system; mesonephric duct system; micro-dilution system; milk drinker's syndrome; Miller-Dieker syndrome; minimum data set; myelodysplastic syndrome; myocardial depressant substance

MDS+ minimum data set (plus)

MDSBP mean daily supine blood pressure

MDSO mentally disturbed sex offender

MDSS medical decision support system

MDT mast [cell] degeneration test; mean dissolution time; median detection threshold; multidisciplinary team; right mentotransverse [fetal position] [Lat. *mento-dextra transversa*]

MDTP multidisciplinary treatment plan

MDTR mean diameter-thickness ratio

MDUO myocardial disease of unknown origin

MDV Marek disease virus; mean dye [bolus] velocity; mucosal disease virus

MDY month, date, year

Mdyn megadyne

ME macular edema; malic enzyme; manic episode; maximum effort; median eminence; medical education; medical examiner; meningoencephalitis; mercaptoethanol; metabolic energy; metabolism; microembolism; microenvironment; middle ear; mouse embryo; mouse epithelial [cell]; myalgic encephalomyelitis; myoepithelial

M/E myeloid/erythroid [ratio]

M+E, M&E monitoring and evaluation

2-ME 2-mercaptoethanol

Me menton; methyl

MEA male-enhanced antigen; Medical Exhibition Association; mercaptoethylamine; monoethanolamine; multiple endocrine adenomatosis

MEA-I multiple endocrine adenomatosis type I

mEAD monophasic action potential early afterdepolarization

meas measurement

MEAP multiphasic environmental assessment procedure

MEB Medical Evaluation Board; muscle-eye-brain [disease]

MeB methylene blue

ME-BH medial eminence of basal hypothalamus

MeBSA methylated bovine serum albumin

MEC median effective concentration; middle ear canal; middle ear cell; minimum effective concentration

mec meconium

MeCCNU methylchloroethylcyclohexylnitrosourea [semustine]

MECG mixed essential cryoglobulinemia

MECP methyl-CpG-binding protein

MECTA mobile electroconvulsive therapy apparatus

MECY methotrexate and cyclophosphamide

MED median erythrocyte diameter; medical, medication, medicine; Medical Entities Dictionary; minimum effective dose; minimum erythema dose; multiple epiphyseal dysplasia

med medial; median; medication; medicine, medical; medium

MEDAC multiple endocrine deficiency, Addison's disease, and candidiasis [syndrome]

MED-ART Medical Automated Records Technology

MEDEVAC, Medevac medical evacuation

MEDEX, Medex extension of physician [Fr. *médicin extension*]

medic military medical corpsman [Lat. *medicus*]

Medi-Cal Medicaid in California

MEDICO Medical International Cooperation

MED-IDDM multiple epiphyseal dysplasia-insulin dependent diabetes mellitus [syndrome]

MEDIHC Military Experience Directed Into Health Careers

MedIndEx medical indexing expert

MEDIPP medical district-initiated planning program

MEDIPRO medical district-initiated peer review organization

MEDLARS Medical Literature Analysis and Retrieval System

MEDLINE MEDLARS On-Line

MEDPAR Medical Provider Analysis and Review; Medicare Provider Analysis and Review

MEdREP Medical Education Reinforcement and Enrichment Program

MEDScD Doctor of Medical Science

MEDSTATS Medical Statistics Expert System

Med-surg medicine and surgery

Med Tech medical technology, medical technologist

MEDTUTOR microcomputer-based tutorial [for MEDLARS]

MEE measured energy expenditure; methylethyl ether; middle ear effusion; multilocus enzyme electrophoresis

MEES medical element engineering and simulation

MEF maximal expiratory flow; middle ear fluid; midexpiratory flow; migration enhancement factor; mouse embryo fibroblast

MEF$_{50}$ mean maximal expiratory flow

MEFR maximal expiratory flow rate

MEFV maximal expiratory flow volume

MEG magnetoencephalogram, magnetoencephalography; megakaryocyte; Megestrol; mercaptoethylguanidine; multifocal eosinophilic granuloma

meg megacycle; megakaryocyte; megaloblast

Meg-CSA megakaryocyte colony-stimulating activity

MEGD minimal euthyroid Graves disease

mEGF mouse epidermal growth factor

MEGX monoethylglycinexylidide

MEI Medicare economic index

MEK methylethylketone

MEL metabolic equivalent level; mouse erythroleukemia

mel melena; melanoma

MELAS mitochondrial encephalomyopathy-lactic acidosis- and stroke-like symptoms [syndrome]

MEL B melarsoprol

MELC murine erythroleukemia cell

mel-CSPG melanoma-specific chondroitin sulfate proteoglycan

MEM macrophage electrophoretic mobility; malic enzyme, mitochondrial; minimal essential medium

memb membrane, membranous

MEM-FBS minimal essential medium with fetal bovine serum

MEMR multiple exostoses-mental retardation [syndrome]

MEN multiple endocrine neoplasia

men meningeal; meningitis; meniscus; menstruation

MEND Medical Education for National Defense

MEN-I multiple endocrine neoplasia, type I

ment mental, mentality

MEO malignant external otitis

5-MeODMT 5-methoxy-N,N-dimethyltryptamine

MeOH methyl alcohol

MEOS microsomal ethanol oxidizing system

MEP maximum expiratory pressure; mean effective pressure; mepiridine; mitochondrial encephalopathy; motor endplate; motor evoked potential

mep meperidine

MEPC miniature end-plate current

MEPP miniature end-plate potential

mEQ, mEq, meq milliequivalent

mEq/l milliequivalents per liter

MER mean ejection rate; medical emergency room; methanol extraction residue; murmur/energy ratio

MERB Medical Examination and Review Board

MERG macular electroretinogram

MERRF myoclonus epilepsy with ragged red fibers [syndrome]

MERRLA myoclonus epilepsy-ragged red fibers-lactic acidosis [syndrome]

MES maintenance electrolyte solution; maximal electroshock; maximal electroshock seizures; myoelectric signal; multiple endocrine syndrome

Mes mesencephalon, mesencephalic

MESA myoepithelial sialadenitis

Mesc mescaline

MESCH Multi-Environment Scheme

MeSH Medical Subject Headings

MESNA [sodium 2-]mercaptoethanesulfonate

MESOR midline estimating statistic of rhythm

MesPGN mesangial proliferative glomerulonephritis

MEST Medical Equipment Technical Society

MET maximal exercise test; metabolic equivalent of the task; metastasis, metastatic; methionine; midexpiratory time; modality examination terminal; multistage exercise test

Met methionine

met metallic [chest sounds]

metab metabolic, metabolism

metas metastasis, metastatic

Met-Enk methionine-enkephalin

METH methicillin

Meth methedrine

meth methyl

Met-Hb methemoglobin

MeTHF methyltetrahydrofolic acid

MetMb metmyoglobin

METS metabolic equivalents [of oxygen consumption]

mets metastases

METT maximum exercise tolerance test

MEU maximum expected utility

MEV maximum exercise ventilation; mevalonate; minimal excursionary ventilation; murine erythroblastosis virus

MeV, mev megaelectron volts

MEWD, MEWDS multiple evanescent white dot [syndrome]

MF magnetic field; meat free; medium frequency; megafarad; membrane filler; merthiolate-formaldehyde [solution]; metacarpal fusion; microfibril; microfilament; microflocculation; microscopic factor; mid frequency; midcavity forceps; mitochondrial fragments; mitogenic factor; mitomycin-fluorouracil; mitotic figure; mucosal fluid; multifactorial; multiplication factor; mutation frequency; mycosis fungoides; myelin figure; myelofibrosis; myocardial fibrosis; myofibrillar

M/F male/female [ratio]

M& F male and female; mother and father

Mf maxillofrontale

mF millifarad

mf microfilaria

MFA master of fine arts [degree]; monofluoroacetate; multifocal functional autonomy; multiple factor analysis

MFAQ multidimensional functional assessment questionnaire

MFAT multifocal atrial tachycardia

MFB medial forebrain bundle; metallic foreign body

MFC minimal fungicidal concentration

MFCM Master, Faculty of Community Medicine

MFCV muscle fiber conduction velocity

MFD mandibulofacial dysostosis; mid-forceps delivery; milk-free diet; minimum fatal dose; multiple fractions per day

mfd microfarad

MFH malignant fibrous histiocytoma

MFHom Member of the Faculty of Homeopathy

MFID multielectrode flame ionization detector

m flac membrana flaccida [Lat.]

MFO medium frequency oscillator; mixed function oxidase

MFOM Master, Faculty of Occupational Medicine

MFP monofluorophosphate; myofascial pain

MFR mean flow rate; mucus flow rate

MFS Marfan syndrome; Medicare fee schedule

MFSS Medical Field Service School

MFST Medical Field Service Technician

MFT multifocal atrial tachycardia; muscle function test

MFV maximal flow-volume [loop]

MFW multiple fragment wounds

MGA master of general administration

MG Marcus Gunn [pupil]; margin; medial gastrocnemius [muscle]; membranous glomerulonephritis; menopausal gonadotropin; mesiogingival; methylglucoside; methylguanidine; monoclonal gammopathy; monoglyceride; mucous granule; muscle group; myasthenia gravis; myoglobin

Mg magnesium

M3G morphine-3-glucuronide

m⁷ᴳ 7-methylguanosine

mg milligram

MGA medical gas analyzer; melengestrol acetate; 3-methylglutaconicaciduria

MgATP magnesium adenosine triphosphate

mγ milligamma

MGB medial geniculate body; myoglobin

MGBG methylglyoxal-bis-(guanylhydrazone)

MGC megacolon; minimal glomerular change

MgC magnocellular neuroendocrine cell

MGCE multifocal giant cell encephalitis

MGCN megalocornea

MGCR meningioma chromosome region

MGCRB Medicare Geographic Classification Review Board

MGD maximal glucose disposal; mixed gonadal dysgenesis

mg/dl milligrams per deciliter

MGDS Member in General Dental Surgery

MGES multiple gated equilibrium scintigraphy

MGF macrophage growth factor; maternal grandfather

MGG May-Grünwald-Giemsa [staining]; molecular and general genetics; mouse gammaglobulin; multinucleated giant cell

MGGH methylglyoxal guanylhydrazone

MGH Massachusetts General Hospital

mgh milligram-hour

mg/kg milligrams per kilogram

MGL minor glomerular lesion

Mgl myoglobin

mg/l milligrams per liter

MGM maternal grandmother; meningioma

mgm milligram

MGMA Medical Group Management Association

MGMT methylguanine-deoxyribonucleic acid methyltransferase

MGN medial geniculate nucleus; membranous glomerulonephritis

MGP marginal granulocyte pool; marginating granulocyte pool; membranous glomerulonephropathy; mucin glycoprotein

MGPS hereditary giant platelet syndrome

MGR modified gain ratio; multiple gas rebreathing

mgr milligram

MGS metric gravitational system

MGSA malignant growth stimulatory activity

MGT multiple glomus tumors

MGUS monoclonal gammopathies of undetermined significance

MGW magnesium sulfate, glycerin, and water

mGy milligray

MH malignant histiocytosis; malignant hyperpyrexia; malignant hypertension; malignant hyperthermia; mammotropic hormone; mannoheptulose; marital history; medial hypothalamus; medical history; melanophore-stimulating hormone; menstrual history; mental health; mental hygiene; moist heat; monosymptomatic hypochondriasis; murine hepatitis; mutant hybrid; myohyoid

mH millihenry

MHA major histocompatibility antigen; May-Hegglin anomaly; Mental Health Association; methemalbumin; microangiopathic hemolytic anemia; microhemagglutination; middle hepatic artery;

mixed hemadsorption; Mueller-Hinton agar

MHAM multiple hamartoma

MHAQ modified health assessment questionnaire

MHA-TP microhemagglutination-*Treponema pallidum*

MHB maximum hospital benefit; Mueller-Hinton base

MHb methemoglobin; myohemoglobin

MHBSS modified Hank balanced salt solution

MHC major histocompatibility complex; mental health care

MHCS Mental Hygiene Consultation Service

MHCU mental health care unit

MHD maintenance hemodialysis; mean hemolytic dose; mental health department; minimum hemolytic dilution; minimum hemolytic dose

MHDP methylene hydroxydiphosphonate

MHDPS Mental Health Demographic Profile System

MHG metropolitan health group

mHg millimeter of mercury

MHI malignant histiocytosis of intestine; Mental Health Index; Mental Health Inventory

MHIQ McMaster health index questionnaire

MHL medial hypothalamic lesion

MHLC Multidimensional Health Locus of Control

MHLS metabolic heat load stimulator

MHN massive hepatic necrosis; Mohs hardness number; morbus hemolyticus neonatorum

MHO microsomal heme oxygenase

mho reciprocal ohm, siemens unit [ohm spelled backwards]

MHP hemiplegic migraine; maternal health program; maternal health program; medical center health plan; 1-mercuri-2-hydroxypropane; metropolitan health plan; monosymptomatic hypochondriacal psychosis; multi-skilled health practitioner

MHPA mild hyperphenylalaninemia

MHPG 3-methoxy-4-hydroxyphenylglycol

MHR major histocompatibility region; malignant hyperthermia resistance; maternal heart rate; maximal heart rate; methemoglobin reductase

MHRI Mental Health Research Institute

MHS major histocompatibility system; malignant hyperthermia in swine; malignant hyperthermia syndrome; malignant hypothermia susceptibility; multiple health screening; multihospital system

MHSA microaggregated human serum albumin

MHT mixed hemagglutination test

MHTS Multiphasic Health Testing Services

MHV magnetic heart vector; middle hepatic vein; mouse hepatitis virus

MHW mental health worker

MHx medical history

MHyg Master of Hygiene

MHz megahertz

MI first meiotic metaphase; maturation index; medical illustrator; medical informatics; medical inspection; melanophore index; menstruation induction; mental illness; mental institution; mercaptoimidazole; mesioincisal; metabolic index; migration index; migration inhibition; mild irritant; mitotic index; mitral incompetence; mitral insufficiency; mononucleosis infectiosa; morphology index; motility index; myocardial infarction; myocardial ischemia; myoinositol

mi mile

MIA Medical Library Association; missing in action

MIAMI Metoprolol in myocardial infarction

MIAs multi-institutional arrangements; medically indigent adults
MIB management information base; Medical Impairment Bureau
MIBG metaiodobenzylguanidine
MIBiol Member of the Institute of Biology
MIBI 2-methoxy-2-methylpropyl isonitrile
MIBK methylisobutyl ketone
MIBT methyl isatin-beta-thiosemicarbazone
MIC maternal and infant care; medical intensive care; Medical Interfraternity Conference; microscopy; minimal inhibitory concentration; minimal isorrheic concentration; minocycline; model immune complex; mononuclear inflammatory cell
MICAM maturation index for colostrum and mature milk
MICC mitogen-induced cellular cytotoxicity
MICG macromolecular insoluble cold globulin
MICR methacholine inhalation challenge response
MICRA Medical Injury Compensation Reform Act
micro microcyte, microcytic; microscopic
microbiol microbiology
microCi microcurie
microg microgram
MICU medical intensive care unit; mobile intensive care unit
MID maximum inhibiting dilution; mesioincisodistal; midinfarct dementia; minimum infective dose; minimum inhibitory dose; minimum irradiation dose; multi-infarct dementia; multiple ion detection
MIDA myocardial ischemia dynamic analysis
mid middle

MIDAS microphthalmia-dermal aplasia-sclerocornea [syndrome]; Multicenter Isradipine Diuretic Arteriosclerosis [study]
MIDCAB minimally invasive direct coronary artery bypass [surgery]
MIDI musical instrument digital interface
MIDS Management Information Decision System
midsag midsagittal
MIF macrophage inhibitory factor; melanocyte[-stimulating hormone]-inhibiting factor; maximum inspiratory flow or force; merthiolate-iodine-formaldehyde [method]; microimmunofluorescence; midinspiratory flow; migration-inhibiting factor; mixed immunofluorescence; müllerian inhibiting factor
MIFC merthiolate-iodine-formaldehyde concentration
MIFR maximal inspiratory flow rate
MIFT microphthalmia-associated transcription factor
MIG measles immune globulin; Medicare Insured Groups
MIg malaria immunoglobulin; measles immunoglobulin; membrane immunoglobulin
MIGT multiple inert gas elimination technique
MIH Master of Industrial Health; migraine with interval headache; minimal intermittent heparin [dose]
MIHA minor histocompatibility antigen
MII second meiotic metaphase
MIKA minor karyotype abnormalities
MIKE mass-analyzed ion kinetic energy
MILP mitogen-induced lymphocyte proliferation
MILS medication information leaflet for seniors
MIME multipurpose Internet mail extension
MIMOSA medical image management in an open system architecture

MIMR minimal inhibitor mole ratio

MIMS medical information management system; medical inventory management system

MIN medial interlaminar nucleus

min mineral; minim; minimum, minimal; minor; minute

MINA monoisonitrosoacetone

MINIA monkey intranuclear inclusion agent

MIO minimum identifiable odor; modular input/output

MiO microorchidism

MIOP magnetic iron oxide particle

MIP macrophage inflammatory protein; major intrinsic protein; maximum inspiratory pressure; maximum intensity projection; mean incubation period; mean intravascular pressure; middle interphalangeal [joint]; minimal inspiratory pressure

MIPA macrophage inflammatory protein alpha

MIPB macrophage inflammatory protein beta

MIPS million of instructions per second

MIR multiple isomorphous replacement

MIRC Market Intelligence Research Corporation; microtubuloreticular complex

MIRD medical internal radiation dose

MIRP myocardial infarction rehabilitation program

MIRU myocardial infarction research unit

MIS management information system; medical information service; meiosis-inducing substance; minimally invasive surgery; motor index score; müllerian inhibiting substance

misc miscarriage; miscellaneous

MISG modified immune serum globulin

MISHAP microcephalus-imperforate anus-syndactyly-hamartoblastoma-abnormal lung lobulation-polydactyly [syndrome]

MISJ Medical Instrument Society of Japan

MISS Medical Interview Satisfaction Scale; Modified Injury Severity Scale

MIST Medical Information Service by Telephone

MIT Massachusetts Institute of Technology; male impotence test; marrow iron turnover; melodic intonation therapy; metabolism inhibition test; miracidial immobilization test; mitomycin; monoiodotyrosine

mit mitral

MITO mitomycin

Mito C mitomycin C

MITT Myers introduction to type

mIU milli-international unit; one-thousandth of an international unit

mix, mixt mixture

MJ Machado-Joseph [disease]; marijuana; megajoule

mJ, mj millijoule

MJA mechanical joint apparatus

MJAD Machado-Joseph Azorean disease

MJD Machado-Joseph disease; Mseleni joint disease

MJRT maximum junctional recovery time

MJT Mead Johnson tube

MK megakaryocyte; monkey kidney; myokinase

Mk monkey

mkat millikatal

mkat/l millikatals per liter

MKB megakaryoblast

MKC monkey kidney cell

m-kg meter-kilogram

MKHS Menkes' kinky hair syndrome

MkK monkey kidney

MkL megakaryoblastic leukemia

MKP monobasic potassium phosphate

MKS, mks meter-kilogram-second

MKSAP medical knowledge self-assessment program

MKTC monkey kidney tissue culture

MKV killed measles vaccine

ML Licentiate in Medicine; Licentiate in Midwifery; malignant lymphoma; marked latency; maximum likelihood; medial leminiscus; mesiolingual; middle lobe; midline; molecular layer; motor latency; mucolipidosis; multiple lentiginosis; muscular layer; myeloid leukemia

ML I, II, III, IV mucolipidosis I, II, III, IV

M/L monocyte/lymphocyte [ratio]

M-L Martin-Lewis [medium]

mL millilambert, milliliter

ml milliliter

MLA left mentoanterior [fetal position] [Lat. *mento-laeva anterior*]; Medical Library Association; mesiolabial; monocytic leukemia, acute

mLa millilambert

MLAA Medical Library Assistance Act

MLAB Multilingual Aphasia Battery

MLAEP middle latency auditory evoked potential

MLaI mesiolabioincisal

MLAP mean left atrial pressure

MLaP mesiolabiopulpal

MLB micro-laryngobronchoscopy; monoaural loudness balance

MLb macrolymphoblast

MLBP mechanical low back pain

MLC minimum lethal concentration; mixed leukocyte culture; mixed ligand chelate; mixed lymphocyte concentration; mixed lymphocyte culture; morphine-like compound; multilamellar cytosome; multileaf collimator; myelomonocytic leukemia, chronic; myosin light chain

MLCK myosin light chain kinase

MLCN multilocular cystic nephroma

MLCO Member of the London College of Osteopathy

MLCP myosin light-chain phosphatase

MLCQ Modified Learning Climate Questionnaire

MLCT metal-to-ligand charge transfer

MLD manual lymph drainage; median lethal dose; metachromatic leukodystrophy; minimal lesion disease; minimum lethal dose

MLD$_{50}$ median lethal dose

ml/dl milliliters per deciliter

MLE maximum likelihood estimation

MLEL malignant lymphoepithelial lesion

MLF medial longitudinal fasciculus; morphine-like factor

MLG mesiolingual groove; mitochondrial lipid glycogen

MLGN minimal lesion glomerulonephritis

ML-H malignant lymphoma, histiocytic

MLI mesiolinguoincisal; mixed lymphocyte interaction

MLL mixed lineage leukemia

ml/l milliliters per liter

MLLT1 mixed lineage leukemia translocated to 1

MLLT2 mixed lineage leukemia translocated to 2

MLN manifest latent nystagmus; membranous lupus nephropathy; mesenteric lymph node; motilin

MLNS minimal lesion nephrotic syndrome; mucocutaneous lymph node syndrome

MLO mesiolinguo-occlusal; *Mycoplasma*-like organism

MLP left mentoposterior [fetal position] [Lat. *mento-laeva posterior*]; mesiolinguopulpal; microsomal lipoprotein; mid-level practitioner

ML-PDL malignant lymphoma, poorly differentiated lymphocytic

MLR mean length response; middle latency response; mixed lymphocyte reaction

MLRD microgastria-limb reduction defects [association]

MLS mean lifespan; median life span; median longitudinal section; microphthalmia-linear skin defects [syndrome]; middle lobe syndrome; mouse leukemia virus; myelomonocytic leukemia, subacute

MLSB migrating long spike burst

MLSI multiple line scan imaging

MLT left mentotransverse [fetal position] [Lat. *mento-laeva transversa*]; mean latency time; median lethal time; Medical Laboratory Technician

MLT-AD medical laboratory technician-associate degree

MLT(ASCP) Medical Laboratory Technician certified by the American Society of Clinical Pathologists

MLTC mixed leukocyte-trophoblast culture; mixed lymphocyte tumor cell

MLT-C medical laboratory technician-certificate

MLTI mixed lymphocyte target interaction

MLU mean length of utterance

MLV Moloney leukemia virus; multilaminar vesicle; murine leukemia virus

MLVAR amphotropic receptor for murine leukemia virus

MLVDP maximum left ventricular developed pressure

mlx millilux

MM macromolecule; Maëlzels metronome; major medical [insurance]; malignant melanoma; manubrium to malleus; Marshall-Marchetti; Master of Management; medial malleolus; mediastinal mass; megamitochondria; melanoma metastasis; meningococcal meningitis; menstrually-related migraine; metastatic melanoma; methadone maintenance; minimal medium; mismatched; morbidity and mortality; mucous membrane; multiple myeloma; muscularis mucosae; myeloid metaplasia; myelomeningocele

M&M morbidity and mortality

mM millimolar; millimole

mm methylmalonyl; millimeter; mucous membrane; muscles

mm^2 square millimeter

mm^3 cubic millimeter

MMA mastitis-metritis-agalactia [syndrome]; medical management analysis; medical materials account; methylmalonic acid; middle meningeal artery; minor morphologic aberration; monomethyladenosine

MMAA mini-microaggregates of albumin

MMAD mass median aerodynamic diameter

MMAP mean maternal arterial blood pressure

MMATP methadone maintenance and aftercare treatment program

MMC migrating myoelectric complex; minimum medullary concentration; mitomycin C; mucosal mast cell

MMD mass median diameter; minimum morbidostatic dose; moyamoya disease; myotonic muscular dystrophy

MME M-mode echocardiography; mobile medical equipment; mouse mammary epithelium

MMED Master of Medicine

MMEF maximum midexpiratory flow

MMEFR maximum midexpiratory flow rate

MMF maxillomandibular fixation; maximum midexpiratory flow; mean maximum flow; Member of the Medical Faculty

MMFR maximum midexpiratory flow rate; maximal midflow rate

MMFV maximum midrespiratory flow volume

MMG mean maternal glucose

MMH monomethylhydrazine

mmHg millimeters of mercury

mmH₂O millimeters of water

MMI macrophage migration inhibition; maximum medical improvement; methylmercaptoimidazole; mucous membrane irritation

MMIF macrophage migration inhibitory factor

MMIH megacystis-microcolon-intestinal hypoperistalsis [syndrome]

MMIHS megacystis-microcolon-intestinal hypoperistalsis syndrome

MMIS Medicaid management information system

MML Moloney murine leukemia; monomethyllysine; myelomonocytic leukemia

mM/l millimoles per liter

MMLV Moloney murine leukemia virus

MMM see 3-M [syndrome]; microsome-mediated mutagenesis; myelofibrosis with myeloid metaplasia; myelosclerosis with myeloid metaplasia

MMMF man-made mineral fibers

MMMT malignant mixed müllerian tumor

MMN morbus maculosus neonatorum; multiple mucosal neuroma

MMNC marrow mononuclear cell

MMO methane monooxygenase

MMOA maxillary mandibular odontectomy alveolectomy

M-mode motion mode

MMoL myelomonoblastic leukemia

mmol millimole

mmol/l millimoles per liter

MMP matrix metalloproteinase; muscle mechanical power

MMPI matrix metalloproteinase specific for collagen type I; Minnesota Multiphasic Personality Inventory

MMPNC Medical Maternal Program for Nuclear Casualties

mmpp millimeters partial pressure

MMPR methylmercaptopurine riboside

MMR mass miniature radiography; masseter muscle rigidity; maternal mortality rate; measles-mumps-rubella [vaccine]; megalocornea-mental retardation [syndrome]; mild mental retardation;

mobile mass x-ray; mono-methylorutin; myocardial metabolic rate

MMS mass mammographic screening; Master of Medical Science; methyl methanesulfonate; Mini-Mental State

MMSA Master of Midwifery, Society of Apothecaries

MMSc Master of Medical Science

MMSE mini-mental status examination

mm/sec millimeters per second

MMSP malignant melanoma of soft parts

mm st muscle strength

MMT alpha-methyl-m-tyrosine; manual muscle test; mouse mammary tumor

MMTA methylmetatyramine

MMTP methadone maintenance treatment program

MMTV mouse mammary tumor virus

MMU medical maintenance unit; mercaptomethyl uracil

mmu millimass unit

mμ millimicron

mμc millimicrocurie

mμg millimicrogram

MMuLV Moloney murine leukemia virus

mμs millimicrosecond

μmμ meson

MMV mandatory minute ventilation; mandatory minute volume

MMVD mixed mitral valve disease

MMWR Morbidity and Mortality Weekly Report

MN a blood group in the MNSs blood group system; malignant nephrosclerosis; Master of Nursing; meganewton; melena neonatorum; melanocytic nevus; membranous nephropathy; membranous neuropathy; mesenteric node; metanephrine; midnight; mononuclear; motor neuron; multinodular; myoneural

M&N morning and night

Mn manganese

mN micronewton; millinormal

mn modal number

MNA maximum noise area

MNAP mixed nerve action potential

MNB mannosidase beta; murine neuroblastoma

5-MNBA 5-mercapto-2-nitrobenzoic acid

MNBCCS multiple nevoid basal-cell carcinoma syndrome

MNC mononuclear cell

MNCV motor nerve conduction velocity

MND minimum necrosing dose; minor neurological dysfunction; modified neck dissection; motor neuron disease

MNG/CRD/DA multinodular goiter/cystic renal disease/digital anomalies [syndrome]

mng morning

MNGIE myo-, neuro-, gastrointestinal encephalopathy

MNJ myoneural junction

MNL marked neutrophilic leukocytosis; maximum number of lamellae; mononuclear leukocyte

MN/m² meganewtons per square meter

MNMS myonephropathic metabolic syndrome

MNNG N-methyl N'-nitro-N-nitrosoguanidine

MNP mononuclear phagocyte

MNR marrow neutrophil reserve

MNS medial nuclear stratum; Melnick-Needles syndrome; moesin

Mn-SOD manganese-superoxide dismutase

MNSs a blood group system consisting of groups M, N, and MN

MNU N-methyl-N-nitrosourea

MO macroorchidism; manually operated; Master of Obstetrics; Master of Osteopathy; medical officer; mesio-occlusal; metastases, zero; mineral oil; minute output; molecular orbital; monooxygenase; month; morbid obesity

MO₂ myocardial oxygen [utilization]

Mo Moloney [strain]; molybdenum; monoclonal

M₀ mitral opening

mo mode; month; morgan

MoA mechanism of action

MoAb monoclonal antibody

MOB mobility [scale]

mob, mobil mobility, mobilization

MOBS Moebius syndrome

MOC maximum oxygen consumption; multiple ocular coloboma

MOD magnetic optic disk; maturity onset diabetes; Medical Officer of the Day; mesio-occlusodistal

mod moderate, moderation; modification

MODEM modulator-demodulator

modem modulator/demodulator

MODM maturity-onset diabetes mellitus

MODS medically oriented data system; multiple-organ dysfunction syndrome

MODY maturity onset diabetes of the young

MOF marine oxidation/fermentation; methotrexate, Oncovin, and fluorouracil; multiple organ failure

MoF moment of force

MOFS multiple organ failure syndrome

MOG myelin-oligodendrocyte glycoprotein

MO&G Master of Obstetrics and Gynaecology

MOH Medical Officer of Health; Ministry of Health

MΩ megohm

mΩ milliohm

MOI maximum oxygen intake; multiplicity of infection

MOIVC membranous obstruction of the inferior vena cava

MOL molecular

mol mole, molecular, molecule

molc molar concentration

molfr mole fraction

mol/kg moles per kilogram

mol/l moles per liter

mol/m³ moles per meter cubed
mol/s moles per second
mol wt molecular weight
MOM milk of magnesia; mucoid otitis media
MoM multiples of the median
Mo-MLV Moloney murine leukemia virus
MOMA methylhydroxymandelic acid
MOMO macrosomia-obesity-macro-cephaly-ocular abnormalities [syndrome]
MO-MOM mineral oil and milk of magnesia
MOMS multiple organ malrotation syndrome
Mo-MSV Moloney murine sarcoma virus
MOMX macroorchidism-marker X chromosome [syndrome]
MON Mongolian [gerbil]
mono monocyte; mononucleosis
MOOW Medical Officer of the Watch
MOP major organ profile; medical out-patient
8-MOP 8-methoxypsoralen
MOPD microcephalic osteodysplastic primordial dwarfism
MOPEG 3-methoxy-4-hydroxyphenyl-glycol
MOPP mechlorethamine, Oncovin, pro-carbazine, prednisone
MOPV monovalent oral poliovirus vaccine
Mor, mor morphine
MORAC mixed oligonucleotides primed amplification of complementary deoxy-ribonucleic acid
MORC Medical Officers Reserve Corps
MORD magnetic optical rotatory dispersion
morphol morphology
mort, mortal mortality
MOS medial orbital sulcus; Medical Outcomes Study; microsomal ethanol-oxidizing system; Moloney murine sarcoma; myelofibrosis osteosclerosis

mOs milliosmolal
mos mosaic
MOSF multiple organ system failure
MOSFET metal oxide semiconductor field effect transistor
mOsm milliosmol
mOsm, MOsm milliosmole
mOsm/kg milliosmoles per kilogram
MOT mouse ovarian tumor
Mot, mot motor
MOTA Manitoba oculo-tricho-anal [syndrome]
MOTT mycobacteria other than tuber-culosis
MOTSA multiple overlapping thin slab acquisition [technique]
MOU memorandum of understanding
MOUS multiple occurrence of unex-plained symptoms
MOV metal-oxide varistor; minimal oc-clusive volume
MOVC membranous obstruction of in-ferior vena cava
MOX moxalactam
MP macrophage; matrix protein; mean pressure; melphalan and prednisone; melting point; membrane potential; men-strual period; mentum posterior; mer-captopurine; mesial pit; mesiopulpal; metacarpophalangeal; metaphalangeal; metatarsophalangeal; methylpredniso-lone; Mibelli porokeratosis; middle pha-lanx; moist pack; monophosphate; mouth piece; mucopolysaccharide; multiparous; multiprogrammable pacemaker; muscle potential; mycoplasmal pneumonia
8-MP 8-methylpsoralen
mp millipond; melting point
M&P managerial and professional [staff]
MPA mean pulmonary arterial [pres-sure]; medial preoptic area; Medical Procurement Agency; medroxyproges-terone acetate; methylprednisolone ac-etate; microscopic polyarteritis; minor physical anomaly

MPa megapascal
MPAP mean pulmonary arterial pressure
MPAS mild perioxic acid Schiff [reaction]
MPB male pattern baldness; meprobamate
MPC marine protein concentrate; maximum permissible concentration; mean plasma concentration; meperidine, promethazine, and chlorpromazine; metallophthalocyanine; minimum mycoplasmacidal concentration
MPCO micropolycystic ovary syndrome
MPCUR maximum permissible concentration of unidentified radionucleotides
MPD main pancreatic duct; maximum permissible dose; mean population doubling; membrane potential difference; minimal perceptible difference; minimal phototoxic dose; multiple personality disorder; myeloproliferative disease; myofascial pain dysfunction
MPDS mandibular pain dysfunction syndrome; myofascial pain dysfunction syndrome
MPE malignant proliferation of eosinophils; maximum permissible exposure; maximum possible error; Medicaid program evaluation
MPEC monopolar electrocoagulation
MPED minimum phototoxic erythema dose
MPEH methylphenylethylhydantoin
MPF maturation promoting factor; mean power frequency
MPG magnetopneumography; mercaptopropionylglycine; methyl green pyronine; 3-methylpurine deoxyribonucleic acid glycosylase
MPGM monophosphoglycerate mutase
MPGN membranoproliferative glomerulonephritis
MPGR multiple planar gradient recalled

MPH male pseudohermaphroditism; Master of Public Health; milk protein hydrolysate
MPharm Master of Pharmacy
MPHD multiple pituitary hormone deficiencies
mphot milliphot
MPhysA Member of Physiotherapists' Association
MPI mannose phosphate isomerase; master patient index; maximum permitted intake; maximum point of impulse; multidimensional pain inventory; Multiphasic Personality Inventory; myocardial perfusion imaging
MPJ metacarpophalangeal joint
MPKC management problem-knowledge coupler
MPL maximum permissible level; melphalan; mesiopulpolingual; myeloproliferative leukemia
MPLa mesiopulpolabial
MPLV myeloproliferative leukemia virus
MPM malignant papillary mesothelioma; medial pterygoid muscle; minor psychiatric morbidity; multiple primary malignancy; multipurpose meal
MPME (5R,8R)-8-(4-p-methoxy-phenyl)-1-piperazynylmethyl-6-methylergolene
MPMP 10[(1-methyl-3-piperidinyl)-methyl]-1OH-phenothiazine
MPMT Murphy punch maneuver test
MPMV Mason-Pfizer monkey virus
MPN most probable number
MPO maximum power output; minimal perceptible odor; myeloperoxidase
MPOA medial preoptic area
MPOD myeloperoxidase deficiency
MPP massive peritoneal proliferation; methyl phenylpyridinium; medical personnel pool; mercaptopyrazide pyrimidine; metacarpophalangeal profile; myelin protein, peripheral

mppcf millions of particles per cubic foot of air

MPPEC mean peak plasma ethanol concentration

MPPG microphotoelectric plethysmography

MPPH p-tolylphenylhydantoin

MPPN malignant persistent positional nystagmus

MPPT methylprednisolone pulse therapy

MPQ McGill Pain Questionnaire

MPR mannose 6-phosphate receptor; marrow production rate; massive preretinal retraction; maximum pulse rate; multiplanar reformatting or reconstruction; myeloproliferative reaction

MP-RAGE magnetization-prepared rapid gradient-echo

MPRD cation-dependent mannose 6-phosphate receptor

MPS meconium plug syndrome; medial premotor system; Member of the Pharmaceutical Society; microbial profile system; mononuclear phagocyte system; Montreal platelet syndrome; movement-produced stimulus; mucopolysaccharide, mucopolysaccharidosis; multiphasic screening; myocardial perfusion scintigraphy; myofascial pain syndrome

MPSoSIS mucopolysaccharidosis

MPSS methylprednisolone sodium succinate; Music Performance Stress Study

MPSV myeloproliferative sarcoma virus

MPsyMed Master of Psychological Medicine

MPT Michigan Picture Test

MPTP 1-methyl-4-phenyl-1,2,3,6-tetrahydropyridine

MPT-R Michigan Picture Test, Revised

MPU Medical Practitioners Union

MPV main portal vein; mean platelet volume; mitral valve prolapse

MPZ myelin protein, zero

mpz millipièze

MQ memory quotient

MQC microbiologic quality control

MQIS Medicare quality indicator system

MQL Medical Query Language [computer]

MR Maddox rods; magnetic resistance; magnetic resonance; mandibular reflex; mannose-resistant; may repeat; measles and rubella; medial raphe; medial rectus [muscle]; medical record; medical release; medium range; megaroentgen; mental retardation; metabolic rate; methemoglobin reductase; methyl red; mitral reflux; mitral regurgitation; modulation rate; mortality rate; mortality ratio; multicentric reticulohistiocytosis; muscle receptor; muscle relaxant

M&R measure and record

M$_r$ relative molecular mass

mR, mr milliroentgen

m/r mass attenuation coefficient

MRA magnetic resonance angiography; main renal artery; marrow repopulation activity; medical record analysis or analyst; medical records administrator; multivariate regression analysis

MRAB machine-readable archives in biomedicine

mrad millirad

MRAP alpha-2-macroglobulin; maximal resting anal pressure; mean right atrial pressure

MRAS main renal artery stenosis

MRBC monkey red blood cell; mouse red blood cell

MRBF mean renal blood flow

MRC maximum recycling capacity; Medical Registration Council; Medical Research Council; Medical Reserve Corps; methylrosaniline chloride

MRCAS medical robotics and computer-assisted surgery

MRCP magnetic resonance cholangiopancreatography

MRD maximum rate of depolarization; measles-rindenpest-distemper [virus group]; medical records department; minimal reacting dose; minimal renal disease; minimal residual disease

mrd millirutherford

MRDD mentally retarded/developmentally disabled [person]

MRE maximal resistive exercise; maximal respiratory effectiveness

MREI mean rate ejection index

mrem millirem

mrep milliroentgen equivalent physical

MRF Markov random field; medical record file; melanocyte-[stimulating hormone]-releasing factor; mesencephalic reticular formation; midbrain reticular formation; mitral regurgitant flow; moderate renal failure; monoclonal rheumatoid factor; müllerian regression factor; muscle regulatory factor

mRF monoclonal rheumatoid factor

MRFC mouse rosette-forming cell

MRFIT Multiple Risk Factor Intervention Trial

MRFT modified rapid fermentation test

MRH melanocyte-stimulating hormone-releasing hormone; multicentric reticulohistiocytosis

MRHA mannose-resistant hemagglutination

mrhm milliroentgens per hour at one meter

MRI machine-readable identifier; magnetic resonance imaging; medical records information; Medical Research Institute; moderate renal insufficiency

MRIF melanocyte[-stimulating hormone] release-inhibiting factor

MRIH melanocyte[-stimulating hormone] release-inhibiting hormone

MRIPHH Member of the Royal Institute of Public Health and Hygiene

MRK Mayer-Rokitansky-Küster [syndrome]

MRL medical records librarian; Medical Research Laboratory

MRM magnetic resonance mammography; modified radical mastectomy

MRMIB Managed Risk Medical Insurance Board

MRMT Minnesota Rate of Manipulation Test

MRN malignant renal neoplasm

mRNA messenger ribonucleic acid

mRNP messenger ribonucleoprotein

MRO master reference oscillator; medical review officer; minimal recognizable odor; muscle receptor organ

MROD Medical Research and Operations Directorate

MRP mean resisting potential; medical reimbursement plan; multidrug resistance-associated protein

MRR marrow release rate; maximum relation rate

MRS magnetic resonance spectroscopy; Mania Rating Scale; medical receiving station; Melkersson-Rosenthal syndrome

MRSA methicillin-resistant *Staphylococcus aureus*

MRSD mental retardation-skeletal dysplasia [syndrome]

MRSH Member of the Royal Society of Health

MRSI magnetic resonance spectroscopy imaging

MRT magnetic resonance tomography; maximum relaxation time; median range score; median reaction time; median recognition threshold; median relapse time; medical records technician; milk ring test; muscle response test

MRU mass radiography unit; minimal reproductive unit

MR/UR Medical Review and Utilization Program

MRV minute respiratory volume; mixed respiratory vaccine

MRVI mixed virus respiratory infection
MRVP mean right ventricular pressure; methyl red, Voges-Proskauer [medium]
MRX mental retardation, X-linked
MRXS mental retardation, X-linked, syndrome
MS Maffuci syndrome; maladjustment score; mandibular series; Marfan syndrome; Marie-Strümpell [syndrome]; mass spectrometry; Master of Science; Master of Surgery; mean square [statistics]; mechanical stimulation; Meckel syndrome; mediastinal shift; medical services; medical staff; medical student; medical supplies; medical survey; Menkes syndrome; menopausal syndrome; mental status; Meretoja syndrome; microscope slide; minimal support; mitral sounds; mitral stenosis; mobile surgical [unit]; modal sensitivity; modified sphygmomanometer; molar solution; Mongolian spot; morphine sulfate; motile sperm; mucosubstance; Münchausen syndrome; multiple sclerosis; muscle shortening; muscle strength; musculoskeletal
3MS modified mini-mental state examination
MS I, II, III, IV medical student–first, second, third, and fourth year
Ms murmurs
ms millisecond; morphine sulfate
m/s meters per second
m/s² meters per second squared
MSA major serologic antigen; male-specific antigen; mannitol salt agar; Medical Services Administration; membrane stabilizing action; membrane-stabilizing activity; metropolitan statistical area; mouse serum albumin; multiple system atrophy; muscle sympathetic activity
MSAA multiple sclerosis-associated agent
MSAFP, MS-AFP maternal serum alpha-fetoprotein
MSAN medical student's admission note

MSAP mean systemic arterial pressure
MSB Master of Science in Bacteriology; mid-small bowel; most significant bit
MSBC maximum specific binding capacity
MSBLA mouse-specific B lymphocyte antigen
MSC marrow stromal cell; Medical Service Corps; Medical Staff Corps
MSc Master of Science
MScD Master of Dental Science
MScMed Master of Science in Medicine
MScN Master of Science in Nursing
MSCP mean spherical candle power
MSCU medical special care unit
MSD material safety data; mean square deviation; mild sickle cell disease; most significant digit; multiple sulfatase deficiency; musculoskeletal dynamic [system]
MSDC Mass Spectrometry Data Centre
MSDI Martin Suicide Depression Inventory
MS-DOS Microsoft Disk Operating System
MSDS material safety data sheet
MSE medical support equipment; mental status examination; muscle-specific enolase
mse mean square error
MSEA Medical Society Executives Association
msec millisecond
m/sec meters per second
MSEL myasthenic syndrome of Eaton-Lambert
MSER mean systolic ejection rate
MSES medical school environmental stress
MSF macrophage slowing factor; macrophage spreading factor; Médicins sans Frontières [Doctors without Borders]; Mediterranean spotted fever; melanocyte-stimulating factor; modified sham feeding

MSG monosodium L-glutamate

MSGQ medical student graduation questionnaire

MSGV mouse salivary gland virus

MSH medical self-help; melanocyte-stimulating hormone; melanophore-stimulating hormone

MSHA mannose-sensitive hemagglutination; Mine Safety and Health Administration

MSHIF melanocyte-stimulating hormone-inhibiting factor

MSHR melanocyte stimulating hormone receptor

MSHRF melanocyte-stimulating hormone-releasing factor

MSHRH melanocyte-stimulating hormone-releasing hormone

MSHSC multiple self-healing squamous carcinoma

MSHyg Master of Science in Hygiene

MSI magnetic source imaging; medium-scale integration

MSIS multi-state information system

MSK medullary sponge kidney

MSKCC Memorial Sloan-Kettering Cancer Center

MSKP Medical Sciences Knowledge Profile

MSL midsternal line; multiple symmetric lipomatosis

MSLA mouse-specific lymphocyte antigen

MSLR mixed skin cell-leukocyte reaction

MSLS Marinesco-Sjögren-like syndrome

MSLT multiple sleep latency test

MSM medium-size molecule; mineral salts medium

MSMAID machine, suction, monitor, airway equipment, intravenous line, drugs [for bronchoscopy]

MSMB microseminoprotein beta

MSN main sensory nucleus; Master of Science in Nursing; mildly subnormal

MSO management service organization; medial superior olive; medical staff organization

MSOF multiple systems organ failure

MSOP medical school objectives project

MSP macrophage stimulating protein; maximum squeeze pressure; median sagittal plane; microseminoprotein; Münchausen syndrome by proxy

msp muscle spasm

MSPB microseminoprotein beta

MSPGN mesangial proliferative glomerulonephritis

MSPH Master of Science in Public Health

MSPhar Master of Science in Pharmacy

MSPN medical student's progress note

MSPQ Modified Somatic Perception Questionnaire

MSPS myocardial stress perfusion scintigraphy

MSQ mental status questionnaire; Minnesota satisfaction questionnaire

MSR macrophage scavenger receptor; Member of the Society of Radiographers; monosynaptic reflex; muscle stretch reflex

MSRPP Multidimensional Scale for Rating Psychiatric Patients

MSRT Minnesota Spatial Relations Test

MSS Marshall-Smith syndrome; massage; Medical Superintendents' Society; Medicare Statistical System; mental status schedule; minor surgery suite; motion sickness susceptibility; mucus-stimulating substance; multiple sclerosis susceptibility; muscular subaortic stenosis

mss massage

MSSA methicillin-sensitive *Staphylococcus aureus*

MSSE multiple self-healing squamous epithelioma

MSSG multiple sclerosis susceptibility gene

MSSVD Medical Society for the Study of Venereal Diseases

MST maximal stimulation test; mean survival time; mean swell time; mercaptopyruvate sulfurtransferase; myeloproliferative syndrome, transient

MSTh mesothorium

MSTI multiple soft tissue injuries

MSTP Medical Scientist Training Program [of NIH]; medical student training program

MSU maple sugar urine; maple syrup urine; medical studies unit; mid-stream urine; monosodium urate; myocardial substrate uptake

MSUD maple syrup urine disease

MSurg Master of Surgery

MSV maximum sustained level of ventilation; mean scale value; mean spatial velocity; Moloney sarcoma virus; murine sarcoma virus

mSv millisievert

MSVC maximal sustained ventilatory capacity

MSW Master of Social Welfare; Master of Social Work; medical social worker; multiple stab wounds

MSWYE modified sea water yeast extract

MT magnetization transfer; malaria therapy; malignant teratoma; mammary tumor; mammilothalamic tract; manual traction; Martin-Thayer [plate, medium]; mastoid tip; maximal therapy; medial thalamus; medial thickness; medical technologist; medical therapy; melatonin; membrana tympani; mesangial thickening; metallothionein; metatarsal; methoxytryptamine; methyltyrosine; microtome; microtubule; mid-trachea; minimal touch; minimum threshold; Monroe tidal drainage; more than; motor threshold; movement time; multiple tics; Muir-Torre [syndrome]; multitest [plate]; muscles and tendons; muscle test; music therapy

M-T macroglobulin-trypsin

M&T *Monilia* and *Trichomonas*

Mt megatonne; *Mycobacterium tuberculosis*

mt mitochondrial

3-MT 3-methoxytyramine

MTA malignant teratoma, anaplastic; medical technical assistant; medical technology assessment; metatarsus adductus; myoclonic twitch activity

mTA meta-tyramine

MTAC mass transfer area coefficient

MTACR multiple tumor-associated chromosome region

MT(ASCP) Medical Technologist certified by the American Society of Clinical Pathologists

MTAD membrana tympana auris dextrae

MTAL medullary thick ascending limb

MTAP methylthioadenosine phosphorylase

MTAS membrana tympana auris sinistrae

MTB methylthymol blue

Mtb *Mycobacterium tuberculosis*

MTBE meningeal tick-borne encephalitis; methyl *tert*-butyl ester

MTBF mean time between (or before) failures

MTC mass transfer coefficient; maximum tolerated concentration; maximum toxic concentration; medical test cabinet; medical training center; medullary thyroid carcinoma; metatarsocuneiform [joint]; mitomycin C

MTD maximum tolerated dose; mean total dose; metastatic trophoblastic disease; Midwife Teacher's Diploma; Monroe tidal drainage; multiple tic disorder

MTDDA Minnesota Test for Differential Diagnosis of Aphasia

MT-DN multitest, dermatophytes and *Nocardia* [plate]

mtDNA mitochondrial deoxyribonucleic acid

MTDT modified tone decay test

MTET modified treadmill exercise test

MTF maximum terminal flow; medical treatment facility; modulation transfer function

MTg mouse thyroglobulin

MTH mithramycin

MTHF, mTHF 5,10-methylene tetrahydrofolate

5-MTHF 5-methyl-tetrahydrofolate

MTHFR 5,10-methylene tetrahydrofolate reductase

MTI malignant teratoma, intermediate; minimum time interval; moving target indicator

MTL mantle zone lymphoma

MTLP metabolic toxemia of late pregnancy

MTM Thayer-Martin, modified [agar]; myotubular myopathy

MT-M multitest, mycology [plate]

MTMX myotubular myopathy, X-linked

MTO Medical Transport Officer; methoxyhydroxyphenylalanine

MTOC microtubule organizing center; mitotic organizing center

MTP maximum tolerated pressure; medial tibial plateau; median time to progression; metacarpophalangeal; metatarsophalangeal; micropayment transfer protocol; microsomal triglyceride transfer protein; microtubule protein

MTPJ metatarsophalangeal joint

MTQ methaqualone

MTR magnetization transfer ratio; Meinicke turbidity reaction; 5-methylthioribose; methyltetrahydrofolate:L-homocysteine S-methyltransferase

MTS Medicare transaction system; magnetization transfer contrast; methotrexate; multicellular tumor spheroid; musculotendinous structure

MTST maximal treadmill stress test

MTT malignant teratoma, trophoblastic; maximal treadmill test; meal tolerance test; mean transit time; methyl-thiazol-diphenyl-tetrazolium; mucous transport time

MTU malignant teratoma, undifferentiated; medical therapy unit; methylthiouracil

MTV mammary tumor virus; metatarsus varus; mouse mammary tumor virus

MTX methotrexate

MT-Y multitest yeast [plate]

MU megaunit; mescaline unit; methyluric [acid]; Montevideo unit; motion unsharpness; motor unit; mouse unit

Mu Mache unit

mU milliunit

mu mouse unit

μ Greek letter *mu*; chemical potential; electrophoretic mobility; heavy chain of immunoglobulin M; linear attenuation coefficient; magnetic moment; mean; micro; micrometer; micron; mutation rate; permeability

μ_o permeability of vacuum

μA microampere

MUA manipulation under anesthesia; middle uterine artery; motor unit activity

MUAP motor unit action potential

μb microbar

μ_B Bohr magneton

μbar microbar

MUC maximum urinary concentration; mucilage; mucosal ulcerative colitis

muc mucilage; mucous, mucus

μC microcoulomb

μc microcurie

μch microcurie-hour

μC-hr microcurie-hour

μCi microcurie

μCi-hr microcurie-hour

μcoul microcoulomb

MUD minimum urticarial dose

MUE motor unit estimated

μF, μf microfarad

MUG MUMPS (see p. 204) Users' Group

μg microgram

MUGA multiple gated acquisition [blood pool scan]

μγ microgamma

MUGEx multigated blood pool image during exercise

μg/kg micrograms per kilogram

μg/l micrograms per liter

MUGR multigated blood pool image at rest

μGy microgray

μH microhenry

μHg micron of mercury

μin microinch

μIU one-millionth of an International Unit

μkat microkatal

μL, μl microliter

mult multiple

Multi-CSF multi-colony-stimulating factor

MultiODA multivariable optimal discriminant analysis

multip multiparous

MuLV, MuLv murine leukemia virus

μM micromolar

μm micrometer; micromilli-

μmg micromilligram [nanogram]

μmHg micrometer of mercury

μmm micromillimeter [nanometer]

μmol micromole

MUMPS Massachusetts General Hospital Utility Multi-Programming System

MuMTv murine mammary tumor virus

μμC micromicrocurie [picocurie]

μμF micromicrofarad [picofarad]

μμg micromicrogram [picogram]

μN nuclear magneton

MUN(WI) Munich Wistar [rat]

MUO myocardiopathy of unknown origin

μΩ microhm

MUP major urinary protein; maximal urethral pressure; motor unit potential

μP microprocessor

μPa micropascal

μR, μr microroentgen

μ/μ mass attenuation coefficient

MURC measurable undesirable respiratory contaminants

MurNAc N-acetylmuramate

MURP Master of Urban and Regional Planning

MUS mouse urologic syndrome

μs microsecond

musc muscle, musculature, muscular

MUSE medicated uretheral system for erection

μsec microsecond

MUST medical unit, self-contained and transportable

MUT mutagen

MUU mouse uterine unit

μU microunit

μV microvolt

μW microwatt

MUWU mouse uterine weight unit

MV measles virus; mechanical ventilation; megavolt; microvascular; microvillus; minute volume; mitral valve; mixed venous; multivessel; veterinary physician [Lat. *Medicus Veterinarius*]

Mv mendelevium

mV, mv millivolt

MVA mechanical ventricular assistance; mevalonic acid; mitral valve area; motor vehicle accident

MV·A megavolt-ampere

mV·A millivolt-ampere

mval millival

MVB multivesicular body

MVC maximum voluntary contraction; motor vehicle crash; mucin; multivane collimator; myocardial vascular capacity

MVD Doctor of Veterinary Medicine; microvascular decompression; mitral valve disease; multivessel coronary disease

MVE mitral valve echo; mitral valve excursion; Murray Valley encephalitis

MVF mitral valve flow

MVH massive vitreous hemorrhage

MVI multivalvular involvement; multivitamin infusion
MVK mevalonate kinase
MVL mitral valve leaflet
MVLS mandibular vestibulolingual sulcoplasty
MVM microvillose membrane; minute virus of mice
MVMT movement
MVN medial ventromedial nucleus
MVO maximum venous outflow; mitral valve opening or orifice
MVO2, MVO₂ myocardial oxygen consumption
mVO₂ minute venous oxygen consumption
MVOA mitral valve orifice area
MVOS mixed venous oxygen saturation
MVP microvascular pressure; mitral valve prolapse
MVPP mustine, vinblastine, procarbazine, and prednisone
MVPS Medicare Volume Performance Standards; mitral valve prolapse syndrome
MVP-SC mitral valve prolapse-systolic click [syndrome]
MVPT Motor-Free Visual Perception Test
MVR massive vitreous reaction; microvitreoretinal; minimal vascular resistance; mitral valve replacement
MVS mitral valve stenosis; multivendor service
mV·s millivolt-second
mvt movement
MVV maximal voluntary ventilation
MW Mallory-Weiss [syndrome]; mean weight; megawatt; microwave; Minot-von Willebrand [syndrome]; molecular weight

mW milliwatt
mWb milliweber
MWD microwave diathermy; molecular weight distribution
MWP mean wedge pressure
MWS Marden-Walker syndrome; Moersch-Woltman syndrome
MWT myocardial wall thickness
MX matrix
Mx maxwell; MEDEX (see p. 189)
M_{xy} transverse magnetization
My myopia; myxedema
my mayer
MYBC myosin-binding protein C
MYBH myosin-binding protein H
MYBP myosin-binding protein
Myco *Mycobacterium*
Mycol mycology, mycologist
MyD myotonic dystrophy
MYEL myelogram
Myel myelocyte
myel myelin, myelinated
MYF myogenic factor
MyG myasthenia gravis
MYH hevy chain myosin
MYHC heavy chain cardiac myosin
MYHCA heavy chain cardiac myosin alpha
MYL light chain myosin
MyMD myotonic muscular dystrophy
MYO myoglobin
Myop myopia
MYX myoxoma
MZ mantle zone; meziocillin; monozygotic
M_z longitudinal magnetization
m/z mass-to-charge ratio
MZA monozygotic twins raised apart
MZT monozygotic twins raised together

N asparagine; Avogadro number; blood factor in the MNS blood group system; loudness; nasal; nasion; nausea; negative; neomycin; neper; nerve; neuraminidase; neurology; neuropathy; neutron number; newton; nicotinamide; nifedipine; nitrogen; nodule; normal [solution]; nucleoside; number; number in sample; number of molecules; number of neutrons in an atomic nucleus; population size; radiance; refractive index; signal size; spin density

0.02N fiftieth-normal [solution]
0.1N tenth-normal [solution]
0.5N half-normal [solution]
NI-NXII first to twelfth cranial nerves
2N double-normal [solution]
N/2 half-normal [solution]
N/10 tenth-normal [solution]
N/50 fiftieth-normal [solution]

n amount of substance expressed in moles; born [Lat. *natus*]; haploid chromosome number; index of refraction; nano; nerve; neuter; neutron; neutron night; number density; normal; nostril [Lat. *naris*]; number; number of density of molecule; principle quantum number; refractive index; rotational frequency; sample size

2n haploid chromosome; diploid
3n triploid
4n tetraploid
ν see *nu*

NA Avogadro constant or number; nalidixic acid; Narcotics Anonymous; network administrator; neuraminidase; neurologic age; neutralizing antibody; neutrophil antibody; nicotinic acid; Nomina Anatomica; nonadherent; noradrenalin; not admitted; not applicable; not available; nuclear antibody; nucleic acid; nucleus ambiguus; numerical aperture; nurse's aide; nursing assistant; nursing auxiliary

N/A not applicable

Na Avogadro number; sodium [Lat. *natrium*]

nA nanoampere

NAA N-acetyl aspartate; naphthaleneacetic acid; neutral amino acid; neutron activation analysis; neutrophil aggregation activity; nicotinic acid amide; no apparent abnormalities

NAACLS National Accrediting Agency for Clinical Laboratory Sciences

NAACOG Nurses Association of the American College of Obstetricians and Gynecologists

NAA/Cr N-acetyl aspartate/creatine [ratio]

NAAP N-acetyl-4-amino-phenazone

NAB novarsenobenzene

NABP National Association of Boards of Pharmacy

NABPLEX National Association of Boards of Pharmacy Licensing Examination

NAC N-acetylcysteine; National Asthma Center; National Audiovisual Center; Noise Advisory Council

NACDS North American Clinical Dermatological Society

NACED National Advisory Council on the Employment of the Disabled

NAC-EDTA N-acetylcysteine EDTA

nAChR nicotinic acetylcholine receptor

NACHRI National Association of Children's Hospitals and Related Institutions

NACOR National Advisory Committee on Radiation

Nacq number of acquisitions

NACSAP National Alliance Concerned with School-Age Parents

NACT National Alliance of Cardiovascular Technologists

NAD neutrophil actin dysfunction; new antigenic determinant; nicotinamide adenine dinucleotide; nicotinic acid dehydrogenase; no abnormal discovery; no active disease; no acute distress; no apparent distress; no appreciable disease; normal axis deviation; not done; nothing abnormal detected

NAD⁺ the oxidized form of NAD

NaD sodium dialysate

NADA New Animal Drug Application

NADABA N-adenoxyldiaminobutyric acid

NADG nicotinamide adenine dinucleotide glycohydrolase

NADH reduced nicotinamide adenine dinucleotide

NADL National Association of Dental Laboratories

NaDodSO₄ sodium dedecyl sulfate

NADP nicotinamide adenine dinucleotide phosphate

NADP⁺ oxidized form of nicotinamide adenine dinucleotide phosphate

NADPH reduced nicotinamide adenine dinucleotide phosphate

NADR National AIDS Demonstration Research; noradrenalin

NAE net acid excretion

NaE, Naₑ exchangeable body sodium

NAEMSP National Association of Emergency Medical Services Physicians

NAEMT National Association of Emergency Medical Technicians

NAEP National Asthma Education Program

NaERC sodium efflux rate constant

NAF nafcillin; National Amputation Foundation; National Ataxia Foundation; net acid flux

NAFEC National Association of Freestanding Emergency Centers

NAG N-acetyl-D-glucosaminidase; narrow-angle glaucoma; nonagglutinable

NAGA N-acetyl-alpha-D-galactosaminidase

NAGO neuraminidase and galactose oxidase

NAGS N-acetylglutamate synthetase

NAH 2-hydroxy-3-naphthoic acid hydrazide

NAHA National Association of Health Authorities

NAHCS National Association of Health Center Schools

NAHDO National Association of Health Data Organizations

NAHG National Association of Humanistic Gerontology

NAHI National Athletic Health Institute

NAHMOR National Association of Health Maintenance Organization Regulators

NAHPA National Association of Hospital Purchasing Agents

NAHQ National Association for Healthcare Quality

NAHSA National Association for Hearing and Speech Action

NAHSE National Association of Health Services Executives

NAHU National Association of Health Underwriters

NAHUC National Association of Health Unit Clerks-Coordinators

NAI net acid input; no accidental injury; no acute inflammation; nonadherence index

NAIC National Association of Insurance Commissioners

NAIR nonadrenergic inhibitory response

Na,K-ATPase sodium-potassium adenosine triphosphatase

NAL nonadherent leukocyte

NALD neonatal adrenoleukodystrophy

NAM N-acetylmuramic acid; natural actomyosin

NAMCS National Ambulatory Medical Care Survey

NAME National Association of Medical Examiners; nevi, atrial myxoma, myxoid neurofibroma, ephelides [syndrome]

NAMH National Association for Mental Health

NAMI National Alliance for the Mentally Ill

NAMN nicotinic acid mononucleotide

NAMP National Alliance for Mental Patients

NAMRU Navy Medical Reserve Unit

NANA N-acetyl neuraminic acid

NANB non-A, non-B [hepatitis]

NANBH non-A, non-B hepatitis

NANC nonadrenergic noncholinergic

NAND not-and

NANDA North American Nursing Diagnosis Association

NAOO National Association of Optometrists and Opticians

NAOP National Alliance for Optional Parenthood

NAP nasion, point A, pogonion [convexity or concavity of the facial profile]; nerve action potential; neutrophil-activating peptide; neutrophil alkaline phosphatase; nodular adrenocortical pathology; nucleic acid phosphatase; nucleosome assembly protein

NAPA N-acetyl-p-aminophenol; N-acetyl procainamide

NAPCA National Air Pollution Control Administration

NAPDP National Association of Prepaid Dental Plans

NaPG sodium pregnanediol glucuronide

NAPH naphthyl; National Association of Public Hospitals; National Asthma Education Program; nicotinamide adenine dinucleotide phosphate

NAPHT National Association of Patients on Hemodialysis and Transplantation

NAPL nucleosome assembly protein-like

NAPM National Association of Pharmaceutical Manufacturers

NAPN National Association of Physicians' Nurses

NAPNAP National Association of Pediatric Nurse Associates and Practitioners

NAPNES National Association for Practical Nursing Education and Services

NAPPH National Association of Private Psychiatric Hospitals

NAPQI N-acetyl-p-benzoquinone imine

NAPT National Association for the Prevention of Tuberculosis

NAQAP National Association of Quality Assurance Professionals

NAR nasal airway resistance; National Association for Retarded [Children, Citizens]; no action required

NARA Narcotics Addict Rehabilitation Act; National Association of Recovered Alcoholics

NARAL National Abortion Rights Action League

NARC narcotic; National Association for Retarded Children; nucleus arcuatus

NARCF National Association of Residential Care Facilities

narco narcotic, narcotic addict, drug enforcement agent

NARD National Association of Retail Druggists

NARES nonallergic rhinitis-eosinophilia syndrome

NARF National Association of Rehabilitation Facilities

NARIC National Rehabilitation Information Center

NARL no adverse response level

NARMC Naval Aerospace and Regional Medical Center

NARMH National Association for Rural Mental Health

NARP neuropathy–ataxia–retinitis pigmentosa [syndrome]

NARS National Acupuncture Research Society

NARSD National Alliance for Research on Schizophrenia and Depression

NAS nasal; National Academy of Sciences; National Association of Sanitarians; neonatal airleak syndrome; neuroallergic syndrome; no added salt

NASA National Aeronautics and Space Administration

NASD National Association of Schools of Dance

NASE National Association for the Study of Epilepsy

NASEAN National Association for State Enrolled Assistant Nurses

NASHS National Adolescent Student Health Survey

NaSIMM National Study of Internal Medicine Manpower

NASM Naval Aviation School of Medicine

NAS-NRC National Academy of Science-National Research Council

NASW National Association of Social Workers

NAT N-acetyltransferase; natal; neonatal alloimmune thrombocytopenia; no action taken; nonaccidental trauma

Nat native; natural

NaT sodium tartrate

NATCO North American Transplant Coordinator Organization

Natr sodium [Lat. *natrium*]

NAVAPAM National Association of Veterans Affairs Physicians and Ambulatory Care Managers

NAVEL naloxone, atropine, Valium, epinephrine, lidocaine

NAZC neutrophil azurocidin

NB nail bed; neuro-Behçcet [syndrome]; neuroblastoma; neurometric battery; newborn; nitrous oxide-barbiturate; normoblast; note well [Lat. *nota bene*]; nutrient broth

Nb niobium

nb newborn; note well [Lat. *nota bene*]

NBA neuron-binding activity

NBC network based computing; non-battle casualty

NBCC nevoid basal cell carcinoma

NBCCS nevoid basal cell carcinoma syndrome

NBCIE nonbullous congential ichthyosiform erythroderma

NBD neurogenic bladder dysfunction; no brain damage

NBF no breast feeding

NBI neutrophil bactericidal index; no bone injury; non-battle injury

NBICU newborn intensive care unit

NBL neuroblastoma

NBM no bowel movement; normal bone marrow; normal bowel movement; nothing by mouth

nbM newborn mouse

nbMb newborn mouse brain

NBME National Board of Medical Examiners; normal bone marrow extract

NBN newborn nursery

NBO non-bed occupancy

NBOME National Board of Osteopathic Medicine Examination

NBP needle biopsy of prostate; neoplastic brachial plexopathy; nucleic acid binding protein

NBRT National Board for Respiratory Therapy

NBS N-bromosuccinimide; National Bureau of Standards; neuroblastoma supressor; nevoid basal cell carcinoma syndrome; Nijmegen breakage syndrome; normal blood serum; normal bowel sounds; normal brain stem; nystagmus blockage syndrome

NBT nitroblue tetrazolium; non-tumor-bearing; normal breast tissue

NBTE nonbacterial thrombotic endocarditis

NBTNF newborn, term, normal, female

NBTNM newborn, term, normal, male

NBT PABA N-benzoyl-L-tyrosyl para-aminobenzoic acid

NBTS National Blood Transfusion Service

n-Bu n-butyl

NBW normal birth weight

NC nasal cannula; nasal clearance; neck complaint; neonatal cholestasis; neural crest; neurologic check; nevus comedonicus; night call; nitrocellulose; no casualty; no change; no charge; no complaints; noise criterion; noncardiac; noncirrhotic; noncontributory; normocephalic; nose cone; not completed; not cultured; nucleocapsid; nursing coordinator

N:C nuclear-cytoplasmic ratio

nC nanocoulomb

nc nanocurie; not counted

NCA National Certification Agency; National Council on Aging; National Council on Alcoholism; neurocirculatory asthenia; neutrophil chemotactic activity; nodulocystic acne; noncontractile area; nonspecific cross-reacting antigen; nuclear cerebral angiogram

n-CAD negative coronoradiographic documentation

NCAE National Council for Alcohol Education

NCAM neural cell adhesion molecule

NCAMI National Committee Against Mental Illness

NCAMLP National Certification Agency for Medical Laboratory Personnel

NcAMP nephrogenous cyclic adenosine monophosphate

NC/AT normal cephalic atraumatic

NCBA National Caucus on Black Aged

NCBI National Center for Biotechnology Information

NCC National Certifying Corporation; noncoronary cusp; nursing care continuity

ncc noncoronary cusp

NCCDC National Center for Chronic Disease Control

NCCEA Neurosensory Center Comprehensive Examination for Aphasia

NCCH National Council of Community Hospitals

NCCIP National Center for Clinical Infant Program

NCCLS National Committee for Clinical Laboratory Standards

NCCLVP National Coordinating Committee on Large Volume Parenterals

NCCMHC National Council for Community Mental Health Centers

NCCPA National Commission on Certification of Physician Assistants

NCCTG North Central Cancer Treatment Group

NCCU newborn convalescent care unit

NCD National Commission on Diabetes; National Council on Drugs; neurocirculatory dystonia; nitrogen clearance delay; normal childhood disorder; not considered disabling

NCDA National Council on Drug Abuse

NCDV Nebraska calf diarrhea virus

NCE negative contrast echocardiography; new chemical entity; nonconvulsive epilepsy

NCEP National Cholesterol Education Program

NCF neutrophil chemotactic factor

NCFA Narcolepsy and Catalepsy Foundation of America

NCF(C) neutrophil chemotactic factor (complement)

NCHC National Council of Health Centers

NCHCA National Commission for Health Certifying Agencies

NCHCT National Center for Health Care Technology

NCHLS National Council of Health Laboratory Services

NCHPD National Council on Health Planning and Development

NCHS National Center for Health Statistics

NCHSR National Center for Health Services Research

NCI National Cancer Institute; noncriterion ischemic [animal]; nuclear contour index; nursing care integration

nCi nanocurie

NCIB National Collection of Industrial Bacteria

NCIC National Cancer Institute of Canada

NCIC CTG National Cancer Institute of Canada Clinical Trial Group

NCIH National Council for International Health

NCJ needle catheter jejunostomy

NCL neuronal ceroid-lipofuscinosis; nucleolin

NCLEX-RN National Council Licensure Examination for Registered Nurses

NCM nailfold capillary microscopy; nurse case manager

N/cm² newtons per square centimeter

NCMC natural cell-mediated cytotoxicity

NCMH National Committee for Mental Health

NCMHI National Clearinghouse for Mental Health Information

NCMI National Committee Against Mental Illness

NCN National Council of Nurses

NCNR National Center for Nursing Research

NCP noncollagen protein

N-CPAP, n-CPAP nasal continuous positive airway pressure

NCPE noncardiac pulmonary edema

NCPIM National Commission to Prevent Infant Mortality

NCPPB National Collection of Plant Pathogenic Bacteria

NCQA National Committee on Quality Assurance

NCR National Research Council; neutrophil chemotactic response; no carbon required; nuclear/cytoplasmic ratio

NCRND National Committee for Research in Neurological Diseases

NCRP National Council on Radiation Protection [and Measurements]

NCRR National Center for Research Resources

NCRV National Committee for Radiation Victims

NCS National Collaborative Study; neocarcinostatin; nerve conduction study; newborn calf serum; no concentrated sweets; noncircumferential stenosis; nystagmus compensation syndrome

NCSBN National Council of State Boards of Nursing

NCSI number of combined spherical irradiation

NCSN National Council for School Nurses

NCT neural crest tumor

NCTC National Cancer Tissue Culture; National Collection of Type Cultures

NCV nerve conduction velocity; noncholera vibrio

NCVS nerve conduction velocity study

NCX sodium-calcium exchanger

NCYC National Collection of Yeast Cultures

ND Doctor of Naturopathy; nasal deformity; natural death; Naval Dispensary; neonatal death; neoplastic disease; neurologic deficit; neuropsychological deficit; neurotic depression; neutral density; new drug; Newcastle disease; no data; no disease; nondetectable; nondiabetic; nondisabling; normal delivery; normal development; Norrie disease; not detected, not determined; not diagnosed; not done; nurse's diagnosis; nutritionally deprived

N/D no defects; not done

N&D nodular and diffuse

N$_D$, n$_D$ refractive index

Nd neodymium

n$_D$ refractive index

NDA National Dental Association; New Drug Application; no data available; no detectable activity; no detectable antibody

NDAC not data accepted

NDATUS National Drug and Alcoholism Treatment Unit Survey

NDC National Data Communications; National Drug Code; Naval Dental Clinic; nondifferentiated cell

NDCD National Drug Code Directory

NDCG Nursing Development Conference Group

NDD no dialysis days

NDE nondestructive evaluation

NDF no diagnostic findings

NDDG National Diabetes Data Group

NDE near-death experience; nondiabetic extremity

NDF neutrophil diffraction factor; new dosage form

NDFDA nonadecafluoro-n-decanoic acid

NDGA nordihydroguaiaretic acid

NDHPCCB non-dihydropyridine calcium channel blocker

NDI nephrogenic diabetes insipidus

NDIR nondispersive infrared analyzer

NDMA nitrosodimethylamine

NDMR nondepolarizing muscle relaxant

nDNA nuclear deoxyribonucleic acid

NDP net dietary protein; nucleoside diphosphate

NDPK nucleoside diphosphate kinase

NDPKA nucleoside diphosphate kinase A

NDPKB nucleoside diphosphate kinase B

NDR neonatal death rate; normal detrusor reflex

NDRI National Disease Research Interchange

NDS Naval Dental School; neurologic deficit score; new drug submission; normal dog serum

NDSB Narcotic Drugs Supervisory Board

NDT neurodevelopmental treatment; noise detection threshold; nondestructive test, nondestructive testing

NDTI National Disease and Therapeutic Index

NDV Newcastle disease virus

Nd/YAG neodymium/yttrium-aluminumgarnet [laser]

NE national emergency; necrotic enteritis; necrotizing enterocolitis; nephropathia epidemica; nerve ending; nerve excitation; neuroendocrine; neuroendocrinology; neuroepithelium; neurological examination; neutrophil elastase; niacin equivalent; no effect; no exposure; nocturnal exacerbation; nonelastic; nonendogenous; norepinephrine; noninvasive evaluation; not elevated; not enlarged; not equal; not evaluated; not examined; nutcracker esophagus

Ne neon

NEA neoplasm embryonic antigen; no evidence of abnormality

NEAS nonerythroid alpha spectrin

NEB nebulin; neuroendocrine body

NEC National Electrical Code; necrotizing enterocolitis; neuroendocrine cell; neuroendocrine convertase; no essential changes; nonesterified cholesterol; not else classified or classifiable; nursing ethics committee

NECHI Northeastern Consortium for Health Information

NECT non-enhanced computed tomography

NED no evidence of disease; no expiration date; normal equivalent deviation

NEDEL no epidemiologically detectable exposure level

NEE needle electrode examination

NEEE Near East equine encephalomyelitis

NEEP negative end-expiratory pressure

NEF nephritic factor

NEFA nonesterified fatty acid

NEFH heavy polypeptide of neurofilament protein

NEFL light polypeptide of neurofilament protein

NEFM medium polypeptide of neurofilament protein

neg negative

NEGF neurite growth-promoting factor

NEHE Nurses for Environmental Health Education

NEI National Eye Institute

NEISS National Electronic Injury Surveillance System

NEJ neuroeffector junction

NEJM New England Journal of Medicine

NEM nemaline; N-ethylmaleimide; no evidence of malignancy

nem nutritional milk unit [Ger. *Nahrungs Einheit Milch*]

NEMA National Eclectic Medical Association

nema nematode

NEMD nonspecific esophageal motor dysfunction

Neo neomycin; neoplasm or neoplastic

neo neoarsphenamine

NEP negative expiratory pressure; nephrology; neutral endopeptidase; no evidence of pathology

nep nephrectomy

Neph nephron; nephritis; nephrosis

NEPHGE nonequilibrated pH gradient electrophoresis

NERHL Northeastern Radiological Health Laboratory

NER no evidence of recurrence

NERD no evidence of recurrent disease

ner nervous

NERO noninvasive evaluation of radiation output

NES not elsewhere specified

NESO Northeastern Society of Orthodontists

NESP Nurse Education Support Program

NEST Nuclear Emergency Search Team

NET nasoendotracheal tube; nerve excitability test; neuroectodermal tumor; neuroendocrine tumor; norepinephrine transporter

NETS Network for Employers for Traffic Safety

NEU, Neu neuraminidase

neu neurilemma

neur, neuro, neurol neurology, neurological, neurologist

neuropath neuropathology

neut neuter, neutral; neutrophil

NEY neomycin egg yolk [agar]

NEYA neomycin egg yolk agar

NF nafcillin; National Formulary; nephritic factor; neurofibromatosis; neurofilament; neutral fraction; neutrophilic factor; noise factor; normal flow; not filtered; not found; nuclear factor

nF nanofarad

NF1 neurofibromatosis type I; nuclear factor 1

NF2 neurofibromatosis type II

NFA nuclear factor A

NFAIS National Federation of Abstracting and Indexing Services

NFAT, NF-AT nuclear factor of activated T [cells]

NFATp pre-existing subunit of nuclear factor of activated T [cells]

NFB National Foundation for the Blind; nonfermenting bacteria

NFC National Fertility Center

NFCE near-fatal choking episode

NFD neurofibrillary degeneration

NFDR neurofaciodigitorenal [syndrome]

NFE nonferrous extract

NFH heavy polypeptide of neurofilament protein; nonfamilial hematuria

NFIC National Foundation for Ileitis and Colitis

NFID National Foundation for Infectious Diseases

NFIRS National Fire Incident Reporting System

NFJ Naegeli-Franceschetti-Jadassohn [syndrome]

NFK nuclear factor kappa

NFKB nuclear factor kappa B

NF-κB nuclear factor-κB

NFL nerve fiber layer; neurofilament protein, light polypeptide

NFLD nerve fiber layer defect

NFLPN National Federation of Licensed Practical Nurses

NFM neurofilament protein, medium polypeptide

NFMD National Foundation for Muscular Dystrophy

NFME National Fund for Medical Education

NFND National Foundation for Neuromuscular Diseases

NFNID National Foundation for Non-Invasive Diagnostics

NFNS neurofibromatosis-Noonan syndrome

NFP not-for-profit [hospital]

NFS National Fertility Study; no fracture seen

NFT neurofibrillary tangle

NFTD normal full term delivery

NFW nursed fairly well

NFX nuclear factor X

NG nasogastric; neoplastic growth; new growth; nitroglycerin; nodose ganglion; no growth; not given

N/G nasogastric

Ng *Neisseria gonorrhoeae*

ng nanogram

NGA nutrient gelatin agar

NGBE neuraminidase/beta-galactosidase expression

NGC nucleus reticularis gigantocellularis

NGF nerve growth factor

NGFA nerve growth factor alpha

NGFB nerve growth factor beta

NGFG nerve growth factor gamma

NGFIA nerve growth factor-induced clone A

NGFIC nerve growth factor-induced clone C

NGFR nerve growth factor receptor

NGGR nonglucogenic/glucogenic ratio

NGI nuclear globulin inclusions

NGL neutral glycolipid

NGPA nursing grade point average

NGR narrow gauze roll; nasogastric replacement

NGS normal goat serum

NGSA nerve growth stimulating activity

NGSF nongenital skin fibroblast

NGT nasogastric tube; nominal group technique; normal glucose tolerance

NGU nongonococcal urethritis

NH natriuretic hormone; Naval Hospital; neonatal hepatitis; neurologically handicapped; nocturnal hypoventilation; nonhuman; nursing home

N(H) proton density

NHA National Health Association; National Hearing Association; National Hemophilia Association; nonspecific hepatocellular abnormality; nursing home administrator

NHAAP National Heart Attack Alert Program

NHANES National Health and Nutrition Examination Survey

NHB National Health Board

NHBE normal human bronchial epithelial [cell]

NHBPCC National High Blood Pressure Coordinating Committee

NHC National Health Council; neighborhood health center; neonatal hypocalcemia; nonhistone chromosomal [protein]; nursing home care

NHCP nonhistone chromosomal protein

NHD normal hair distribution

NHDC National Hansen's Disease Center

NHDF normal human diploid fibroblast

NHDL non-n-high-density lipoprotein

NHDS National Health Data System; National Hospital Discharge Survey

NHE sodium-hydrogen exchanger

NHF National Health Federation; National Hemophilia Foundation; nonimmune hydrops fetalis

NHG normal human globulin

NHGJ normal human gastric juice

NHH neurohypophyseal hormone

NHI National Health Institute

NHIF National Head Injury Foundation

NHIS National Health Interview Survey

NHK normal human kidney

NHL nodular histiocytic lymphoma; non-Hodgkin lymphoma

NHLA National Health Lawyers Association

NHLBI National Heart, Lung, and Blood Institute

NHML non-Hodgkin malignant lymphoma

NHMRC National Health and Medical Research Council

NHP nonhemoglobin protein; nonhistone protein; normal human pooled plasma; Nottingham Health Profile; nursing home placement

NHPC National Health Planning Council

NHPF National Health Policy Forum

NHPIC National Health Planning Information Center

NHPPN National Health Professions Placement Network

NHQRA Nursing Home Quality Reform Act

NHR net histocompatibility ratio

NHRA Nursing Home Reform Act

NHRC National Health Research Center

NHS Nance-Horan syndrome; National Health Service; National Hospice Study; normal horse serum; normal human serum

NHSAS National Health Service Audit Staff

NHSC National Health Service Corps

NHS CCC National Health Service Centre for Coding and Classification [UK]

NHSR National Hospital Service Reserve

NHT nonpenetrating head trauma

NHTSA National Highway Traffic Safety Administration

NI neuraminidase inhibition; neurological improvement; neutralization index; no information; noise index; not identified; not isolated; nucleus intercalatus

Ni nickel

NIA National Institute on Aging; nephelometric inhibition assay; niacin; no information available; Nutritional Institute of America

nia niacin

NIAAA National Institute of Alcohol Abuse and Alcoholism

NIADDK National Institute of Arthritis, Diabetes, Digestive and Kidney Diseases

NIAID National Institute of Allergy and Infectious Diseases

NIAMDD National Institute of Arthritis, Metabolism, and Digestive Diseases

NIAMS National Institute of Arthritis, Musculoskeletal and Skin Diseases

NIB National Institute for the Blind

NIBP noninvasive blood pressure [monitoring]

NIBSC National Institute for Biological Standards and Control

NIC National Informatics Center; neurogenic intermittent claudication; neurointensive care; nursing interim care; Nursing Interventions Classification

NICET National Institute of Certification in Engineering Technologies

NICHHD National Institute of Child Health and Human Development

NICU neonatal intensive care unit; neurological intensive care unit; neurosurgical intensive care unit; nonimmunologic contact urticaria

NID nidogen; nonimmunological disease

NIDA National Institute of Drug Abuse

NIDD non-insulin-dependent diabetes

NIDDM non-insulin-dependent diabetes mellitus

NIDDY non-insulin-dependent diabetes in the young

NIDM National Institute for Disaster Mobilization

NIDR National Institute of Dental Research

NIDS nonionic detergent soluble

NIEHS National Institutes of Environmental Health Sciences

NIF negative inspiratory force; neutrophil immobilizing factor; nonintestinal fibroblast

Nig non-immunoglobulin

nig black [Lat. *niger*]

NIGMS National Institute of General Medical Sciences

NIH National Institutes of Health

NIHL noise-induced hearing loss

NIHR National Institute of Handicapped Research

NIHS National Institute of Hypertension Studies

NII National Information Infrastructure; National Insurance Institute

NIIC National Injury Information Clearinghouse

NIIS National Institute of Infant Services

NIL noise interference level

NIMBY not in my backyard

NIMH National Institute of Mental Health

NIMP National Intern Matching Program

NIMR National Institute for Medical Research

NIMS National Infant Mortality Surveillance

NINCDS National Institute of Neurological and Communicative Disorders and Stroke

NINCDS/ADRDA National Institute of Neurological and Communicative Diseases and Stroke/Alzheimer's Disease and Related Disorders Association

NINDB National Institute of Neurological Diseases and Blindness

NIOSH National Institute for Occupational Safety and Health

NIP nipple; no infection present; no inflammation present

NIPH National Institute of Public Health

NIPPV noninvasive positive pressure ventilation

NIPS neuroleptic-induced Parkinson syndrome

NIPTS noise-induced permanent threshold shift

NIR near infrared

nIR non-insulin-resistance

NIRA nitrite reductase

NIRD nonimmune renal disease

NIRMP National Intern and Resident Matching Program

NIRNS National Institute for Research in Nuclear Science

NIRS near-infrared spectroscopy; normal inactivated rabbit serum

NIS nationwide impatient sample; near-infrared intracranial spectroscopy; N-iodosuccinimide; no inflammatory signs

NISO National Information Standards Organization

NIT National Intelligence Test

NITD noninsulin-treated disease

nit nitrous

nitro nitroglycerin

NIV nodule-inducing virus

NJ nasojejunal

NJPC National Joint Practice Commission

NK Commission on [Anatomical] Nomenclature [Ger. *Nomenklatur Kommission*]; natural killer [cell]; neurokinin; not known

n/k not known

NK2 neurokinin 2

NKA neurokinin A; no known allergies

nkat nanokatal

NKB neurokinin B

NKC nonketotic coma

NKCA natural killer cell activity

NKCF natural killer cytotoxic factor

NKDA no known drug allergies

NKFA no known food allergies

NKH nonketogenic hyperglycemia; nonketotic hyperosmotic

NKHA nonketotic hyperosmolar acidosis

NKHS nonketotic hyperosmolar syndrome; normal Krebs-Henseleit solution

NKN neurokinin

NKNA neurokinin A

NKNAR neurokinin A receptor

NKNB neurokinin B

NKSF natural killer cell stimulatory factor

NKTR natural killer triggering receptor

NL neural lobe; neutral lipid; nodular lymphoma; normal; normal libido, normal limits

nl nanoliter; normal [value]

NLA National Leukemia Association; neuroleptoanesthesia; normal lactase activity

NLB needle liver biopsy

NLD nasolacrimal duct; necrobiosis lipoidica diabeticorum

NLDL normal low-density lipoprotein

NLE neonatal lupus erythematosus

Nle norleucine

NLF neonatal lung fibroblast; nonlactose fermentation

NLK neuroleukin

NLL nonlymphoblastic leukemia

NLM National Library of Medicine; noise level monitor

NLNE National League for Nursing Education

NLP no light perception; nodular liquefying panniculitis; normal light perception; normal luteal phase

NLS Names Learning Test; Neu-Laxova syndrome; nonlinear least squares; normal lymphocyte supernatant

NLT normal lymphocyte transfer; not less than; nucleus lateralis tuberis

NLTCS National Long Term Care Survey

NLX naloxone; nephrolithiasis, X-linked

NM near-miss; neomycin; neuromedin; neuromuscular; neutrophil migration; nictitating membrane; nitrogen mustard; nocturnal myoclonus; nodular melanoma; nonmotile; normetanephrine; not malignant; not measurable, not measured; not mentioned; not motile; nuclear medicine, technologist in nuclear medicine

N&M nerves and muslces; night and morning

N/m newtons per meter

N-m newton-meter

N/m² newtons per square meter

N x m newtons by meter

nM nanomolar

nm nanometer; night and morning [Lat. *nocte et mane*]

NMA National Malaria Association; National Medical Association; neurogenic muscular atrophy; *N*-nitroso-*N*-methylalanine

NMAC National Medical Audiovisual Center

NM(ASCP) Technologist in Nuclear Medicine certified by the American Society of Clinical Pathologists

NMB neuromedin B; neuromuscular blockade; neuromuscular blocking; neuromuscular blocker/blocking [drug, agent]

NMBA neuromuscular blocking agent

NMBR neuromedin B receptor

NMC National Medical Care; Naval Medical Center; neuromuscular control; nonmotor condition; nucleus reticularis magnocellularis

NMCES National Medical Care Expenditure Survey

NMCUES National Medical Care Utilization and Expenditure Survey

NMD neuromyodysplasia

NMDA N-methyl-D-aspartate

NMDAR N-methyl-D-aspartate receptor

NmDG N-methyl-D-glutamine

NMDS nursing minimum data set

NME National Medical Enterprises; neuromyeloencephalopathy

NMES neuromuscular electrical stimulation

NMF N-methylformamide; National Medical Fellowship; National Migraine Foundation; nonmigrating fraction

NMFI National Master Facility Inventory

NMHCA National Mental Health Consumers' Association

NMI no mental illness; normal male infant

NMIS nursing management information system

NMJ neuromuscular junction

NML nodular mixed lymphoma

NMM nodular malignant melanoma

NMN nicotinamide mononucleotide; normetanephrine

NMNRU National Medical Neuropsychiatric Research Unit

nmol nanomole

NMOR nemadione oxidoreductase; N-nitrosomorpholine

NMOS N-type metal oxide semiconductor

NMP normal menstrual period; nucleoside monophosphate

NMPCA nonmetric principal component analysis

NMPTP N-methyl-4-phenyl-1,2,3,6-tetrahydropyridine

NMR neonatal mortality rate; nictitating membrane response; nuclear magnetic resonance

NMRD nuclear magnetic relaxation dispersion

NMRDC Naval Medical Research and Development Command

NMRI Naval Medical Research Institute; nuclear magnetic resonance imaging

NMRL Naval Medical Research Laboratory

NMRS nuclear magnetic resonance spectroscopy

NMRU Naval Medical Research Unit

NMS Naval Medical School; neuroleptic malignant syndrome; neuromuscular spindle; normal mouse serum

N·m/s newton meters per second

NMSE normalized mean square error

NMSIDS near-miss sudden infant death syndrome

NMSS National Multiple Sclerosis Society

NMT neuromuscular tension; neuromuscular transmission; N-methyltransferase; N-myristoyltransferase; no more than; nuclear medicine technology or technologist

NMTS neuromuscular tension state

NMTCB Nuclear Medicine Technology Certification Board

NMTD nonmetastatic trophoblastic disease

NMU neuromuscular unit; nitrosomethylurea

NN neonatal; nevocellular nevus; normally nourished; normal nutrition; nurse's notes

nn nerves; new name [Lat. *nomen novum*]

NNAS neonatal narcotic abstinence syndrome

NNC National Nutrition Consortium

NND neonatal death; New and Non-official Drugs; nonspecific nonerosive duodenitis

NNDC National Naval Dental Center

NNE neonatal necrotizing enterocolitis; nonneuronal enolase

NNEB National Nursery Examination Board

NNG nonspecific nonerosive gastritis

NNHS National Nursing Home Survey

NNI noise and number index

NNIS National Nosocomial Infections Study

NN/LM National Network of Libraries of Medicine

NNM neonatal mortality

NNMC National Naval Medical Center

NNN Novy-MacNeal-Nicolle [medium]

NNNMU N-nitroso-N-methylurethane

NNO no new orders

n nov new name [Lat. *nomen novum*]

NNP neonatal nurse practitioner; nerve net pulse

NNR New and Nonofficial Remedies

NNS nonneoplastic syndrome

NNT nuclei nervi trigemini

NNU neonatal unit

NNWI Neonatal Narcotic Withdrawal Index

NO narcotics officer; nitric or nitrous oxide; none obtained; nonobese; nurse's office

No nobelium

No, no number [Lat. *numero*]

NOA National Optometric Association

NOABX no antibiotics

NOAEL no observed adverse effect level

NOAPP National Organization of Adolescent Pregnancy and Parenting

NOBT nonoperative biopsy technique

NOC not otherwise classified

noc, noct at night [Lat. *nocte*]

NOCDQ nursing organizational climate description questionnaire

NOD Naito-Oyanagi disease; National Organization on Disability; nodular melanoma; nonobese diabetic; notify of death

NOE nuclear Overhauser effect

NOEL no observed effect level

NOESY nuclear Overhauser effect spectroscopy

NOF National Osteopathic Foundation; National Osteoporosis Foundation

NOFT nonorganic failure-to-thrive

NOII nonocclusive intestinal ischemia

NOK next of kin

nom dub a doubtful name [Lat. *nomen dubium*]

NOMI nonocclusive mesenteric infarction

non-REM non-rapid eye movement [sleep]

NOP not otherwise provided for

NOPHN National Organization for Public Health Nursing

NOR noradrenaline; normal; nortriptyline; nucleolar organizer region

NORC National Opinion Research Center

NOR-EPI norepinephrine

norleu norleucine

norm normal

NORML National Organization for the Reform of Marijuana Laws

NOS network operating system; nitric oxide synthetase; non-organ-specific; not on staff; not otherwise specified

NOSAC nonsteroidal anti-inflammatory compound

NOSIC Neurologic Outcome Scale for Infants and Children

NOSIE Nurses' Observation Scale for Inpatient Evaluation

NOSTA Naval Ophthalmic Support and Training Activity

NOT nocturnal oxygen therapy

NOTB National Ophthalmic Treatment Board

NOTT nocturnal oxygen therapy trial

NOV Novantrone

nov n new name [Lat. *novum nomen*]

NOVS National Office of Vital Statistics

nov sp new species [Lat. *novum species*]

NP nasopharynx, nasopharyngeal; near point; necrotizing pancreatitis; neonatal-perinatal; neuritic plague; neuropathology; neuropeptide; neurophysin; neuropsychiatry; new patient; newly presented; Niemann-Pick [disease]; nitrogen-phosphorus; nitrophenol; no pain; no pressure; nonpalpable; nonparalytic; nonpathogenic; nonphagocytic; normal plasma; normal pressure; nonpracticing; not perceptible; not performed; not pregnant; not present; nucleoplasmic; nucleoprotein; nucleoside phosphorylase; nurse practitioner; nursed poorly; nursing procedure; proper name [Lat. *nomen proprium*]

N-P need-persistence

Np neper; neptunium; neurophysin

np nucleotide pair

NPA National Pharmaceutical Association; National Pituitary Agency; near point accommodation; Nurse Practice Act

NPA-NIHHDP National Pituitary Agency-National Institutes of Health Hormone Distribution Program

NPB nodal premature beat; nonprotein bound

NPBF nonplacental blood flow

NPBV negative pressure body ventilator

NPC nasopharyngeal carcinoma; near point of convergence; nodal premature contractions; nonparenchymal [liver] cell; nonproductive cough; nucleus of posterior commissure

NPCa nasopharyngeal carcinoma

NPCP National Prostatic Cancer Project; non-*Pneumocystis* pneumonia

NP cult nasopharyngeal culture

NPD narcissistic personality disorder; natriuretic plasma dialysate; negative pressure device; Niemann-Pick disease; nitrogen-phosphorus detector; nonpathologic diagnosis; normal protein diet

NPDB National Practitioner Data Bank

NPDC neurofibromatosis-pheochromocytoma-duodenal carcinoma [syndrome]

NPDL nodular poorly differentiated lymphocytic

NPDR nonproliferative diabetic retinopathy

NPE neurogenic pulmonary edema; neuropsychologic examination; no palpable enlargement; normal pelvic examination

NPF nasopharyngeal fiberscope; National Parkinson Foundation; National Pharmaceutical Foundation; National Psoriasis Foundation; no predisposing factor

NPFT Neurotic Personality Factor Test

NPH neutral protamine Hagedorn (insulin) [not used anymore]; normal pressure hydrocephalus; nucleus pulposus herniation

NPhx nasopharynx

NPI Narcissistic Personality Inventory; neuropsychiatric institution; no present illness; nucleoplasmic index

NPIC neurogenic peripheral intermittent claudication

NPII Neonatal Pulmonary Insufficiency Index

NPJT nonparoxysmal atrioventricular junctional tachycardia

NPK neuropeptide K

NPL National Physics Laboratory; neoproteolipid

NPM nothing per mouth

NPN nonprotein nitrogen

NPO nothing by mouth [Lat. *nulla per os*]; nucleus preopticus

NPO/HS nothing by mouth at bedtime [Lat. *nulla per os hora somni*]

NPOS nurses professional orientation scale

NPP nitrophenylphosphate; normal pool plasma; nucleus tegmenti pedunculopontinus

NPPase nucleotide pyrophosphatase
NPPC Nursing Professional Practice Council
NPPE negative pressure pulmonary edema
NPPH nucleotide pyrophosphohydrolase
NPPNG nonpenicillinase-producing *Neisseria gonorrhoeae*
NP polio nonparalytic poliomyelitis
NPR net protein ratio; normal pulse rate; nucleoside phosphoribosyl
NPRL Navy Prosthetics Research Laboratory
NPS nail-patella syndrome
NPSA normal pilosebaceous appartus
NPSH nonprotein sulhydryl [group]
NPT neoprecipitin test; nocturnal penile tumescence; normal pressure and temperature; sodium phosphate transport
NPU net protein utilization
NPUI nursing process utilization inventory
NPV negative predictive value; pressure value; negative pressure ventilation; net present value; nuclear polyhidrosis virus; nucleus paraventricularis
NPY neuropeptide Y
NPYR neuropeptide Y receptor
NQA nursing quality assurance
NQO NAD(P)H:quinone oxidoreductase
4NQO 4-nitroquinoline 1-oxide
NQR nuclear quadruple resonance
NR do not repeat [Lat. *non repetatur*]; nerve root; neural retina; neutral red; noise reduction; nonreactive; nonrebreathing; no radiation; no reaction; no recurrence; no refill; no report; no respiration; no response; no result; nonresponder; nonretarded; normal range; normal reaction; normotensive rat; not readable; not recorded; not resolved; nurse; nursing [service]; nutrition ratio; Reynold's number
N/R not remarkable
N$_R$ Reynold's number

nr near
NRA nitrate reductase; nucleus retroambigualis
NRB nonrejoining break
NRBC National Rare Blood Club; normal red blood cell; nucleated red blood cell
NRbc nucleated red blood cell
NRC National Research Council; National Response Center; normal retinal correspondence; not routine care; Nuclear Regulatory Commission
NRCC National Registry in Clinical Chemistry; National Research Council of Canada
NRCL nonrenal clearance
NRDL Naval Radiological Defense Laboratory
NREH normal renin essential hypertension
NREM nonrapid eye movement [sleep]
NREMT-P nationally registered emergency medical technician-paramedic
NREN National Research and Education Network
NRF Neurosciences Research Foundation; normal renal function
NRFC nonrosette-forming cell
NRFD not ready for data
NRG nursing resources grouping
NRGC nucleus reticularis gigantocellularis
NRH nodular regenerative hyperplasia
NRHA National Rural Health Association
NRI nerve root involvement; nerve root irritation; nonrespiratory infection
NRK normal rat kidney
NRL nucleus reticularis lateralis
NRM National Registry of Microbiologists; normal range of motion; nucleus reticularis magnocellularis
NRMP National Resident Matching Progam
nRNA nuclear ribonucleic acid

nRNP nuclear ribonucleoprotein

NROM normal range of motion

NRP nucleus reticularis parvocellularis

NRPC nucleus reticularis pontis caudalis

NRPG nucleus reticularis paragiganto-cellularis

NRR net reproduction rate

NRRL Northern Regional Research Laboratory

NRS neurobehavioral rating scale; normal rabbit serum; normal reference serum; numerical rating scale

NRSA National Research Service Award [of NIH]

NRSCC National Reference System in Clinical Chemistry

NRSFPS National Reporting System for Family Planning Services

NRT near-real time

NRU neutral red uptake

NRV nucleus reticularis ventralis

NS natural science; Neosporin; nephro-sclerosis; nephrotic syndrome; nervous system; neurological surgery, neuro-surgery; neurosecretion, neurosecretory; neurosyphilis; neurotic score; nodular sclerosis; nonsmoker; nonspecific; non-stimulation; nonstructural; nonsympto-matic; Noonan syndrome; normal saline [solution]; normal serum; normal so-dium [diet]; Norwegian scabies; no sam-ple; no sequelae; no specimen; not seen; not significant; not specified; not suffi-cient; not symptomatic; nuclear sclero-sis; nursing services; Nursing Sister

N/S normal saline [solution]

Ns nasospinale; nerves

ns nanosecond; nonspecific; no seque-lae; no specimen; not significant; nylon suture

NSA Neurological Society of America; normal serum albumin; no salt added; no significant abnormality; no significant anomaly; number of signals averaged

nsa no salt added

NSABP National Surgical Adjuvant Breast Project

NSAD no signs of acute disease

NSAE nonsupported arm exercise

NSAI nonsteroidal anti-inflammatory [drug]

NSAIA nonsteroidal anti-inflammatory agent

NSAID nonsteroidal anti-inflammatory drug

NSAM Naval School of Aviation Med-icine

NSC neurosecretory cell; no significant change; nonservice connected; nonspe-cific suppressor cell; normal child with short stature

nsc nonservice connected; no significant change

NSCC National Society for Crippled Children

NSCD nonservice connected disability

NSCLC non-small-cell lung cancer

NSCS night shift call system

NSCT National Society of Cardiovas-cular Technologists

NSD Nairobi sheep disease; neonatal staphylococcal disease; neurosecretory dysfunction; night sleep deprivation; nominal single dose; nominal standard dose; normal standard dose; no signifi-cant defect; no significant deficiency; no significant deviation; no significant dif-ference; no significant disease; normal spontaneous delivery

NSE neuron-specific enolase; nonspe-cific esterase; normal saline enema

nsec nanosecond

NSF National Science Foundation; nod-ular subepidermal fibrosis

NSFTD normal spontaneous full-term delivery

NSG neurosecretory granule

nsg nursing

NSGCT nonseminomatous germ cell tumor

NSGCTT nonseminomatous germ-cell tumor of the testis

NSG Hx nursing history

NSGI nonspecific genital infection

NSH National Society for Histotechnology

NSHD nodular sclerosing Hodgkin disease

NSHPT neonatal severe hyperparathyroidism

NSI negative self-image; no signs of infection/inflammation; non-syncytium-inducing

NSICU neurosurgical intensive care unit

NSIDS near sudden infant death syndrome

NSILA nonsuppressible insulinlike activity

NSILP nonsuppressible insulinlike protein

NSJ nevus sebaceus of Jadassohn

NSM neurosecretory material; neurosecretory motor neuron; nonantigenic specific mediator; nutrient sporulation medium

N·s/m² newton seconds per square meter

NSMR National Society for Medical Research

NSN nephrotoxic serum nephritis; nicotine-stimulated neurophysin

NSNA National Student Nurse Association

NSND nonsymptomatic and nondisabling

NSO Neosporin ointment; nucleus supraopticus

NSP neuron specific protein; nonstructural protein

NSPB National Society for the Prevention of Blindness

NSPH neonatal severe hyperparathyroidism

NSPN neurosurgery progress note

NSQ Neuroticism Scale Questionnaire; not sufficient quantitiy

NSR nasal septal reconstruction; non-specific reaction; normal sinus rhythm; no sign of recurrence; not seen regularly

NSR/M no sign of recurrence or metastases

NSS normal saline solution; normal size and shape; not statistically significant; nutrition support services

NSSQ Norbeck social support questionnaire

NSSTT nonspecific ST and T [wave]

NST neospinothalamic [tract]; nonshivering thermogenesis; nonstress test; nutritional support team

NSTT nonseminomatous testicular tumor

NSU neurosurgical unit; nonspecific urethritis

NSurg neurosurgery, neurosurgeon

NSV nonspecific vaginitis/vaginosis

NSVD normal spontaneous vaginal delivery

NSVT nonsustained ventricular tachycardia

NSX neurosurgical examination

nsy nursery

NT nasotracheal; neotetrazolium; neurotensin; neurotrophic; neutralization test; nicotine tartrate; nontender; nontumoral; normal temperature; normal tissue; normotensive; nortriptyline; not tested; N-terminal [fragment]; nucleotidase; nucleotide

5'NT 5'-nucleotidase

Nt amino terminal

nt nucleotide

N&T nose and throat

NTA natural thymocytotoxic autoantibody; nitrilotriacetic acid; Nurse Training Act

NTAB nephrotoxic antibody

NTBR not to be resuscitated

NTC neotetrazolium chloride

NTCC National Type Culture Collection

NTCP noninvasive transcutaneous cardiac pacing; normal tissue complication probability

NTD neural tube defect; nitroblue tetrazolium dye; noise tone difference; 5'-nucleotidase

NTE neuropathy target esterase; neurotoxic esterase; not to exceed

NTF neurotrophic factor; normal throat flora

NTFOM normal tissue complication-based figure-of-merit

NTG nitroglycerin; nitrosoguanidine; nontoxic goiter; normal triglyceridemia

NTGO nitroglycerin ointment

Nth normothermia

NTHH nontumorous, hypergastrinemic hyperchlorhydria

NTI nonthyroid illness

NTIA National Telecommunications and Information Administration

NTIG nontreated immunoglobulin

NTIS National Technical Information Service

NTKR neurotrophic tyrosine kinase receptor

NTLI neurotensin-like immunoreactivity

NTM nontuberculous mycobacteria

NTMI nontransmural myocardial infarction

NTN nephrotoxic nephritis

NTOS neurogenic thoracic outlet syndrome

NTP National Toxicology Program; nitroprusside; normal temperature and pressure; nucleoside triphosphate

NT&P normal temperature and pressure

NTR negative therapeutic reaction; normotensive rat; nutrition

ntr nutriton

NTRC National Toxins Research Center

NTS nasotracheal suction; nephrotoxic serum; neurotensin; nontropical sprue; nucleus tractus solitarius

NTT nearly total thyroidectomy

NTU Navy Toxicology Unit

NTV nerve tissue vaccine

nt wt net weight

NTX naltrexone

NTZ normal transformation zone

NU name unknown

nU nanounit

nu nude [mouse]

v Greek letter *nu*; degrees of freedom; frequency; kinematic velocity; neutrino

NUC nonspecific ulcerative colitis; sodium urate crystal

Nuc nucleoside

nuc nucleated

NUCARE nursing care research

nucl nucleus

NUD nonucler dyspepsia

NUG necrotizing ulcerative gingivitis

NUI number user identification

nullip nulliparous

NUMA nuclear mitotic apparatus

numc number concentration

NURB Neville upper reservoir buffer

Nut nutrition

NUV near ultraviolet

NV nausea and vomiting; negative variation; neovascularization; next visit; nonveteran; normal value; not vaccinated; not venereal; not verified; not volatile

Nv naked vision

N&V nausea and vomiting

NVA near visual acuity

NVB neurovascular bundle

NVD nausea, vomiting, and diarrhea; neck vein distention; neovascularization of the disk; neurovesicle dysfunction; nonvalvular disease; normal vaginal delivery; no venereal disease; Newcastle virus disease; number of vessels diseased

N/V/D nausea, vomiting, diarrhea

NVE native valve endocarditis

NVG neovascular glaucoma; nonventilated group

NVL no visible lesion

NVM neovascular membrane; nonvolatile matter

NVS neurologic vital signs

NVSS normal variant short stature
NW naked weight; nasal wash
NWB nonweightbearing
NWDA National Wholesale Druggists Association
NWR normotensive Wistar rat
NWTS National Wilms' Tumor Study
NX naloxane
NXG necrobiotic xanthogranuloma
ny, nyst nystagmus
NYC New York City [medium]

NYD not yet diagnosed; not yet discovered
NYHA New York Heart Association
NYHAFC New York Heart Association Functional Class
NZ normal zone
NZB New Zealand black [mouse]
NZC New Zealand chocolate [mouse]
NZO New Zealand obese [mouse]
NZR New Zealand red [rabbit]
NZW New Zealand white [mouse]

O blood type in the ABO blood group; eye [Lat. *oculus*]; nonmotile strain of microorganisms [Ger. *ohne Hauch*]; objective findings; observed frequency in a contingency table; obstetrics; obvious; occipital electrode placement in electroencephalography; occiput; occlusal; [doctor's] office; often; ohm; old; opening; operator; operon; opium; oral, orally; orange [color]; orderly respirations [anesthesia chart]; ortho-; orthopedics; osteocyte; other; output; ovine; oxygen; pint [Lat. *octarius*]; respirations [anesthesia chart]; zero

O₂ both eyes; diatomic oxygen; molecular oxygen

O₃ ozone

o eye [Lat. *oculus*]; opening; ovary transplant; pint [Lat. *octarius*]; see *omicron*

ō negative; without

Ω see *ohm*

Ω see *omega*

ω see *omega*

OA obstructive apnea; occipital artery; occipito-anterior; occiput anterior; octanoic acid; ocular albinism; [o]esophageal atresia; old age; oleic acid; opiate analgesia; opsonic activity; optic atrophy; oral alimentation; orotic acid; osteoarthritis; osteoarthrosis; ovalbumin; overall assessment; Overeaters Anonymous; oxalic acid

O&A observation and assessment

O₂a oxygen availability

OAA Old Age Assistance; Older Americans Act; Opticians Association of America; oxaloacetic acid

OAAD ovarian ascorbic acid depletion

OAB ABO blood group; old age benefits

OABP organic anion binding protein

OA/BVM oral airway/bag-valve-mask

OAD obstructive airway disease; organic anionic dye

OADC oleate-albumin-dextrose-catalase [medium]

OAE otoacoustic emission

OAF open air factor; osteoclast activating factor

OAG open angle glaucoma

OAH ovarian androgenic hyperfunction

OAISO overaction of the ipsilateral superior oblique

OAK Kjer optic atrophy

OALF organic acid labile fluid

OALL ossification of anterior longitudinal ligament

OAM outer acrosomal membrane

OAP Office of Adolescent Pregnancy; old age pension, old age pensioner; ophthalmic artery pressure; osteoarthropathy; oxygen at atmospheric pressure; precocious osteoarthrosis

OAPP Office of Adolescent Pregnancy Programs

OAR organ at risk

OARS older Americans resources and services

OAS old age security; oral allergy syndrome; osmotically active substance

OASD ocular albinism-sensorineural deafness [syndrome]

OASDHI Old Age, Survivors, Disability and Health Insurance

OASDI Old Age Survivors and Disability Insurance

OASI Old Age and Survivors Insurance

OASP organic acid soluble phosphorus

OAT ornithine aminotransferase

OATL ornithine aminotransferase-like

OAV oculoauriculovertebral [dysplasia]

OAVD oculoauriculovertebral dysplasia

OAW oral airways

OB obese [mouse]; obese, obesity; objective benefit; obliterative bronchiolitis; obstetrics, obstetrician; occult bacteremia; occult bleeding; olfactory bulb; oligoclonal band

O&B opium and belladonna

OBB own bed bath

OBD organic brain disease

OBE Office of Biological Education

OBF organ blood flow

OBG, ObG obstetrics and gynecology, obstetrician-gynecologist

OBGS obstetrical and gynecological surgery

OB-GYN, ob-gyn obstetrics and gynecology, obstetrician-gynecologist

obj objective

obl oblique

ob/ob obese [mouse]

OBP odorant-binding protein; ova, blood, parasites [in stool]

OBRA Omnibus Reconciliation Act

OBS obesity; obstetrical service; organic brain syndrome

Obs observation, observed; obstetrics, obstetrician

obs obsolete

Obst obstetrics, obstetrician

obst, obstr obstruction, obstructed

OB-US obstetrical ultrasound [examination of the fetus]

OC obstetrical conjugate; occlusocervical; office call; on call; only child; optic chiasma; oral contraceptive; order communication [system]; original claim; organ culture; outer canthal [distance]; ovarian cancer; oxygen consumed

O&C onset and course

OCA oculocutaneous albinism; olivopontocerebellar atrophy; oral contraceptive agent

OCa ovarian carcinoma

OCAD occlusive carotid artery disease

O₂cap oxygen capacity

OCBF outer cortical blood flow

OCC object-centered coordinate [method]; oral cholecystography

occ occasional; occiput, occipital; occlusion; occlusive; occupation; occurrence

occas occasional

occip occiput, occipital

occl occlusion, occlusive

OccTh occupational therapy, occupational therapist

occ ther occupational therapist or therapy

occup occupation, occupational

occup Rx occupational therapy

OCD obsessive compulsive disorder; Office of Child Development; Office of Civil Defense; osteochondritis dissecans; ovarian cholesterol depletion; oxygen cost diagram

OCG omnicardiogram; oral cholecystogram

OCH oral contraceptive hormone

OCHS Office of Cooperative Health Statistics

OCIS Oncology Center Information System

OCLC online computer library center

OCM oral contraceptive medication

OCN oculomotor nucleus; oncology certified nurse

OCP octacalcium phosphate; ocular cicatricial pemphigoid; oral case presentation; oral contraceptive pill

OC&P ova, cysts, and parasites

OCPD obsessive compulsive personality disorder

OCR oculocardiac reflex; oculocerebrorenal [syndrome]; optical character recognition

oCRF ovine corticotropin-releasing factor

OCRG oxycardiorespirography

oCRH ovine corticotropin-releasing hormone

OCRL Lowe's oculocerebrorenal [syndrome]

OCRS oculocerebrorenal syndrome

OCS occipital condyle syndrome; Ondine's curse syndrome; open canalicular system; oral contraceptive steroid; outpatient clinic substation

OCSD oculocraniosomatic disease

OCSI orthostatic change in shock index

OCT object classification test; optimal cutting temperature; oral contraceptive therapy; ornithine carbamoyltransferase; orthotopic cardiac transplantation; oxytocin challenge test

OCTD overlap connective tissue disease

OCU observation care unit

OCV ordinary conversational voice

OD Doctor of Optometry; obtained absorbance; occipital dysplasia; occupational dermatitis; occupational disease; oculodynamic; Ollier disease; on duty; once a day; open drop [anesthesia]; optical density; optimal dose; originally derived; out-of-date; outside diameter; overdose, overdosage; right eye [Lat. *oculus dexter*]

O-D obstacle-dominance

O₂D oxygen delivery

ODA right occipitoanterior [fetal position] [Lat. *occipito-dextra anterior*]

ODB opiate-directed behavior

ODC oritidine decarboxylase; ornithine decarboxylase; oxygen dissociation curve

Odc ornithine decarboxylase

ODCP ornithine decarboxylase pseudogene

ODD oculodentodigital [dysplasia]; oppositional defiant disorder

OD'd overdosed [drug]

ODE Office of Device Evaluation [of FDA]

ODED oculo-digito-esophago-duodenal [syndrome]

ODM ophthalmodynamometer, ophthalmodynamometry

ODOD oculo-dento-osseous dysplasia

Odont odontogenic

ODP offspring of diabetic parents; right occipitoposterior [fetal position] [Lat. *occipito-dextra posterior*]

ODPHP Office of Disease Prevention and Health Promotion

ODQ on direct questioning

ODS organized delivery system; osmotic demyelination syndrome

ODSG ophthalmic Doppler sonogram

ODT oculodynamic tract; right occipitotransverse [fetal position] [Lat. *occipito-dextra transversa*]

ODTS organic dust toxic syndrome

ODU optical density unit

OE on examination; order entry [system]; orofacial cleft; orthopedic examination; otitis externa; out-stationed enrollment

O/E observed/expected [ratio]

O&E observation and examination

Oe oersted

OEE osmotic erythrocyte enrichment; outer enamel epithelium

OEF oil immersion field; oxygen extraction fraction

OEIS omphalocele, exstrophy, imperforate anus, spinal defects [complex]

OEL occupational exposure limit

OEM opposite ear masked; original electronic manufacturer

OER osmotic erythrocyte [enrichment]; oxygen enhancement ratio

O₂ER oxygen extraction ratio

OERP Office of Education and Regional Programming

OES oral esophageal stethoscope; optical emission spectroscopy

oesoph esophagus [oesophagus]

OET oral endotracheal tube; oral esophageal tube

OF occipitofrontal; open field [test]; optical fundus; orbitofrontal; osmotic fragility; osteitis fibrosa; oxidation-fermentation

O/F oxidation-fermentation
OFA oncofetal antigen
OFAGE orthogonal field alternation gel electrophoresis
OFBM oxidation-fermentation basal medium
OFC occipitofrontal circumference; orbitofacial cleft; osteitis fibrosa cystica
OFCTAD occipito-facio-cervico-thoraco-abdomino-digital dysplasia
OFD object-film distance; occipital frontal diameter; oro-facial-digital [syndrome]
ofd object-film distance
Off official
OFHA occipitofrontal headache
OFM orofacial malformation
OFNE oxygenated fluorocarbon emulsion [delivery system]
OG obstetrics and gynecology; occlusogingival; oligodendrocyte; optic ganglion; orange green; orogastric
O&G obstetrics and gynecology
OGC oculogyric crisis
OGD [o]esophago-gastro-duodenoscopy
OGDH oxoglutarate dehydrogenase
OGF ovarian growth factor; oxygen gain factor
OGH ovine growth hormone
OGI oxygen-glucose index
OGJ [o]esophagogastric junction
OGS oxygenic steroid
OGTT oral glucose tolerance test
OH hydroxycorticosteroid; obstructive hypopnea; occipital horn; occupational health; occupational history; oligomer hybridization; open heart [surgery]; osteopathic hospital; out of hospital; outpatient hospital
17-OH 17-hydroxycorticosteroid
oh every hour [Lat. *omni hora*]
OHA oral hypoglycemic agents
OHAHA ophthalmoplegia-hypotonia-ataxia-hypacusis-athetosis [syndrome]
OHB$_{12}$ hydroxycobalamin
O$_2$Hb oxyhemoglobin

OHC occupational health center; outer hair cell
OHCA out-of-hospital cardiac arrest
OH-Cbl hydroxycobalamin
OHCC hydroxycalciferol
OHCOB hydroxycobalamin
OHCS hydroxycorticosteroid
OHD hydroxyvitamin D; Office of Human Development; Ondine-Hirschsprung disease; organic heart disease
25-OH-D 25-hydroxyvitamin D
OHDA hydroxydopamine
16-OH-DHAS 16-alpha-hydroxydehydroepiandrosterone sulfate
8-OH-DPAT 8-hydroxy-2-(di-n-propylamino)tetralin
OHDS Office of Human Development Services
OHE other hospital employee
OHF Omsk hemorrhagic fever
OHFA hydroxy fatty acid
OHFT overhead frame trapeze
OHI Occupational Health Institute; operative hypertension indicator; oral hygiene index; Oral Hygiene Instruction
OHIAA hydroxyindoleacetic acid
OHIPD Office of Health Information Programs Development
OHI-S Oral Hygiene Instruction-Simplified
OHL oral hairy leukoplakia
OHMO Office of Health Maintenance Organizations
OHN occupational health nurse
OHP hydroxyprogesterone; hydroxyproline; occupational health plan; Oregon Health Plan; oxygen under high pressure
17-OHP 17-hydroxyprogesterone
OHR occupational health research; Office of Health Research
OHS obesity hypoventilation syndrome; occipital Horn syndrome; occupational health service; ocular histoplasmosis syndrome; open heart surgery; ovarian hyperstimulation syndrome

OHSD hydroxysteroid dehydrogenase

OHSS ovarian hyperstimulation syndrome

OHT ocular hypertension

OHTA Office of Health Technology Assessment

OI obturator internus; occasional insomnia; opportunistic infection; opsonic index; orgasmic impairment; orientation inventory; orthoiodohippurate; osteogenesis imperfecta; oubain insensitivity; oxygen intake

O-I outer and inner

OIC osteogenesis imperfecta congenita

OID optimal immunomodulating dose; Organism Identification Number; oxygen insufflation device

OIF observed intrinsic frequency; oil immersion field; Osteogenesis Imperfecta Foundation

OIG Office of the Inspector General

OIH Office of International Health; orthoiodohippurate; ovulation-inducing hormone

OILD occupational immunologic lung disease

oint ointment

OIP organizing interstitial pneumonia

OIR Office of Information Resources; Office of International Research

OIT organic integrity test

OJ orange juice

OKC odontogenic keratocyst

OKN optokinetic nystagmus

OKT ornithine ketoacid amino-transferase

ol left eye [Lat. *oculus laevus*]

OLA left occipitoanterior [fetal position] [Lat. *occipito-laeva anterior*]; oligonucleotide ligation assay

OLAS oligoisoadenylate synthetase

OLB olfactory bulb; open liver biopsy; open lung biopsy

OLD obstructive lung disease; orthochromatic leukodystrophy

OLE object linking and embedding

olf olfactory

OLFR olfactory receptor

OLH ovine lactogenic hormone

oLH ovine luteinizing hormone

OLIDS open loop insulin delivery system

ol oliv olive oil [Lat. *oleum olivea*]

OLP left occipitoposterior [fetal position] [Lat. *occipito-laeva posterior*]

OLR otology, laryngology, and rhinology

OLRx orthotopic liver transplantation

ol res oleoresin

OLS oubain-like substance

OLT left occipitotransverse [fetal position] [Lat. *occipito-laeva transversa*]; orthotopic liver transplantation

OM obtuse mental; occipitomental; occupational medicine; ocular movement; oculomotor; Osborne Mendel [rat]; osteomalacia; osteomyelitis; osteopathic manipulation; otitis media; outer membrane; ovulation method

om every morning [Lat. *omni mane*]

OMAC otitis media, acute catarrhal

OMAR Office of Medical Applications of Research

OMAS occupational maladjustment syndrome

OMB Office of Management and Budget

OMC office of managed care; orientation-memory-concentration [test]

OMCT Orientation-Memory-Concentration Test

OMD ocular muscle dystrophy; oculomandibulodyscephaly; organic mental disorder; oromandibular dystonia

OME office of medical examiner; otitis media with effusions

Ω Greek capital letter *omega*

Ω ohm

Ω^{-1} ohm-1, siemens

ω Greek lower case letter *omega*; angular velocity

OMERACT Outcome Measures in Rheumatoid Arthritis Clinical Trial

OMFAQ older Americans resources and services (OARS) multidimensional functional assessment questionnaire

OMG oligodendrocyte-myelin glyco-protein

OMGP oligodendrocyte-myelin glyco-protein

OMH Office of Mental Health

OMG osteopathic medical school graduate

OMI office of medical investigator; old myocardial infarction

o Greek letter *omicron*

OMIM Online Mendelian Inheritance in Man [database]

OML orbitomental line

OMM outer mitochondrial membrane

OMN oculomotor nerve

OMNI Organizing Medical Networked Information [UK]

OMP olfactory marker protein; ornithine monophosphate; outer membrane protein

OMPA octamethyl pyrophosphora-mide; otitis media, purulent, acute

OMPC, OMPCh otitis media, purulent, chronic

OMR oligomycin-resistant; online medical record

OMS organic mental syndrome; oto-mandibular syndrome

OM&S osteopathic medicine and surgery

OMSA otitis media, suppurative, acute

OMSC otitis media secretory (or suppurative) chronic

OMT object modeling technique; ocular microtremor; O-methyltransferase; ophthalmic medical technician or technologist; osteopathic manipulative therapy

OMVC open mitral valve commissurotomy

ON occipitonuchal; office nurse; onlay; optic nerve; orthopedic nurse; osteonecrosis; osteonectin; overnight

ONC oncogene; oncology; Orthopaedic Nursing Certificate; over-the-needle catheter

OND Ophthalmic Nursing Diploma; orbitonasal dislocation; other neurological disorders

ONG optic nerve glioma

ONMRS onychotrichodysplasia-neutropenia-mental retardation syndrome

ONP operating nursing procedure; orthonitrophenyl

ONPG o-nitrophenyl-beta-D-galactopyranoside

ONS Oncology Nursing Society

ONTG oral nitroglycerin

ONTR orders not to resuscitate

OO oophorectomy

O&O on and off

OOA outer optic anlage

OOB out of bed

OOH out-of-hospital

OOH/CA out-of-hospital cardiac arrest

OOLR ophthalmology, otology, laryngology, and rhinology

OOM, oom oogonial metaphase

OOR out-of-room

OORR orbicularis oculi reflex response

OOW out of wedlock

OOWS objective opiate withdrawal scale

OP occipitoparietal; occipitoposterior; occiput posterior; octapeptide; olfactory peduncle; opening pressure; operation, operative; operative procedure; ophthalmology; opponens pollicis; organophosphorus; oropharynx; orthostatic proteinuria; osmotic pressure; osteoporosis; outpatient; ovine prolactin

O&P ova and parasites

O/P outpatient

Op ophthalmology; opisthocranion

op operation; operator

OPA open procurement agency

op-amp operational amplifier

OPB outpatient basis

OPC oculopalatocerebral [syndrome]; outpatient clinic

OPCA olivopontocerebellar atrophy

OPCD olivopontocerebellar degeneration

OPCOS oligomenorrheic polycystic ovary syndrome

OPD obstetric prediabetic; optical path difference; otopalatodigital [syndrome]; outpatient department; outpatient dispensary; p-phenylenediamine

O'p-DDD mitotane

OpDent operative dentistry

OPDG ocular plethysmodynamography

OPG ocular pneumoplethysmography; orthopantomogram; oxypolygelatin

opg opening

OPH obliterative pulmonary hypertension; ophthalmia

OPH, Oph ophthalmology; ophthalmoscopy, ophthalmoscope

OPHC Office of Prepaid Health Care

OphD Doctor of Ophthalmology

Ophth ophthalmology

OPI oculoparalytic illusion; Omnibus Personality Inventory

OPIDN organophosphorus-induced delayed neuropathy

OPK optokinetic

OPL other party liability; outer plexiform layer; ovine placental lactogen

OPLL ossification of posterior longitudinal ligament

OPM occult primary malignancy; Office of Personnel Management; ophthalmoplegic migraine

OPN ophthalmic nurse; osteopontin

OPO Organ Procurement Organization

OPP osmotic pressure of plasma; oxygen partial pressure

opp opposite

OPPA vincristine, procarbazine, prednisone, Adriamycin

OPPG oculopneumoplethysmography

OPRD opiate receptor delta

OPRK opiate receptor kappa

OPRR Office of Protection from Research Risks

OPRT orotate phosphoribosyltransferase

OPRTase orotate phosphoribosyltransferase

OPS operations; optical position sensor; osteoporosis-pseudolipoma syndrome; outpatient service; outpatient surgery

OPSA ovarian papillary serous adenocarcinoma

OpScan optical scanning

OPSI overwhelming postsplenectomy infection

OPSR Office of Professional Standards Review

OPT outpatient; outpatient treatment

opt best [Lat. *optimus*]; optics, optician

OPTHD optimal hemodialysis

OPV oral polio vaccine

OPWL opiate withdrawal

OR a logical binary relation that is true if any argument is true, and false otherwise; [o]estrogen receptor; odds ratio; oil retention [enema]; open reduction; operating room; optic radiation; oral rehydration; orosomucoid; orthopedic; orthopedic research

O-R oxidation-reduction

O$_R$ rate of outflow

Or orbitale

ORA opiate receptor agonist

ORALABX oral antibiotics

ORANS Oak Ridge Analytical System

ORBC ox red blood cell

ORC oculo-reno-cerebellar [syndrome]

orch orchitis

ORD optical rotatory dispersion; oral radiation death

ORDS Office of Research, Demonstration, and Statistics

ORE oil retention enema

OREF Orthopedic Research and Education Foundation

ORF open reading frame
OR&F open reduction and fixation
orf open reading frame
Org, org organic
ORIF open reduction with internal fixation
OrJ orange juice
ORL otorhinolaryngology
ORM orosomucoid; other regulated material; oxygen ratio monitor
ORMC oxygen ratio monitor controller
ORN operating room nurse; orthopedic nurse
Orn ornithine
ORNL Oak Ridge National Laboratory
ORO oil red O
OROS oral osmotic
ORP oxidation-reduction potential
ORPM orthorhythmic pacemaker
ORS olfactory reference syndrome; oral rehydration solution; oral surgery, oral surgeon; Orthopaedic Research Society; orthopedic surgeon, orthopedic surgery; oxygen radical scavengers
ORSA osteoclast resorption stimulating activity
ORT object relations technique; operating room technician; oral rehydration therapy
orth, ortho orthopedics, orthopedic
ORW Osler-Rendu-Weber [syndrome]
OS left eye [Lat. *oculus sinister*]; occipitosacral; occupational safety; office surgery; Omenn syndrome; opening snap; operating system; oral surgery; organ-specific; orthopedic surgeon, orthopedic surgery; Osgood-Schlatter [disease]; osteogenic sarcoma; osteosarcoma; osteosclerosis; oubain sensitivity; overall survival; oxygen saturation
Os osmium
OSA obstructive sleep apnea; Office of Services to the Aging; Optical Society of America; ovarian sectional area
OSAS obstructive sleep apnea syndrome
osc oscillation

OSCAR on-line survey, certification and reporting system
OSCC oral squamous cell carcinoma
OSCE objective structured clinical examination
OSF organ system failure; osteoclast-stimulating factor; outer spiral fiber; overgrowth stimulating factor
OSHA Occupational Safety and Health Adminstration
OSH Act Occupational Safety and Health Act of 1970
OSI open systems interconnection [reference model]
OSM ovine submaxillary mucin; oxygen saturation meter
osm osmole; osmosis, osmotic
OSMED otospondylometaphyseal dysplasia
Osm/kg osmoles per kilogram
Osm/l osmoles per liter
osmol osmole
OSRD Office of Scientific Research and Development
OSS over-the-shoulder strap
oss osseous
OST object sorting test; Office of Science and Technology
osteo osteoarthritis; osteomyelitis; osteopathy
OSUK Ophthalmological Society of the United Kingdom
OT objective test; oblique talus; occlusion time; occupational therapist, occupational therapy; ocular tension; office therapy; old term (in anatomy); old tuberculin; olfactory threshold; optic tract; orientation test ; original tuberculin; ornithine transcarbamylase; orotracheal; orthopedic treatment; otolaryngology; otology; oxytocin; oxytryptamine
Ot otolaryngology
OTA occupational therapy assistant; Office of Technology Assessment; ornithine transaminase; orthotoluidine arsenite

OTC ornithine transcarbamylase; oval target cell; over-the-counter; oxytetracycline

OTCD ornithine carbomoyltransferase deficiency

OTD oculotrichodysplasia; oral temperature device; organ tolerance dose

OTE optically transparent electrode

OTF octamer-binding transcription factor; oral transfer factor

OTFC oral transmucosal fenatyl citrate

OTI ovomucoid trypsin inhibitor

OTM orthotoluidine manganese sulfate

OTO otology; otorhinolaryngology

Otol otology, otologist

OTPS other than personal services

OTR Ovarian Tumor Registry; Occupational Therapist, Registered

OTReg Occupational Therapist, Registered

OTS occipital temporal sulcus; orotracheal suction

OTT orotracheal tube

OTU olfactory tubercle; operational taxonomic unit

OTZ oxathiozolidine

OU observation unit; Oppenheimer-Urbach [syndrome]

ou both eyes together [Lat. *oculi unitas*]

OUB oubain

OUBR oubain resistance

OULQ outer upper left quadrant

OURQ outer upper right quadrant

OUS overuse syndrome

OV oculovestibular; office visit; osteoid volume; outflow volume; ovalbumin; ovary; overventilation; ovulation

Ov ovary

ov ovum

OVA ovalbumin

ova ovariectomy

OVC ovarian cancer

OVD occlusal vertical dimension

OvDF ovarian dysfunction

OVX ovariectomized

OW once weekly; open wedge; outer wall; oval window

O/W oil in water

OWI Office of Worksite Initiatives

OWR Osler-Weber-Rendu [syndrome]; ovarian wedge resection

OWS outerwear syndrome

OX optic chiasma; oxacillin; oxalate; oxide; orthopedic examination; oxytocin

Ox oxygen

OXA oxaprotiline

OXP oxypressin

OXT oxytocin

OXTR oxytocin receptor

OXY, oxy oxygen

OYE old yellow enzyme

oz ounce

oz ap apothecaries' ounce (U.S.)

oz apoth apothecaries' ounce (U.K.)

oz t ounce troy (U.S.)

oz tr ounce troy (U.K.)

P an electrocardiographic wave corresponding to a wave of depolarization crossing the atria; by weight [Lat. *pondere*]; father [Lat. *pater*]; near [Lat. *proximum*]; near point [Lat. *punctum proximum*]; pain; parietal electrode placement in electroencephalography; parity; part; partial pressure; *Pasteurella*; paternal; patient; penicillin; percent; percussion; perforation; permeability; peta-; pharmacopeia; phenophthalein; phenylalanine; phosphate group; phosphorus; physiology; pig; pint; placebo; plan; plasma; *Plasmodium*; *Pneumocystis*; point; poise; poison, poisoning; polarity; polarization; pole; polymyxin; pons; population; porcelain; porcine; porphyrin; position; positive; posterior; postpartum; power; precipitin; precursor; prednisone; premolar; presbyopia; pressure; primary; primipara; probability; product; progesterone; prolactin; proline; properdin; propionate; protein; *Proteus*; proximal; *Pseudomonas*; psychiatry; pulmonary; pulse; pupil; radiant power; significance probability [value]; sound power; weight [Lat. *pondus*]

P₁, P-one first parental generation

P₂ pulmonic second sound

P₃ proximal third

P-50 oxygen half-saturation pressure

p atomic orbital with angular momentum quantum number 1; freeze preservation; the frequency of the more common allele of a pair; momentum; papilla; phosphate; pico-; pint; pond; pressure; probability; proton; pupil; short arm of chromosome; sound pressure

p after; pulse

p- para

p24 HIV antigen

Π see *pi*

π see *pi*

ψ see *psi*

φ see *phi*

PA panic attack; pantothenic acid; paralysis agitans; paranoia; passive aggressive; pathology; patient's advocate; peak amplitude; periarteritis; peridural artery; periodic acid; periodontal abscess; pernicious anemia; phakic-aphakic; phenylalkylamine; phosphatidic acid; phenylalanine; phosphoarginine; photoallergy; phthalic anhydride; physician advisor; physician assistant; pituitary-adrenal; plasma adsorption; plasma aldosterone; plasminogen activator; platelet adhesiveness; platelet aggregation; platelet-associated; polyamine; polyarteritis; polyarthritis; post-aural; posteroanterior; prealbumin; predictive accuracy; pregnancy-associated; presents again; primary aldosteronism; primary amenorrhea; primary anemia; prior to admission; proactivator; proanthocyanidin; procainamide; professional association; prolonged action; propionic acid; prostate antigen; protective antigen; proteolytic action; prothrombin activity; protrusio acetabuli; pseudoaneurysm; *Pseudomonas aeruginosa;* psychoanalysis; psychogenic aspermia; pulmonary arterial [pressure]; pulmonary artery; pulmonary atresia; pulpoaxial; puromycin aminonucleoside; pyruvic acid; pyrrolizidine alkaloid; yearly [Lat. *per annum*]

Pₐ alveolar pressure

P-A posteroanterior

P&A percussion and auscultation

Pa pascal; pathologist, pathology; protactinium; *Pseudomonas aeruginosa;* pulmonary arterial [pressure]

P$_A$ partial pressure of arterial fluid

pA picoampere

pa through the anus [Lat. *per anum*]; yearly [Lat. *per annum*]

PAA partial agonist activity; phenylacetic acid; phosphonoacetic acid; physical abilities analysis; plasma angiotensinase activity; polyacrylamide; polyamino acid; pyridine acetic acid

PAB para-aminobenzoate; performance assessment battery; pharmacologic autonomic block; poly(A)-binding [protein]; premature atrial beat; purple agar base

PABA para-aminobenzoic acid

PABD predeposit autologous blood donation

PABP pulmonary artery balloon pump

PABV percutaneous aortic balloon valvuloplasty

PAC papular acrodermatitis of childhood; parent-adult-child; pericarditis-arthropathy-camptodactyly [syndrome]; phenacetin, aspirin, and caffeine; physical activity [scale]; plasma aldosterone concentration; platelet-associated complement; Policy Advisory Committee; preadmission certification; premature atrial contraction; product of ambulatory care; pulmonary artery catheterization

pac pachytene

PACAP pituitary adenylate cyclase activating polypeptide

PACC primary ambulatory care center; promoting aphasics' communicative competence

PACE Pacing and Clinical Electrophysiology; paired basic amino acid cleaving enzyme; personalized aerobics for cardiovascular enhancement; Program of All-inclusive Care for the Elderly; pulmonary angiotensin I converting enzyme

PA$_{CO}$ mean alveolar gas volume

P$_{ACO_2}$ partial pressure of carbon dioxide in alveolar gas

P$_{aCO2}$ partial pressure of carbon dioxide in arterial blood

PACP pulmonary alveolar-capillary permeability; pulmonary artery counterpulsation

PACS patient care and services; picture archiving and communication system

PACS DB picture archiving and communication system data base

PACT papillary carcinoma of thyroid; precordial acceleration tracing; prepaid accountable care term

PACU postanesthetic care unit

PACWP pulmonary arterial capillary wedge pressure

PAD pain and distress; patient surface axis depth; percutaneous abscess drainage; percutaneous automated discectomy; peripheral artery disease; phenacetin, aspirin, and desoxyephedrine; photon absorption densitometry; primary affective disorder; psychoaffective disorder; pulmonary artery diastolic; pulsatile assist device

PADL personal activities of daily living

PADP pulmonary artery diastolic pressure

PADUA progressive augmentation by dilating the urethra anterior

PAE progressive assistive exercise

paed pediatrics, pediatric [*paediatrics, paediatric*]

PAEDP pulmonary artery end-diastolic pressure

PAEP progestagen-associated endometrial protein

PAES popliteal artery entrapment syndrome

PAF paroxysmal atrial fibrillation; peroxisomal assembly factor; phosphodiesterase-activating factor; plain abdominal film; platelet-activating factor; platelet-aggregating factor; pollen adherence factor; premenstrual assessment form; progressive autonomic failure; pulmonary arteriovenous fistula

PA&F percussion, auscultation, and fremitus

PAFA priority based assessment of foot additives

PAF-A platelet-activating factor of anaphylaxis

PAFAMS Pan-American Federation of Associations of Medical Schools

PAFD percutaneous abscess and fluid drainage; pulmonary artery filling defect

PAFI platelet-aggregation factor inhibitor

PAFIB paroxysmal atrial fibrillation

PAFP pre-Achilles fat pad

PAG periaqueductal gray [matter]; polyacrylamide gel; pregnancy-associated globulin; proliferation-associated gene

pAg protein A-gold [technique]

PAGA proliferation-associated gene A

PAGE polyacrylamide gel electrophoresis

PAGIF polyacrylamide gel isoelectric focusing

PAGMK primary African green monkey kidney

PAGOD pulmonary hypoplasia-hypoplasia of pulmonary artery-agonadism-omphalocele/diaphragmatic defect-dextrocardia [syndrome]

PAH para-aminohippurate; phenylalanine hydrolase; polycyclic aromatic hydrocarbon; predicted adult height [by Bayley-Pinneau]; pulmonary alveolar hypoventilation; pulmonary artery hypertension; pulmonary artery hypotension

PAHA para-aminohippuric acid; procainamide-hydroxylamine

PAHO Pan-American Health Organization

PAHVC pulmonary alveolar hypoxic vasoconstrictor

PAI patient assessment instrument; plasminogen activator inhibitor

PAI-1 plasminogen-activator inhibitor-1

PAIC procedures, alternatives, indications, and complications

PAICS phosphoribosylaminoimidazole carboxylase

PAID problem areas in diabetes [scale]

PAIDS paralyzed academic investigator's disease syndrome; pediatric acquired immunodeficiency syndrome

PAIgG platelet-associated immunoglobulin G

PAIN pyoderma gangrenosum, aphthous stomatitis, inflammatory eye disease, erythema nodosum [disorders associated with inflammatory bowel disease]

PAIRS Pain and Impairment Relationship Scale

PAIS partial androgen insensitivity syndrome; phosphoribosylaminoimidazole synthetase; psychosocial adjustment to illness scale

PAIS-SR psychosocial adjustment to illness scale-self reported

PAJ paralysis agitans juvenilis

PAL pathology laboratory; peptidyl-alpha-hydroxyglycine alpha-amidating lysine phase alteration plane; posterior axillary line; product of activated lymphocytes; pyogenic abscess of the liver

pal palate

PALA N-(phosphonacetyl)-L-aspartate

PALP placental alkaline phosphatase

palp palpation, palpate

palpi palpitation

PALS parietolateral lymphocyte sheath; pediatric advanced life support; prison-acquired lymphoproliferative syndrome

PAM pancreatic acinar mass; penicillin aluminum monostearate; peptidylglycine alpha-amidating monooxygenase; phenylalaline mustard; physical agent modality; p-methoxyamphetamine; post-auricular myogenic; pralidoxime; pre-arrest morbidity [index]; pregnancy-associated α-macroglobulin; primary amebic meningoencephalitis; principles of ambulatory medicine; professions allied to medicine; pulmonary alveolar macrophage; pulmonary alveolar microlithiasis; pulse amplitude modulation; pyridine aldoxime methiodide

PAMC pterygoarthromyodysplasia congenital

PAMD primary adrenocortical micronodular dysplasia

PAME preanesthesia medical examination; primary amebic meningoencephalitis

PAMIE physical and mental impairment of function evaluation

PAMP pulmonary artery mean pressure

PAN periarteritis nodosa; periodic alternating nystagmus; peroxyacylnitrate; polyarteritis nodosa; positional alcohol nystagmus; puromycin aminonucleoside

pan pancreas, pancreatic, pancreatectomy

Panc pancreas or pancreatic

P-ANCA perinuclear anti-neutrophilic cytoplasmic antibody

PAND primary adrenocortical nodular dysplasia

PANS puromycin aminonucleoside

PANSS Positive and Negative Syndrome Scale

PAO peak acid output; peripheral airway obstruction; plasma amine oxidase; polyamine oxidase; pulmonary artery occlusion; pustulotic arthroosteitis

PAo airway opening pressure; ascending aortic pressure; pulmonary artery occlusion pressure

PAO$_2$ alveolar oxygen partial pressure

PaO$_2$ partial oxygen tension in arterial blood; partial pressure of oxygen in arterial blood

PAOD peripheral arterial occlusive disease; peripheral arteriosclerotic occlusive disease

PAOP pulmonary artery occlusion pressure

PAP pancreatitis-associated protein; Papanicolaou [test]; papaverine; passive-aggressive personality; patient assessment program; peak airway pressure; phosphoadenosine phosphate; peroxidase antibody to peroxidase; peroxidase-antiperoxidase [method]; placental acid/alkaline phosphatase; positive airway pressure; primary atypical pneumonia; prostatic acid phosphatase; pseudoallergic reaction; pulmonary alveolar proteinosis; pulmonary artery pressure; purified alternate pathway

Pap Papanicolaou test

pap papilla

PAPF platelet adhesiveness plasma factor

papova papilloma-polyoma-vacuolating agent [virus]

PAPP para-aminopropiophenone; pregnancy-associated plasma protein

PAPPA pregnancy-associated plasma protein A

PAPPC pregnancy-associated plasma protein C

PAPS 3'-phosphoadenosine-5'-phosphosulfate; primary antiphospholipid antibody syndrome

Paps papillomas

Pap sm Papanicolaou smear

PAPUFA physiologically active polyunsaturated fatty acid

pa-pv pulmonary arterial pressure-pulmonary venous pressure

PAPVC partial anomalous pulmonary venous connection

PAPVD partial anomalous pulmonary venous drainage

PAPVR partial anomalous pulmonary venous return

PAQ Personal Attitudes Questionnaire

PAR participating provider; passive avoidance reaction; perennial allergic rhinitis; photosynthetically active radiation; Physical Activity Recall [Questionnaire]; physiological aging rate; plain abdominal radiograph; platelet aggregate ratio; postanesthesia recovery; postanesthesia room; posterior wall or aortic root; Program for Alcohol Recovery; proximal alveolar region; pseudoautosomal region; pulmonary arteriolar resistance

par paraffin; paralysis

PARA, Para, para number of pregnancies producing viable offspring

para paraplegic; parathyroid, parathyroidectomy

para 0 nullipara

para I primipara

para II secundipara

para III tripara

para IV quadripara

parasit parasitology; parasite, parasitic

parasym parasympathetic

parent parenteral

parox paroxysm, paroxysmal

PARR postanesthesia recovery room

PARS Personal Adjustment and Role Skills Scale

PARU postanesthetic recovery unit

PAS para aminosalicylate; Parent Attitude Scale; patient administration system; patient appointments and scheduling; periodic acid-Schiff [reaction]; peripheral anterior synechia; persistent atrial standstill; Personality Assessment Scale; photoacoustic spectroscopy; phosphatase acid serum; physician-assisted suicide; posterior airway space; pre-admission screening; pregnancy advisory service; premature atrial stimulus; professional activity study; progressive accumulated stress; pulmonary arterial stenosis; pulmonary artery systolic

Pas pascal-second

Pa x s pascals per second

PASA para-aminosalicylic acid; primary acquired sideroblastic anemia; proximal articular set angle

PASARR pre-admission screening and resident review

PASAT Paced Auditory Serial Addition Task

PAS-C para-aminosalicylic acid crystallized with ascorbic acid

PASD after diastase digestion

PASG pneumatic antishock garment

PASH periodic acid-Schiff hematoxylin

PASM periodic acid-silver methenamine

PASP pancreas-specific protein; pulmonary artery systolic pressure

pass passive

pass ROM passive range of motion

PASSOR Physiatric Association for Spine, Sports, and Occupational Rehabilitation

PAST periodic acid-Schiff technique

Past *Pasteurella*

PASVR pulmonary anomalous superior venous return

PASW personal assistance service worker

PAT Pain Apperception Test; paroxysmal atrial tachycardia; patient; phenylaminotetrazole; physical abilities test; picric acid turbidity; platelet aggregation test; polyamine acetyltransferase; preadmission assessment team/test; preadmission testing; predictive ability test; pregnancy at term; psychoacoustic test

pat patella; patent; paternal origin; patient

PATE psychodynamic and therapeutic education; pulmonary artery thromboembolism

PATH pathology, pathological; pituitary adrenotropic hormone; physicians at teaching hospitals

path pathogenesis, pathogenic; pathology, pathological

Patm atmospheric pressure

PAT-SED pseudoachondroplastic dysplasia

PA-T-SP periodic acid-thiocarbo-hydrazide-silver proteinate

PAU phenol-acetic acid-urea

PAV percutaneous aortic valvuloplasty; poikiloderma atrophicans vasculare; posterior arch vein; proportional assist ventilation

pavex passive vascular exercise

PAVF pulmonary arteriovenous fistula

PAVM pulmonary arteriovenous malformation

PAVNRT paroxysmal atrioventricular nodal reciprocal tachycardia

PAW peripheral airways; pulmonary artery wedge

Paw mean airway pressure

PAWP pulmonary arterial wedge pressure

PAWS primary withdrawal syndrome

PB British pharmacopeia [*Pharmacopoeia Britannica*]; paraffin bath; Paul-Bunnell [antibody]; periodic breathing; peripheral blood; peroneus brevis; phenobarbital; phenoxybenzamine phonetically balanced; pinealoblastoma; polymyxin B; premature beat; pressure breathing; protein binding; punch biopsy

Pb lead [Lat. *plumbum*]; phenobarbital; presbyopia

P&B pain & burning; phenobarbital and belladonna

PBA polyclonal B-cell activity; pressure breathing assist; prolactin-binding assay; prune belly anomaly; pulpobuccoaxial

PBAL protected bronchoalveolar lavage

PBB polybrominated biphenyl

Pb-B lead in blood

PBBs polybrominated biphenyls

PBC peripheral blood cell; point of basal convergence; pre-bed care; primary biliary cirrhosis; progestin-binding complement

PBD postburn day

PBE tuberculin from *Mycobacterium tuberculosis bovis* [Ger. *Perlsucht Bacillenemulsion*]

PBF peripheral blod flow; placental blood flow; pulmonary blood flow

PBFE peroxisomal bifunctional enzyme

PBFe protein-bound iron

PBG porphobilinogen

PBGD porphobilinogen deaminase

PBGS, PBG-S porphobilinogen synthase

PBH pulling boat hands

PBHB poly-beta-hydroxybutyrate

PBI parental bonding instrument; penile pressure/brachial pressure index; protein-bound iodine

PbI lead intoxication

PBIgG platelet surface bound immunoglobulin G

PBK phosphorylase B kinase

PBL peripheral blood leukocyte; peripheral blood lymphocyte; problem-based learning

PBLC peripheral blood lymphocyte count; premature birth living child; problem-based learning curriculum

PBLT peripheral blood lymphocyte transformation

PBM peak bone mass; peripheral basement membrane; peripheral blood mononuclear [cell]; placental basement membrane

PBMC peripheral blood mononuclear cell; pharmaceutical benefit management company

PBMNC peripheral blood mononuclear cell

PBMV pulmonary blood mixing volume

PBN paralytic brachial neuritis; peripheral benign neoplasm; polymyxin B sulfate, bacitracin, and neomycin

PBNA partial body neutron activation

PBO penicillin in beeswax and oil; placebo

PBP penicillin-binding protein; porphyrin biosynthesis pathway; prostate-binding protein; pseudobulbar palsy; pulsatile bypass pump

PBPI penile-brachial pulse index

PBPK physiologically based pharmacokinetic [model]

PBPV percutaneous balloon pulmonary valvuloplasty

PBS perfusion-pressure breakthrough syndrome; phenobarbital sodium; phosphate-buffered saline; planar bone scan; primer binding site; prune belly syndrome; pulmonary branch stenosis

PBSC peripheral blood stem cell

PBSP prognostically bad signs during pregnancy

PBT Paul-Bunnell test; phenacetin breath test; piebald trait; profile-based therapy

PBT₄ protein-bound thyroxine

PBV predicted blood volume; pulmonary blood volume

PBW posterior bite wing

PBZ personal breathing zone; phenylbutazone; phenoxybenzamine; pyribenzamine

PC avoirdupois weight [Lat. *pondus civile*]; packed cells; paper chromatography; paracortex; parent cell; particulate component; partition coefficient; penicillin; pentose cycle; peritoneal cell; personal care; pharmacology; phase contrast; pheochromocytoma; phosphate cycle; phosphatidylcholine; phosphocreatine; phosphorylcholine; photoconduction; physicians' corporation; pill counter; piriform cortex; plasma concentration; plasma cortisol; plasmacytoma; plasmin complex; plastocyanin; platelet concentrate; platelet count; pneumotaxic center; polycentric; polyposis coli; poor condition; poor coordination; portacaval; portal cirrhosis; postcoital; posterior cervical; posterior chamber; posterior commissure; posterior cortex; potential complications; preconditioning; precordial; prenatal care; present complaint; primary closure; printed circuit; procollagen; productive cough; professional corporation; prohormone convertase; prostatic carcinoma; protein C; protein convertase;

proximal colon; pseudocyst; pubococcygeus [muscle]; pulmonary capillary; pulmonary circulation; pulmonary compliance; pulmonic closure; Purkinje cell; pyloric canal; pyruvate carboxylase

pc parsec; percent; picocurie

p/c presenting complaint

PCA para-chloramphetamine; parietal cell antibody; passive cutaneous anaphylaxis; patient care assistant/aide; patient care audit; patient-controlled analgesia; perchloric acid; percutaneous carotid angiography; personal care assistant; Physicians Corporation of America; polyclonal antibody; porous coated anatomic [prosthesis]; portacaval anastomosis; posterior cerebral artery; posterior communicating aneurysm/artery; precoronary care area; President's Council on Aging; principal components analysis; procoagulant activity; prostatic carcinoma; pyrrolidine carboxylic acid

PCAS patient care algorithm system

PCAST President's Committee of Advisors on Science and Technology

PCB paracervical block; polychlorinated biphenyl; portacaval bypass; postcoital bleeding; procarbazine

PcB near point of convergence to the intercentral base line [*punctum convergens basalis*]

PC-BMP phosphorylcholine-m-binding myeloma protein

PCC Pasteur Culture Collection; percutaneous cecostomy; pheochromocytoma; phosphate carrier compound; plasma catecholamine concentration; platinum-containing compound; pneumatosis cystoides coli; Poison Control Center; precoronary care; premature chromosome condensation; primary care clinic or center; primary care continuum; primary care curriculum; protein C cofactor; prothrombin complex concentration

PCc periscopic concave

pcc premature chromosome condensation

PCCAP physicians' continued competence assessment program

PCCF protein C cofactor

PCCM pediatric critical care medicine; primary care case management; primary care case manager

PCCU post-coronary care unit

PCD pacer-cardioverter-defibrillator; papillary collecting duct; paraneoplastic cerebellar degeneration; paroxysmal cerebral dysrhythmia; percutaneous catheter drainage; phosphate-citrate-dextrose; plasma cell dyscrasia; polycystic disease; posterior corneal deposits; premature centromere division; primary ciliary dyskinesia; prolonged contractile duration; pterin-4a-carbinolamine dehydratase; pulmonary clearance delay

PCDC plasma clot diffusion chamber

PCDF polychorinated dibenzofuran

PCE physical capacity evaluation; pseudocholinesterase

PCEA patient-controlled epidural anesthesia

PCF peripheral circulatory failure; pharyngoconjunctival fever; platelet complement fixation; posterior cranial fossa; prothrombin conversion factor

pcf pounds per cubic feet

PCFIA particle concentration of fluorescence immunoassay

PCFT platelet complement fixation test

PCG pancreatico-cholangiography; paracervical ganglion; phonocardiogram; preventive care group; primate chorionic gonadotropin; pubococcygeus [muscle]

PCH paroxysmal cold hemoglobinuria; polycyclic hydrocarbon

PCHE pseudocholinesterase

PCI patient classification index; pneumatosis cystoides intestinales; prophylactic cranial irradiation; protein C inhibitor

pCi picocurie

PCIC Poison Control Information Center

PC-IRV pressure-controlled inverted ratio ventilation

PCIS Patient-Care Information System; postcardiac injury syndrome

PCK phosphoenolpyruvate carboxykinase; polycystic kidney

PCKD polycystic kidney disease

PCL pacing cycle length; persistent corpus luteum; plasma cell leukemia; posterior chamber lens; posterior cruciate ligament; primary care loan

PCLI plasma cell labeling index

PCM patient care manager or management; patient classification system; primary cutaneous melanoma; process control monitor; protein-calorie malnutrition; protein carboxymethylase

PCMB parachloromercuribenzoate

PCMO Principal Clinical Medical Officer

PCMS patient care management system

PCMs patient care management categories

PCMT pacemaker circus movement tachycardia; protein carboxyl methyltransferase

PCN penicillin; primary care nursing

PCNA proliferating cell nuclear antigen

PCNB pentachloronitrobenzene

PCNL percutaneous nephrostolithotomy

PCNV postchemotherapy nausea and vomiting; Provisional Committee on Nomenclature of Viruses

PCO patient complains of; polycystic ovary; predicted cardiac output

P_{CO} partial pressure of carbon monoxide

P_{CO_2}, pCO_2 partial pressure of carbon dioxide

PCOC Primary Care Organization Consortium

PCOD polycystic ovarian disease

PCOM posterior communicating [artery]

PCON Primary Care Organization Network

PCOS polycystic ovary syndrome
PCP parachlorophenate; patient care plan; pentachlorophenol; 1-(1-phenylcyclohexyl)piperidine; peripheral coronary pressure; persistent cough and phlegm; phencyclidine; *Pneumocystis carinii* pneumonia; postoperative constrictive pericarditis; primary care physician; primary care provider; prochlorperazine; procollagen peptide; prolylcarboxypeptidase; pulmonary capillary pressure; pulse cytophotometry
PCPA para-chlorophenylalanine
PCPB procarboxypeptide B
PCPL pulmonary capillary protein leakage
pcpn precipitation
PCQ polychloroquaterphenyl
PCR patient contact record; phosphocreatinine; plasma clearance rate; polymerase chain reaction; post-compression remodeling; protein catabolism rate
PCr phosphocreatine
PCRV polycythemia rubra vera
PCS palliative care service; Patient Care System; patterns of care study; pelvic congestion syndrome; pharmacogenic confusional syndrome; portacaval shunt; post-cardiac surgery; postcardiotomy syndrome; postcholecystectomy syndrome; postconcussion syndrome; premature centromere separation; primary cancer site; prolonged crush syndrome; proportional counter spectrometry; proximal coronary sinus; pseudotumor cerebri syndrome
pcs preconscious
PCSM percutaneous stone manipulation
PCSW personal care service worker
PCT peripheral carcinoid tumor; plasma clotting time; plasmacrit test; plasmacytoma; polychlorinated triphenyl; polychlorinated triphenyl; porphyria cutanea tarda; portacaval transposition; positron computed tomography; postcoital test;

progesterone challenge test; prothrombin consumption time; proximal convoluted tubule
pct percent
PCU pain control unit; primary care unit; patient care unit; pulmonary care unit
PCV packed cell volume; polycythemia vera; postcapillary venule; pressure-control ventilation
PCV-M polycythemia vera with myeloid metaplasia
PCW pericanalicular web; personal care worker; primary capillary wedge; pulmonary capillary wedge; purified cell walls
PCWP pulmonary capillary wedge pressure
PCx periscopic convex
PCZ procarbazine; prochlorperazine
PD Doctor of Pharmacy; Dublin Pharmacopoeia; interpupillary distance; Paget disease; pancreatic duct; papilla diameter; paralyzing dose; Parkinson disease; parkinsonian dementia; paroxysmal discharge; pars distalis; patent ductus; patient day; pediatric, pediatrics; percentage difference; percutaneous drain; peritoneal dialysis; personality disorder; phenyldichlorarsine; phosphate dehydrogenase; phosphate dextrose; photosensitivity dermatitis; Pick disease; plasma defect; poorly differentiated; posterior descending; posterior division; postnasal drainage; postural drainage; potential difference; pregnanediol; present disease; pressor dose; prism diopter; problem drinker; program director; progression of disease; protein degradation; problem degradation; protein diet; psychotic depression; pulmonary disease; pulpodistal; pulse duration; pulsed diastolic; pulsed Doppler [wave]; pupillary distance; pyloric dilator
2-PD two-point discrimination
Pd palladium; pediatrics

PDA patent ductus arteriosus; personal digital assistant; posterior descending artery; pulmonary disease anemia

PdA pediatric allergy

PDAB para-dimethylaminobenzaldehyde

PD-AB-SAAP pulsed diastolic autologous blood selective aortic arch perfusion

PDAP Palmer drug abuse program

PD/AR photosensitivity dermatitis and actinic reticuloid syndrome

PDB Paget disease of bone; paradichlorobenzene; patient's database; phosphorus-dissolving bacteria; preventive dental [health] behavior

PDC parkinsonism dementia complex; pediatric cardiology; penta-decylcatechol; phosducin; physical dependence capacity; plasma dioxin concentration; preliminary diagnostic clinic; private diagnostic clinic

PdC pediatric cardiology

PDCA plan-do-check-act

PDCD primary degenerative cerebral disease

PD-CSE pulsed Doppler cross-sectional echocardiography

PDD pervasive developmental disorder; platinum diamminodichloride [cisplatin]; primary degenerative dementia; pyridoxine-deficient diet

PDDR pseudovitamin D-dependent rickets

PDE paroxysmal dyspnea on exertion; phosphodiester; progressive dialysis encephalopathy; pulsed Doppler echocardiography

PdE pediatric endocrinology

PDEB phosphodiesterase beta

PD-ECGF platelet-derived endothelial cell growth factor

PDEG phosphodiesterase gamma

PDF Parkinson's Disease Foundation; peritoneal dialysis fluid; Portable Document Format; pyruvate dehydrogenase

PDG parkinsonism-dementia complex of Guam; phosphogluconate dehydrogenase

PDGA pteroyldiglutamic acid

PDGF platelet-derived growth factor

PDGFA platelet-derived growth factor, A chain

PDGFR platelet-derived growth factor receptor

PDGFRB platelet-derived growth factor receptor beta

PDGS partial form of DiGeorge syndrome

PDH past dental history; phosphate dehydrogenase; position-of-the-dynamometer-handle [test]; progressive disseminated histoplasmosis; pyruvate dehydrogenase

PDHA pyruvate dehydrogenase alpha

PDHa pyruvate dehydrogenase in active form

PDHB pyruvate dehydrogenase beta

PDHC pyruvate dehydrogenase complex

PdHO pediatric hematology-oncology

PDI pain disability index; periodontal disease index; plan-do integration; psychomotor development index

Pdi transdiaphragmatic pressure

Pdi$_{max}$ maximum transdiaphragmatic pressure

PDIE phosphodiesterase

P-diol pregnanediol

PDL pancreatic duct ligation; periodontal ligament; poorly differentiated lymphocyte; population doubling level; progressive diffuse leukoencephalopathy

pdl poundal; pudendal

PDLC poorly differentiated lung cancer

PDLD poorly differentiated lymphocytic-diffuse

PDLL poorly differentiated lymphocytic lymphoma

PDLN poorly differentiated lymphocytic-nodular

PDM point distribution model

PDMS patient data management system; pharmacokinetic drug monitoring service; polydimethylsiloxane

PDN prednisone; private duty nurse

PdNEO pediatric neonatology

PdNEP pediatric nephrology

PDP pattern disruption point; piperidinopyrimidine; platelet-derived plasma; primer-dependent deoxynucleic acid polymerase; Product Development Protocol; programmed data processor

PDPD prolonged-dwell peritoneal dialysis

PDPDM protein-deficient pancreatic diabetes mellitus

PDPH postdural puncture headache

PDPI primer-dependent deoxynucleic acid polymerase index

PDQ Personality Diagnostic Questionnaire; physician's data query; Premenstrual Distress Questionnaire; prescreening developmental questionnaire; protocol data query

PDR pediatric radiology; peripheral diabetic retinopathy; *Physicians' Desk Reference*; postdelivery room; primary drug resistance; proliferative diabetic retinopathy

PdR pediatric radiology

pdr powder

PDRB Permanent Diability Rating Board

PDRT Portland Digit Recognition

PDS pain-dysfunction syndrome; paroxysmal depolarizing shift; patient data system; Patient-Doctor Society; pediatric surgery; penile Doppler study; peritoneal dialysis system; plasma-derived serum; polydioxanone sutures; predialyzed serum; proteodermatan sulfate

PdS pediatric surgery

PDSG pigment dispersion syndrome glaucoma

PDSIP Physician-Delivered Smoking Intervention Project

PDSRS Panic Disorder Self-Rating Scale

PDT photodynamic therapy; population doubling time

PDUF pulsed Doppler ultrasonic flowmeter

PDUFA Prescription Drug User Fee Act

PDUR Predischarge Utilization Review

PDV peak disatolic velocity

PDW platelet distribution width

PDWHF platelet-derived wound-healing factor

PDYN prodynorphin

PE Edinburgh Pharmacopoeia; pancreatic extract; paper electrophoresis; partial epilepsy; pelvic examination; penile erection; pericardial effusion; peritoneal exudate; pharyngoesophageal; phase-encoded; phenylethylamine; phenylephrine; phenytoin equivalent; phosphatidyl ethanolamine; photographic effect; phycoerythrin; physical education; physical engineering; physical examination; physical exercise; physician extender; physiological ecology; pigmented epithelium; pilocarpine-epinephrine; placental extract; plant engineering; plasma exchange; platinum etoposide; pleural effusion; point of entry; polyethylene; potential energy; powdered extract; preeclampsia; preexcitation; present evaluation; pressure equalization; presumptive eligibility; prior to exposure; probable error; professional engineer; program evaluation; pseudoexfoliation; pulmonary edema; pulmonary embolism; pyrogenic exotoxin

Pe pressure on expiration

PEA pelvic examination under anesthesia; phenylethyl alcohol; phenylethylamine; polysaccharide egg antigen; pulseless electrical activity

PEAP positive end-airway pressure

PEAR phase encoded artifact reduction

PEBG phenethylbiguanide

PEBP patient escorted by police

PEC pelvic cramps; peritoneal exudate cell; pyrogenic exotoxin C

PECAM platelet-endothelial cell adhesion molecule

PECS patient evaluation and conference system; pediatrics evaluation in community setting

PED patient examined by doctor; pediatric emergency department; pink-eyed dilution

PED, ped pediatrics

PEDF pigment epithelium-derived factor

PeDS Pediatric Drug Surveillance

PEE phosphate-eliminating enzyme

PEEK polyetheretherketone

PEEP positive end-expiratory pressure, peak end-expiratory pressure

PEEPi intrinsic peak end-expiratory pressure

PEF peak expiratory flow; Psychiatric Evaluation Form; pulmonary edema fluid

PEFR peak expiratory flow rate

PEFV partial expiratory flow volume

PEG Patient Evaluation Grid; percutaneous endoscopic gastrostomy; pneumoencephalogram, pneumoencephalography; polyethylene glycol

PEI Patient Exit Interview; phosphate excretion index; physical efficiency index; polyethyleneimine

PEJ percutaneous endoscopic jejunostomy

PEL peritoneal exudate lymphocyte; permissible exposure limit

PEM pediatric emergency medicine; peritoneal exudate macrophage; polymorphic epithelial mucin; prescription event monitoring; primary enrichment medium; probable error of measurement; protein energy malnutrition

PEMA phenylethylmalonamide

PE$_{max}$ maximum expiratory pressure

PEN pharmacy equivalent name

Pen penicillin

PENK proenkephalin

PENT phenylethanolamine N-methyltransferase

Pent pentothal

PEO progressive external ophthalmoplegia

PEP peptidase; phospho(enol)pyruvate; peer evaluation program; phosphoenolpyruvate; pigmentation, edema, and plasma cell dyscrasia [syndrome]; polyestradiol phosphate; pore-forming protein; postencephalitic parkinsonism; pre-ejection period; protein electrophoresis

Pep peptidase

PEPA peptidase A

PEPB peptidase B

PEPC peptidase C

PEPc corrected pre-ejection period

PEPCK phosphoenolpyruvate carboxykinase

PEPD peptidase D

PEPE peptidase E

PEPI pre-ejection period index

PEPP positive expiratory pressure plateau

PEPS peptidase S

PER peak ejection rate; periodogram; protein efficiency ratio

per perineal; periodicity, periodic

percus percussion

Perf perfusion or perfusionist

perf perforation

PERG pattern electroretinogram

PERI Psychiatric Epidemiology Research Interview

periap periapical

Perio periodontics

PERK prospective evaluation of radial keratotomy [protocol]

PERLA pupils equal, react to light and accommodation

PerNET peripheral neuroectodermal tumor

perp perpendicular

PERRLA pupils equal, round, and reactive to light and accommodation

PERS Patient Evaluation Rating Scale
PERT program evaluation review technique
PES Patient Escort Service; photoelectron spectroscopy; physicians' equity services; polyethylene sulfonate; postextrasystolic; preepiglottic space; preexcitation syndrome; primary empty sella [syndrome]; pseudoexfoliative syndrome; psychiatric emergency services
Pes esophageal pressure
PESP postextrasystolic potentiation
PESS problem, etiology, signs and symptoms
Pess pessary
PET peak ejection time; polyethylene terphthalate; poor exercise tolerance; positron emission tomography; preeclamptic toxemia; pressure equilization tube; progressive exercise test; psychiatric emergency team
PET$_{CO2}$ end-tidal pressure of carbon dioxide
PETH pink-eyed, tan-hooded [rat]
PETN pentaerythritol tetranitrate
petr petroleum
PETQI patient education total quality improvement
PETT pendular eye-tracking test; positron emission transverse tomography
PEU plasma equivalent unit
PEV peak expiratory velocity
pev peak electron volts
PEW pulmonary extravascular water
PEWV pulmonary extravascular water volume
PEx physical examination
Pex peak exercise
PF pair feeding; peak flow; perfusion fluid; pericardial fluid; periosteal fibroblast; peritoneal fluid; permeability factor; personality factor; picture-frustration [study]; plantar flexion; plasma factor; platelet factor; pleural fluid; power factor; primary fibrinolysin; prostatic fluid; pulmonary factor; pulmonary function; Purkinje fiber; purpura fulminans; push fluids
P-F picture-frustration [test]
P$_f$ final pressure
PF$_{1-4}$ platelet factors 1 to 4
Pf *Plasmodium falciparum*
pF picofarad
PFA p-fluorophenylalanine; phosphonoformate
PFAS performic acid-Schiff [reaction]
PFC pair-fed control [mice]; patient-focused care; pelvic flexion contracture; perfluorocarbon; pericardial fluid culture; persistent fetal circulation; plaque-forming cell
pFc noncovalently bonded dimer of the C-terminal immunoglobulin of the Fc fragment
PFD polyostotic fibrous dysplasia; pseudoinflammatory fundus disease
PFDA perfluoro-decanoic acid
PFE pelvic floor exercise
PFFD proximal focal femoral deficiency
PFG peak flow gauge; pulsed-field gel electrophoresis
PFGE pulsed field gel electrophoresis
PFGS phosphoribosyl formylglycinamide synthetase
PFIB perfluoroisobutylene
PFK phosphofructokinase; 6-phosphofructo-2-kinase
PFKF 6-phosphofructo-2-kinase, fibroblast type
PFKL phosphofructokinase, liver type; 6-phosphofructo-2-kinase, liver type
PFKM phosphofructokinase, muscle type
PFKP phosphofructokinase, platelet type; 6-phosphofructo-2-kinase, platelet type
PFKX 6-phosphofructo-2-kinase X
PFL profibrinolysin
PFM peak flow meter

PFN partially functional neutrophil; profilin

PFO patent foramen ovale

PFOB perfluorocytylbromide

PFP peripheral facial paralysis; platelet-free plasma

PFPS patellofemoral pain syndrome

PFQ personality factor questionnaire

PFR parotid flow rate; peak flow rate

PFRC predicted functional residual capacity

PFS patellofemoral syndrome; primary fibromyalgia syndrome; protein-free supernatant; pulmonary function score

PFT pancreatic function test; parafascicular thalamotomy; posterior fossa tumor; prednisone, fluorouracil, and tamomifen; pulmonary function test

PFTBE progressive form of tick-borne encephalitis

PFU plaque-forming unit; pock-forming unit

PFUO prolonged fever of unknown origin

PFV physiologic full value

PG paregoric; parotid gland; pentagastrin; pepsinogen; peptidoglycan; Pharmacopoeia Germanica; phosphate glutamate; phosphatidylglycerol; phosphogluconate; pigment granule; pituitary gonadotropin; plasma glucose; plasma triglyceride; polyfalacturonate; postgraduate; pregnanediol glucuronide; pregnant; progesterone; prolyl hydrolase; propylene glycol; Prospect Hill [virus]; prostaglandin; proteoglycan; pyoderma gangrenosum

2PG 2-phosphoglycerate

3PG 3-phosphoglycerate

Pg nasopharyngeal electrode placement in electroencephalography; gastric pressure; pogonion; pregnancy, pregnant

pg picogram; pregnant

PGA pepsinogen A; phosphoglyceric acid; polyglandular autoimmune [syndrome]; prostaglandin A; pteroylglutamic acid

PGA$_{1-3}$ prostaglandins A$_1$ to A$_3$

PGAP pilot geriatric arthritis program

PGAS persisting galactorrhea-amenorrhea syndrome; polyglandular autoimmune syndrome

PGB porphobilinogen; prostaglandin B

PGC progastricin; primordial germ cell

PGD phosphogluconate dehydrogenase; phosphoglyceraldehyde dehydrogenase; prostaglandin D

PGD$_2$ prostaglandin D$_2$

6-PGD 6-phosphogluconate dehydrogenase

PGDH phosphogluconate dehydrogenase

PGDR plasma glucose disappearance rate

PGE platelet granule exract; posterior gastroenterostomy

PGE, PGE$_1$, PGE$_2$ prostaglandins E, E$_1$, E$_2$

PGF, PGF$_1$, PGF$_2$ prostaglandins F, F$_1$, F$_2$

PGFT phosphoribosylglycinamide formyltransferase

PG prostaglandin G

PGG polyclonal gamma globulin

PGG$_2$ prostaglandin G$_2$

PGH pituitary growth hormone; porcine growth hormone; prostaglandin H

PGH$_2$ prostaglandin H$_2$

PGHS prostaglandin G/H synthase

PGI phosphoglucose isomerase; potassium, glucose, and insulin; prostaglandin I

PGI$_2$ prostaglandin I$_2$

PGK phosphoglycerate kinase

PGL persistent generalized lymphadenopathy; phosphoglycolipid; 6-phosphogluconolactonase

PGlyM phosphoglyceromutase

PGM phosphoglucomutase; phosphoglycerate mutase

PGMA phosphoglycerate mutase A
PGMB phosphoglycerate mutase B
PGN proliferative glomerulonephritis
PGO ponto-geniculo-occipital [spike]
PGP phosphoglyceroyl phosphatase; postgamma proteinuria; prepaid group practice; progressive general paralysis
PGR progesterone receptor; psychogalvanic response
PgR progesterone receptor
PGS peristent gross splenomegaly; Pettigrew syndrome; plant growth substance; postsurgical gastroparesis syndrome; prostaglandin synthetase
PGSI prostaglandin synthetase inhibitor
PGSR phosphogalvanic skin response
PGTR plasma glucose tolerance rate
PGTT prednisolone glucose tolerance test
PGU peripheral glucose uptake; postgonococcal urethritis
PGUT phosphogalactose uridyl transferase
PGV proximal gastric vagotomy
PGWB psychological general well-being [index]
PGX prostacyclin
PGY postgraduate year
PGYE peptone, glucose yeast extract
PH parathyroid hormone; partial hepatectomy; partial hysterectomy; passive hemagglutination; past history; patient's history; persistent hepatitis; personal history; pharmacopeia; pharmacy, pharmacist, or pharmaceutical; physical history; porphyria hepatica; posterior hypothalamus; previous history; primary hyperoxaluria; primary hyperparathyroidism; prostatic hypertrophy; pseudohermaphroditism; public health; pulmonary hypertension; pulmonary hypoplasia
Ph pharmacopeia; phenyl; Philadelphia [chromosome]; phosphate
Ph^1 Philadelphia chromosome
pH hydrogen ion concentration
pH$_1$ isoelectric point

ph phial; phot
PHA passive hemagglutination [test]; peripheral hyperalimentation; phenylalanine; phytohemagglutinin; phytohemagglutinin antigen; pseudohypoaldosteronism; public health agency; pulse-height analyzer
pH$_A$ arterial blood hydrogen tension
PHAF peripheral hyperalimentation formula
PHAL phytohemagglutinin-stimulated lymphocyte
phal phalangeal
PHA-LCM phytohemagglutinin-stimulated leukocyte conditioned medium
PHA-NSP passive hemagglutination to nonstructural protein
PHAP phytohemagglutinin protein
phar pharmaceutical; pharmacy; pharynx
Pharm B Bachelor of Pharmacy [Lat. *Pharmaciae Baccalaureus*]
Phar C pharmaceutical chemist
Pharm pharmacy
Pharm D Doctor of Pharmacy [Lat. *Pharmaciae Doctor*]
Pharm M Master of Pharmacy [Lat. *Pharmaciae Magister*]
pharm pharmacist; pharmacology; pharmacopeia; pharmacy
PHAVER pterygia-heart defects-autosomal recessive inheritance-vertebral defects-ear anomalies-radial defects [syndrome]
PHB polyhydroxybutyrate; preventive health behavior; prohibitin
PhB, Phb Pharmacopoeia Britannica
PHBB propylhydroxybenzyl benzimidazole
PHBQ Physicians' Humanistic Behaviors Questionnaire
PHC personal health costs; posthospital care; premolar hypodontia, hyperhidrosis, [premature] canities [syndrome]; primary health care; primary hepatic carcinoma; proliferative helper cell

PhC pharmaceutical chemist

Ph¹ᶜ Philadelphia chromosome

PHCC primary hepatocellular carcinoma

PHCP prehospital care provider

PHD pathological habit disorder; personal health data; post-heparin plasma diamine oxidase; potentially harmful drug

PhD Doctor of Pharmacy [Lat. *Pharmaciae Doctor*]; Doctor of Philosophy [Lat. *Philosophiae Doctor*]

PHE periodic health examination; phenylephrine

Phe phenylalanine

PhEEM photoemission electron microscopy

Pheo pheochromocytoma; pheophytin

PHF paired helical filament; personal hygiene facility

PHFG primary human fetal glia

PhG Graduate in Pharmacy; Pharmacopoeia Germanica

phgly phenylglycine

PHHI persistent hyperinsulinemic hypoglycemia of infancy

PHI passive hemagglutination inhibition; past history of illness; phosphohexose isomerase; physiological hyaluronidase inhibitor; prehospital index

PhI Pharmacopoeia Internationalis

φ Greek letter *phi*; magnetic flux; osmotic coefficient

PHIHM prehospital invasive hemodynamic monitoring

PHIM posthypoxic intention myoclonus

PHK phosphohexokinase; phosphorylase kinase; postmortem human kidney

PHKA phosphorylase kinase, alpha

PHKB phosphorylase kinase, beta

PHKD phosphorylase kinase, delta

PHKG phosphorylase kinase, gamma

PHLA postheparin lipolytic activity

PHLOP polymerase-halt-mediated linkage of primers

PHLS Public Health Laboratory Service

PHM peptide histidine methionine; peptidylglycine alpha-hydroxylating monooxygenase; posterior hyaloid membrane; pulmonary hyaline membrane

PhM Master of Pharmacy [Lat. *Pharmaciae Magister*]; pharyngeal muscle

PhmG Graduate in Pharmacy

PHN paroxysmal noctural hemoglobinuria; passive Heymann nephritis; postherpetic neuralgia; public health nursing, public health nurse

PHO physician-hospital organization

PH₂O partial pressure of water vapor

phos phosphate

PHOX paired mesoderm homeobox [gene]

PHP panhypopituitarism; postheparin phospholipase; prehospital program; prepaid health plan; primary hyperparathyroidism; pseudohypoparathyroidism

p-HPPO p-hydroxyphenyl pyruvate oxidase

PHPT primary hyperparathyroidism; pseudohypoparathyroidism

pHPT primary hyperparathyroidism

PHPV persistent hyperplastic primary vitreous

PHR peak heart rate; photoreactivity

PHS Physicians' Health Study; pooled human serum; posthypnotic suggestion; Public Health Service

PHSC pleuripotent hemopoietic stem cell

pH-stat apparatus for maintaining the pH of a solution

PHT phenytoin; portal hypertension; primary hyperthyroidism; pulmonary hypertension

PhTD Doctor of Physical Therapy

PHTLS prehospital trauma life support

PHV peak height velocity; Prospect Hill virus

PHX pulmonary histiocytosis X

Phx past history; pharynx

PHY pharyngitis; physical; physiology

PHYS physiology
PhyS physiologic saline [solution]
phys physical; physician
Phys Ed physical education
physio physiology; physiotherapy
Phys Med physical medicine
PhysPRC Physician's Payment Review Commission
Phys Ther physical therapist or therapy
PI first meiotic prophase; isoelectric point; pacing impulse; package insert; pancreatic insufficiency; parainfluenza; pars intermedia; patient's interest; performance intensity; perinatal injury; periodontal index; permeability index; personal injury; personality inventory; Pharmacopoeia Internationalis; phosphatidylinositol; physically impaired; pineal body; plaque index; plasmin inhibitor; pneumatosis intestinalis; poison ivy; ponderal index; postictal immobility; postinfection; postinfluenza; postinjury; postinoculation; preinduction [examination]; premature infant; prematurity index; preparatory interval; present illness; primary infarction; primary infection; principal investigator; product information; proinsulin; prolactin inhibitor; protamine insulin; protease inhibitor; proximal intestine; pulmonary incompetence; pulmonary index; pulmonary infarction; pulsatility index
P_I inspiratory pressure
Pi, P_i inorganic phosphate
Pi parental generation; pressure in inspiration; protease inhibitor
pI isoelectric point
pi post-injection
Π Greek capital letter *pi*
π Greek lower case letter *pi;* the ratio of circumference to diameter, 3.1415926536
PIA photoelectric intravenous angiography; plasma insulin activity; preinfarction angina; Psychiatric Institute of America; *R*-phenylisopropyladenosine

PIAT Peabody Individual Achievement Test
PIAVA polydactyly-imperforate anus-vertebral anomalies [syndrome]
PIBC percutaneous intraaortic balloon counterpulsation [catheter]
PIC Personality Inventory for Children; polymorphism information content
PICA percutaneous transluminal coronary angioplasty; Porch Index of Communicative Abilities; posterior inferior cerebellar artery; posterior inferior communicating artery
PICC peripherally inserted central catheter
PICD primary irritant contact dermatitis
PICFS postinfective chronic fatigue syndrome
PICSO pressure-controlled intermittent coronary sinus occlusion
PICU pediatric intensive care unit; pulmonary intensive care unit
PID pain intensity difference [score]; pelvic inflammatory disease; photoionization detector; picture image directory; plasma iron disappearance; postinertia dyskinesia; prolapsed/protruded intervertebral disk
PIDRA portable insulin dosageregulating apparatus
PIDS primary immunodeficiency syndrome
PIDT plasma iron disappearance time
PIE postinfectious encephalomyelitis preimplantation embryo; prosthetic infectious endocarditis; pulmonary infiltration with eosinophilia; pulmonary interstitial emphysema
PIF paratoid isoelectric focusing variant protein; peak inspiratory flow; proinsulin-free; prolactin-inhibiting factor; prolactin release-inhibiting factor; proliferation-inhibiting factor; prostatic interstitial fluid
PIFG poor intrauterine fetal growth

PIFR peak inspiratory flow rate
PIFT platelet immunofluorescence test
PIG polymeric immunoglobulin
PIGA phosphatidylinositol glycan A
pigm pigment, pigmented
PIGR polymeric immunoglobulin receptor
PIH periventricular-intraventricular hemorrhage; phenyl isopropylhydrazine; pregnancy-induced hypertension; prolactin-inhibiting hormone
PII plasma inorganic iodine; primary irritation index
PIIP portable insulin infusion pump
PIIS posterior inferior iliac spine
PIL patient information leaflet
π**m** pi meson
PILBD paucity of interlobular bile ducts
PILL Pennebaker Inventory of Limbic Languidness
PIM penicillamine-induced myasthenia
PI$_{max}$ maximum inspiratory pressure at residual volume
PIN product identification number
PINN proposed international nonproprietary name
PINV postimperative negative variation
PIO$_2$ partial pressure of inspired oxygen
PION posterior ischemic optic neuropathy
PIOPED Prospective Investigation of Pulmonary Embolism Diagnosis [database]
PIP paralytic infantile paralysis; peak inflation pressure, peak inspiratory pressure; periodic interim payment; piperacillin; pressure inversion point; prolactin-inducible protein; proximal interphalangeal; Psychotic Inpatient Profile; psychosis, intermittent hyponatremia, polydipsia [syndrome]; posterior interphalangeal; probable intrauterine pregnancy
PIP$_2$ phosphatidylinositol 4,5-biphosphate or diphosphate

PI-P phosphatidylinositol-4-phosphate
PIPE persistent interstitial pulmonary emphysema
PIPIDA p-isopropylacetanilido imidodiacetic acid
PIPJ proximal interphalangeal joint
PI-PP phosphatidylinositol-4,5-biphosphate
PIQ Performance Intelligence Quotient
PIR postinhibition rebound; protein identification resource
PIRI plasma immunoreactive insulin
PIRS plasma immunoreactive secretion
PIS preinfarction syndrome; primary immunodeficiency syndrome; Provisional International Standard
pIs isoelectric point
PISCES percutaneously inserted spinal cord electrical stimulation
PIT pacing-induced tachycardia; patella inhibition test; picture identification test; pitocin; pitressin; plasma iron turnover
pit pituitary
PITC phenylisothiocyanate
PITR plasma iron turnover rate
PIU polymerase-inducing unit
PIV parainfluenza virus; polydactyly-imperforate anus-vertebral anomalies [syndrome]; projective image visualization
PIVD protruded intervertebral disk
PIVH peripheral intravenous hyperalimentation; periventricular-intraventricular hemorrhage
PIVKA protein induced by vitamin K absence or antagonism
P/I/X patients, indicators, external bodies
PIXE particle-induced x-ray emission; proton-induced x-ray emission
Pixel picture element
PJ pancreatic juice; Peutz-Jeghers [syndrome]
PJB premature junctional beat
PJC premature junctional contractions
PJM positive joint mobilization

PJP pancreatic juice protein

PJS peritoneojugular shunt; Peutz-Jeghers syndrome

PJT paroxysmal junctional tachycardia

PK penetrating keratoplasty; pericardial knock; pharmacokinetics; pig kidney; Prausnitz-Küstner [reaction]; protein kinase; psychokinesis; pyruvate kinase

pK negative logarithm of the dissociation constant; plasma potassium

pK' apparent value of a pK; negative logarithm of the dissociation constant of an acid

pk peck

PkA prekallikrein activator

pK$_a$ negative logarithm of the acid ionization constant

PKAR protein kinase activation ratio

PKase protein kinase

PKC problem-knowledge coupler; protein kinase C

PKCA protein kinase C alpha

PKCB protein kinase C beta

PKCE protein kinase C epsilon

PKCG protein kinase C gamma

PKCSH protein kinase C heavy chain

PKCSL protein kinase C light chain

PKCZ protein kinase C zeta

PKD polycystic kidney disease; proliferative kidney disease

PKI potato kallikrein inhibitor

PKK plasma prekallikrein

PKL pyruvate kinase, liver type

PKM pyruvate kinase, muscle

PKN parkinsonism

PKP penetrating keratoplasty

PKR phased knee rehabilitation; Prausnitz-Küstner reaction

PKS protein kinase sequence

PKT Prausnitz-Küstner test

PKU phenylketonuria

PKV killed poliomyelitis vaccine

pkV peak kilovoltage

PL palmaris longus; pancreatic lipase; perception of light; peroneus longus; phospholipase; phospholipid; photoluminescence; placebo; placental lactogen; plantar; plasmalemma; plastic surgery; platelet lactogen; polarized light; preleukemia; programming language; prolactin; prolymphocytic leukemia; pulpolingual; Purkinje layer

Pl poiseuille

P$_L$ transpulmonary pressure

pl picoliter; placenta; plasma; platelet

PL/I programming language I (one)

PLA peripheral laser angioplasty; phenyl lactate; phospholipase A; phospholipid antibody; placebo therapy; plasminogen activator; platelet antigen; polylactic acid; potentially lethal arrhythmia; procaine/lactic acid; Product License Application; pulp linguoaxial

P$_{La}$ left atrial pressure

PLa pulpolabial

Pla left atrial pressure

PLA2 phospholipase A2

PLAP placental alkaline phosphatase

PLAT plasminogen activator, tissue-type

Plat platelet

PLAU plasminogen activator, urinary

PLAUR plasminogen activator receptor, urokinase type

PLB parietal lobe battery; phospholamban; phospholipase B; porous layer bead

PLC phospholipase C; primary liver cancer; proinsulin-like component; protein-lipid complex; pseudolymphocytic choriomeningitis

PLCC primary liver cell cancer

PLCO postoperative low cardiac output

PLCx posterolateral circumflex branch [of coronary artery]

PLD peripheral light detection; phospholipase D; platelet defect; polycystic liver disease; posterior latissimus dorsi [muscle]; potentially lethal damage

PLDH plasma lactic dehydrogenase

PLDR potentially lethal damage repair

PLE paraneoplastic limbic encephalopathy; protein-losing enteropathy; pseudolupus erythematosus

PLED periodic lateral epileptiform discharge

PLES parallel-line equal space

PLET polymyxin, lysozyme, EDTA, and thallous acetate [in heart infusion agar]

PLEVA pityriasis lichenoides et varioliformis acuta

PLF perilymphatic fistula; posterior lung fiber

PLFS perilymphatic fistula syndrome

PLG plasminogen; L-propyl-L-leucyl-glucinamide

PLGL plasminogen-like

P-LGV psittacosis-lymphogranuloma venereum

PLH placental lactogenic hormone

PLI professional liability insurance

PlIgG surface IgG

PLISSIT permission to be sexual, limited information, specific suggestions, intensive therapy

PLL peripheral light loss; phase-locked loop; poly-L-lysine; pressure length loop; posterior longitudinal ligament; prolymphocytic leukemia

PLM percent labeled mitoses; periodic leg movement; plasma level monitoring; polarized light microscopy

PLMV posterior leaf mitral valve

PLN peripheral lymph node; phospholamban

PLND pelvic lymph node dissection

PLO polycystic lipomembranous osteodysplasia

PLOD procollagen-lysine 2-oxoglutarate 5-dioxygenase

PLP phospholipid; plasma leukapheresis; polypeptide; polystyrene latex particles; posterior lobe of pituitary [gland]; proteolipid protein; pyridoxal phosphate

PLPH post-lumbar puncture headache

PLR pupillary light reflex

PLS Papillon-Lefèvre syndrome; polydactyly-luxation syndrome; preleukemic syndrome; primary lateral sclerosis; prostaglandin-like substance; pulmonary leukostasis syndrome

PLSD protected least significant difference

PLST progressively lowered stress threshold

Pl Surg plastic surgeon or surgery

PLT pancreatic lymphocytic infiltration; platelet; primed lymphocyte test; primed lymphocyte typing; psittacosis-lympho-granuloma venereum-trachoma [group]

PLTC Partnership for Long Term Care

plumb lead [Lat. *plumbum*]

PLUT Plutchnik [geriatric rating scale]

PLV partial liquid ventilation; poliomyelitis live vaccine; panleukopenia virus; phenylalanine, lysine, and vasopressin; posterior light ventricle

PLWA person living with acquired immune deficiency syndrome

PLWS Prader-Labhart-Willi syndrome

plx plexus

PLZ phenelzine

PLZF promyelocytic leukemia zinc finger

PM after death (Lat. *post mortem*); after noon [Lat. *post meridiem*]; mean pressure; pacemaker; pantomography; papillary muscle; papular mucinosis; partial meniscectomy; perinatal mortality; peritoneal macrophage; petit mal epilepsy [Fr. *petit mal*]; photomultiplier; physical medicine; plasma membrane; platelet membrane; platelet microsome; pneumomediastinum; poliomyelitis; polymorph, polymorphonuclear; polymyositis; porokeratosis of Mibelli; posterior mitral; postmenstrual; postmortem; premarketing [approval]; premenstrual; premolar; premotor; presystolic murmur;

pretibial myxedema; preventive medicine; primary motivation; prostatic massage; protein methylesterase; protocol management; pterygoid muscle; pubertal macromastia; pulmonary macrophage; pulpomesial

Pm paratid midle [band protein]; promethium

pM picomolar

pm picometer

PMA index of prevalence and severity of gingivitis, where P = papillary gingiva, M = marginal gingiva, and A = attached gingiva; papillary, marginal, attached [gingiva]; para-methoxyamphetamine; Pharmaceutical Manufacturers Association; phenylmercuric acetate; phorbol myristate acetate; phosphomolybdic acid; premarket approval; primary mental abilities; progressive muscular atrophy; pyridylmercuric acetate

PMB papillomacular bundle; para-hydroxymercuribenzoate; polychrome methylene blue; polymorphonuclear basophil; polymyxin B; postmenopausal bleeding

PMC paramyotonia congenita; patient management category; phenylmercuric chloride; physical medicine clinic; pleural mesothelial click; premature mitral closure; pseudomembranous colitis

PMCC product-moment correlation coefficient [Pearson]

PMCH pro-melanin-concentrating hormone

PMCHL pro-melanin-concentrating hormone-like

PMCS patient management computer stimulation

PMD Pelizaeus-Merzbacher disease; posterior mandibular depth; primary myocardial disease; private medicine doctor; programmed multiple development; progressive muscular dystrophy

PMDD premenstrual dysphoric disorder

PM/DM polymyositis/dermatomyositis

PM-DRG pediatric modified diagnosis-related group

PMDS peristent müllerian duct syndrome; primary myelodysplastic syndrome

PME periodic monitoring examination; phosphomonoester; polymorphonuclear eosinophil; progressive myoclonus epilepsy

PMEA 9-(2-phosphomethoxyethyl) adenine

PMF platelet membrane fluidity; progressive massive fibrosis; proton motive force; pterygomaxillary fossa

pmf proton motive force

PMG primary medical group

PMGCT primary mediastinal germ-cell tumor

PMH past medical history; posteromedial hypothalamus

PMHR predicted maximum heart rate

PMI pain management inventory; past medical illness; patient medication instruction; perioperative myocardial infarction; point of maximal impulse; point of maximal intensity; posterior myocardial infarction; postmyocardial infarction; present medical illness; previous medical illness

PMIS postmyocardial infarction syndrome; PSRO (see p. 251) Management Information System

PML peripheral motor latency; polymorphonuclear leukocyte; posterior mitral leaflet; progressive multifocal leukodystrophy; progressive multifocal leukoencephalopathy; prolapsing mitral leaflet; promyelocytic leukemia; pulmonary microlithiasis

PMLE polymorphous light eruption

PMM pentamethylmelamine; protoplast maintenance medium

PMMA polymethylmethacrylate

PMN polymorphonuclear; polymorphonuclear neutrophil; polymorphonucleotide

PMNC percentage of multinucleated cells; peripheral blood mononuclear cell
PMNG polymorphonuclear granulocyte
PMNL peripheral blood monocytes and polymorphonuclear leukocytes; polymorphonuclear leukocyte
PMNN polymorphonuclear neutrophil
PMNR periadenitis mucosa necrotica recurrens
PMO postmenopausal osteoporosis; Principal Medical Officer
pmol picomole
PMP pain management program; patient management program; patient medication profile; peripheral myelin protein; peroxisomal membrane protein; persistent mentoposterior [fetal position]; previous menstrual period
PMPM, pmpm per member per month
PMPS postmastectomy pain syndrome
PMPY per member per year
PMQ phytylmenaquinone
PMR patient meta-record; perinatal mortality rate; periodic medical review; physical medicine and rehabilitation; polymyalgia rheumatica; prior medical record; progressive muscular relaxation; proportionate morbidity/mortality ratio; proton magnetic resonance
PM&R physical medicine and rehabilitation
PMRS physical medicine and rehabilitation service
PMS patient management system; perimenstrual syndrome; periodic movements during sleep; phenazine methosulfate; polydactyly-myopia syndrome; postmarketing surveillance; postmenstrual stress; postmitochondrial supernatant; pregnant mare serum; premenstrual syndrome, premenstrual symptoms; psychotic motor syndrome
PMSC pediatric medical special care; pluripotent myeloid stem cell
PMSF phenylmethylsulfonyl fluoride

PMSG pregnant mare serum gonadotropin
PMT parent management training; phenol O-methyltransferase; photomultiplier tube; Porteus maze test; premenstrual tension; pyridoxyl-methyl-tryptophan
PMTS premenstrual tension syndrome
PMTT pulmonary mean transit time
PMV paramyxovirus; percutaneous mitral balloon valvotomy; prolapse of mitral valve
PMVL, pMVL posterior mitral valve leaflet
PMW pacemaker wires
PMX paired mesoderm homeobox [gene]
PN papillary necrosis; parenteral nutrition; penicillin; perceived noise; percussion note; periarteritis nodosa; peripheral nerve; peripheral neuropathy; phrenic nerve; plaque neutralization; pneumonia; polyarteritis nodosa; polyneuritis; polyneuropathy; polynuclear; positional nystagmus; posterior nares; postnatal; practical nurse; predicted normal; primary nurse; progress note; protease nexin; psychiatry and neurology; psychoneurotic; pyelonephritis; pyridine nucleotide
P/N positive/negative
P&N psychiatry and neurology
P-5'-N pyridine-5'-nucleosidase
P$_{N2}$ partial pressure of nitrogen
Pn pneumatic; pneumonia
pn pain
PNA Paris Nomina Anatomica; peanut agglutinin; pentosenucleic acid
P$_{Na}$ plasma sodium
PNAvQ positive-negative ambivalent quotient
PNB p-nitrobiphenyl; perineal needle biopsy; peripheral nerve block; premature nodal beat
PNBT p-nitroblue tetrazolium
PNC penicillin; peripheral nucleated cell; pneumotaxic center; premature nodal contracture

PND paroxysmal nocturnal dyspnea; partial neck dissection; postnasal drainage; postnasal drip; postnatal death; principal neutralizing determinant; purulent nasal drainage

PNdb perceived noise decibel

PNE peripheral neuroepithelioma; plasma norepinephrine; pneumoencephalography; pseudomembranous necrotizing enterocolitis

PNEM paraneoplastic encephalomyelitis

PNET peripheral neuroepithelioma; primitive neuroectodermal tumor

pneu, pneum pneumonia

PNF proprioceptive neuromuscular facilitation

PNG penicillin G

PNH paroxysmal nocturnal hemoglobinuria; polynuclear hydrocarbon

PNHA Physicians National Housestaff Association

PNI peripheral nerve injury; postnatal infection; prognostic nutritional index

PNID Peer Nomination Inventory for Depression

PNK polynucleotide kinase; pyridoxine kinase

PNK(H) pyridoxine kinase, high

PNK(L) pyridoxine kinase, low

PNL peripheral nerve lesion; polymorphonuclear neutrophilic leukocyte

PNLA percutaneous needle lung aspiration

PNM perinatal mortality; peripheral dysostosis, nasal hypoplasia, and mental retardation [syndrome]; peripheral nerve myelin

PNMR postnatal mortality risk

PNMT phenyl-ethanolamine-N-methyltransferase

PNO Principal Nursing Officer

p-NO₂ p-nitrosochloramphenicol

PNP pancreatic polypeptide; para-nitrophenol; peak negative pressure; pediatric nurse practitioner; peripheral neuropathy; pneumoperitoneum; polyneuropathy; predictive value of negative results; psychogenic nocturnal polydipsia; purine nucleoside phosphorylase

P-NP para-nitrophenol

PNPase polynucleotide phosphorylase

PNPB positive-negative pressure breathing

PNPP para-nitrophenylphosphate

PNPR positive-negative pressure respiration

PNS paraneoplastic syndrome; parasympathetic nervous system; partial nonprogressive stroke; peripheral nerve stimulation; peripheral nervous system; posterior nasal spine; practical nursing student

PNT partial nodular transformation; patient

Pnt patient

Pnthx pneumothorax

PNU protein nitrogen unit

Pnx pneumothorax

PNZ posterior necrotic zone

PO by mouth, orally [Lat. *per os*]; parieto-occipital; parietal operculum; period of onset; perioperative; posterior; postoperative; predominant organism; pulse oximetry

P₀ opening pressure

PO₂, P_{O2}, pO2 partial pressure of oxygen

Po polonium; porion

po by mouth [Lat. *per os*]

p/o postoperative

POA pancreatic oncofetal antigen; phalangeal osteoarthritis; preoptic area; primary optic atrophy

POAG primary open-angle glaucoma

POA-HA preoptic anterior hypothalamic area

POB penicillin, oil, beeswax; phenoxybenzamine; place of birth

POC particulate organic carbon; point of care; postoperative care; probability of chance; product of conception; pro-opiomelanocortin

POD peroxidase; place of death; podiatry; polycystic ovary disease; pool of doctors; postoperative day; pouch of Douglas
PODx preoperative diagnosis
POE pediatric orthopedic examination; physician order entry; point of entry; polyoxyethylene; postoperative endophthalmitis; proof of eligibility
POEMS polyneuropathy, organomegaly, endocrinopathy, M protein, skin changes [syndrome]
POF pattern of failure; position of function; premature ovarian failure; primary ovarian failure; pyruvate oxidation factor
PofE portal of entry
POFX X-linked premature ovarian failure
POG pediatric oncology group; polymyositis ossificans generalisata
Pog pogonion
pOH hydroxide ion concentration in a solution
POHI physically or otherwise health-impaired
POHS presumed ocular histoplasmosis syndrome
POI Personal Orientation Inventory
poik poikilocyte, poikilocytosis
POIS Parkland On-Line Information Systems
pois poison, poisoning, poisoned
pol polish, polishing
POLA polymerase alpha
polio poliomyelitis
POLIP polyneuropathy-ophthalmoplegia-leukoencephalopathy-intestinal pseudoobstruction [syndrome]
Poly polymorphonuclear
poly-A, poly(A) polyadenylic acid
poly-C, poly(C) polycytidylic acid
poly-G, poly(G) polyguanylic acid
poly-I, poly(I) polyinosinic acid
poly-IC, poly-I:C copolymer of polyinosinic and polycytidylic acids; synthetic RNA polymer
polys polymorphonuclear leukocytes

poly-T, poly(T) polythymidylic acid
poly-U, poly(U) polyuridylic acid
POM pain on motion; prescription only medicine
POMC proopiomelanocortin
POMONA pregnancy and postpartum, osteoporosis, mastectomy rehabilitation, osteoarthritis, nerve pain, athletic injuries
POMP phase-offset multiplanar [pulse sequence in magnetic resonance imaging]; principal outer material protein
POMR problem-oriented medical record
POMS Profile of Mood States
PON paraoxonase; particulate organic nitrogen
pond by weight [Lat. *pondere*]; heavy [Lat. *ponderosus*]
POP diphosphate group; pain on palpation; paroxypropione; persistent occipitoposterior [fetal position]; pituitary opioid peptide; plasma osmotic pressure; plaster of Paris; polymyositis ossificans progressiva
Pop popliteal; population
POPLINE Population Information On-line
poplit popliteal
POPOP 1,4-bis-(5-phenoxazol-2-yl)benzene
POR patient-oriented research; physician of record; postocclusive oscillatory response; prevalence odds ratio; problem-oriented record
PORC porphyria, Chester type
PORH postoperative reactive hyperemia
PORP partial ossicular replacement prosthesis
PORT Patient Outcome Research Team; postoperative respiratory therapy
POS periosteal osteosarcoma; physician order set; point of service; polycystic ovary syndrome; psychoorganic syndrome

pos position; positive
POSC problem-oriented system of charting
POSM patient-operated selector mechanism
POSS proximal over-shoulder strap
POSSUM Pictures of Standard Syndromes and Undiagnosed Malformations
post posterior
postgangl postganglionic
postop, post-op postoperative
Post Pit posterior pituitary [gland]
POT periostitis ossificans toxica; postoperative treatment
pot potassium; potential
potass potassium
POU placenta, ovary, and uterus
PoV portal vein
POW Powassan [encephalitis]
powd powder
POX point of exit
PP diphosphate group; emphysema [pink puffers]; near point of accommodation [Lat. *punctum proximum*]; pacesetter potential; palmoplantar; pancreatic polypeptide; paradoxical pulse; paraplatin; parietal pulse; partial pressure; perfusion pressure; peritoneal pseudomyxoma; persisting proteinuria; Peyer patches; pinprick; placental protein; placenta previa; planned parenthood; plasma pepsinogen; plasmapheresis; plasma protein; plaster of Paris; polypropylene; polystyrene agglutination plate; population planning; posterior papillary; posterior pituitary; postpartum; postprandial; precocious puberty; preferred provider; primapara; primary provider; private practice; proactivator plasminogen; protoporphyria; protoporphyrin; proximal phalanx; pseudomyxoma peritonei; pterygoid process; pulmonary pressure; pulse pressure; pulsus paradoxus; purulent pericarditis; pyrophosphatase; pyrophosphate

P-P prothrombin proconvertin
P-5'-P pyridoxal-5'-phosphate
PP$_1$ free pyrophosphate
pp near point of accommodation [Lat. *punctum proximum*]; postprandial; postpartum
PPA palpation, percussion, auscultation; pepsin A; phenylpropanolamine; phenylpyruvic acid; Pittsburgh pneumonia agent; polyphosphoric acid; posterior margin of pulmonary artery; posterior pulmonary artery; postpartum amenorrhea; postpill amenorrhea; preferred provider arrangement; pure pulmonary atresia
PP&A palpation, percussion, and auscultation
Ppa pulmonary artery pressure
PPAR peroxisome proliferator activated receptor
PPAS peripheral pulmonary artery stenosis
Ppaw pulmonary artery wedge pressure
PPB platelet-poor blood; pneumococcal pneumonia and bacteremia; positive pressure breathing
PPb postparotid basic protein
ppb parts per billion
PPBP pro-platelet basic protein
PPBS postprandial blood sugar
PPC pentose phosphate cycle; peripheral posterior curve; plasma prothrombin conversion; pneumopericardium; progressive patient care; proximal palmar crease
PPCA plasma prothrombin conversion accelerator; proserum prothrombin conversion accelerator
PPCD polymorphous posterior corneal dystropy
PPCE postproline cleaving enzyme
PPCF peripartum cardiac failure; plasma prothrombin conversion factor
PPCM postpartum cardiomyopathy
PPCRA pigmented paravenous chorioretinal atrophy

PPD packs per day; paraphenylenediamine; percussion and postural drainage; permanent partial disability; phenyldiphenyloxadiazole; postpartum day; primary physical dependence; progressive perceptive deafness; purified protein derivative; Siebert purified protein derivative of tuberculin

PPDS phonologic programming deficit syndrome

PPD-S purified protein derivative-standard

PPE palmoplantar erythrodysesthesia; personal protective equipment; polyphosphoric ester; porcine pancreatic elastase; protective personal equipment; pulmonary permeability edema

PPES palmar-plantar erythrodysesthesia syndrome

PPF pellagra preventive factor; phagocytosis promoting factor; phosphonoformate; plasma protein fraction

PPFA Planned Parenthood Federation of America

PPG photoplethysmography; platelet proteoglycan; portal pressure gradient

ppg picopicogram

PPGA postpill galactorrhea-amenorrhea

PPGB protective protein of beta-galactosidase

PPGF polypeptide growth factor

PPGP prepaid group practice

ppGpp 3'-pyrophosphoryl-guanosine-5'-diphosphate

PPH past pertinent history; persistent pulmonary hypertension; phosphopyruvate hydratase; postpartum hemorrhage; primary pulmonary hypertension; protocollagen proline hydroxylase

pphm parts per hundred million

PPHN persistent pulmonary hypertension of the newborn

PPHP pseudopseudohypoparathyroidism

ppht parts per hundred thousand

PPI partial permanent impairment; patient package insert; present pain intensity; purified porcine insulin

PPi, PP$_i$ inorganic pyrophosphate

PPID peak pain intensity difference [score]

PPIE prolonged postictal encephalopathy

PPK palmoplantar keratosis; prekallikrein

PPL penicilloyl polylysine; posterior pulmonary leaflet

Ppl intrapleural pressure

PPLO pleuropneumonia-like organism

PPM permanent pacemaker; phosphopentomutase; physician practice management; pigmented pupillary membrane; posterior papillary muscle; pulse position modulated

ppm parts per million; pulses per minute

PPMA progressive postmyelitis muscular atrophy

PPMS Performax's Personal Matrix System

PPN partial parenteral nutrition; pedunculopontine nucleus

PPNA peak phrenic nerve activity

PPNAD primary pigmented nodular adrenocortical disease

PPNG penicillinase-producing *Neisseria gonorrhoeae*

PPO platelet peroxidase; preferred provider option; preferred provider organization

PPP pain perception profile; palatopharyngoplasty; palmoplantar pustulosis; pentose phosphate pathway; peripheral pulse present; photostimulable phosphor plate; Pickford projective pictures; platelet-poor plasma; pluripotent progenitor; point-to-point protocol; polyphoretic phosphate; porcine pancreatic polypeptide; portal perfusion pressure; protein phosphatase; purified placental protein

PPPA protein phosphatase alpha

PPPBL peripheral pulses palpable both legs

PPPI primary private practice insurance

PPPP porokeratosis punctata palmaris et plantaris

PPR physician-patient relation; physician payment reform; posterior primary ramus; Price precipitation reaction

PPr paraprosthetic

PPRC Physician Payment Review Commission

PPRF paramedian pontine reticular formation; postpartum renal failure

PPROM preterm premature rupture of fetal membranes

PPRP polyadenosine diphosphate-ribose polymerase

PPRWP poor precordial R-wave progression

PPS Personal Preference Scale; physician, patient and society [course]; polyvalent pneumococcal polysaccharide; popliteal pterygium syndrome; postpartum sterilization; postperfusion syndrome; postpericardiotomy syndrome; postpolio syndrome; postpump syndrome; primary acquired preleukemic syndrome; prospective payment system; prospective pricing system; protein plasma substitute; pulse per second

PPSH pseudovaginal perineoscrotal hypospadias

PPT parietal pleural tissue; partial prothrombin time; peak-to-peak threshold; Pfeiffer-Palm-Teller [syndrome]; plant protease test; polypurine tract; postpartum thyroiditis; pulmonary platelet trapping; pulmonary physical therapy

ppt parts per trillion; precipitation, precipitate; prepared

pptd precipitated

PPTL postpartum tubul ligation

PPV pneumococcal polysaccharide vaccine; porcine parvovirus; positive predictive value; positive pressure ventilation; progressive pneumonia virus; pulmonary plasma volume

PPVr regional pulmonary plasma volume

PPVT Peabody Picture Vocabulary Test

PPVT-R Peabody Picture Vocabulary Test, Revised

Ppw pulmonary wedge pressure

PPY pancreatic polypeptide

PQ paraquat; parent questionnaire; permeability quotient; physician's questionnaire; plastoquinone; pronator quadratus; pyrimethamine-quinine

PQOL Perceived Quality of Life [scale]

PQRST provocative and palliative factors, quality of pain, radiation of pain, severity of pain, timing of pain [pain characteristics in low back pain syndrome]

PR by way of the rectum [Lat. *per rectum*]; far point [of accommodation] [Lat. *punctum remotum*]; palindromic rheumatism; parallax and refraction; partial reinforcement; partial remission; partial response; particular respirator; peer review; perfusion rate; peripheral resistance; per rectum; phenol red; photoreaction; physical rehabilitation; pityriasis rosea; posterior root; postmyalgia rheumatica; postural reflex; potency ratio; preference record; pregnancy; pregnancy rate; preretinal; pressoreceptor; pressure; prevention; Preyer reflex; proctology; production rate; profile; progesterone receptor; progressive relaxation; progressive resistance; progress report; prolactin; prolonged remission; propranolol; prosthion; protein; public relations; pulmonary rehabilitation; pulse rate; pulse repetition; pyramidal response

P-R the time between the P wave and the beginning of the QRS complex in electrocardiography [interval]

P&R pelvic and rectal [examination]; pulse and respiration

Pr praseodymium; prednisolone; presbyopia; primary; prism; production rate [of steroid hormones]; prolactin; propyl

pr far point of accommodation [Lat. *punctum remotum*]; pair; per rectum; prism

PRA panel-reactive antibody; phosphoribosylamine; physician recognition award; plasma renin activity; progesterone receptor assay

prac, pract practice, practitioner

PRAGMATIC pregnancy, rheumatoid arthritis, acromegaly, glucose metabolism disorders, mechanical injury, amyloid, thyroid disease, infectious disease, crystals in gout or pseudogout [disorders associated with carpal tunnel syndrome]

PrA-HPA protein A hemolytic plaque assay

PRAISE Prospective Randomized Amlodipine Survival Evaluation

PRAS pre-reduced anaerobically sterilized [medium]; pseudo-renal artery syndrome

PRB basic proline-rich protein; Prosthetics Research Board

PRBC packed red blood cells; placental residual blood volume

PRBS pseudorandom binary sequence

PRBV placental residual blood volume

PRC packed red cells; peer review committee; phase response curve; plasma renin concentration; professional review committee

PRCA pure red cell aplasia

pRCA posterior right coronary artery

PRD partial reaction of degeneration; physician relations department; postradiation dysplasia

PRE photoreacting enzyme; physician's report of examination; pigmented retinal epithelium; preplacement examination; progressive resistive exercise; proton relaxation enhancement

pre preliminary; preparation or prepare; pretreatment

pre-AIDS pre-acquired immune deficiency syndrome

pre-amp preliminary amplifier

PRECEDE predisposing, reinforcing, and enabling causes in educational diagnosis and evaluation [model]

precip precipitate, precipitated, precipitation

PRED prednisone

PREDICT Prospective Randomized Evaluation of Diltiazem CD Trial

prefd preferred

preg, pregn pregnancy, pregnant

prelim preliminary

prem premature, prematurity

PreMACE prednisone, methotrexate, Adriamycin, cyclophosphamide, etoposide

pre-mRNA precursor messenger ribonucleic acid

preop, pre-op preoperative

PREP phosphoribosylpyrophosphate; Physician Review and Enhancement Program

prep, prepd prepare, prepared

preserv preserve, preserved, preservation

press pressure

prev prevention, preventive; previous

PREVMEDU preventive medicine unit

PRF partial reinforcement; patient report form; perforin; plasma recognition factor; pontine reticular formation; progressive renal failure; prolactin releasing factor; pulse repetition frequency

pRF polyclonal rheumatoid factor

PRFM premature rupture of fetal membranes

PRG phleborheography; purge

PRGS phosphoribosylglycineamide synthetase

PRH past relevant history; prolactin releasing hormone

PRI Pain Rating Index; phosphate reabsorption index; phosphoribose isomerase; placental ribonuclease inhibitor

PRIAS Packard radioimmunoassay system

PRICE protection, relative rest, ice, compression, elevation

PRICEMM protection, relative rest, ice, compression, elevation, modalities, medication

PRICES protection, rest, ice, compression, elevation, support [primary treatment of tendinitis and overuse injury]; physician modalities, rehabilitation, injections, cross-training, evaluation, salicylates [secondary treatment of tendinitis and overuse injury]

PRIDE Parents Resource Institute for Drug Education

PRIH prolactin release-inhibiting hormone

PRIM primase

PRIME Prematriculation Program in Medical Education

PRIMEX primary care extender

primip primipara

PRIND prolonged reversible ischemic neurologic deficit

PRI(S) pain rating intensity score

PRIST paper radioimmunosorbent test

PRK photorefractive keratectomy; primary rabbit kidney

PRKAR protein kinase, cyclic adenosine monophosphate-dependent, regulatory

PRKAR1A protein kinase, cyclic adenosine monophosphate-dependent, regulatory, type 1 alpha

PRKC protein kinase C

PRKCA protein kinase C alpha

PRL, Prl prolactin

PRLR prolactin receptor

PRM phosphoribomutase; photoreceptor membrane; premature rupture of membranes; Primary Reference Material; protamine

PrM preventive medicine

PRN Physicians Research Network; polyradiculoneuropathy; prion

prn as required [Lat. *pro re nata*]

PRNP prion protein

PRNT plaque reduction neutralization test

PRO peer review organization; physician review organization; Professional Review Organization; pronation; protein

Pro proline; prophylactic; prothrombin

pro protein

ProACT professionally advanced care team

prob probable

PROC protein C

proc proceedings, procedure; process

PROC GLM general linear model procedure

proct, procto proctology, proctologist, proctoscopy

prod production, product

prog progress, progressive

progn prognosis

PROH propyl-4-hydrolase

PROHB propyl-4-hydrolase, beta

PROLOG programming in logic

prolong prolongation, prolonged

PROM passive range of motion; premature rupture of fetal membranes; prolonged rupture of fetal membranes; programmable read only memory; prosthetic range of motion

PROMIS Problem-Oriented Medical Information System

pron pronator, pronation

PROP propranolol

ProPAC Prospective Payment Assessment Commission

PRO-PBP pro-platelet basic protein

proph prophylactic, prophylaxis

PROS protein S

pros prostate, prostatic

PROSP protein S pseudogene

prosth prosthesis, prosthetic

PROTO protoporphyrin

prov provisional

prox proximal

PRP physiologic rest position; pityriasis rubra pilaris; platelet-rich plasma; polyribosyl ribitol phosphate; postural rest position; pressure rate product; primary Raynaud phenomenon; progressive rubella panencephalitis; proliferative retinopathy photocoagulation; proline-rich protein; Psychotic Reaction Profile; pulse repetition period

Prp prion protein

PRPH peripherin

PRPP phosphoribosyl pyrophosphate

PRPS prostatic secretory protein

PRQ personal resources questionnaire

PRR proton relaxation rate; pulse repetition rate

PrR progesterone receptor

PRRB Provider Reimbursement Review Board

PRRE pupils round, regular, and equal

PRRF paramedian pontine reticular formation

PR-RSV Prague Rous sarcoma virus

PRS Personality Rating Scale; Pierre Robin syndrome; plasma renin substrate; proctorectosigmoidoscopy

PRSIS Prospective Rate Setting Information System

PRT *Penicillium roqueforti* toxin; pharmaceutical research and testing; phosphoribosyl transferase; postoperative respiratory therapy; prospective randomized trial

PRTH pituitary resistance to thyroid hormone

PRTH-C prothrombin time control

PRTN proteinase

PRTS Partington syndrome

PRU peripheral resistance unit

PRV polycythemia rubra vera; pseudorabies virus

PRVEP pattern reversal visual evoked potential

PRW polymerized ragweed

PRX pseudoexfoliation

Prx prognosis

prx proximal

PRZF pyrazofurin

PS pacemaker syndrome; paired stimulation; paradoxical sleep; paraspinal; parasympathetic; Parkinson syndrome; parotid sialography; partial saturation; partial seizure; pathological stage; patient's serum; pediatric surgery; performing scale [I.Q.]; periodic syndrome; pferdestärke (German for horsepower); phosphate saline [buffer]; phosphatidyl serine; photosensitivity, photosensitization; photosynthesis; phrenic stimulation; physical status; physiologic saline; plastic surgery; polysaccharide; polystyrene; population sample; Porter-Silber [chromogen]; prescription; presenting symptom; prostatic secretion; proteasome; protein synthesis; protamine sulfate; protein S; Proteus syndrome; psychiatric; pulmonary stenosis; pyloric stenosis

P/S polisher-stimulator; polyunsaturated/saturated [fatty acid ratio]

P&S paracentesis and suction

Ps prescription; *Pseudomonas;* psoriasis

ps per second; picosecond

PSA parasternal short axis; pleomorphic salivary gland adenoma; polyethylene sulfonic acid; polysaccharide adhesin; posterior spinal artery; professional services agreement; progressive spinal ataxia; prolonged sleep apnea; prostate specific antigen; protein S alpha; psoriatic arthritis

Psa systemic blood pressure

PSAC President's Science Advisory Committee

PSACH pseudoachondrodysplasia

PSAD prostate-specific antigen density

PSAG pelvic sonoangiography

PSAGN poststreptococcal acute glomerulonephritis

PSAn psychoanalysis
PSAP primary public safety answering point; prosaposin; pulmonary surfactant apoprotein
PSB protected specimen brush; protein S beta
PSbetaG pregnancy-specific beta-1-glycoprotein
PSBG pregnancy-specific beta-1-glycoprotein
PSC patient services coordination; Porter-Silber chromogen; posterior subcapsular cataract; primary sclerosing cholangitis; professional service corporation; proteasome component; pulse synchronized contractions
PsChE pseudocholinesterase
PSCI Primary Self Concept Inventory
Psci pressure at slow component intercept
PSCT peripheral stem cell transplantation
PSD particle size distribution; peptone, starch, and dextrose; periodic synchronous discharge; phase-sensitive detector; poststenosis dilation; postsynaptic density; power spectrum density
PSDA Patient Self-Determination Act; psychoactive substance abuse and dependence
PSDES primary symptomatic diffuse esophageal spasm
PSE paradoxical systolic expansion; penicillin-sensitive enzyme; portal systemic encephalopathy; Present State Examination; purified spleen extract
psec picosecond
PSEK progressive symmetrical erythrokeratoderma
PSF peak scatter factor; peptide supply factor; point spread function; pseudosarcomatous fasciitis
PSG peak systolic gradient; phosphate, saline, and glucose; polysomnogram; presystolic gallop; pregnancy-specific glycoprotein

PSGN poststreptococcal glomerulonephritis
PSH past surgical history; postspinal headache
PsHD pseudoheart disease
PSI posterior sagittal index; problem solving information; prostaglandin synthetic inhibitor; psychological services index; psychosomatic inventory
psi pounds per square inch
ψ Greek letter *psi*; wave function
psia pounds per square inch absolute
PSICU pediatric surgical intensive care unit
pSIDS partially unexplained sudden infant death syndrome
PSIFT platelet suspension immunofluorescence test
PSIL preferred frequency speech interference level
PSIS posterior sacroiliac spine
PSK protein serine kinase
PSL parasternal line; photostimulable luminescence; potassium, sodium chloride, and sodium lactate [solution]; prednisolone
PSM postmitochondrial supernatant; presystolic murmur
PSMA proximal spinal muscular atrophy
PSMed psychosomatic medicine
PSMF protein-sparing modified fast
PSMT psychiatric services management team
PSMS physical self-maintenance scale
PSN provider-sponsored network
PSO proximal subungual onychomycosis
PSP pancreatic spasmolytic peptide; paralytic shellfish poisoning; parathyroid secretory protein; periodic short pulse; phenolsulfonphthalein; phosphoserine phosphatase; photostimulable phosphor plate; positive spike pattern; posterior spinal process; postsynaptic potential; prednisone sodium phosphate; progressive supranuclear palsy; prostatic

secretory protein; pseudopregnancy; pulmonary surfactant apoprotein

PSPS secretory pancreatic stone protein

PSQ Parent Symptom Questionnaire; Patient Satisfaction Questionnaire

PSR pain sensitivity range; perspective surface rendering; portal systemic resistance; proliferative sickle retinopathy; pulmonary stretch receptor

PSRC Plastic Surgery Research Council

PSRO Professional Standards Review Organization

PSS painful shoulder syndrome; physiologic saline solution; porcine stress syndrome; primary Sjögren syndrome; progressive systemic scleroderma; progressive systemic sclerosis; psoriasis severity scale; Psychiatric Status Schedule; pure sensory stroke

pSS primary Sjögren syndrome

PST pancreatic suppression test; paroxysmal supraventricular tachycardia; penicillin, streptomycin, and tetracycline; peristimulus time; phenolsulfotransferase; platelet survival time; poststenotic; poststimulus time; prefrontal sonic treatment; protein-sparing therapy; proximal straight tubule

PSTI pancreatic secretory trypsin inhibitor

PSTV potato spindle tuber virus

PSU photosynthetic unit; primary sampling unit

PSurg plastic surgery

PSV pressure-support ventilation

PSVER pattern shift visual evoked response

PSVT paroxysmal supraventricular tachycardia

PSW primary surgical ward; positive sharp wave; psychiatric social worker

PSWT psychiatric social work training

PSX pseudoexfoliation

Psy psychiatry; psychology

psych psychology, psychological

psychiat psychiatry, psychiatric

psychoan psychoanalysis, psychoanalytical

psychol psychology, psychological

psychopath psychopathology, psychopathological

psychosom psychosomatic

psychother psychotherapy

psy-path psychopathic

Ps-ZES pseudo-Zollinger-Ellison syndrome

PT pain threshold; parathormone; parathyroid; paroxysmal tachycardia; part time; patient; pericardial tamponade; permanent and total; pharmacy and therapeutics; phenytoin; photophobia; phototoxicity; physical therapy, physical therapist; physical training; physiotherapy; pine tar; plasma thromboplastin; pneumothorax; polyvalent tolerance; position tracking; posterior tibial [artery pulse]; posttetanic; posttransfusion; posttransplantation; posttraumatic; premature termination [of pregnancy]; preoperative therapy; preterm; propylthiouracil; protamine; prothrombin time; proton density; pulmonary tuberculosis; psychotherapy; pulmonary thrombosis; pyramidal tract; temporal plane

P&T permanent and total [disability]; pharmacy and therapeutics

Pt patient; platinum

pt part; patient; pint; point

PTA parallel tubular arrays; parathyroid adenoma; percutaneous transluminal angioplasty; peroxidase-labeled antibody; persistent truncus arteriosus; phosphotungstic acid; physical therapy assistant; plasma thromboplastin antecedent; posttraumatic amnesia; pretreatment anxiety; prior to admission; prior to arrival; prothrombin activity

PTAF platelet activating factor

PTAFR platelet activating factor receptor

PTAH phosphotungstic acid hematoxylin

PTAP purified diphtheria toxoid precipitated by aluminum phosphate

PTAT pure tone average threshold

PTB patellar tendon bearing; prior to birth

PTb pulmonary tuberculosis

PTBA percutaneous transluminal balloon angioplasty

PTBD percutaneous transhepatic biliary drainage; percutaneous transluminal balloon dilatation

PTBE pyretic tick-borne encephalitis

PTBNA protected transbronchial needle aspirate

PTBPD posttraumatic borderline personality disorder

PTBS posttraumatic brain syndrome

PTC papillary thyroid carcinoma; percutaneous transhepatic cholangiography; phase transfer catalyst; phenothiocarbazine; phenylthiocarbamide; phenylthiocarbamoyl; plasma thromboplastin component; posttetanic count; premature tricuspid closure; prior to conception; prothrombin complex; pseudotumor cerebri

PTCA percutaneous transluminal coronary angioplasty

PtcCO$_2$ transcutaneous partial pressure of carbon dioxide

PTCER pulmonary transcapillary escape rate

PtcO$_2$ transcutaneous oxygen tension

PTCR percutaneous transluminal coronary recanalization

PTCRA percutaneous transluminal coronary rotational ablation

PTD percutaneous transluminal dilatation; permanent total disability; personality trait disorder; preterm delivery; prior to delivery

PTE parathyroid extract; posttraumatic epilepsy; pretibial edema; proximal tibial epiphysis; pulmonary thromboembolism

PTED pulmonary thromboembolic disease

PteGlu pteroylglutamic acid

PTEN pentaerythritol tetranitrate

pter end of short arm of chromosome

PTF patient treatment file; plasma thromboplastin factor; posterior talofibular [ligament]; proximal tubular fragment

PTFA prothrombin time fixing agent

PTFE polytetrafluoroethylene

PTFNA percutaneous transthoracic fine-needle aspiration

PTFS posttraumatic fibromyalgia syndrome

PTG parathyroid gland; prostaglandin

PTGE prostaglandin E

PTGER prostaglandin E receptor

PTH parathormone; parathyroid; parathyroid hormone; percutaneous transhepatic drainage; phenylthiohydantoin; plasma thromboplastin component; posttransfusion hepatitis

PTHC percutaneous transhepatic cholangiography

PTHL parathyroid hormone-like

PTHLP parathyroid-hormone-like protein

PTHR parathyroid hormone receptor

PTHRP, PTHrP parathyroid-hormone-related peptide; parathyroid-hormone-related protein

PTHS parathyroid hormone secretion [rate]

PTI pancreatic trypsin inhibitor; persistent tolerant infection; Pictorial Test of Intelligence; placental thrombin inhibitor; pulsatility transmission index

PTK protein-tyrosine kinase

PTL peritoneal telencephalic leukoencephalomyopathy; pharyngotracheal lumen; plasma thyroxine level posterior tricuspid leaflet; preterm labor

PTLA pharyngeal tracheal lumen airway

PTLC precipitation thin-layer chromatography

PTLD posttransplanatation lymphoproliferative disorder; prescribed tumor lethal dose

PTM posterior trabecular meshwork; posttransfusion mononucleosis; posttraumatic meningitis; prothymosin; pulse time modulation

Ptm pterygomaxillary [fissure]

PTMA phenyltrimethylammonium; prothymosin alpha

PTMDF pupils, tension, media, disc, fundus

PTMPY per thousand members per year

PTMS parathymosin

PTN pain transmission neuron; pleiotrophin; posterior tibial nerve

pTNM TNM (see p. 383) staging of tumors as determined by correlation of clinical, pathologic, and residual findings

PTO Klemperer's tuberculin [Ger. *Perlsucht Tuberculin Original*]

PTP pancreatic thread protein; percutaneous transhepatic portography; physical treatment planning; posterior tibial pulse; posttetanic potential; posttransfusion purpura; protein-tyrosine phosphatase; proximal tubular pressure

Ptp transpulmonary pressure

PTPC protein-tyrosine phosphatase C

PTPG protein-tyrosine phosphatase gamma

PTPI posttraumatic pulmonary insufficiency

PTPM post-traumatic progressive myelopathy

PTPN protein-tyrosine phosphatase, non-receptor

PTPRA protein-tyrosine phosphatase receptor alpha

PTPRB protein-tyrosine phosphatase receptor beta

PTPRF protein-tyrosine phosphatase receptor F

PTPRG protein-tyrosine phosphatase receptor gamma

PTPS postthrombophlebitis syndrome; 6-pyruvoyl tetrahydropterin synthase

PTPT protein-tyrosine phosphatase, T-cell

PTQ parent-teacher questionnaire

PTR patellar tendon reflex; patient termination record; patient to return; peripheral total resistance; plasma transfusion reaction; prothrombin time ratio; psychotic trigger reaction

PTr porcine trypsin

Ptr intratracheal pressure

PTRA percutaneous transluminal renal angioplasty

PT Rep patient's representative

PTRIA polystyrene-tube radioimmunoassay

Ptrx pelvic traction

PTS para-toluenesulfonic acid; postthrombotic syndrome; posttraumatic syndrome; Pressure and Tension Scale; prior to surgery; 6-pyruvoyl tetrahydropterin synthase

Pts, pts patients

PTSD posttraumatic stress disorder

PTSH poststimulus time histogram

PTSM Plant, Technology and Safety Management

PTSS posttraumatic stress syndrome

PTT partial thromboplastin time; particle transport time; posterior tibial tendon (transfer); prothrombin time; pulmonary transit time; pulse transmission time

ptt partial thromboplastin time

PTU propylthiouracil

PTV planning target volume; posterior tibial vein

PTV$_2$ planning target volume 2

PTX pentoxifylline; picrotoxinin; pneumothorax

PTx parathyroidectomy; pelvic traction

Ptx pneumothorax

PTZ pentylenetetrazol

PU palindromic unit; passed urine; pepsin unit; peptic ulcer; pregnancy urine; 6-propyluracil; prostatic urethra

Pu plutonium; purine; purple

PUA patient unit assistant

pub public

PUBS percutaneous umbilical blood sampling; purple urine bag syndrome

PUC pediatric urine collector; premature uterine contractions

PUD peptic ulcer disease; pudendal

PuD pulmonary disease

PUF pure ultrafiltration

PUFA polyunsaturated fatty acid

PUH pregnancy urine hormones

PUI platelet uptake index

PUJO pelvi-ureteric junction obstruction

PUL percutaneous ultrasonic lithotripsy

PUL, pul, pulm pulmonary

PULHEMS physique, upper extremity, lower extremity, hearing and ears, eyes and vision, mental capacity, emotional stability [profile]

PULSES physical condition, upper limb function, lower limb function, sensory component, excretory function, mental and status (or support factors in revised version) [profile]

PUM peanut-reactive urinary mucin

PUMP putative metalloproteinase

PUMS patient utility measurement set; permanently unfit for military service

PUN plasma urea nitrogen

PUO pyrexia of unknown origin

PUPPP pruritic urticarial papules and plaques of pregnancy

PUR polyurethrane

Pur purple

pur purulent

purg purgative

PUT provocative use test; putamen

PUU puumala [virus]

PUV posterior urethral valve

PUVA psoralen ultraviolet A-range

PV pancreatic vein; papillomavirus; paraventricular; paravertebral; pemphigus vulgaris; peripheral vascular; peripheral vein; peripheral vessel; pityriasis versicolor; plasma viscosity; plasma volume; polio vaccine; polycythemia vera; polyoma virus; polyvinyl; portal vein; postvasectomy; postvoiding; predictive value; pressure velocity; process variable; pulmonary valve; pulmonary vein

P-V pressure-volume [curve]

P&V pyloroplasty and vagotomy

Pv *Proteus vulgaris*; venous pressure

PVA Paralyzed Veterans of America; peripheral venous alimentation; polyvinyl acetate; polyvinyl alcohol; pressure volume area

PVAc polyvinyl acetate

PVALB parvalbumin

PVB cis-platinum, vinblastine, bleomycin; paravertebral block; premature ventricular beat

PVC peripheral venous catheterization; persistent vaginal cornification; polyvinyl chloride; postvoiding cystogram; predicted vital capacity; premature ventricular contraction; primary visual cortex; pulmonary venous confluence; pulmonary venous congestion

PVCM paradoxical vocal cord motion

PV$_{CO2}$ partial pressure of carbon dioxide in mixed venous blood

PVD patient very disturbed; peripheral vascular disease; portal vein dilation; posterior vitreous detachment; postural vertical dimension; premature ventricular depolarization; pulmonary vascular disease

PVDF polyvinylidene difluoride; polyvinyl diisopropyl fluoride

PVE premature ventricular extrasystole; prosthetic valve endocarditis

P-VEP pattern visual evoked potential

PVF peripheral visual field; portal venous flow; primary ventricular fibrillation

PVFS postviral fatigue syndrome
PVG pulmonary valve gradient
PVH periventricular hemorrhage; pulmonary venous hypertension
PVI patient video interview; peripheral vascular insufficiency; perivascular infiltration; positron volume imaging
PVK penicillin V potassium
PVL perivalvular leakage; permanent vision loss
PVM pneumonia virus of mice; proteins, vitamins, and minerals
PVMed preventive medicine
PVN paraventricular nucleus; predictive value negative
PVNPS post-Viet Nam psychiatric syndrome
PVNS pigmented villonodular synovitis
PVO pulmonary venous obstruction
PV$_{O2}$ partial oxygen pressure in mixed venous blood
PVOD pulmonary vascular obstructive disease; pulmonary veno-occlusive disease
PVP penicillin V potassium; peripheral vein plasma; peripheral venous pressure; polyvinylpyrrolidone; portal venous pressure; predictive value of positive results; pulmonary venous pressure
PVP-I polyvinylpyrrolidone-iodine
PVR peripheral vascular resistance; perspective volume rendering; poliovirus receptor; postvoiding residual; pulpulmonary valve replacement or repair; monary vascular resistance; pulse volume recording
PVRI pulmonary vascular resistance index
PVS percussion, vibration, suction; persistent vegetative state; persistent viral syndrome; Plummer-Vinson syndrome; poliovirus susceptibility; polyvinyl sponge; premature ventricular systole; programmed ventricular stimulation; pulmonary valvular stenosis

PVT paroxysmal ventricular tachycardia; portal vein thrombosis; pressure, volume, and temperature; private patient; psychomotor vigilance task
PVW posterior vaginal wall
PVY potato virus Y
pvz pulverization
PW peristaltic wave; plantar wart; posterior wall [of the heart]; pressure wave; psychological warfare; pulmonary wedge [pressure]; pulsed wave
Pw progesterone withdrawal
PWB partial weight bearing
PWBC peripheral white blood cell
PWBRT prophylactic whole brain radiation therapy
PWC peak work capacity; physical work capacity
PWCA pure white cell aplasia
PWCR Prader-Willi chromosome region
pwd powder
PWDS postweaning diarrhea syndrome
PWE posterior wall excursion
PWI posterior wall infarct
PWLV posterior wall of left ventricle
PWM pokeweed mitogen; pulse with modulation
PWP pulmonary wedge pressure
PWS port wine stain; Prader-Willi syndrome
PWT physician waiting time; posterior wall thickness
pwt pennyweight
PWV pulse wave velocity
PX pancreatectomized; peroxidase; physical examination
Px past history; physical examination; pneumothorax; prognosis
PXA pleomorphic xanthoastrocytoma
PXE pseudoxanthoma elasticum
PXM projection x-ray microscopy; pseudoexfoliation material
PXMP peroxysomal membrane protein
PXS pseudoexfoliation syndrome
PXT piroxantrone

Py phosphopyridoxal; polyoma [virus]; pyridine; pyridoxal
PYA psychoanalysis
PyC pyogenic culture
PYCR pyrroline-5-carboxylate reductase
PYE peptone yeast extract
PYG peptone-yeast extract-glucose [broth]
PYGM peptone-yeast-glucose-maltose [broth]
PYLL potential years of life lost
PYM psychosomatic
PYP pyrophosphate
Pyr pyridine; pyruvate

PyrP pyridoxal phosphate
PZ pancreozymin; pregnancy zone; proliferative zone; protamine zinc
Pz 4-phenylazobenzylcarbonyl; parietal midline electrode placement in electroencephalography
pz pièze
PZA pyrazinamide
PZ-CCK pabcreozymin-cholecystokinin
PZE piezoelectric
PZI protamine zinc insulin
PZP pregnancy zone protein
PZQ praziquantel
PZT lead zirconate titanate

Q cardiac output; coulomb [electric quantity]; electric charge; flow; 1,4-glucan branching enzyme; glutamine; heat; qualitative; quality; quantity; quart; quartile; Queensland [fever]; query [fever]; question; quinacrine; quinidine; quinone; quotient; radiant energy; reactive power; reaction energy; temperative coefficient; see QRS [wave]

Q_{10} temperature coefficient

q each, every [Lat. *quaque*]; electric charge; long arm of chromosome; quart; quintal

QA quality assessment; quality assurance

QAC quaternary ammonium compound

QACC quality assurance coordination committee

QAF quality adjustment factor

QA&I quality assessment and improvement

QALE quality-adjusted life expectancy

QALPACS quality patient care scale

QALY quality-adjusted life year

QAM quality assurance monitoring

QAP quality assurance program or professional; quinine, atabrine, and pamaquine

QAR quantitative autoradiography

QARANC Queen Alexandra's Royal Army Nursing Corps

QARNNS Queen Alexandra's Royal Naval Nursing Service

QAS quality assurance standard

QAUR quality assurance and utilization review

QB whole blood

Q_B total body clearance

QBIC query by image content

QBV whole blood volume

QC quality characteristics; quality control; quinine colchicine

Qc pulmonary capillary blood flow

QCIM Quarterly Cumulative Index Medicus

Q_{CO_2} carbon dioxide evolution by a tissue

QCT quantitative computed tomography

QD Qi deficiency

qd every day [Lat. *quaque die*]

QDPR quinoid dihydropteridine reductase

qds to be taken four times a day [Lat. *quater die sumendum*]

QED quantum electrodynamics

QEE quadriceps extension exercise

QEEG, qEEG quantitative electroencephalography

QEF quail embryo fibroblasts

QENF quantifying examination of neurologic function

QEONS Queen Elizabeth's Overseas Nursery Service

QEW quick early warning

QF quality factor; query fever; quick freeze; relative biological effectiveness

QFES Quality Feedback Expert System

Q fever query fever

qh every hour [Lat. *quaque hora*]

q2h every two hours [Lat. *quaque secunda hora*]

q3h every three hours [Lat. *quaque tertia hora*]

q4h every four hours [Lat. *quaque quarta hora*]

QHDS Queen's Honorary Dental Surgeon

QHNS Queen's Honorary Nursing Sister

QHP Queen's Honorary Physician

QHS Queen's Honorary Surgeon

qhs every hour of sleep [Lat. *quaque hora somni*]

QI quality improvement; quality indicator

qid four times daily [Lat. *quater in die*]
QIDN Queen's Institute of District Nursing
QIN quality improvement network
QIP quality improvement project
QJ quadriceps jerk
QL quality of life
ql as much as desired [Lat. *quantum libet*]
Q-LES-Q Quality of Life Enjoyment and Satisfaction Questionnaire
QLQ quality of life questionnaire
QLQ-C quality of life questionnaire-cancer
QLS Quality of Life Scale; quasielastic light-scattering spectroscopy
QM quality management; quinacrine mustard
qm every morning [Lat. *quaque mane*]
QMB qualified Medicare beneficiary
QMF quadrature mirror filter
QMI Q-wave myocardial infarction
QMP Quality Management Program
QMR quick medical reference
QMT quantitative muscle test
QMWS quasi-morphine withdrawal syndrome
qn every night [Lat. *quaque nocte*]
QNB quinuclidinyl benzilate
QNS Queen's Nursing Sister
qns quantity not sufficient
Qo oxygen consumption
Q$_{O_2}$ oxygen quotient; oxygen utilization
Q$_o$ flow at origin
qod every other day [Lat. *quaque altera die*]
qoh every other hour [Lat. *quaque altera hora*]
qon every other night [Lat. *quaque altera nocte*]
QOL quality of life
QOLI quality of life index
QOLI-P quality of life index-Padilla
QLOQ quality of life questionnaire
QoS quality of service

QP quanti-Pirquet [reaction]
Qp pulmonary blood flow
qp as much as desired [Lat. *quantum placeat*]
QPC quality of patient care
Qpc pulmonary capillary blood flow
QPEEG quantitative pharmaco-electroencephalography
qPM every night
qq each, every [Lat. *quoque*]
qqd every day [Lat. *quoque die*]
qqh every four hours [Lat. *quaque quarta hora*]
qq hor every hour [Lat. *quaque hora*]
QR quality review; quantity is correct [Lat. *quantum rectum*]; quieting response; quinaldine red
qr quadriradial; quantity is correct [Lat. *quantum rectum*]; quarter
QRB Quality Review Bulletin
QRM quality and resource management
QRS in electrocardiography, the complex consisting of Q, R, and S waves, corresponding to depolarization of ventricles [complex]; in electrocardiography, the loop traced by QRS vectors, representing ventricular depolarization [interval]
QRS-ST the junction between the QRS complex and the ST segment in the electrocardiogram [junction]
QRS-T the angle between the QRS and T vectors in vectorcardiography [angle]
QRZ wheal reaction time [Ger. *Qaddel Reaktion Zeit*]
QS question screening; quiet sleep
Qs systemic blood flow
Q$_s$ systemic blood flow
qs as much as will suffice [Lat. *quantum sufficit*]; sufficient quantity [Lat. *quantum satis*]
QSAR quantitative structure-activity relationship
QSART quantitative sudomotor axon reflex testing

QSPV quasistatic pressure volume
QSS quantitative sacroiliac scintigraphy
QST quantitative sensory test
QT cardiac output; Quick test
Q-T in electrocardiography, the time from the beginning of the QRS complex to the end of the T wave [interval]
qt quantity; quart; quiet
QTc Q-T interval corrected for heart rate
Q-Tc corrected Q-T [interval]
qter end of long arm of chromosome
Q-TWIST quality-adjusted time without symptoms of disease and subjective toxic effects of treatment
quad quadrant; quadriceps; quadriplegic
quadrupl four times as much [Lat. *quadruplicato*]
qual quality, qualitative
quant quantity, quantitative

quar quarintine
QUART quadrantectomy, axillary dissection, radiotherapy
Quat, quat four [Lat. *quattuor*]
QUEST Quality, Utilization, Effectiveness, Statistically Tabulated
QUICHA quantitative inhalation challenge apparatus
quinq five [Lat. *quinque*]
quint fifth, quintan [Lat. *quintus*]
quot quotient
quotid daily, quotidian [Lat. *quotidie*]
quot op sit as often as necessary [Lat. *quoties opus sit*]
qv as much as you desire [Lat. *quantum vis*]; which see [Lat. *quod vide*]
QWB quality of well-being [questionnaire, scale, or index]
QYD Qi and Yin deficiency

R arginine; Behnken unit; Broadbent registration point; a conjugative plasmid responsible for resistance to various elements; any chemical group (particularly an alfyl group); electrical resistance; far point [Lat. *remotum*]; in electrocardiography, the first positive deflection during the QRS complex [wave]; gas constant; organic radical; race; racemic; radioactive; radiology; radius; ramus; Rankine [scale]; rate; ratio; reaction; Réaumur [scale]; rectal; rectified; red; registered trademark; regression coefficient; regular; regular insulin; regulator [gene]; rejection factor; relapse; relaxation; release [factor]; remission; remote; repressor; residue; resistance; respiration; respiratory exchange ratio; response; responder; rest; restricted; reverse [banding]; rhythm; ribose; *Rickettsia*; right; Rinne [test]; roentgen; rough [colony]; rub

R′ in electrocardiography, the second positive deflection during the QRS complex

R+ Rinne test positive

+R Rinne test positive

−R Rinne test negative

°R degree on the Rankine scale; degree on the Réaumur scale

R1, R2, R3, etc. years of resident study

r correlation coefficient; density; radius; ratio; recombinant; regional; ribose; ribosomal; ring chromosome; roentgen; sample correlation coefficient

r^2 coefficient of determination

ρ see *rho*

RA radioactive; ragocyte; ragweed antigen; rapidly adapting [receptors]; reactive arthritis; reciprocal asymmetrical; refractory anemia; refractory ascites; renal artery; renin-angiotensin; repeat action; residual air; retinoic acid; rheumatoid arthritis; right angle; right arm; right atrium; right auricle; rotation angiography; Roy adaptation [model]

R_A airway resistance

Ra radial; radium; radius

rA riboadenylate

RAA renin-angiotensin-aldosterone [system]

RAAMC Royal Australian Army Medical Corps

RAAS renin-angiotensin-aldosterone system

RAB remote afterloading brachytherapy

RABA rabbit antibladder antibody

Rab rabbit

RAC research appraisal checklist

rac racemate, racemic

RACE rapid amplification of complementary deoxyribonucleic acid ends

RAD radial artery catheter; radiation absorbed dose; radical; radiography or radiographic; reactive airways disease; right atrium diameter; right axis deviation; roentgen administered dose

Rad radiology; radiotherapy; radium

rad radiation absorbed dose; radial; radian; radical; radius; root [Lat. *radix*]

RADA rosin amine-D-acetate

RADAI rheumatoid arthritis disease activity index

RADAR rapid assessment of disease activity in rheumatology

RADC Royal Army Dental Corps

RADIO radiotherapy

radiol radiology

RadLV radiation leukemia virus

RADP right acromiodorsoposterior

RADS reactive airways dysfunction syndrome; retrospective assessment of drug safety

rad/s rad per second; radian per second

rad ther radiation therapy

RADTS rabbit antidog thymus serum

RADTT radiation therapy technologist

RAE right atrial enlargement

RAEB refractory anemia with excess blasts

RAEBiT, RAEB-T refractory anemia with excess blasts in transformation

RAEM refractory anemia with excess myeloblasts

RAF repetitive atrial firing; rheumatoid arthritis factor

RAFMS Royal Air Force Medical Services

RAFW right atrial free wall

RAG ragweed; recombination activating gene

RAGE rapid gradient echo

Ragg rheumatoid agglutinin

RAH regressing atypical histiocytosis; right atrial hypertrophy

RAHO rabbit antibody to human ovary

RAHTG rabbit antihuman thymocyte globulin

RAI radioactive iodine; radioactive isotope; resident assessment instrument; resting ankle index; right atrial inversion; right atrial involvement

RAID radioimmunodetection

RAIS reflection-absorption infrared spectroscopy

RAITI right atrial inversion time index

RAIU radioactive iodine uptake

RALPH renal-anal-lung-polydactyly-hamartoblastoma [syndrome]

RALT routine admission laboratory tests

RAM random-access memory; rapid alternating movements; rectus abdominis muscle; rectus abdominis myocutaneous [flap]; reduced acquisition matrix; research aviation medicine; resource allocation methodology; right anterior measurement

RAMC Royal Army Medical Corps

RAM-FAST reduced acquisition matrix-Fourier acquired steady state

RAMP radioactive antigen microprecipitin; right atrial mean pressure

RAMT rabbit antimouse thymocyte

RANA rheumatoid arthritis nuclear antigen

RAN resident's admission notes

rANP rat atrial natriuretic peptide

RAO right anterior oblique

RaONC radiation oncology

RAP recurrent abdominal pain; regression-associated protein; renal artery pressure; resident assessment protocol; rheumatoid arthritis precipitin; right atrial pressure

RAPD relative afferent pupillary defect

RAPK reticulate acropigmentation of Kitamura

RAPM refractory anemia with partial myeloblastosis

RAPO rabbit antibody to pig ovary

RAPs radiologists, anesthesiologists, and pathologists

RAR rapidly adapting receptor; rat insulin receptor; retinoic acid receptor; right arm reclining; right arm recumbent

RARA retinoic acid receptor alpha

RARB retinoic acid receptor beta

RARE rapid acquisition with relaxation enhancement

RARG retinoic acid receptor gamma

RARLS rabbit anti-rat lymphocyte serum

RARS refractory anemia with ring sideroblasts

RARTS rabbit anti-rat thymocyte serum

RAS rapid atrial stimulation; recurrent aphthous stomatitis; reflex activating stimulus; reliability, availability, serviceability; renal artery stenosis; renin-angiotensin system; residency application service; reticular activating system; rheumatoid arthritis serum

RA-S refractory anemia with ringed sideroblasts

ras retrovirus-associated DNA sequence

RASS rheumatoid arthritis and Sjögren syndrome

RAST radioallergosorbent test

RAT repeat action tablet; rheumatoid arthritis test

RATG rabbit antithymocyte globulin

RATHAS rat thymus antiserum

rAT-P recombinant antitrypsin Pittsburgh

RATx radiation therapy

RAU radioactive uptake

RAV Rous-associated virus

RAVC retrograde atrioventricular conduction; Royal Army Veterinary Corps

RAVLT Rey Auditory Verbal Learning Test

RAW right atrial wall

Raw airway resistance

R$_{AW}$ airway resistance

RAWTS ribonucleic acid amplification with transcript sequencing

RAZ razoxane

RB radiation burn; rating board; rebreathing; reticulate body; retinoblastoma; right bronchus; right bundle

Rb retinoblastoma; rubidium

RBA relative binding affinity; rescue breathing apparatus; right basilar artery; right brachial artery; rose bengal antigen

RBAP repetitive bursts of action potential

RBAS rostral basilar artery syndrome

RBB right bundle branch

RBBB right bundle-branch block

RBBP retinoblastoma binding protein

RBBsB right bundle-branch system block

RBBx right breast biopsy

RBC red blood cell; red blood corpuscle; red blood count

rbc red blood cell

RBCD right border cardiac dullness

rBCG recombinant bacille Calmette-Guérin [vaccine]

RBCM red blood cell mass

RBCV red blood cell volume

RBD recurrent brief depression; relative biological dose; right border of dullness

RBE relative biological effectiveness

RBF regional blood flow; regional bone mass; renal blood flow

RBI radiographic baseline

Rb Imp rubber base impression

RBL rat basophilic leukemia; Reid baseline; retinoblastoma-like

RBN retrobulbar neuritis

RBNA Royal British Nurses Association

RBOW rupture of the bag of waters

RBP retinol-binding protein; riboflavin-binding protein

RBPC cellular retinol-binding protein

RBPI intestinal retinol-binding protein

RBRVS resource-based relative value scale

RBS random blood sugar; Roberts syndrome; Rutherford backscattering

RbSA rabbit serum albumin

RBTN rhombotin

RBTNL rhombotin-like

RBV right brachial vein

RBW relative body weight

RBZ rubidazone

RC an electronic circuit containing a resistor and capacitor in series; radiocarpal; reaction center; recrystallization; red cell; red cell casts; red corpuscle; Red Cross; referred care; regenerated cellulose; rehabilitation counseling; residential care; respiration ceases; respiratory care; respiratory center; respiratory compensation; rest cure; retention catheter; retrograde cystogram; rib cage; root canal; routine cholecystography

R&C resistance and capacitance

Rc conditioned response; receptor

RCA red cell agglutination; relative chemotactic activity; renal cell carcinoma; right carotid artery; right coronary artery

RCAMC Royal Canadian Army Medical Corps

rCBF regional cerebral blood flow

rCBV regional cerebral blood volume

RCC radiological control center; rape crisis center; ratio of cost to charges; receptor-chemoeffector complex; red cell cast; red cell count; regulator of chromosome condensation; renal cell carcinoma; right common carotid

rcc right coronary cusp

RCCM Regional Committee for Community Medicine

RCCP renal cell carcinoma, papillary

RCCT randomized controlled clinical trial

RCD relative cardiac dullness

RCDA recurrent chronic dissecting aneurysm

RCDP rhizomelic chondrodysplasia punctata

RCDR relative corrected death rate

RCE reasonable compensation equivalent

RCF red cell ferritin; red cell folate; relative centrifugal field/force; ristocetin cofactor

RCG radioelectrocardiography

RCGP Royal College of General Practitioners

RCH rectocolic hemorrhage

RCHF right congestive heart failure

RCHMS Regional Committee for Hospital Medical Services

RCI respiratory control index

RCIA red cell immune adherence

RCIRF radiologic contrast-induced renal failure

RCIT red cell iron turnover

RCITR red cell iron turnover rate

RCL renal clearance

RCM radial contour model; radiographic contrast medium; red cell mass; reinforced clostridial medium; replacement culture medium; right costal margin; Royal College of Midwives

rCMRGlc regional cerebral metabolic rate for glucose

rCMRO$_2$ regional cerebral metabolic rate for oxygen

RCN right caudate nucleus; Royal College of Nursing

RCoF ristocetin cofactor

RCOG Royal College of Obstetricians and Gynaecologists

RCP red cell protoporphyrin; retrocorneal pigmentation; riboflavin carrier protein; Royal College of Physicians

rCP regional cerebral perfusion

rcp reciprocal translocation

RCPath Royal College of Pathologists

RCPH red cell peroxide hemolysis

RCPSGlas Royal College of Physicians and Surgeons, Glasgow

RCR relative consumption rate; replication-competent retrovirus; respiratory control ratio

RCRA Resource Conservation and Recovery Act

RCS rabbit aorta-contracting substance; red cell suspension; reticulum cell sarcoma; right coronary sinus; Royal College of Science; Royal College of Surgeons

RCSE Royal College of Surgeons, Edinburgh

RCSSS resource coordination system for surgical service

RCT radiotherapy and chemotherapy; randomized clinical trial; randomized controlled trial; registered care technologist; retrograde conduction time; root canal therapy; Rorschach content test; rotator cuff tear

rct a marker showing the ability of virulent strains to replicate at 40°C, while vaccine strain shows no replication

RCU respiratory care unit

RCV recoverin; red cell volume

RCVS Royal College of Veterinary Surgeons

RD radial deviation; radiology department; rate difference; Raynaud disease; reaction of degeneration; registered dietitian; Reiter disease; related donor; renal disease; resistance determinant; respiratory disease; retinal degeneration; retinal detachment; Reye disease; rheumatoid disease; right deltoid; Riley-Day [syndrome]; Rolland-Desbuquois [syndrome]; rubber dam; ruminal drinking; ruptured disk

Rd rate of disappearance

rd rutherford

R&D research and develpment

RDA recommended daily allowance; recommended dietary allowance; Registered Dental Assistant; right dorsoanterior [fetal position]

RDB random double-blind [trial]

RDBMS relational database management system

RDBP RD [gene] binding protein

RDC research diagnostic criteria

RDDA recommended daily dietary allowance

RDDP ribonucleic acid-dependent deoxynucleic acid polymerase

RDE receptor-destroying enzyme

RDE_D radiation dose required

RDES remote data entry system

RDFC recurring digital fibroma of childhood

RDH Registered Dental Hygienist

RDHBF regional distribution of hepatic blood flow

RDI recommended daily intake; respiratory disturbance index; rupture-delivery interval

RDLBBB rate-dependent left bundle-branch block

RDM readmission

rDNA recombinant (or ribosomal) deoxyribonucleic acid

RDOG radiology diagnostic oncology group

RDP right dorsoposterior [fetal position]

RDQ respiratory disease questionnaire

RDRS rapid disability rating scale

RDS Raskin Depression Scale; respiratory distress syndrome; reticuloendothelial depressing substance; rhodanese; slow retinal degeneration

RDT retinal damage threshold; routine dialysis therapy

RDV rice dwarf virus

RDW red blood cell distribution width index

RDX radixin

RE radium emanation; readmission; rectal examination; reference emitter; reflux esophagitis; regional enteritis; renal and electrolyte; resistive exercise; resting energy; restriction endonuclease; reticuloendothelial; retinol equivalent; right ear; right eye

R_E respiratory exchange ratio

R&E research and education

Re rhenium

R_e Reynold number

REA radiation emergency area; radioenzymatic assay; renal anastomosis; right ear advantage

rea rearrangement

REAB refractory anemia with excess of blasts

REACH rural efforts to assist children at home

readm readmission

REALM rapid estimate of adult literacy in medicine

REAR renal, ear, anal, and radial [malformation syndrome]

REAS reasonably expected as safe; retained, excluded antrum syndrome

REAT radiological emergency assistance team

REB roentgen-equivalent biological

REC receptor; recombination, recombinant [chromosome]

rec fresh [Lat. *recens*]; recessive; recombinant chromosome; record; recovery; recurrence, recurrent

RECA recombination protein A

RECG radioelectrocardiography
recip recipient; reciprocal
recon the smallest unit of DNA capable of recombination [recombination + Gr. *on* quantum]
recond reconditioned, reconditioning
recumb recumbent
recryst recrystallization
rect rectal; rectification, rectified; rectum; rectus [muscle]
Rec Ther recreational therapy
recur recurrence, recurrent
RED radiation experience data; rapid erythrocyte degeneration
red reduction
redox oxidation-reduction
REE rapid extinction effect; rare earth element; resting energy expenditure
REEDS retention of tears, ectrodactyly, ectodermal dysplasia, and strange hair, skin and teeth [syndrome]
REEG radioelectroencephalography
R-EEG resting electroencephalography
ReEND reproductive endocrinology
REEP right end-expiratory pressure
reev re-evaluate
reex re-examine
REF ejection fraction at rest; referred; refused; renal erythropoietic factor
ref reference; reflex
Ref Doc referring doctor
REFI regional ejection fraction image
ref ind refractive index
refl reflex
Ref Phys referring physician
REFRAD released from active duty
REG radiation exposure guide; radioencephalogram, radioencephalography
Reg registered
reg region; regular
regen regenerated, regenerating, regeneration
reg rhy regular rhythm
regurg regurgitation
REH renin essential hypertension

rehab rehabilitation, rehabilitated
REL rate of energy loss; recommended exposure limit; resting expiratory level
rel relative
RELAY relayed correlation spectroscopy
RELE resistive exercise of lower extremities
RELP restriction fragment length polymorphism
RelTox Relational Toxicology [Project]
RELV restriction fragment length variant
REM rapid eye movement; recent-event memory; reticular erythematous mucinosis; return electrode monitor; roentgen-equivalent-man
rem removal
REMA repetitive excess mixed anhydride
REMAB radiation-equivalent-manikin absorption
REMCAL radiation-equivalent-manikin calibration
remit remittent
REMP roentgen-equivalent-man period
REMS rapid eye movement sleep
REN renal; renin
REO respiratory enteric orphan [virus]
REP replication protein; rest-exercise program; retrograde pyelogram; roentgen equivalent-physical
rep let it be repeated [Lat. *repetatur*]; replication; roentgen equivalent-physical
REPA replication protein A
repol repolarization
REPS reactive extensor postural synergy
rept let it be repeated
req request, requested
RER renal excretion rate; respiratory exchange ratio; rough endoplasmic reticulum
RERF Radiation Effects Research Foundation
RES radionuclide esophageal scintigraphy; reticuloendothelial system

res research; resection; resident; residue; resistance
RESNA Rehabilitation Engineering Society of North America
resp respiration, respiratory; response
Resp Ther respiratory therapy
REST Raynaud's phenomenon, esophageal motor dysfunction, sclerodactyly, and telangiectasia [syndrome]; regressive electroshock therapy
RESTT respiratory therapy technician
resusc resuscitation
RET reticular; reticulocyte; retina; retention; retained; right esotropia
ret rad equivalent therapeutic
retard retardation, retarded
ret cath retention catheter
retic reticulocyte
REV reticuloendotheliosis virus
ReV regulator of virion
rev reverse; review; revolution
re-x reexamination
Rex regulator x
RF radial fiber; radio frequency; receptive field; regurgitant fraction; Reitland-Franklin [unit]; relative flow; relative fluorescence; release factor; renal failure; replicative form; resistance factor; resonant frequency; respiratory failure; reticular formation; retroperitoneal fibromatosis; rheumatic fever; rheumatoid factor; riboflavin; risk factor; root canal filling; rosette formation
R^F rate of flow
Rf respiratory frequency; rutherfordium
R$_f$ in paper or thin-layer chromatography, the distance that a spot of a substance has moved from the point of application
rf radiofrequency; rapid filling
RFA resident functional atlas; right femoral artery; right frontoanterior [fetal position]
RFB retained foreign body
RFC request for comments; retrograde femoral catheter; rosette-forming cell

RFE relative fluorescence efficiency
RFFIT rapid fluorescent focus inhibition test
RFH right femoral hernia
RFI radiofrequency interference; recurrence-free interval; renal failure index
RFL right frontolateral [fetal position]
RFLA rheumatoid-factor-like activity
RFLP restriction fragment length polymorphism
RFLS rheumatoid-factor-like substance
Rfm rifampin
RFP recurrent facial paralysis; request for proposal; right frontoposterior [fetal position]
RFPS (Glasgow) Royal Faculty of Physicians and Surgeons of Glasgow
RFR rapid fluid resuscitation; refraction
RFS relapse-free survival; renal function study; rotating frame spectroscopy
RFT respiratory function test; rod-and-frame test; right frontotransverse [fetal position]
RFV right femoral vein
RFW rapid filling wave
RG right gluteal
rG regular gene
RGBMT renal glomerular basement membrane thickness
RGC radio-gas chromatography; remnant gastric cancer; retinal ganglion cell; right giant cell
RGD range-gated Doppler
RGE relative gas expansion
RGEA right gastroepiploic artery
RGH rat growth hormone
RGI recovery from growth inhibition
RGM right gluteus medius
rGM-CSF recombinant granulocyte-macrophage colony-stimulating factor
RGN Registered General Nurse
RGO reciprocating gait orthosis
RGP retrograde pyelography
RGR relative growth rate

RGS Rieger syndrome

RGU regional glucose utilization

RH radiant heat; radiation hybrid; radiological health; reactive hyperemia; recurrent herpes; regulatory hormone; rehabilitation; relative humidity; releasing hormone; renal hemolysis; retinal hemorrhage; right hand; right heart; right hemisphere; right hyperphoria; room humidifier

Rh rhesus [factor]; rhinion; rhodium

Rh+ rhesus positive

Rh– rhesus negative

rh rheumatic

r/h roentgens per hour

RHA Regional Health Authority; right hepatic artery

RhA rheumatoid arthritis

RHB right heart bypass

RHBF reactive hyperemia blood flow

RHBs Regional Hospital Boards

RHC resin hemoperfusion column; respiration has ceased; right heart catheterization; right hypochondrium

RHCSA Regional Hospitals Consultants' and Specialists' Association

RHD radiological health data; relative hepatic dullness; renal hypertensive disease; rheumatic heart disease

RHE retinohepatoendocrinologic [syndrome]

RHEED reflection high-energy electron diffraction

rheo rheology

rheu, rheum rheumatic, rheumatoid

RHF right heart failure

Rh F rheumatic fever

RHG right hand grip

rhG-CSF recombinant human granulocyte colony-stimulating factor

rhGM-CSF recombinant human granulocyte macrophage colony-stimulating factor

RHI Rural Health Initiative

Rhin rhinology

rhino rhinoplasty

RHJSC Regional Hospital Junior Staff Committee

RHL recurrent herpes labialis; right hepatic lobe

RHLN right hilar lymph node

rhm roentgens per hour at 1 meter

RhMK rhesus monkey kidney

RhMk rhesus monkey

RhMkK rhesus monkey kidney

RHMV right heart mixing volume

RHN Rockwell hardness number

RHO rhodopsin; right heeloff

ρ Greek letter *rho*; correlation coefficient; electric charge density; electrical resistivity; mass density; reactivity

RHOM rhombosine

RHR renal hypertensive rat; resting heart rate

r/hr roentgens per hour

RHS Ramsay Hunt syndrome; Rapp-Hodgkin syndrome; reciprocal hindlimb-scratching [syndrome]; right hand side; right heelstrike

RHT renal homotransplantation

rH-TNF recombinant human tumor necrosis factor

rh-tPA recombinant tissue plasminogen activator

RHU registered health underwriter; rheumatology

rHuEpo recombinant human erythropoietin

rHuTNF recombinant human tumor-necrosing factor

RHV right hepatic vein

RI radiation intensity; radioactive isotope; radioimmunology; recession index; recombinant inbred [strain]; refractive index; regenerative index; regional ileitis; regular insulin; relative intensity; release inhibition; remission induction; renal insufficiency; replicative intermediate; resistive index; respiratory illness; respiratory index; retroactive inhibition; retroactive interference; ribosome; rosette index (or inhibition)

r_i intraclass correlation coefficient

RIA radioimmunoassay; reversible ischemic attack

RIA-DA radioimmunoassay double antibody [test]

RIAS Roter Interactional Analysis System

Rib riboflavin; ribose

RIBA recombinant immunoblot assay

RIBS Rutherford ion backscattering

RIC right internal carotid [artery]; Royal Institute of Chemistry

RICE rest, ice, compression, and elevation

RICM right intercostal margin

RiCoF ristocetin cofactor

RICP recurrent intrahepatic cholestasis of pregnancy

RICU respiratory intensive care unit

RID radial immunodiffusion; remission-inducing drug; ruptured intervertebral disc

RIF radiological interface; release-inhibiting factor; rifampin; right iliac fossa; rosette-inhibiting factor

RIFA radioiodinated fatty acid

RIFC rat intrinsic factor concentrate

rIFN recombinant interferon

RIG rabies immune globulin; rat insuloma gene

RIGH rabies immune globulin, human

RIH right inguinal hernia

RIHSA radioactive iodinated human serum albumin

rIL recombinant interleukin

RILT rabbit ileal loop test

RIM radioisotope medicine; recurrent induced malaria; relative-intensity measure

RIMA right internal mammary artery

riMLF rostral interstitial median longitudinal fasciculus

RIMR Rockefeller Institute for Medical Research

RIMS resonance ionization mass spectrometry

RIN radioisotope nephrography; rat insulinoma

RINB Reitan-Indiana Neuropsychological Battery

RIND reversible ischemic neurologic deficit

RINN recommended international nonproprietary name

RIO right inferior oblique

RIP radioimmunoprecipitation; reflex inhibiting pattern; respiratory inductance plethysmography

RIPA radioimmunoprecipitation assay

RIPH Royal Institute of Public Health

RIPHH Royal Institute of Public Health and Hygiene

RIPP resistive-intermittent positive pressure

RIR relative incidence rates; right interior rectus [muscle]

RIRB radioiodinated rose bengal

RIS radiology information system; rapid immunofluorescence staining; resonance ionization spectroscopy

RISA radioactive iodinated serum albumin; radioimmunosorbent assay

RISC reduced-instruction-set computer

RIST radioimmunosorbent test

RIT radioimmune trypsin; radioiodinated triolein; radioiodine treatment; rosette inhibition titer

RITA Randomised Intervention Treatment of Angina [UK]; right internal thoracic artery

RITC rhodamine isothiocyanate

RIU radioactive iodine uptake

RIVC right inferior vena cava

RIVD ruptured intervertebral disc

RJA regurgitant jet area

RK rabbit kidney; radial keratotomy; reductase kinase; rhodopsin kinase; right kidney

RKG radiocardiogram

RKH Rokitansky-Küster-Hauser [syndrome]
RKM rokitamycin
RKV rabbit kidney vacuolating [virus]
RKY roentgen kymography
RL radial line; radiation laboratory; reduction level; renal dysplasia-limb defects [syndrome]; resistive load; reticular lamina; right lateral; right leg; right lung; Ringer lactate [solution]
R&L right and left
RLC residual lung capacity
RLD related living donor; ruptured lumbar disc
RLE right lower extremity
RLF retrolental fibroplasia; right lateral femoral
RLL right lobe of liver; right lower limb; right lower lobe
RLM right lower medial
RLN recurrent laryngeal nerve; regional lymph node; relaxin
RLNC regional lymph node cell
RLND regional lymph node dissection
RLO residual lymphatic output
RLP radiation leukemia protection; ribosome-like particle
RLPV right lower pulmonary vein
RLQ right lower quadrant
RLR right lateral rectus [muscle]
RLS recursive least square; restless leg syndrome; Ringer lactate solution; Roussy-Levy syndrome
RLSB right lower scapular border
R-Lsh right-left shunt
RLSL recursive least square lattice
RLV Rauscher leukemia virus
RLWD routine laboratory work done
RLX relaxin
RLXH relaxin H
RLZ right lower zone
RM radical mastectomy; random migration; radon monitor; range of movement; red marrow; reference material; relative mobility; rehabilitation medicine; rein-

forced maneuver; resistive movement; respiratory movement; Riehl melanosis; risk management; routine management; ruptured membranes
Rm relative mobility; remission
rm remission; room
RMA rapid membrane assay; refuses medical advice; Registered Medical Assistant; relative medullary area; right mentoanterior [fetal position]
RMANOVA repeated measures analysis of variance
RMB right mainstem bronchus
RMBF regional myocardial blood flow
RMC reticular magnocellular [nucleus]; right middle cerebral [artery]
RMCA right middle cerebral artery
RMCH rod monochromacy or monochromatism
RMCL right midclavicular line
RMD retromanubrial dullness
RMDP Resource Mothers Development Project
RME rapid maxillary expansion; resting metabolic expenditure; right mediolateral episiotomy
RMEC regional medical education center
RMED rural medical education [program]
RMF right middle finger
RMK rhesus monkey kidney
RML radiation myeloid leukemia; regional medical library; right mediolateral; right middle lobe
RMLB right middle lobe bronchus
RMLS right middle lobe syndrome
RMLV Rauscher murine leukemia virus
RMM rapid micromedia method
RMN Registered Mental Nurse
RMO Regional Medical Officer; Resident Medical Officer
RMP rapidly miscible pool; regional medical program; regional myocardial infarction; resting membrane potential; ribulose monophosphate pathway; rifampin; right mentoposterior [fetal position]

RMPA Royal Medico-Psychological Association

RMR relative maximum respone; resting metabolic rate; right medial rectus [muscle]

RMS rectal morphine sulfate [suppository]; red man syndrome; repetitive motion syndrome; respiratory muscle strength; rhabdomyosarcoma; rheumatic mitral stenosis; rhodomyosarcoma; rigid man syndrome; root-mean-square

rms root-mean-square

RMSA regulator of mitotic spindle assembly; rhabdomyosarcoma, alveolar

RMSa rhabdomyosarcoma

RMSCR rhabdomyosarcoma chromosomal region

RMSD root-mean-square deviation

RMSF Rocky Mountain spotted fever

RMSS Ruvalcaba-Myhre-Smith syndrome

RMT Registered Music Therapist; relative medullary thickness; retromolar trigone; right mentotransverse [fetal position]

RMUI relief medication unit index

RMuLV Rauscher murine leukemia virus

RMV respiratory minute volume

RMZ right midzone

RN radionuclide; red nucleus; Registered Nurse; registry number; residual nitrogen; reticular nucleus

Rn radon

RNA radionuclide angiography; Registered Nurse Anesthetist; ribonucleic acid; rough, noncapsulated, avirulent [bacterial culture]

RNAA radiochemical neutron activation analysis

RNAse, RNase ribonuclease

RN-C registered nurse-certification

RND radical neck dissection; radionuclide dacryography; reactive neurotic depression

RNFP Registered Nurse Fellowship Program

RNIB Royal National Institute for the Blind

RNICU regional neonatal intensive care unit

RNID Royal National Institute for the Deaf

RNP ribonucleoprotein

RNR ribonucleotide reductase

RNS reference normal serum; repetitive nerve stimulation; ribonuclease

RNSC radionuclide superior cavography

Rnt roentgenology

RNTMI transfer ribonucleic acid initiator methionine

RNV radionuclide venography

rNTP ribonuclease-5;pr-triphosphate

RNVG radionuclide ventriculography

RO radiation oncology; radiation output; ratio of; relative odds; renal osteodystrophy; reverse osmosis; Ritter-Oleson [technique]; routine order; rule out

ro radius of orifice

R/O rule out

ROA right occipitoanterior [fetal position]

ROAD reversible obstructive airways disease

ROAT repeat open application test

ROATS rabbit ovarian antitumor serum

rob robertsonian translocation

ROC receiver operating characteristic; receptor-operated channels; relative operating characteristic; resident on call; residual organic carbon

ROCF Rey-Osterrieth Complex Figure

rOEF regional oxygen extraction fraction

roent roentgenology

ROESY rotating frame Overhauser effect spectroscopy

ROH rat ovarian hyperemia [test]

ROI reactive oxygen intermediate; region of interest; right occipitolateral [fetal position]

ROIH right oblique inguinal hernia

ROJM range of joint motion

ROM range of motion; read only memory; reduction of movement; regional office manual; removal of metal [pins or plates in orthopedic surgery]; rupture of membranes

Rom Romberg [sign]

rom reciprocal ohm meter

ROM CP range of motion complete and painfree

ROP removal of pins or plates; removal of plaster [of Paris]; retinopathy of prematurity; right occipitoposterior [fetal position]

RO PACS radiation oncology picture archiving and communication system

ROPE respiratory-ordered phase encoding

ROPS rollover protective structure

Ror Rorschach [test]

ROS reactive oxygen species; review of systems; rod outer segment

RoS rostral sulcus

ROSC return to spontaneous circulation

ROSP rod outer segment protein

ROSS review of subjective symptoms

ROT real oxygen transport; remedial occupational therapy; right occipitotransverse [fetal position]

rot rotating, rotation

ROU recurrent oral ulcer

ROW Rendu-Osler-Weber [syndrome]; rest of the world

RP radial pulse; radiopharmaceutical; rapid processing [of film]; Raynaud phenomenon; reactive protein; readiness potential; recreation and passtime; rectal prolapse; refractory period; regulatory protein; relapsing polychondritis; reperfusion; replication protein; respiratory rate; rest pain; resting potential; resting pressure; retinitis pigmentosa; retrograde pyelogram; retroperitoneal; reverse phase; rheumatoid polyarthritis;

ribonucleoprotein; ribose phosphate; ribosomal protein

R5P ribose-5-phosphate

R/P respiratory pulse [rate]

R$_p$ pulmonary resistance

RPA radial photon apsorptiometry; replication protein A; resultant physiologic acceleration; reverse passive anaphylaxis; right pulmonary artery

RPase ribonucleic acid polymerase

RPC reactive perforating collagenosis; relapsing polychondritis; relative proliferative capacity

RPCF, RPCFT Reiter protein complement fixation [test]

RPCGN rapidly progressive crescenting glomerulonephritis

RPCH rural primary care hospital

RPD removable partial denture

RPE rate of perceived exertion; recurrent pulmonary embolism; retinal pigment epithelium; ribulose 5-phosphate 3-epimerase

RPEP rabies post-exposure prophylaxis

RPF relaxed pelvic floor; renal plasma flow; retroperitoneal fibrosis

RPG radiation protection guide; Report Program Generator[PC language]; retrograde pyelogram; rheoplethysmography

RPGMEC Regional Postgraduate Medical Education Committee

RPGN rapidly progressive glomerulonephritis

RPh Registered Pharmacist

RPHA reversed passive hemagglutination

RPHAMFCA reversed passive hemagglutination by miniature centrifugal fast analysis

RP-HPLC reverse phase-high performance liquid chromatography

RPI regional perfusion index; relative percentage index; reticulocyte production index, ribose 5-phosphate isomerase

RPIPP reverse phase ion-pair partition

RPK ribosephosphate kinase

RPLAD retroperitoneal lymphadenectomy

RPLC reverse phase liquid chromatography

RPLD repair of potentially lethal damage

RPM, rpm rapid processing mode; revolutions per minute

RPMD rheumatic pain modulation disorder

RPMI Roswell Park Memorial Institute [medium]

RPO right posterior oblique

RPP heart rate-systolic blood pressure product; retropubic prostatectomy

RPPI role perception picture inventory

RPPR red cell precursor production rate

RPR rapid plasmin reagin [test]

RPr retinitis proliferans

RPRC regional primate research center

RPRF rapidly progressive renal failure

RPRCT rapid plasma reagin cord test

RPS renal pressor substance; revolutions per second

rps revolutions per second

RPSM residency program in social medicine

RPSP reference preparation for serum proteins

RPS4Y ribosomal protein S4, Y-linked

RPT rapid pull-through; refractory period of transmission; Registered Physical Therapist; renal parenchymal thickness

RPTA renal percutaneous transluminal angioplasty

RPTC regional poisoning treatment center

Rptd ruptured

RPV right portal vein; right pulmonary vein

RPVP right posterior ventricular pre-excitation

RQ recovery quotient; [Hazardous Substance] Reportable Quantities [List]; reportable quantity; respiratory quotient

RQDS Revised Quantified Denver Scale of Communication

RR radiation reaction; radiation response; rate ratio; rational recovery [group]; recovery room; relative response; relative risk; renin release; respiratory rate; respiratory reserve; response rate; results reporting [system]; retinal reflex; rheumatoid rosette; ribonucleotide reductase; risk ratio; Riva-Rocci [sphygmomanometer]

R&R rate and rhythm; rest and recuperation

RRA radioreceptor assay; registered record administrator

RRAC Research Realignment Advisory Committee

RRC residency review committee; risk reduction component; routine respiratory care; Royal Red Cross; rural referral center

RRE radiation-related eosinophilia

RRE, RR&E round, regular, and equal [pupils]

RRF residual renal function

RR-HPO rapid recompression-high pressure oxygen

RRI recurrent respiratory infection; reflex relaxation index; relative response index

RRIS recurrent respiratory infection syndrome

RRL Registered Record Librarian

RRM ribonucleotide reductase M

RRN returning [for advanced studies] registered nurse

rRNA ribosomal ribonucleic acid

rRNP ribosomal ribonucleoprotein

RRP relative refractory period

RRpm respiratory rate per minute

RRR regular rhythm and rate; renin release rate (or ratio)

RR&R regular rate and rhythm

RRS retrorectal space; Richards-Rundle syndrome

RRT random response technique; Registered Respiratory Therapist; relative retention time

RRU respiratory resistance unit

RS radioscaphoid; random sample; rating schedule; Raynaud syndrome; recipient's serum; rectal sinus; rectal suppository; rectosigmoid; reducing substance; Reed-Steinberg [cell]; reinforcing stimulus; Reiter syndrome; relative stimulus; renal specialist; respiratory syncytial [virus]; response to stimulus; resting subject; reticulated siderocyte; retinoschisis; Rett syndrome; review of symptoms; Reye syndrome; right sacrum; right septum; right side; right stellate [ganglion]; Ringer solution; Roberts syndrome; Rous sarcoma

Rs *Rauwolfia serpentina*; systemic resistance

R/s roentgens per second

r$_s$ rank correlation coefficient

RSA rabbit serum albumin; regular spiking activity; relative specific activity; relative standard accuracy; reticulum cell sarcoma; right sacroanterior [fetal position]; right subclavian artery; roentgenographic stereogrammetric analysis

Rsa systemic arterial resistance

RSB reticulocyte standard buffer; right sternal border

RSC rat spleen cell; rested state contraction; reversible sickle-cell; right subclavian

RScA right scapuloanterior [fetal position]

RSCN Registered Sick Children's Nurse

RScP right scapuloposterior [fetal position]

RSD reflex sympathetic dystrophy; relative standard deviation

RSDS reflex sympathetic dystrophy syndrome

RSE rapid spin-echo

RSEP right somatosensory evoked potential

RSES Rosenberg Self-Esteem Scale

RSH Royal Society of Health

RSI rapid-sequence induction; rapid sequence intubation; repetition strain injury

RSIC Radiation Shielding Information Center

R-SIRS Revised Seriousness of Illness Rating Scale

RSIVP rapid-sequence intravenous pyelography

RSL right sacrolateral [fetal position]

RSLD repair of sublethal damage

RSM risk screening model; Royal Society of Medicine

RSMR relative standard mortality rate

RSN restin; right substantia nigra

RSNA Radiological Society of North America

RSO radiation safety officer; Resident Surgical Officer; right superior oblique [muscle]

rSO$_2$ regional oxygen saturation

RSP removable silicone plug; ribose-5-phosphatase; right sacroposterior [fetal position]

RSPCA Royal Society for the Prevention of Cruelty to Animals

RS$_3$PE remitting seronegative symmetrical synovitis with pitting edema

RSPH Royal Society for the Promotion of Health

RSPK recurrent spontaneous psychokinesis

RSR regular sinus rhythm; relative survival rate; right superior rectus [muscle]

rSr an electrocardiographic complex

RSS rat stomach strip; rectosigmoidoscopy; Russell-Silver syndrome

RSSE Russian spring-summer encephalitis

RSSR relative slow sinus rate

RST radiosensitivity test; reagin screen test; right sacrotransverse [fetal position]; rubrospinal tract

R_{st} in paper or thin layer chromatography, the distance that a spot of a substance has moved, relative to a reference standard spot

RSTI Radiological Service Training Institute

RSTL relaxed skin tension lines

RSTMH Royal Society of Tropical Medicine and Hygiene

RSTS retropharyngeal soft tissue space

RSU radiological sciences unit

RSV respiratory syncytial virus; right subclavian vein; Rous sarcoma virus

RSVC right superior vena cava

RSVP retired senior volunteer program

RT radiologic technologist; radiotelemetry; radiotherapy; radium therapy; rapid tranquilization; reaction time; reading test; reciprocating tachycardia; recreational therapy; rectal temperature; reduction time; Registered Technician; renal transplantation; resistance transfer; respiratory therapist/therapy; response time; rest tremor; retransformation; reverse transcriptase; reverse transcription; right; right thigh; room temperature; Rubinstein-Taybi [syndrome]

RT3, rT$_3$ reverse triiodothyronine

Rt right; total resistance

rT ribothymidine

rt right

RTA ray tracing algorithm; renal tubular acidosis; reverse transcriptase assay; road traffic accident

RTAD renal tubular acidification defect

RT(ARRT) Radiologic Technologist certified by the American Registry of Radiologic Technologists

RTC random control trial; rape treatment center; renal tubular cell; residential treatment center; return to clinic

rtc return to clinic

RT-CT radiotherapy dedicated computed tomography

RTD renal tubular defect; routine test dilution

Rtd retarded

RTECS Registry of Toxic Effects of Chemical Substances

RTF resistance transfer factor; respiratory tract fluid

RTG-2 rainbow trout gonadal tissue cells

rTHF recombinant tumor necrosis factor

RTI respiratory tract infection; reverse transcriptase inhibition

RTK receptor-tyrosine kinase; rhabdoid tumor of the kidney

rtl rectal

rt lat right lateral

RTM registered trademark

RTN renal tubular necrosis

RT(N)(ARRT) Radiologic Technologist (Nuclear Medicine) certified by the American Registry of Radiologic Technologists

RTO return to office; right toeoff

RTOG radiation therapy oncology group

RTP radiation treatment planning; renal transplantation patient; reverse transcriptase-producing [agent]

rTPA/rtPA recombinant tissue plasminogen activator

rt-PA recombinant tissue plasminogen activator

RT-PCR reverse transcriptase-polymerase chain reaction

RTR Recreational Therapist, Registered; red blood cell turnover rate; retention time ratio

RT(R)(ARRT) Registered Technologist, Radiography certified by the American Registry of Radiologic Technologists)

RTS real time scan; Rett syndrome; revised trauma score; right toestrike; Rothmund-Thomson syndrome; Rubinstein-Taybi syndrome

RT(T)(ARRT) Radiologic Technologist (Radiation Therapy) certified by the American Registry of Radiologic Technologists

RTRR return to recovery room

RTTP radiation therapy treatment planning

RTU real-time ultrasonography; relative time unit; renal transplantation unit

RT₃U resin triiodothyronine uptake

RTW return to work

RTV room temperature vulcanization

RU radioulnar; rat unit; reading unit; residual urine; resin uptake; resistance unit; retrograde urogram; right upper; roentgen unit

Ru ruthenium

ru radiation unit

RU-1 human embryonic lung fibroblasts

RU-486 mifepristone

RUA reduced under anesthesia

RUD recurrent ulcer of the duodenal bulb

RUE right upper extremity

RUG resource utilization group

RUL right upper eyelid; right upper lateral; right upper limb; right upper lobe

RuMP ribulose monophosphate pathway

RUOQ right upper outer quadrant

Ru1,5P ribulose-1,5-biphosphate

Ru5P ribulose-5-phosphate

rupt ruptured

RUP right upper pole

RUPV right upper pulmonary vein

RUQ right upper quadrant

RUR resin-uptake ratio

RURTI recurrent upper respiratory tract infection

RUS radioulnar synostosis

RUSB right upper sternal border

RUSP right ventricular systolic pressure

RUV residual urine volume

RUX right upper extremity

RUZ right upper zone

RV random variable; rat virus; Rauscher virus; rectovaginal; reinforcement value; renal vein; residual volume; respiratory volume; retroversion; return visit; rheumatoid vasculitis; rhinovirus; right ventricle, right ventricular; rubella vaccine; rubella virus; Russell viper

R_V radius of view

RVA re-entrant ventricular arrhythmia; right ventricle activation; right vertebral artery

RVAD right ventricular assist device

RVAW right ventricle anterior wall

RVB red venous blood

RVC rectovaginal constriction

RVD relative vertebral density; right ventricular dysplasia

RVDC right ventricular diastolic collapse

RVDO right ventricular diastolic overload

RVDV right ventricular diastolic volume

RVE right ventricular enlargement

RVECP right ventricular endocardial potential

RVEDD right ventricular end-diastolic diameter

RVEDP right ventricular end-diastolic pressure

RVEDV right ventricular end-diastolic volume

RVEDVI right ventricular end-diastolic volume index

RVEF right ventricular ejection fraction; right ventricular end-flow

RVET right ventricular ejection time

RVF renal vascular failure; Rift Valley fever; right ventricular failure; right visual field

RVFP right ventricular filling pressure

RVG right ventral glutens [muscle]; right visceral ganglion

RVH renovascular hypertension; right ventricular hypertrophy

RVHD rheumatic valvular heart disease

RVI relative value index; right ventricle infarction

RVID ventricular internal dimension

RVIT right ventricular inflow tract

RV-IVRT right ventricular isovolumic relaxation time

RVL right vastus lateralis
RVLG right ventrolateral gluteal
RVM right ventricular mean
RVO Regional Veterinary Officer; relaxed vaginal outlet; right ventricular outflow
RVOT right ventricular outflow tract
RVP red veterinary petrolatum; resting venous pressure; right ventricular pressure
RVPEP right ventricular pre-ejection period
RVPFR right ventricular peak filling rate
RVPRA renal vein plasma renin activity
RVR reduced vascular response; renal vascular resistance; repetitive ventricular response; resistance to venous return
RVRA renal vein rein activity; renal venous renin assay
RVRC renal vein renin concentration
RVS rectovaginal space; relative value scale/study; reported visual sensation; retrovaginal space
RVSO right ventricular stroke output
RVSW right ventricular stroke work
RVSWI right ventricular stroke work index
RVT renal vein thrombosis
RVTE recurring venous thromboembolism
RV/TLC residual volume/total lung capacity
RVU relative value unit
RVV right ventricular volume; rubella vaccine-like virus; Russell viper venom

RVVO right ventricular volume overload
RVVT Russell viper venom time
RVWT right ventricle wall thickness
RW radiological warfare; ragweed; respiratory work; Romano-Ward [syndrome]; round window
R-W Rideal-Walker [coefficient]
RWAGE ragweed antigen E
RWIS restraint and water immersion stress
RWJF Robert Wood Johnson Foundation
RWM regional wall motion
RWMA regional wall motion abnormality
RWP ragweed pollen; R-wave progression
RWS radiology work station; ragweed sensitivity
RWT relative wall thickness
RX reaction
Rx drug; medication; pharmacy; prescribe, prescription, prescription drug; take [Lat. *recipe*]; therapy; treatment
RXLI recessive X-linked ichthyosis
RXN reaction
RXR retinoid X receptor
RXRA retinoid X receptor alpha
RXRG retinoid X receptor gamma
RXT right exotropia
R-Y Roux-en-Y [anastomosis]
RYD ryanodine
RYR ryanodine receptor

S apparent power; in electrocardiography, a negative deflection that follows an R wave [wave]; entropy; exposure time; half [Lat. *semis*]; left [Lat. *sinister*]; mean dose per unit cumulated activity; the midpoint of the sella turcica [point]; sacral; saline; *Salmonella*; saturated; *Schistosoma*; schizophrenia; second; section; sedimentation coefficient; sella [turcica]; semilente [insulin]; senile, senility; sensation; sensitivity; septum; serine; serum; *Shigella*; siderocyte; siemens; sigmoid; signature [prescription]; silicate; single; small; smooth [colony]; soft [diet]; solid; soluble; solute; sone [unit]; space; spatial; specificity; spherical; *Spirillum*; spleen; standard normal deviation; *Staphylococcus*; stem [cell]; stimulus; *Streptococcus*; streptomycin; subject; subjective findings; substrate; sulfur; sum of an arithmetic series; supravergence; surface; surgery; suture; Svedberg [unit]; swine; Swiss [mouse]; synthesis; systole; without [Lat. *sine*]

S1-S5 first to fifth sacral nerves

S_1-S_4 first to fourth heart sounds

s atomic orbital with angular momentum quantum number 0; distance; left [Lat. *sinister*]; length of path; sample standard deviation; satellite [chromosome]; scruple; second; section; sedimentation coefficient; sensation; series; signed; suckling

s specific heat capacity; without (Lat. *sine*]

s^{-1} cycles per second

s^2 sample variance

Σ see *sigma*

σ see *sigma*

SA salicylic acid; saline [solution]; salt added; sarcoidosis; sarcoma; scalenus anticus; secondary amenorrhea; secondary anemia; secondary arrest; self-analysis; semen analysis; sensitizing antibody; serum albumin; serum aldolase; sexual addict; sexual assault; simian adenovirus; sinoatrial; sinus arrest; sinus arrhythmia; skin-adipose [unit]; sleep apnea; slightly active; slowly adapting [receptor]; soluble in alkaline medium; specific activity; spectrum analysis; spiking activity; standard accuracy; status asthmaticus; stimulus artifact; Stokes-Adams [syndrome]; subarachnoid; succinylacetone; suicide attempt; surface antigen; surface area; sustained action; sympathetic activity; systemic aspergillosis

S-A sinoatrial; sinoauricular

S&A sickness and accident [insurance]; sugar and acetone

Sa the most anterior point of the anterior contour of the sella turcica [point]; saline; *Staphylococcus aureus*

sA statampere

SAA serum amyloid A; severe aplastic anemia

SAAP selective aortic arch perfusion

SAARD slow-acting antirheumatic drug

SAAS Substance Abuse Attitude Survey

SAAST self-administered alcohol screening test

SAB Scientific Advisory Board; serum albumin; significant asymptomatic bacteriuria; sinoatrial block; Society of American Bacteriologists; spontaneous abortion; subarachnoid block

SAb spontaneous abortion

SABP spontaneous acute bacterial peritonitis

SAC saccharin; sacrum; screening and acute care; Self-Assessment of Communication [scale]; short-arm cast; social activity [scale]; subarea advisory council

sacch saccharin

SACD subacute combined degeneration

SACE serum angiotensin-converting enzyme

SACH small animal care hospital; solid ankle cushioned heel

SACNAS Society for the Advancement of Chicanos and Native Americans in Science

SACS secondary anticoagulation system

SACSF subarachnoid cerebrospinal fluid

SACT sinoatrial conduction time

SAD Scale of Anxiety and Depression; seasonal affective disorder; Self-Assessment Depression [scale]; severe aortic stenosis; small airway disease; source-to-axis distance; sugar, acetone, and diacetic acid; suppressor-activating determinant

SADD Short-Alcohol Dependence Data [questionnaire]; standardized assessment of depressive disorders; Students Against Drung Driving

SADL simulated activities of daily living

SADR suspected adverse drug reaction

SADS Schedule for Affective Disorders and Schizophrenia

SADS-C Schedule for Affective Disorders and Schizophrenia-Change

SADS-L Schedule for Affective Disorders and Schizophrenia-Lifetime

SADT Stetson Auditory Discrimination Test

SAE serious adverse event; short above-elbow [cast]; specific action exercise; subcortical arteriosclerotic encephalopathy; supported arm exercise

SAEB sinoatrial entrance block

SAEM Society for Academic Emergency Medicine

SAEP *Salmonella abortus equi* pyrogen

SAF scrapie-associated fibrils; self-articulating femoral; serum accelerator factor; simultaneous auditory feedback

SAFA soluble antigen fluorescent antibody

SAFTEE-GI systematic assessment for treatment emergent events-general inquiry

SAFTEE-SI systematic assessment for treatment emergent events-systematic inquiry

SAG salicyl acyl glucuronide; sonoangiography; Swiss agammaglobulinemia

sag sagittal

SAGM sodium chloride, adenine, glucose, mannitol

SAH S-adenosyl-L-homocysteine; subarachnoid hemorrhage

SAHA seborrhea-hypertrichosis/hirsutism-alopecia [syndrome]

SAHH S-adenosylhomocysteine hydrolase

SAHIGES *Staphylococcus aureus* hyperimmunoglobulinemia E syndrome

SAHS sleep apnea-hypersomnolence [syndrome]

SAI Self-Analysis Inventory; Sexual Arousability Inventory; Social Adequacy Index; suppressor of anchorage independence; systemic active immunotherapy

SAICAR sylaminoimidazole carboxylase

SAID specific adaptation to imposed demand [principle]

SAIDS sexually acquired immunodeficiency syndrome; simian acquired immune deficiency syndrome

SAIMS student applicant information management system

SAL sensorineural activity level; sterility assurance level; suction-assisted lipectomy

Sal salicylate, salicylic; *Salmonella*

sAl serum aluminum [level]

sal salicylate, salicylic; saline; saliva

Salm *Salmonella*

SALP salpingectomy; salpingography; serum alkaline phosphatase

Salpx salpingectomy

SAM S-adenosyl-L-methionine; scanning acoustic microscope; senescence accelerated mouse; sex arousal mechanism; short-arc motion; staphylococcal absorption method; substrate adhesion molecule; sulfated acid mucopolysaccharide; surface active material; systolic anterior motion

SAMA Student American Medical Association

SAMD S-adenosyl-L-methionine decarboxylase

SAM-DC S-adenosyl-L-methionine decarboxylase

SAMe S-adenosyl-L-methionine

SAMO Senior Administrative Medical Officer

S-AMY serum amylase

SAN sinoatrial node; sinoauricular node; slept all night; solitary autonomous nodule

Sanat sanatorium

SANDR sinoatrial nodal reentry

sang sanguinous

sanit sanitary, sanitation

SANS scale for the assessment of negative symptoms

SANWS sinoatrial node weakness syndrome

SAO small airway obstruction; splanchnic artery occlusion; subvalvular aortic obstruction

S$_{AO2}$ oxygen saturation in alveolar gas

S$_{aO2}$ oxygen saturation in arterial blood

SAP sensory action potential; serum acid phosphatase; serum alkaline phosphatase; serum amyloid P; situs ambiguus with polysplenia; sphingolipid activator protein; *Staphylococcus aureus* protease; surfactant-associated protein; systemic arterial pressure; systolic arterial pressure

SAPD sphingolipid activator protein deficiency

SAPF simultaneous anterior and posterior [spinal] fusion

saph saphenous

SAPHO synovitis-acne-pustulosis hyperostosis-osteomyelitis [syndrome]

SAPK stress-activated protein kinase

SAPX salivary peroxidase

SAQ short arc quadriceps [muscle]

SAQC statistical analysis of quality control

SAR scatter/air ratio; seasonal allergic rhinitis; sexual attitude reassessment; slowly adapting receptor; specific absorption rate; structure-activity relationship; supra-aortic ridge; supra-aortic ring

Sar sulfarsphenamine

SARA sexually acquired reactive arthritis; Superfund Amendments and Reauthorization

SAS sarcoma amplified sequence; self-rating anxiety scale; short arm splint; Sklar Aphasia Scale; sleep apnea syndrome; small animal surgery; small aorta syndrome; social adjustment scale; sodium amylosulfate; space-adaptation syndrome; specific activity scale; statistical analysis system; sterile aqueous solution; sterile aqueous suspension; subaortic stenosis; subarachnoid space; sulfasalazine; supravalvular aortic stenosis; surface-active substance; synchronous atrial stimulation

SASE self-addressed stamped envelope

SASMAS skin-adipose superficial musculoaponeurotic system

SASP salicylazosulfapyridine

SASPP syndrome of absence of septum pellucidum with preencephaly

SAS-SR social adjustment scale, self-report

SAST Self-administered Alcoholism Screening Test; selective arterial secretin injection test; serum aspartate aminotransferase

SAT saliva alcohol test; satellite; serum antitrypsin; single-agent chemotherapy;

slide agglutination test; sodium ammonium thiosulfate; spermatogenic activity test; spontaneous activity test; subacute thyroiditis; symptomless autoimmune thyroiditis; systematic assertive therapy; systolic acceleration time

Sat, sat saturation, saturated

SATA spatial average, temporal average

SATB special aptitude test battery

satd saturated

SATL surgical Achilles tendon lengthening

SATP spatial average temporal peak

SATS substance, amount ingested, time ingested, symptoms

SAU statistical analysis unit

SAV sequential atrioventricular [pacing]

SAVD spontaneous assisted vaginal delivery

SAVE saved-young-life equivalent; sudden A-ventilatory event; survival and ventricular enlargement [trial]

SAX short axis; surface antigen, X-linked

SAx short axis

SAX-APEX short-axis plane, apical

SAX-MV short-axis, mitral valve

SAX-PM short-axis plane, papillary muscle

SB Bachelor of Science; Schwartz-Bartter [syndrome]; serum bilirubin; shortness of breath; sick bay; sideroblast; single blind [study]; single breath; sinus bradycardia; small bowel; sodium balance; sodium bisulfite; soybean; spina bifida; spontaneous blastogenesis; spontaneous breathing; Stanford-Binet [Intelligence Scale]; stereotyped behavior; sternal border; stillbirth; surface binding

Sb antimony [Lat. *stibium*]; strabismus

sb stilb

SBA serum bile acid; soybean agglutinin; spina bifida aperta

SBAHC school-based adolescent health care

SBB stimulation-bound behavior

SBC school-based clinic; serum bactericidal concentration; strict bed confinement

SBD senile brain disease

S-BD seizure-brain damage

SbDH sorbitol dehydrogenase

SBE breast self-examination; short below-elbow [cast]; shortness of breath on exertion; small bowel enema; subacute bacterial endocarditis

SBET Society for Biomedical Engineering Technicians

S/ß sickle cell beta-thalassemia

SBF serologic-blocking factor; specific blocking factor; splanchnic blood flow

SBFT small bowel follow-through

SBG selenite brilliant green

SBH sea-blue histiocyte

SBHC school-based health center

SBI soybean trypsin inhibitor

SBIS Stanford-Binet Intelligence Scale

SBL soybean lecithin

sBL sporadic Burkitt lymphoma

SBLA sarcoma, breast and brain tumors, leukemia, laryngeal and lung cancer, and adrenal cortical carcinoma

SB-LM Stanford-Binet Intelligence Test-Form LM

SBM Solomon-Bloembergen-Morgan [equation]

SBMA spinal bulbar muscular atrophy

SBN State Board of Nursing

SBN$_2$ single-breath nitrogen test]

SBNS Society of British Neurological Surgeons

SBNT single-breath nitrogen test

SBNW single-breath nitrogen washout

SBO small bowel obstruction; spina bifida occulta

SBOM soybean oil meal

SBP schizobipolar; serotonin-binding protein; spontaneous bacterial peritonitis; steroid-binding plasma [protein]; sulfobromophthalein; systemic blood pressure; systolic blood pressure

SBQ Smoking Behavior Questionnaire

SBR small bowel resection; spleen-to-body [weight] ratio; strict bed rest; styrene-butadiene rubber

SBRN sensory branch of radial nerve

SBRT split beam rotation therapy

SBS shaken baby syndrome; short bowel syndrome; sick building syndrome; sinobronchial syndrome; small bowel series; social breakdown syndrome; straight back syndrome

SBSS Seligmann's buffered salt solution

SBT serum bactericidal titer; single-breath test; sulbactam

SBTI soybean trypsin inhibitor

SBTPE State Boards Test Pool Examination

SBTT small bowel transit time

SBV singular binocular vision

SC conditioned stimulus; sacrococcygeal; Sanitary Corps; scalenus [muscle]; scapula; Schwann cell; sciatica; science; sclerosing cholangitis; secondary cleavage; secretory component; self care; semicircular; semilunar valve closure; serum complement; serum creatinine; service-connected; sex chromatin; Sézary cell; short circuit; sick call; sickle cell; sigmoid colon; siliconecoated; single chemical; skin conduction; slow component; Snellen chart; sodium citrate; soluble complex; special care; spinal canal; spinal cord; squamous carcinoma; start conversion; statistical control; sternoclavicular; stratum corneum; subcellular; subclavian; subcorneal; subcortical; subcostal; subcutaneous; succinylcholine; sugar-coated; superior colliculus; supportive care; supraclavicular; surface colony; systemic candidiasis; systolic click

S/C subcutaneous, sugar-coated [pill]

S-C sickle cell

S&C sclerae and conjunctivae

Sc scandium; scapula; science, scientific; screening

sC statcoulomb

sc subcutaneous

SCA self-care agency; severe congenital anomaly; sickle-cell anemia; single-camera autostereoscopic [imaging]; single-channel analyzer; sperm-coating antigen; spinocerebellar ataxia; steroidal-cell antibody; subclavian artery; superior cerebellar artery; suppressor cell activity

SCAA Skin Care Association of America; sporadic cerebral amyloid angiopathy

SCABG single coronary artery bypass

SCAD short chain acyl-coenzyme A dehydrogenase

SCAG Sandoz Clinical Assessment-Geriatric [Rating]

SCH student contact hour; succinylcholine

SCAMIA Symposium on Computer Applications in Medical Care

SCAMIN Self-Concept and Motivation Inventory

SCAN suspected child abuse and neglect; systolic coronary artery narrowing

SCAP scapula

SCARF skeletal abnormalities, cutis laxa, craniostenosis, psychomotor retardation, facial abnormalities [syndrome]

SCAT sheep cell agglutination test; sickle cell anemia test; Sports Competition Anxiety Test

SCAVF spinal cord arteriovenous fistula

SCAVM spinal cord arteriovenous malformation

SCB strictly confined to bed

SCBA self-contained breathing apparatus

SCBE single contrast barium enema

SCBF spinal cord blood flow

SCBG symmetric calcification of the basal cerebral ganglia

SCBH systemic cutaneous basophil hypersensitivity

SCBP stratum corneum basic protein

SCC self-care center; sequential combination chemotherapy; services for crippled children; short-course chemotherapy; small-cell carcinoma; small cleaved cell; spinal cord compression; squamous cell carcinoma

SC4C subcostal four-chamber [view]

SCCA single-cell cytotoxicity assay

SCCB small-cell carcinoma of the bronchus

SCCC squamous cell cervical carcinoma

SCCH sternocostoclavicular hyperostosis

SCCHN squamous cell carcinoma of the head and neck

SCCHO sternocostoclavicular hyperostosis

SCCL small cell carcinoma of the lung

SCCM Sertoli cell culture medium; Society of Critical Care Medicine

SCCT severe cerebrocranial trauma

SCD scleroderma; service-connected disability; sickle-cell disease; spinocerebellar degeneration; subacute combined degeneration; subacute coronary disease; sudden cardiac death; systemic carnitine deficiency

ScD Doctor of Science

SCDA situational control of daily activities [scale]

ScDA right scapuloanterior [fetal position] [Lat. *scapulodextra anterior*]

SCDF skin condition data form

ScDP right scapuloposterior [fetal position] [Lat. *scapulodextra posterior*]

SCE secretory carcinoma of the endometrium; sister chromatid exchange; split hand-cleft lip/palate ectodermal [dysplasia]; subcutaneous emphysema

SCe somatic cell

SCEP sandwich counterelectrophoresis; spinal cord evoked potential

SCER sister chromatid exchange rate

SCF Skin Cancer Foundation; stem cell factor; subcostal frontal [view]

SCFA short-chain fatty acid

SCFE slipped capital femoral epiphysis

SCG serum chemistry graft; serum chemogram; sodium cromoglycate; superior cervical ganglion

SCh succinylchloride; succinylcholine

SChE serum cholinesterase

schiz schizophrenia

SCHL subcapsular hematoma of the liver

SCI Science Citation Index; spinal cord injury; structured clinical interview

Sci science, scientific

SCID severe combined immunodeficiency [syndrome]; soft copy image display; Structured Clinical Interview for DSM-IV [diagnosis]

SCIDS severe combined immunodeficiency syndrome

SCIDX severe combined immunodeficiency disease, X-linked

SCII Strong-Campbell Interest Inventory

SCIM spinal cord injury medicine

SCINT, scint scintigraphy

SCIS spinal cord injury service

SCIU spinal cord injury unit

SCIV subcutaneous intravenous

SCIWORA spinal cord injury without radiographic abnormality

SCJ squamocolumnar junction; sternoclavicular joint; sternocostal joint

SCK serum creatine kinase

SCL scleroderma; serum copper level; sinus cycle length; soft contact lens; stromal cell line; subcostal lateral [view]; symptom check list; syndrome checklist

SCL-90 symptom checklist 90

scl sclerosis, sclerotic, sclerosed

ScLA left scapuloanterior [fetal position] [Lat. *scapulolaeva anterior*]

SCLC small cell lung carcinoma

SCLD sickle-cell chronic lung disease

SCLE subacute cutaneous lupus erythematosus

scler sclerosis, scleroderma

ScLP left scapuloposterior [fetal position] [Lat. *scapulolaeva posterior*]

SCL-90-R symptom checklist 90, revised

SCLS systemic capillary leak syndrome

SCM Schwann cell membrane; sensation, circulation, and motion; Society of Computer Medicine; soluble cytotoxic medium; spleen cell-conditioned medium; split cord malformation; spondylitic caudal myelopathy; State Certified Midwife; streptococcal cell membrane; sternocleidomastoid; surface-connecting membrane

SCMC spontaneous cell-mediated cytotoxicity

SCMO Senior Clerical Medical Officer

SCN special care nursing; suprachiasmatic nucleus

SCN1A sodium channel, neuronal alpha-subunit type 1

SCNS subcutaneous nerve stimulation

SCO sclerocystic ovary; somatic crossing-over; subcommissural organ

SCOP scopolamine

SCOR Specialized Center of Research [NIH]

SCOT subcostal [right ventricle] outflow [view]

SCP single-celled protein; standard care plan; sodium cellulose phosphate; soluble cytoplasmic protein; specialty care physician; sterol carrier protein; submucous cleft palate; superior cerebral peduncle

scp spherical candle power

SCPR standard cardiopulmonary resuscitation

SCPK serum creatine phosphokinase

SCPN serum carboxypeptidase N

SCPNT Southern California Postrotary Nystagmus Test

S-CPR standard post-compression remodeling

SCPT schizophrenic chronic paranoid type

SCR Schick conversion rate; short consensus repeat; silicon-controlled rectifier; skin conductance response; slow-cycling rhodopsin; spondylitic caudal radiculopathy

SCr serum creatinine

scr scruple

SCRAM speech-controlled respirometer for ambulation measurement

SCRF surface coil rotating frame

scRNA small cytoplasmic ribonucleic acid

SCS Saethre-Chotzen syndrome; shared computer system; silicon-controlled switch; Society of Clinical Surgery; spinal cord stimulation; Splint Classification System [of ASHT]; systolic click syndrome

SCSA subcostal shoert axis

SCSB static charge sensitive bed

SCSIT Southern California Sensory Integration Test

SCT secretin; sex chromatin test; sexual compatibility test; sickle-cell trait; sperm cytotoxicity; spinal computed tomography; spinocervicothalamic; staphylococcal clumping test; sugar-coated tablet

S$_{CT}$ serum creatinine

SCTAT sex cord tumor with annular tubules

SCTR secretin receptor

SCTx spinal cervical traction

SCU self-care unit; special care unit

SCUBA self-contained underwater breathing apparatus

SCUD septicemic cutaneous ulcerative disease

SCUF slow continuous ultrafiltration therapy

SCU-PA single-chain urokinase plasminogen activator

SCUT schizophrenic chronic undifferentiated type

SCV sensory nerve conduction velocity; smooth, capsulated, virulent; subclavian vein; squamous-cell carcinoma of the vulva

SCV-CPR simultaneous compression ventilation-cardiopulmonary resuscitation
SCVIR Society of Cardiovascular and Interventional Radiology
SCWM subcortical white matter
SD Sandhoff disease; senile dementia; septal defect; serologically defined; serologically detectable; serologically determined; serum defect; Shine-Dalgarno [sequence]; short dialysis; shoulder disarticulation; Shy-Draper [syndrome]; skin destruction; skin dose; somatization disorder; sphincter dilatation; spontaneous delivery; sporadic depression; Sprague-Dawley [rat]; spreading depression; stable disease; standard deviation; statistical documentation; Stensen duct; Still disease; stone disintegration; straight drainage; strength duration; streptodornase; sudden death; superoxide dismutase; systolic discharge
S-D sickle-cell hemoglobin D; suicide-depression
S/D sharp/dull; systolic/diastolic
Sd stimulus drive
S^d discriminative stimulus
SDA right sacroanterior [fetal position] [Lat. *sacrodextra anterior*]; sialodacryoadenitis; specific dynamic action; succinic dehydrogenase activity
SDAT senile dementia of Alzheimer type
SDAVF spinal dural arteriovenous fistula
SDB sleep-disordered breathing
SDBP seated (or standing, or supine) diastolic blood pressure
SDC serum digoxin concentration; Smith delay compensator; sodium deoxycholate; subacute combined degeneration; subclavian hemodialysis catheter; succinyldicholine; syndectan
SDCL symptom distress check list
SDCN N-syndectan, neural syndectan
SDD sporadic depressive disease; sterile dry dressing

SDDS 2-sulfamoyl-4,4;pr-diaminodiphenylsulfone
SDE specific dynamic effect; subdural empyema
SDEEG sterotactic depth electroencephalography
SDES symptomatic diffuse esophageal spasm
SDF slow death factor; stress distribution factor
SDG sucrose density gradient
SDGF schwannoma-derived growth factor
SDH serine dehydratase; sorbitol dehydrogenase; spinal dorsal horn; subdural hematoma; succinate dehydrogenase
SDHD sudden death heart disease
SDI standard deviation interval; survey diagnostic instrument
SDIHD sudden death ischemic heart disease
SDILINE Selective Dissemination of Information On-Line [data bank]
SDL serum digoxin level; speech discrimination level
sdl sideline; subline
SDM sensory detection method; standard deviation of the mean
SDMS Society of Diagnostic Medical Sonographers
SDN sexually dimorphic nucleus
SDO sudden dosage onset
SDP shared decision-making program; right sacroposterior [fetal position] [Lat. *sacrodextra posterior*]
SDR spontaneously diabetic rat; surgical dressing room
SDRS social dysfunction rating scale
SDS same day surgery; school dental services; self-rating depression scale; sensory deprivation syndrome; sexual differentiation scale; short depression screen; Shy-Drager syndrome; single-dose suppression; sodium dodecylsulfate; specific diagnosis service; standard

deviation score; sudden death syndrome; sulfadiazine silver; sustained depolarizing shift

SDSEM spinocerebellar degeneration-slow eye movements [syndrome]

SD-SK streptodornase-streptokinase

SDSL symmetrical digital single line

SDS/PAGE, SDS-PGE sodium dodecylsulfate-polyacrylamide gel electrophoresis

SDT sensory detection theory; right sacrotransverse [fetal position] [Lat. *sacrodextra transversa*]; signal detection theory; single-donor transfusion; speech detection threshold

SD$_t$ standard deviation of total scores

SDU standard deviation unit; step-down unit

SDUB short double upright brace

SDW spin density-weighted

SDYS Simpson dysmorphia syndrome

SE saline enema; sanitary engineering; side effect; smoke exposure; solid extract; sphenoethmoidal; spin-echo; spongiform encephalopathy; Spurway-Eddowes [syndrome]; standard error; standard error of measurement; staphylococcal endotoxin; staphylococcal enterotoxin; starch equivalent; Starr-Edwards [prosthesis]; status epilepticus; subendothelial; subependymal nodule

S&E safety and efficiency

Se secretion; selenium

$_s$E early systolic wave

SEA sheep erythrocyte agglutination; shock-elicited aggression; soluble egg antigen; spontaneous electrical activity; staphylococcal enterotoxin A

SEAT sheep erythrocyte agglutination test

SEB seborrhea; staphylococcal enterotoxin B

SEBA staphylococcal enterotoxin B antiserum

SEBL self-emptying blind loop

SEBM Society of Experimental Biology and Medicine

SEC secretin; Singapore epidemic conjunctivitis; soft elastic capsule

Sec Seconal

sec second; secondary; section

sec-Bu sec-butyl

SECG stress electrocardiography

SECRET stiffness of joint, elderly individuals, constitutional symptoms, arthritis, elevated erythrocyte sedimentation rate, temporal arthritis [in polymyalgia rheumatica]

SECSY spin echo correlated spectroscopy

sect section

SED sedimentation rate; skin erythema dose; spondyloepiphyseal dysplasia; standard error of deviation; staphylococcal enterotoxin D

sed sedimentation; stool [Lat. *sedes*]

SEDL spondyloepiphyseal dysplasia, late

sed rt sedimentation rate

SEDT spondyloepiphyseal dysplasia tarda

SEDT-PA spondyloepiphyseal dysplasia tarda-progressive arthropathy

SEE standard error of estimate

SEEG stereotactic electroencephalography

SEER Surveillance Epidemiology and End Results [Program]

SEF somatically-evoked field; staphylococcal enterotoxin F

SEG segment; soft elastic gelatin; sonoencephalogram

segm segment, segmented

SEGNE secretory granules of neural and endocrine [cells]

SEH subependymal hemorrhage

SEI Self-Esteem Inventory

SEL serum ethanol level

SELF Self-Evaluation of Life Function [scale]

SEM sample evaluation method; scanning electron microscopy; secondary enrichment medium; standard error of measurement; standard error of the mean; systolic ejection murmur

sem one-half [Lat. *semis*]; semen, seminal

SEMD spondyloepimetaphyseal dysplasia

SEMDIT spondyloepimetaphyseal dysplasia, Irapa type

SEMG semenogelin

sEMG surface electromyography

SEMI subendocardial myocardial infarction

SEMDJL spondyloepimetaphyseal dysplasia with joint laxity

SEN scalp-ear-nipple [syndrome*]*; State Enrolled Nurse

sen sensitive, sensitivity

SENIC study of the efficacy of nosocomial infection control

SENS sensitivity or sensitization; Stewart evaluation of nursing scale

SENSOR Sentinel Event Notification System for Occupational Risks

sens sensation, sensorium, sensory

SEP self-evaluation process; sensory-evoked potential; septum; somatosensory evoked potential; sperm entry point; spinal evoked potential; surface epithelium; systolic ejection period

sEP single evoked potential

separ separation, separation

SEQ side effects questionnaire

seq sequence; sequel, sequela, sequelae; sequestrum

SER sebum excretion rate; sensitizer enhancement ratio; sensory evoked response; service; smooth endoplasmic reticulum; smooth-surface endoplasmic reticulum; somatosensory evoked response; supination, external rotation [fracture]; surgical emergency room; systolic ejection rate

Ser serine; serology; serous; service

sER smooth endoplasmic reticulum

ser series, serial

SER-IV supination external rotation, type 4 fracture

SerCl serum chloride

SERHOLD National Biomedical Serials Holding Database

SERLINE Serials on Line

sero, serol serological, serology

SERPIN serpine protease inhibitor

SERS Stimulus Evaluation/Response Selection [test]

SERT sustained ethanol release tube

serv keep, preserve [Lat. *serva*]; service

SERVHEL Service and Health Records

SES Society of Eye Surgeons; socioeconomic status; spatial emotional stimulus; sphenoethmoidal suture; subendothelial space

SESAP Surgical Educational and Self-Assessment Program

SET surrogate embryo transfer; systolic ejection time

SET-N software evaluation tool for nursing

SETTS subjective experience of therapeutic touch survey

sev severe; severed

SEWHO shoulder-elbow-wrist-hand orthosis

SF Sabin-Feldman [test]; safety factor; salt-free; scarlet fever; screen film; seminal fluid; serosal fluid; serum factor; serum ferritin; serum fibrinogen; sham feeding; shell fragment; shunt flow; sickle cell-hemoglobin F [disease]; simian foam-virus; skin fibroblast; soft feces; spinal fluid; spontaneous fibrillation; stable factor; steel factor; sterile female; stress formula; sugar-free; superior facet; suppressor factor; suprasternal fossa; surviving fraction; Svedberg flotation [unit]; swine fever; symptom-free; synovial fluid

SF-36 short-form health survey [36 items]
Sf *Streptococcus faecalis*
S$_f$ Svedberg flotation unit
SFA saturated fatty acid; seminal fluid assay; serum folic acid; stimulated fibrinolytic activity; superior femoral artery
SFAP single-fiber action potential
SFB Sanfilippo syndrome type B; saphenofemoral bypass; surgical foreign body
SFBL self-filling blind loop
SFC soluble fibrin complex; soluble fibrin-fibrinogen complex; spinal fluid count
SFD silo filler's disease; skin-film distance; small for dates; spectral frequency distribution
SFE slipped femoral epiphysis
SFEMG single fiber electromyography
SFFA serum free fatty acid
SFFF sedimentation field flow fractionation
SFFV spleen focus-forming virus
SFG subglottic foreign body
SFH schizophrenia family history; serum-free hemoglobin; stroma-free hemoglobin
SFI Sexual Function Index; Social Function Index
SFIS structural family interaction scale
SFL synovial fluid lymphocyte
SFM Schimmelpenning-Fuerstein-Mims [syndrome]; serum-free medium; solution-focused management
SFMC soluble fibrin monomer complex
SFP screen filtration pressure; simultaneous foveal perception; spinal fluid pressure; stopped flow pressure
SFR screen filtration resistance; stroke with full recovery
SFS serial foveal seizures; skin and fascia stapler; social functioning schedule; spatial frequency spectrum; split function study
SFT Sabin-Feldman test; sensory feedback therapy; skinfold thickness
SFU surgical follow-up

SFV Semliki Forest virus; shipping fever virus; Shope fibroma virus; squirrel fibroma virus
SFW sexual function of women; shell fragment wound; slow-filling wave
SG Sachs-Georgi [test]; salivary gland; serum globulin; serum glucose; signs; skin graft; soluble gelatin; specific gravity; subgluteal; substantia gelatinosa; Surgeon General
sg specific gravity
SGA small for gestational age
SG$_{AW}$ specific airway conductance
SGB Simpson-Golabi-Behmel [syndrome]; sparsely granulated basophil
SGBS Simpson-Golabi-Behmel syndrome
SGC spermicide-germicide compound
SGCA subependymal giant cell astrocytoma
SGD specific granule deficiency
SGE secondary generalized epilepsy
SGF sarcoma growth factor; skeletal growth factor
SGH subgluteal hematoma
SGL salivary gland lymphocyte
SGLT sodium-glucose transporter
SGM Society for General Microbiology
SGML standard generalized markup language [of ISO]
SGNE secretory granule neuroendocrine [protein]
SGO Surgeon General's Office; surgery, gynecology, and obstetrics
SGOT serum glutamate oxaloacetate transaminase (aspartate aminotransferase)
SGP serine glycerophosphatide; sialoglycoprotein; Society of General Physiologists; soluble glycoprotein; sulfated glycoprotein
SGPA salivary gland pleomorphic adenoma
SGPT serum glutamate pyruvate transaminase (alanine aminotransferase)

SGR Sachs-Georgi reaction; Shwartzman generalized reaction; skin galvanic reflex; submandibular gland renin; substantia gelatinosa Rolandi
SGSG Scandinavian Glioma Study Group
S-Gt Sachs-Georgi test
SGTT standard glucose tolerance test
SGV salivary gland virus; selective gastric vagotomy
SGVHD syngeneic graft-versus-host disease
SH Salter-Harris [fracture]; Schönlein-Henoch [purpura]; self-help; serum hepatitis; sexual harassment; sex hormone; Sherman [rat]; sick in hospital; sinus histiocytosis; social history; somatotropic hormone; spontaneously hypertensive [rat]; standard heparin; state hospital; sulfhydryl; surgical history; symptomatic hypoglycemia; syndrome of hyporeninemic hypoaldosteronism; systemic hyperthermia
S/H sample and hold
S&H speech and hearing
Sh sheep; Sherwood number; *Shigella*; shoulder
sh shoulder
SHA staphylococcal hemagglutinating antibody
sHa suckling hamster
SHAA serum hepatitis associated antigen; Society of Hearing Aid Audiologists
SHAA-Ab serum hepatitis associated antigen antibody
SHAFT sad, hostile, anxious, frustrating, tenacious [patient] syndrome
SHARP school health additional referral program
SHB sequential hemibody [irradiation]
S-Hb sulfhemoglobin
SHBD serum hydroxybutyric dehydrogenase
SHBG sex hormone binding globulin
SHCC State Health Coordinating Council
SHCO sulfated hydrogenated castor oil

SHD sudden heart death
SHE Syrian hamster embryo
SHEENT skin, head, eyes, ears, nose, and throat
SHEP Systolic Hypertension in the Elderly Program
SHF simian hemorrhagic fever
shf super-high frequency
SHFD split hand/foot deformity
SHG synthetic human gastrin
SHH syndrome of hyporeninemic hypoaldosteronism
SHHD Scottish Home and Health Department
SHHH self-help for hard of hearing
SHHV Society for Health and Human Values
SHI significant head injury
Shig *Shigella*
SHL sensorineural hearing loss
SHLA soluble human lymphocyte antigen
SHLD shoulder
SHMC sinus histiocytosis with massive lymphadenopathy
SHML sinus histiocytosis with massive lymphadenopathy
SHMO, S/HMO social health maintenance organization
SHMP Senior Hospital Medical Officer
SHMT serine-hydroxymethyl transferase
SHN spontaneous hemorrhagic necrosis; subacute hepatic necrosis
SHO secondary hypertrophic osteoarthropathy; Senior House Officer
SHORT, S-H-O-R-T short stature, hyperextensibility of joints or hernia or both, ocular depression, Rieger anomaly, teething delayed
short-FRAME short stature-facial anomalies-Rieger anomaly-midline anomalies-enamel defects [syndrome]
SHP Schönlein-Henoch purpura; secondary hyperparathyroidism; state health plan

SHPDA State Health Planning and Development Agency

sHPT secondary hyperparathyroidism

SHR spontaneously hypertensive rat

SHS Sayre head sling; sheep hemolysate supernatant

SHSP spontaneously hypertensive stroke-prone [rat]

SHSS Stanford Hypnotic Susceptibility Scale

SHT simple hypocalcemic tetany; subcutaneous histamine test

SHTTP secure hypertext transport protocol

SHUR System for Hospital Uniform Reporting

SHV simian herpes virus

SI International System of Units [Fr. *le Système International d'Unités*]; sacroiliac; saline infusion; saline injection; saturation index; self-inflicted; sensory integration; septic inflammation; serious illness; serum iron; severity index; sex inventory; signal intensity; Singh Index; single injection; small intestine; social interaction; soluble insulin; spirochetosis icterohaemorrhagica; stimulation index; stress incontinence; stroke index; sucrase isomaltase; suppression index

Si the most anterior point on the lower contour of the sella turcica [point]; silicon

S&I suction and irrigation

SIA serum inhibitory activity; stress-induced analgesia; stress-induced anesthesia; subacute infectious arthritis

SIADH syndrome of inappropriate secretion of antidiuretic hormone

SIB self-injurious behavior

sib, sibs sibling, siblings

SIC serum insulin concentration; Standard Industrial Classification

SICD serum isocitrate dehydrogenase

SICU spinal intensive care unit; surgical intensive care unit

SID single intradermal [test]; Society for Investigative Dermatology; sucrase-isomaltase deficiency; sudden inexplicable death; sudden infant death; suggested indication of diagnosis; systemic inflammatory disease

SIDAM structured interview for the diagnosis of dementia of the Alzheimer type

SIDS sudden infant death syndrome; sulfo-iduronate sulfatase

SIE stroke in evolution

SIECUS Sex Information and Education Council of the United States

SIF serum-inhibition factor

SIFT selector ion flow tube

SIG small inducible gene

SIg, sIg surface immunoglobulin

sig sigmoidoscopy; significant

S-IgA secretory immunoglobulin A

SIGH-D structured interview for the Hamilton Depression Scale

Σ Greek capital letter *sigma*; syphilis; summation of series

σ Greek lower case letter *sigma*; conductivity; cross section; millisecond; molecular type or bond; population standard deviation; stress; surface tension; wave number

sigmo sigmoidoscope or sigmoidoscopy

SIH stimulation-induced hypalgesia; stress-induced hyperthermia; suction-induced hypoxemia

SIHE spontaneous intramural hematoma of the esophagus

SI-HRDS structured interview Hamilton rating scale for depression

SII self-inflicted injury

SIJ sacroiliac joint

SIL soluble interleukin; speech interference level

SILD Sequenced Inventory of Language Development

SIM selected ion monitoring; Society of Industrial Microbiology

SIMA single internal mammary artery

SIMP Schmele instrument to measure the process of nursing care

SIMP-C Schmele instrument to measure the process of nursing care

SIMP-H Schmele instrument to measure the process of nursing care in home care

SIMS secondary ion mass spectroscopy

simul simultaneously

SIMV synchronized intermittent mandatory ventilation; synchronized intermittent mechanical ventilation

SIN salpingitis isthmica nodosa

SIO sacroiliac orthosis

SIOP International Society of Pediatric Oncology

SIP Sickness Impact Profile; slow inhibitory potential; surface inductive plethysmography

sIPTH serum immunoreactive parathyroid hormone

SIQ Symptom Interpretation Questionnaire

SIQR semi-interquartile range

SIR single isomorphous replacement; specific immune release; standardized incidence ratio; syndrome of immediate reactivities

SIRA Scientific Instrument Research Association

SIREF specific immune response enhancing factor

SIRF severely impaired renal function

SIRS soluble immune response suppressor; Structured Interview of Reported Symptoms; systemic inflammatory response syndrome

SIS semantic indexing system; serotinin irritation syndrome; simian sarcoma; simulator-induced syndrome; social information system; spontaneous interictal spike; sterile injectable solution; sterile injectable suspension

SISH Stage I Systolic Hypertension in the Elderly [study]

SISI short increment sensitivity index

SISS Sentinel Injury Surveillance System [for Gunshot and Stab Wounds] small inducible secreted substances

SISV, SiSV simian sarcoma virus

SIT serum inhibiting titer; Slosson Intelligence Test; sperm immobilization test; suggested immobilization test

SITS supraspinatus, infraspinatus, teres minor, subscapularis [shoulder muscles comprising the rotator cuff]

SIV simian immunodeficiency virus; Sprague-Dawley-Ivanovas [rat]

SIVagm simian immunodeficiency virus from African green monkeys

SIVMAC simian immunodeficiency virus of macaques

SIW self-inflicted wound

SIWIP self-induced water intoxication and psychosis

SIWIS self-induced water intoxication and schizophrenic disorders

S_J Jaccard coefficient

SJA Schwartz-Jampel-Aberfeld [syndrome]

SjO_2 jugular bulb venous oxygen saturation

SJR Shinowara-Jones-Reinhart [unit]

SJS Stevens-Johnson syndrome; stiff joint syndrome; Swyer-James syndrome

SjS Sjögren syndrome

$SjVO_2$ jugular venous oxygen saturation

SK seborrheic keratosis; senile keratosis; Sloan-Kettering [Institute for Cancer Research]; spontaneous killer [cell]; streptokinase; swine kidney

Sk skin

SKA supracondylar knee-ankle [orthosis]

SKALP skin-derived antileukoproteinase

SKAT Sex Knowledge and Attitude Test

skel skeleton, skeletal

SKI Sloan-Kettering Institute

SKL serum killing level

SKSD, SK-SD streptokinase-streptodornase

sk trx skeletal traction

SL sarcolemma; sclerosing leukoencephalopathy; secondary leukemia; segment length; sensation level; sensory latency; septal leaflet; short-leg [brace]; Sibley-Lehninger [unit]; signal level; Sinding Larsen [syndrome]; Sjögren-Larsson [syndrome]; slit lamp; small lymphocyte; sodium lactate; solidified liquid; sound level; Stein-Leventhal [syndrome]; streptolysin; sublingual

S_L systolic wave, latent

S/L sublingual

Sl Steel [mouse]

sl in a broad sense [Lat. *sensu lato*]; stemline; sublingual

SLA left sacroanterior [fetal position] [Lat. *sacrolaeva anterior*]; single-cell liquid cytotoxic assay; slide latex agglutination; soluble liver antigen; superficial linear array; surfactant-like activity

SL_A segment length, anterior

SLAC scapholunate advanced collapse [wrist]

SLAM scanning laser acoustic microscope; systemic lupus erythematosus activity measure

SLAP serum leucine aminopeptidase

SLAT simultaneous laryngoscopy and abdominal thrusts

SLB short-leg brace

SLC short-leg cast

SLCC short-leg cylinder cast

SLD, SLDH serum lactate dehydrogenase; sublethal damage

SLDR sublethal damage repair

SLE slit lamp examination; St. Louis encephalitis; systemic lupus erythematosus

SLEA sheep erythrocyte antibody

SLEDAI systemic lupus erythematosus disease activity index

SLEP short latent evoked potential

SLEV St. Louis encephalitis virus

SLHR sex-linked hypophosphatemic rickets

SLI selective lymphoid irradiation; somatostatin-like immunoreactivity; splenic localization index

SL_I segment length, inferior

SLIC scanning liquid ionization chamber

SLIDRC Student Loan Interest Deduction Restoration Coalition

SLIP serial line interface protocol

SLIR somatostatin-like immunoreactivity

SLK superior limbic keratoconjunctivitis

SLKC superior limbic keratoconjunctivitis

SLL small lymphocytic lymphoma

SL_L segment length, lateral

SLM sound level meter

SLMC spontaneous lymphocyte-mediated cytotoxicity

SLN sublentiform nucleus; superior laryngeal nerve

SLNWBC short-leg nonweightbearing cast

SLNWC short-leg nonwalking cast

SLO Smith-Lemli-Opitz syndrome; streptolysin O

SLOS Smith-Lemli-Opitz syndrome

SLP left sacroposterior [fetal position] [Lat. *sacrolaeva posterior*]; segmental limb systolic pressure; sex-limited protein; short luteal phase; subluxation of the patella

SLPI secretory leukocyte protease inhibitor

SLPP serum lipophosphoprotein

SLR Shwartzman local reaction; single lens reflex; straight leg raising

SLRT straight leg raising test

SLS segment long-spacing; short-leg splint; single limb support; Sjögren-Larsson syndrome; stagnant loop syndrome; Stein-Leventhal syndrome

SL_S segment length, septal

SLT left sacrotransverse [fetal position] [Lat. *sacrolaeva transversa*]; single lung transplantation; smokeless tobacco; solid logic technology

SLUD salivation, lacrimation, urination, defecation

SLUDGE salivation, lacrimation, urination, defecation, gastrointestinal upset, emesis

SLWC short-leg walking cast

SM Master of Science; sadomasochism; self-monitoring; silicon microphysiometer; simple mastectomy; skim milk; smooth muscle; somatomedin; space medicine; sphingomyelin; splenic macrophage; sports medicine; streptomycin; Strümpell-Marie [syndrome]; submandibular; submaxillary; submucous; suckling mouse; sucrose medium; suction method; superior mesenteric; surgical microscope; surrogate mother; sustained medication; symptoms; synaptic membrane; synovial membrane; systolic motion; systolic murmur

S/M sudomasochism

Sm samarium; *Serratia marcescens*, Smith [antigen]

sm smear

sM suckling mouse

SMA sequential multiple analysis or analyzer; sequential multichannel autoanalyzer; simultaneous multichannel autoanalyzer; smooth muscle antibody; Society for Medical Anthropology; somatomedin A; spinal muscular atrophy; spontaneous motor activity; standard method agar; superior mesenteric artery; supplementary motor area

SM-A somatomedin A

SMA-6 Sequential Multiple Analysis-m-six different serum tests

SMABF superior mesenteric artery blood flow

SMAC Sequential Multiple Analyzer Computer

SMAE superior mesenteric artery embolism

SMAF smooth muscle activating factor; specific macrophage arming factor

SMAG Special Medical Advisory Group

SMAL serum methyl alcohol level

sm an small animal

SMAO superior mesenteric artery occlusion

SMART simultaneous multiple angle reconstruction technique

SMAS submuscular aponeurotic system; superficial musculo-aponeurotic system; superior mesenteric artery syndrome

SMAST Short Michigan Alcoholism Screening Test

SMB selected mucosal biopsy; standard mineral base

sMb suckling mouse brain

SMBFT small bowel follow-through

SMC Scientific Manpower Commission; smooth muscle cell; somatomedin C; succinylmonocholine

SM-C, Sm-C somatomedin C

SMCA smooth muscle contracting agent; suckling mouse cataract agent

SMCD senile macular choroidal degeneration; systemic mast cell disease; systemic meningococcal disease

SM-C/IGF somatomedin C/insulin-like growth factor

SMCR Smith-Magenis chromosome region

SMD senile macular degeneration; spondylometaphyseal dysplasia; submanubrial dullness

SMDA Safe Medical Devices Act [of 1990]; starch methylenedianiline

SMDC sodium-N-methyl dithiocarbamate; standards for medical device communication

SMDM Society for Medical Decision Making

SMDS secondary myelodysplastic syndrome

SME severe myoclonic epilepsy

SMED spondylometaphyseal dysplasia

SMEDI stillbirth-mummification, embryonic death, infertility [syndrome]

SMEI severe myoclonic epilepsy of infancy

SMEM supplemented Eagle minimum essential medium

SMF streptozocin, mitomycin C, and 5-fluorouracil

smf sodium motive force

SMFP state medical facilities plan

SMG specialty medical group; submandibular gland

SMH state mental hospital; strongyloidiasis with massive hyperinfection

SMHA state mental health agency

SMHC smooth muscle heavy chain myosin

SMI Self-Motivation Inventory; senior medical investigator; severe mental impairment; silent myocardial infarction; small volume infusion; stress myocardial image; Style of Mind Inventory; supplementary medical insurance; sustained maximum inspiration

SmIg surface membrane immunoglobulin

SML smouldering leukemia

SMM smoldering multiple myeloma

SMMD specimen mass measurement device

SMMSE Standardized Mini-Mental State Examination

SMN second malignant neoplasm; stathmin

SMNB submaximal neuromuscular block

SMO Senior Medical Officer

SMOH Senior Medical Officer of Health; Society of Medical Officers of Health

SMON subacute myeloopticoneuropathy

SMP slow moving protease; standard medical practice; submitochondrial particle; sulfamethoxypyrazine; sympathetically maintained pain

SMPR small mannose 6-phosphate receptor

SMR senior medical resident; sensorimotor rhythm; severe mental retardation; sexual maturity rating; skeletal muscle relaxant; somnolent metabolic rate; standardized mortality ratio; stroke with minimum residuum; submucosal resection

SMRR submucosal resection and rhinoplasty

SMRV squirrel monkey retrovirus

SMS senior medical student; serial motor seizures; Shared Medical Systems; Smith-Magenis syndrome; somatostatin; stiff-man syndrome; supplemental minimum sodium

SMSA standard metropolitan statistical area

SMSV San Miguel sea lion virus

SMT spontaneous mammary tumor; stereotactic mesencephalic tractomy

S-MUAP surface-detected motor unit action potential

SMuLV Scripps murine leukemia virus

SMV superior mesenteric vein

SMX, SMZ sulfamethoxazole

SN sclerema neonatorum; scrub nurse; sensorineural; sensory neuron; serum neutralization; sinus node; spontaneous nystagmus; staff nurse; student nurse; subnormal; substantia nigra; supernatant; suprasternal notch

S/N signal/noise [ratio]

Sn subnasale

SNA specimen not available; Student Nurses Association

SNa serum sodium concentration

SNagg serum normal agglutinator

SNAP sensory nerve action potential; S-nitroso-N-acetylpenicillamine

SNB scalene node biopsy

SNC spontaneous neonatal chylothorax

SNCL sinus node cycle length

SNCS sensory nerve conduction studies

SNCV sensory nerve conduction velocity

SND sinus node dysfunction; striatonigral degeneration

SNDA Student National Dental Association

SNDO Standard Nomenclature of Diseases and Operations

SNE sinus node electrogram; subacute necrotizing encephalomyelography

SNES suprascapular nerve entrapment syndrome

SNF sinus node formation; skilled nursing facility

SNGBF single nephron glomerular blood flow

SNGFR single nephron glomerular filtration rate

SNHL sensorineural hearing loss

SNIPA seronegative inflammatory polyarthritis

SNIVT Society of Non-Invasive Vascular Technology

SNM Society of Nuclear Medicine; sulfanilamide

SNMA Student National Medical Association

SNMT Society of Nuclear Medical Technologists

SNOBOL String-Oriented Symbolic Language

SNODO Standard Nomenclature of Diseases and Operations

SNOMED Systematized Nomenclature of Medicine

SNOP Systematized Nomenclature of Pathology

SNP school nurse practitioner; sinus node potential; sodium nitroprusside

SNR selective nerve root [block]; signal-to-noise ratio; substantia nigra zona reticulata; supernumerary rib

SNRB selective nerve root block

snRNA small nuclear ribonucleic acid

snRNP small nuclear ribonucleoprotein particle

snRP small nuclear ribonucleoprotein polypeptide

snRPB small nuclear ribonucleoprotein polypeptide B

snRPN small nuclear ribonucleoprotein polypeptide N

SNRT sinus node recovery time

SNRTd sinus node recovery time, direct measuring

SNRTi sinus node recovery time, indirect measuring

SNS Senior Nursing Sister; Society of Neurological Surgeons; sympathetic nervous system

SNSA seronegative spondyloarthropathy

S-NSE serum neuron-specific enolase

SNST sciatic nerve stretch test

SNT sinuses, nose, and throat

SNU skilled nursing unit

SNV spleen necrosis virus

SNW slow negative wave

SO salpingo-oophorectomy; Schlatter-Osgood [test]; second opinion; sex offender; spheno-occipital [synchondrosis]; sphincter of Oddi; standing orders; superior oblique [muscle]; supraoptic; supraorbital

S&O salpingo-oophorectomy

SO$_2$ oxygen saturation

SOA stimulus onset asynchrony; swelling of ankles

SoA symptoms of asthma

SOAA signed out against advice

SOAMA signed out against medical advice

SOA-MCA superficial occipital artery to middle cerebral artery

SOAP subjective, objective, assessment, and plan [problem-oriented record]

SOAPIE subjective, objective, assessment, plan, implementation, and evaluation [problem-oriented record]

SOB see order blank; shortness of breath

SOBOE shortness of breath on exertion

SOC sequential oral contraceptive; Standard Occupational Classification; standards of care; synovial osteochondromatosis; syphilitic osteochondritis

SoC state of consciousness

SocSec Social Security

SocServ social services

S-OCT serum ornithine carbamyl transferase

SOD septo-optic dysplasia; superoxide dismutase

sod sodium

sod bicarb sodium bicarbonate

SODAS spheroidal oral drug absorption system

SODF sperm outer defense fiber

SODH sorbitol dehydrogenase

SOF superior orbital fissure

SOH sympathetic orthostatic hypotension

SOHN supraoptic hypothalamic nucleus

SOI severity of illness

SOL solution; space-occupying lesion

sol soluble, solution

SOLEC stand on one leg eyes closed

Soln, sol'n solution

SOLVD studies of left ventricular dysfunction

SOM secretory otitis media; sensitivity of method; serous otitis media; somatotropin; state operations manual; superior oblique muscle; suppurative otitis media

SOMA Student Osteopathic Medical Association

somat somatic

SOMI sternal occipital mandibular immobilization

SON superior olivary nucleus; supraoptic nucleus

SONH spontaneous osteonecrosis of the hip

SONK spontaneous osteonecrosis of the knee

SOO structured office oral [examination]

SOP service–object pair; standard operating procedure

SoP standard of performance

SOPA Survey of Pain Attitudes; syndrome of primary aldosteronism

SOPCA sporadic olivopontocerebellar ataxia

SOPI service object pair instance

SOQ Suicide Opinion Questionnaire

SOR stimulus-organism response; superoxide release

SOr supraorbitale

sOR stratified odds ratio

Sorb, sorb sorbitol

SORD sorbitol dehydrogenase

SOREM sleep onset rapid eye movement

SOS self-obtained smear; supplemental oxygen system

SOSA Student Osteopathic Surgical Association

SOSF single organ system failure

SOT sensory organization test; systemic oxygen transport

SOWS subjective opiate withdrawal scale

SP sacroposterior; sacrum to pubis; salivary progesterone; schizotypal personality; semi-private [room]; senile plaque; sepiaopterin; septum pellucidum; seropositive; serum protein; shunt pressure; shunt procedure; silent period; skin potential; sleep deprivation; soft palate; solid phase; speech pathology; spleen; spontaneous proliferation; standard practice; standard procedure; standardized patient; standardized-patient [assessment]; staphylococcal protease; status post; stool preservative; storage phosphor [radiography]; subliminal perception; substance P; suprapatellar; suprapubic; surface polypeptide; surfactant protein; symphysis pubis; systolic pressure

Sp the most posterior point on the posterior contour of the sella turcica; species; specific; specimen; sphenoid; spine; *Spirillum*; summation potential

S/P, s/p status, post[operative]

S7P sedoheptulose-7-phosphate

sP senile parkinsonism

sp space; species; specific; spine, spinal; spirit

SPA salt-poor albumin; sheep pulmonary adenomatosis; sperm penetration assay; spinal progressive amyotrophy; spondyloarthropathy; spontaneous platelet aggregation; staphylococcal protein A; student progress assessment; suprapubic aspiration; surface polypeptide, anonymous

SP-A surfactant protein A

SPACE single potential analysis of cavernous electrical activity

sp act specific activity

SPAD stenosing peripheral arterial disease

SPAF spontaneous paroxysmal atrial fibrillation

SPAG small particle aerosol generator

SPAI steroid protein activity index

SPAM scanning photoacoustic microscopy

SPAMM spatial modulation of magnetization

sp an spinal anesthesia

SPAR sensitivity prediction by acoustic reflex

SPARC cysteine-rich acidic secreted protein

SPAT slow paroxysmal atrial tachycardia

SPB sinking pre-beta-lipoprotein

SP-B surfactant protein B

SPBI serum protein-bound iodine

SPC salicylamide, phenacetin, and caffeine; seropositive carrier; single palmar crease; single photoelectron count; spleen cell; statistical process control; synthetizing protein complex

SPCA serum prothrombin conversion accelerator; Society for Prevention of Cruelty to Animals

SPCC Spill Prevention, Control, and Countermeasure [plan]

SPCD syndrome of primary ciliary dyskinesia

Sp Cd, sp cd spinal cord

SPD schizotypal personality disorder; sociopathic personality disorder; specific paroxysmal discharge; spermidine; standard peak dilution; storage pool deficiency

SPDC strio-pallido-dentate calcinosis

SPE septic pulmonary edema; serum protein electrolytes; serum protein electrophoresis; streptococcal pyrogenic exotoxin; sucrose polyester; sustained physical exercise

SPEAR selective parenteral and enteral anti-sepsis regimen

SPEC specificity

SPE-C streptococcal pyrogenic exotoxin type C

Spec specialist, specialty

spec special; specific; specimen

spec gr specific gravity

SPECT single photon emission computed tomography

sPEEP spontaneous peak end-expiratory pressure

SPEG serum protein electrophoretogram

SPEL syndactyly-polydactyly-earlobe [syndrome]

SPEM smooth pursuit eye movement

SPEP serum protein electrophoresis

SPERM spastic paraplegia-epilepsy-mental retardation [syndrome]

SPF skin protection factor; specific-pathogen free; spectrophotofluorometer; S-phase fraction; split products of fibrin; standard perfusion fluid; Stuart-Prower factor; sun protection factor; systemic pulmonary fistula

Sp Fl, sp fl spinal fluid

SPG serine phosphoglyceride; spastic paraplegia; splenoportography; sucrose, phosphate, and glutamate; symmetrical peripheral gangrene

SpG specific gravity

spg sponge

SPGA Bovarnik solution; sucrose

SpGr, sp gr specific gravity

SPGX spastic paraplegia, X-linked

SPH secondary pulmonary hemosiderosis; severely and profoundly handicapped; spherocyte; spherocytosis; sphingomyelin

Sph sphenoidale; sphingomyelin

sph spherical; spherical lens; spheroid

sp ht specific heat

SPI Self-Perception Inventory; serum precipitable iodine; serum protein index; Shipley Personal Inventory; standardized-patient instructor

SPIA solid-phase immunoabsorption; solid-phase immunoassay

SPICU surgical pulmonary intensive care unit

SPID summed pain intensity difference

SPIF solid-phase immunoassay fluorescence

SPIH superimposed pregnancy-induced hypertension

spin spine, spinal

spir spiral; spirit

SPJ saphenopopliteal junction

SPK serum pyruvate kinase; superficial punctate keratitis

SPL skin potential level; sound pressure level; splanchnic; spontaneous lesion; staphylococcal phage lysate; superior parietal lobule; surfactant proteolipid

SPLATT split anterior tibial tendon

sPLM sleep-related periodic leg movements

SPLV serum parvovirus-like virus

SPM shocks per minute; spermine; subhuman primate model; suspended particulate matter; synaptic plasma membrane

SpM spiriformis medialis [nucleus]

spm spermatogonial metaphase

SPMA spinal progressive muscular atrophy

SPMR standard proportionate mortality ratio (or rate)

SPMSQ Short Portable Mental Status Questionnaire

SPN senior plan network; sialophorin; solitary pulmonary nodule; supplemental parental nutrition; sympathetic preganglionic neuron

SpnCbT spinocerebellar tract

SpO₂ pulse oximetry

SPOCS surgical planning and orientation computer system

SPOD spouse's perception of disease

spon, spont spontaneous

SPONASTRIME spondylar and nasal alterations with striated metaphyses

SPOOL simultaneous peripheral operation on-line

SPP plural of *species*; Sexuality Preference Profile; skin perfusion pressure; suprapubic prostatectomy

spp plural of *species*

Sp Pn, Sp Pnx spontaneous pneumothorax

SPPP, sppp plural of *subspecies*

SPPS solid phase peptide synthesis; stable plasma protein solution

SPPT superprecipitation response

SPR sepiapterin reductase; serial probe recognition; specific pathogen free; Society for Pediatric Radiology; Society for Pediatric Research; solid phase radioimmunoassay

Spr scan projection radiography

spr sprain

SPRIA solid phase radioimmunoassay

SPROM spontaneous premature rupture of membrane

SPRR small proline-rich protein

SPRRA small proline-rich protein A

SPRRB small proline-rich protein B

SPRRC small proline-rich protein C

SPS scapuloperoneal syndrome; shoulder pain and stiffness; simple partial seizures; slow-progressive schizophrenia; Society of Pelvic Surgeons; sodium polyanethol sulfonate; sodium polystyrene; sound production sample; spermidine synthase; stimulated protein synthesis; Suicide Probability Scale; systemic progressive sclerosis

SpS sphenoid sinus

spSHR stroke-prone spontaneously hypertensive rat

SPST Symonds Picture-Story Test

SPT secretin-pancreazymin [test]; single patch technique; sleep period time; spectrin; station pull-through [technique]

SpT spinal tap

SPTA spectrin alpha

SPTAN spectrin alpha, nonerythroid

Sp tap spinal tap

SPTI systolic pressure time index

SPTS subjective posttraumatic syndrome

SPTx static pelvic traction

SPU short procedure unit; Society of Pediatric Urology; standardized photometric unit

SPV selective proximal vagotomy; Shope papilloma virus; sulfophosphovanillin

SPW subxiphoid pericardial window

SPZ sulfinpyrazone

SQ social quotient; status quo; subcutaneous; survey question; symptom questionnaire

Sq subcutaneous

sq square; squamous

SQC statistical quality control

sq cell ca squamous cell carcinoma

SQL structured query language

SQUID superconducting quantum interference device

SR sarcoplasmic reticulum; saturation recovery; scanning radiometer; screen; secretion rate; sedimentation rate; seizure resistant; senior resident; sensitivity response; sensitization response; service record; sex ratio; shorthair [guinea pig]; short range; side rails; sigma reaction; sinus rhythm; skin resistance; sleep and rest; slow release; smooth-rough [colony]; specific release; specific response; spontaneous respiration; steroid resistance; stimulus response; stomach rumble; stress related; stretch reflex; sulfonamide-resistant; superior rectus; sustained release; synchronization ratio; systemic resistance; systems research; systems review

S-R smooth-rough [bacteria]

Sr strontium

sr steradian

SRA segmental renal artery; serum renin activity; spleen repopulating activity

SRAM static random access memory

SR$_{AW}$, SR$_{aw}$ specific airway resistance

SRBC sheep red blood cells

SRBD sleep-related breathing disorder

SRC sedimented red cells; sheep red cells

src Rous sarcoma oncogene

SRCA specific red cell adherence

SRCBC serum reserve cholesterol binding capacity

SR/CP schizophrenic reaction, chronic paranoid

SRD service-related disability; Society for the Relief of Distress; Society for the Right to Die; sodium-restricted diet; specific reading disability

SRDS severe respiratory distress syndrome

SRDT single radial diffusion test

SRE Schedule of Recent Experiences; sterol regulatory element

SREBP sterol regulatory element binding protein

sREM stage rapid eye movement

SRF severe renal failure; skin reactive factor; somatotropin-releasing factor; split renal function; subretinal fluid

SRF-A slow-reacting factor-anaphylaxis

SRFS split renal function study

SRG specialty review group

SRH single radial hemolysis; somatotropin-releasing hormone; spontaneously responding hyperthyroidism; stigmata of recent hemorrhage

SRI serotonin reuptake inhibitor; severe renal insufficiency; sorcin; Stanford Research Institute; structured review instrument

SRID single radial immunodiffusion

SRIF somatotropin-release inhibiting factor

SRM spontaneous rupture of membranes; Standard Reference Material; superior rectus muscle

SMRD stress-related mucosal damage

SRN State Registered Nurse

sRNA soluble ribonucleic acid

SRNG sustained release nitroglycerin

SRNS steroid-responsive nephrotic syndrome

SRO sex-ratio organism; single room occupancy; smallest region of overlap; Steele-Richardson-Olszewski [syndrome]

SROC summary receiver operating characteristic

SROM spontaneous rupture of membrane

SRP short rib-polydactyly [syndrome]; signal recognition particle; Society for Radiological Protection; State Registered Physiotherapist; synchronized retroperfusion

SRPR signal recognition particle receptor

SRPS short rib-polydactyly syndrome

SRQ Self-Reporting Questionnaire

SRR standardized rate ratio; surgery recovery room

SRRS Social Readjustment Rating Scale

SR-RSV Schmidt-Ruppin strain Rous sarcoma virus

SRS schizophrenic residual state; sex reassignment surgery; Silver-Russell syndrome; simple repeat sequence; slow-reacting substance; Social and Rehabilitation Service; social relationship scale; spermidine synthase; standard rating scale; Symptom Rating Scale

SRSA, SRS-A slow-reacting substance of anaphylaxis

SRT sedimentation rate test; simple reaction time; sinus node recovery time; sitting root test; speech reception test; speech reception threshold; spontaneously resolving thyrotoxicosis; surfactant replacement therapy; sustained-release theophylline; symptom rating test

SRU sample ratio units; side rails up; solitary rectal ulcer; structural repeating unit

SRUS solitary rectal ulcer syndrome

SRV Schmidt-Ruppin virus; simian retrovirus; superior radicular vein

SRVT sustained re-entrant ventricular tachyarrhythmia

SRW short ragweed [test]

SRWS super radiology work station

SS disulfide; sacrosciatic; saline soak; saline solution; saliva sample; saliva substitute; *Salmonella-Shigella* [agar]; salt substitute; saturated solution; Schizophrenia Subscale; seizure-sensitive; selective shunt; serum sickness; Sézary syndrome; short sleep; short stature; siblings; sickle cell; side-to-side; signs and symptoms; single-stranded; Sjögren syndrome; skull series [radiographs]; soap suds; Social Security; social services; somatostatin; sparingly soluble; stainless steel; standard score; statistically significant; steady state; sterile solution; steroid sensitivity; Stickler syndrome; subaortic stenosis; subscapular; subspinale; substernal; suction socket; sum of squares; supersaturated; support and stimulation; Sweet syndrome; systemic sclerosis

S/S salt substitute; signs/symptoms

S&S signs and symptoms
Ss *Shigella sonnei*; subjects
SSA salicylsalicylic acid; sicca syndrome A; skin-sensitizing antibody; skin sympathetic activity; Sjögren syndrome A; Smith surface antigen; Social Security Administration; sperm-specific antiserum; sulfosalicylic acid
SSA1 Smallest Space Analysis
SSAA sicca syndrome associated antigen A; Sjögren syndrome-associated antigen A; syringomyelia secondary to arachnoid adhesions
SSAV simian sarcoma-associated virus
SSB short spike burst; sicca syndrome B; single-strand break; single-stranded binding [protein]; stereospecific binding
SS-B Sjögren syndrome B
SSBG sex steroid-binding globulin; social services block grant
SSC single-strand conformational [analysis]; sister strand crossover; somatosensory cortex; standard saline citrate; standard sodium citrate; syngeneic spleen cell
SSc systemic scleroderma; systemic sclerosis
SSCA spontaneous suppressor cell activity
SSCCS slow spinal cord compression syndrome
ss(c)DNA single-stranded circular deoxyribonucleic acid
SSCF sleep stage change frequency
SSCP single-stranded conformational polymorphism
SSCr stainless steel crown
SSCT stereotactic subcaudate tractotomy
SSD shaded surface display; single saturating dose; Social Security disability; source-skin distance; source-surface distance; speech-sound discrimination; succinate semialdehyde dehydrogenase; sum of square deviations; syndrome of sudden death

SSDBS symptom schedule for the diagnosis of borderline schizophrenia
SSDD steroid sulfatase deficiency disease
SSDI Social Security Disability Income; Supplemental Security Disability Income
ssDNA single-stranded DNA
SSE saline solution enema; skin self-examination; soapsuds enema; steady state exercise; subacute spongiform encephalopathy
SSEA stage-specific embryonic antigen
SSEP somatosensory evoked potential
SSER somatosensory evoked response
SSES Sexual Self-Efficacy Scale
SSF soluble suppressor factor; supplemental sensory feedback
SSFP steady state free procession
SSG sublabial salivary gland
SSHL severe sensorineural hearing
SSI segmental sequential irradiation; shoulder subluxation inhibition; small-scale integration; Social Security increment; Somatic Symptom Inventory; subshock insulin; supplemental security income; surgical site infection; System Sign Inventory
SSI 4,6 Somatic Symptom Index [of DIS]
SSIDS sibling of sudden infant death syndrome [victim]
SSIE Smithsonian Science Information Exchange
SSKI saturated solution of potassium iodide
SSL secure sockets layer; skin surface lipid; sufficient sleep
SSLI serum sickness-like illness
SSM subsynaptic membrane; superficial spreading melanoma
SSMS saturated solution of magnesium iodide
SSN severely subnormal; subacute sensory neuropathy; suprasternal notch
SSNHL sudden sensorineural hearing loss

SSNS steroid-sensitive nephrotic syndrome

SSO sequence-specific oligonucleotide [probe]; Society of Surgical Oncology; special sense organ

SSOP Second Surgical Opinion Program; sequence-specific oligonucleotide probe

SSP Sanarelli-Shwartzman phenomenon; subacute sclerosing panencephalitis; slice sensitivity profile; subspecies; supersensitivity perception

ssp subspecies

SSPCP service-specific practice cost percentage

SSPE subacute sclerosing panencephalitis

SSPG steady state plasma glucose

SSPI steady state plasma insulin

SSPL saturation sound pressure level

SSPP subsynaptic plate perforation

SSPS side-to-side portacaval shunt

SS-PSE Schizophrenic Subscale of the Present State Examination

SSQ Social Support Questionnaire

SSR site-specific recombination; somatosensory response; surgical supply room

SSRI selective serotonin reuptake inhibitor

ssRNA single-stranded ribonucleic acid

SSS scalded skin syndrome; secondary Sjögren syndrome; sick sinus syndrome; specific soluble substance; Stanford Sleepiness Scale; sterile saline soak; subscapular skinfold; superior sagittal sinus; systemic sicca syndrome

SSSI Siegel Scale of Support for Innovation

SSSS staphylococcal scalded skin syndrome

SSST superior sagittal sinus thrombosis

SSSV superior sagittal sinus velocity

SST sodium sulfite titration; somatostatin

SSTR somatostatin receptor

SSU self-service unit; sterile supply unit

SSV Schoolman-Schwartz virus; simian sarcoma virus

SSX sulfisoxazole

ST esotropia; scala tympani; scaphotrapezoid; sclerotherapy; sedimentation time; semitendinosus; sensory threshold; shock therapy; sickle [cell] thalassemia; sincerity test; sinus tachycardia; sinus tympani; skin test; skin thickness; slight trace; slow twitch; spastic torticollis; speech therapist; sphincter tone; stable toxin; standard test; starting time; sternothyroid; stimulus; store; stress test; stria terminalis; striation; subtalar; subtotal; sulfotransferase; surface tension; surgical technologist; surgical treatment; survival time; syndrome of the trephined; systolic time

S-T [*segment*] in electrocardiography, the portion of the segment between the end of the S wave and the beginning of the T wave; sickle-cell thalassemia

St, st let it stand [Lat. *stet*]; let them stand [Lat. *stent*]; stage [of disease]; status; stere; sterile; stimulation; stokes; stone [unit]; straight; stroke; stomach; stomion; subtype

STA second trimester abortion; serum thrombotic accelerator; superficial temporal artery

Sta staphylion

stab stabilization; stabnuclear neutrophil

STAG slow-target attaching globulin; split-thickness autogenous graft

STA-MCA superficial temporal artery to middle cerebral artery

STAI State Trait Anxiety Inventory

STANDOUT soft thresholding and depth cueing of unspecified techniques

StanPsych standard psychiatric [nomenclature]

Staph, staph *Staphylococcus*, staphylococcal

STAR Specialty Training and Advanced Research [NIH]

STAS sporadic testicular agenesis syndrome

STAT immediately (Lat. *statim*); signal transducer and activator of transcription

stat immediately [Lat. *statim*]; radiation emanation unit [German]

STATH statherin

Stb stillborn

STC serum theophylline concentration; soft tissue calcification; stroke treatment center; subtotal colectomy

STD selective T-cell defect; sexually transmitted disease; skin-to-tumor distance; skin test dose; sodium tetradecyl sulfate; standard test dose

std saturated; standardized

STDH skin test for delayed hypersensitivity

STE Scholars for Teaching Excellence

STEAM stimulated echo acquisition mode

STEL short-term exposure limit

STEM scanning transmission electron microscope; Society of Teachers of Emergency Medicine

STEN staphylococcal toxic epidermal necrolysis

sten stenosis, stenosed

STEP Sequential Test of Educational Programs

stereo stereogram

STESS self-rating treatment emergent symptom scale

STET submaximal treadmill exercise test

STF serum thymus factor; slow-twitch fiber; special tube feeding; specialized treatment center; stefin; sudden transient freezing

STFM Society of Teachers of Family Medicine

STFT short-time Fourier transform

STEV short-term exposure value

STG split-thickness graft

STH somatotropic hormone; subtotal hysterectomy

STh sickle cell thalassemia

STHRF somatotropic hormone releasing factor

STI Scientific and Technical Information; serum trypsin inhibitor; soybean trypsin inhibitor; systolic time interval

STIC Science and Technology Information Center; serum trypsin inhibition capacity; solid-state transducer intracompartment

stillb stillborn

stim stimulated, stimulation; stimulus

STIR short tau inversion recovery

STK stem cell tyrosine kinase; streptokinase

STL serum theophylline level; status thymicolymphaticus; stereolithography; swelling, tenderness and limited motion

STLI subtotal lymphoid irradiation

STLOM swelling, tenderness, and limitation of motion

STLS subacute thyroiditis-like syndrome

STLV simian T-lymphotropic virus

STM scanning tunneling microscope; short-term memory; streptomycin

STMS short test of mental status

STMY stromelysin

STN streptozocin; subthalamic nucleus; supratrochlear nucleus

sTNM TNM (see p. 383) staging of tumors as determined by surgical procedures

STNR symmetric tonic neck reflex

STNV satellite tobacco necrosis virus

STO store

stom stomach

STONE Shanghai Trial of Nifedipine in the Elderly

STOP Study of Hypertension in the Elderly [Sweden] or Swedish Trial in Old Patients with Hypertension; surgical termination of pregnancy

STOP 2 Swedish Trial in Old Patients with Hypertension 2

STORCH syphilis, toxoplasmosis, rubella, cytomegalovirus, and herpesvirus

STP phenol-preferring sulfotransferase; scientifically treated petroleum; sodium thiopental; standard temperature and pressure; standard temperature and pulse; strategic technology planning

STPD a volume of gas at standard temperature and pressure that contains no water vapor

STPS specific thalamic projection system

STQ superior temporal quadrant

STR soft tissue relaxation; statherin; stirred tank reactor

Str, str *Streptococcus*, streptococcal

strab strabismus

Strep *Streptococcus;* streptomycin

STRT skin temperature recovery time

struct structure, structural

STS sequence tagged site; serologic test for syphilis; sodium tetradecyl sulfate; sodium thiosulfate; standard test for syphilis; steroid sulfatase

STSA Southern Thoracic Surgical Association

STSE split-thickness skin excision

STSG split-thickness skin graft

STSS staphylococcal toxic shock syndrome

STT scaphotrapeziotrapezoid [joint]; serial thrombin time; skin temperature test

STU skin test unit

STUR Student Team Utilizing Research [project]

STV superior temporal vein

STVA subtotal villose atrophy

STVS short-term visual storage

STX saxitoxin; syntaxin

STZ streptozocin; streptozyme

SU salicyluric acid; secretory unit; sensation unit; solar urticaria; sorbent unit; spectrophotometric unit; status uncertain; subunit; sulfonamide; sulfonylurea; supine

Su sulfonamide

SUA serum uric acid; single umbilical artery; single unit activity

subac subacute

subclav subclavian; subclavicular

subcut subcutaneous

subling sublingual

SubN subthalamic nucleus

subq subcutaneous

subsp subspecies

substd substandard

suc suction

Succ succinate, succinic

SUD skin unit dose; sudden unexpected death

SUDH succinyldehydrogenase

SUDI sudden unexpected death in infancy

SUFE slipped upper femoral epiphysis

SUI stress urinary incontinence

SUID sudden unexplained infant death

sulf sulfate

sulfa sulfonamide

SULF-PRIM sulfamethoxazole and trimethoprim

SUMA sporadic ulcerating and mutilating acropathy

SUMIT streptokinase-urokinase myocardial infarct test

SUMMIT Stanford University Medical Media and Information Technology

SUMSE stroke unit mental status examination

SUN standard unit of nomenclature; serum urea nitrogen

SUO syncope of unknown origin

SUP schizo-unipolar; supination

sup above [Lat. *supra*]; superficial; superior; supinator; supine

supin supination, supine

supp suppository

suppl supplement, supplementary

SUPPORT Study to Understand Prognoses and Preferences for Outcomes and Risks of Treatment

suppos suppository

SURF surfeit

SURG, Surg surgery, surgical, or surgeon

SURS solitary ulcer of rectum syndrome; surveillance and utilization review

SUS Saybolt Universal Seconds; solitary ulcer syndrome; stained urinary sediment; suppressor sensitive

susp suspension, suspended

SUTI symptomatic urinary tract infection

SUUD sudden unexpected unexplained death

SUV small unilamellar vessel

SUX succinylcholine

SV saphenous vein; sarcoma virus; satellite virus; selective vagotomy; semilunar valve; seminal vesicle; severe; sigmoid volvulus; simian virus; single ventricle; sinus venosus; snake venom; splenic vein; spontaneous ventilation; stroke volume; subclavian vein; subventricular; supravital; synaptic vesicle

S/V surface/volume ratio

SV2 synaptic vesicle protein 2

SV40 simian vacuolating virus 40

Sv sievert

sv sievert; single vibration

SVA selective vagotomy and antrectomy; selective visceral angiography; sequential ventriculoatrial [pacing]; subtotal villous atrophy

SVAS supravalvular aortic stenosis; supraventricular aortic stenosis

SVAT synaptic vesicle amine transformer

SVB saphenous vein bypass

SVBG saphenous vein bypass grafting

SVC saphenous vein cutdown; segmental venous capacitance; selective venous catheterization; slow vital capacity; subclavian vein catheterization; superior vena cava; supraventricular extrasystole

SVCCS superior vena cava compression syndrome

SVCG spatial vectorcardiogram

SVCO superior vena-caval obstruction

SVCP Special Virus Cancer Program

SVCR segmental venous capacitance ratio

SVCS superior vena cava syndrome

SVD single vessel disease; singular value decomposition; small vessel disease; spontaneous vaginal delivery; spontaneous vertex delivery; swine vesicular disease

SVE slow volume encephalography; soluble viral extract; sterile vaginal examination

SVG saphenous vein graft

SVI slow virus infection; stroke volume index; systolic velocity integral

SVL superficial vastus lateralis

SVM seminal vesicle microsome; syncytiovascular membrane

SVMT synaptic vesicle monoamine transformer

SVN sinuvertebral nerve; small volume nebulizer

SvO$_2$ venous oxygen saturation

SVOM sequential volitional oral movement

SVP selective vagotomy and pyloroplasty; small volume parenteral [infusion]; standing venous pressure; superior vascular plexus

SVPB supraventricular premature beat

SVR sequential vascular response; systemic vascular resistance

SVRI systemic vascular resistance index

SVS slit ventricle syndrome; Society for Cardiovascular Surgery

SVT sinoventricular tachycardia; subclavian vein thrombosis; supraventricular tachyarrhythmia; supraventricular tachycardia

SVTh subvalvular thickening

SW seriously wounded; short waves; sinewave; slow wave; soap and water; social worker; spike wave; spiral wound; stab wound; sterile water; stroke work; Sturge-Weber [syndrome]; Swiss Webster [mouse]

S/W spike wave

Sw swine

SWA seriously wounded in action; slow-wave activity

SWC submaximal working capacity

SWCM social work case manager

SWD short wave diathermy

SWE slow wave encephalography

SWG silkworm gut; standard wire gauge

SWI sterile water for injection; stroke work index; surgical wound infection

SWIM sperm-washing insemination method

SWIORA spinal cord injury without radiologic abnormality

SWM segmental wall motion

SWMF Semmes-Weinstein monofilament

SWO superficial white onychomycosis

SWOG South West Oncology Group

SWR serum Wassermann reaction; surgical wound infection rate

SWS slow-wave sleep; spike-wave stupor; steroid-wasting syndrome; Sturge-Weber syndrome

SWT sine-wave threshold

SWU septic work-up

Sx suction

Sx, S$_x$ signs; symptoms

SXCT spiral x-ray computed tomography

SXR skull x-ray [examination]

Sxs serological sex-specific [antigen]

SXT sulfamethoxazole-trimethoprim [mixture]

SY spectroscopy; syphilis, syphilitic

SYA subacute yellow atrophy

SYB synaptobrevin

SYDS stomach yin deficiency syndrome

sym symmetrical; symptom

sympath sympathetic

symph symphysis

sympt symptom

SYN synapse; synovitis

syn synergistic; synonym; synovial

synd syndrome

SYP synaptophysin

syph syphilis, syphilitic

SYR Syrian [hamster]

syr syrup [Lat. *syrupus*]; syringe

SYS stretching-yawning syndrome

sys system, systemic

SYS-BP systolic blood pressure

syst system, systemic; systole, systolic

SYST-EUR Systolic Hypertension in Europeans Study

SYT synaptotagmin

SZ streptozocin

Sz seizure; schizophrenia

SZN streptozocin

T absolute temperature; an electrocardiographic wave corresponding to the repolarization of the ventricles [wave]; life [time]; period [time]; ribosylthymine; tablespoonful; *Taenia*; tamoxifen; telomere or terminal banding; temperature; temporal electrode placement in electroencephalography; temporary; tenderness; tension [intraocular]; tera; tesla; testosterone; tetra; tetracycline; theophylline; therapy; thoracic; thorax; threatened [animal]; threonine; thrombosis; thrombus; thymidine; thymine; thymus [cell]; thymus-derived; thyroid; tidal gas; tidal volume; time; tincture; tocopherol; topical; torque; total; toxicity; training [group]; transition; transmittance; transverse; treatment; *Treponema*; *Trichophyton*; tritium; tryptamine; *Trypanosoma*; tuberculin; tuberculosis; tumor; turnkey system; type

$T_{1/2}$, $t_{1/2}$ half-life

T1 longitudinal relaxation time

T1-T12 first to twelfth thoracic vertebrae

T_1 spin-lattice or longitudinal relaxation time; tricuspid first sound

T + 1, T + 2, T + 3 first, second, and third stages of increased intraocular tension

T-1, T-2, T-3 first, second, and third stages of decreased intraocular tension

T2 transverse relaxation time

T_2 diiodothyronine; spin-spin or transverse relaxation time

T2* effective transverse relaxation time

T_2^* effective transverse relaxation time

2,4,5-T 2,4,5-trichlorophenoxyacetic acid

T_3 triiodothyronine

T_4 thyroxine

T-7 free thyroxine factor

T_{90} time required for 90% mortality in a population of microorganisms exposed to a toxic agent

t duration; Student t test; teaspoonful; temperature; temporal; terminal; tertiary; test of significance; three times [Lat. *ter*]; time; tissue; tonne; translocation

TA alkaline tuberculin; arterial tension; axillary temperature; tactile afferent; Takayasu arteritis; teichoic acid; temporal arteritis; terminal antrum; therapeutic abortion; thermophilic *Actinomyces*; thymocytotoxic autoantibody; thyroglobulin autoprecipitation; thyroid antibody; thyroid autoimmunity; tibialis anterior; titratable acid; total alkaloids; total antibody; toxic adenoma; toxin-antitoxin; traffic accident; transactional analysis; transaldolase; transantral; transplantation antigen; transposition of aorta; trapped air; triamcinolone acetonide; tricuspid atresia; trophoblast antigen; true anomaly; truncus arteriosus; tryptamine; tryptose agar; tube agglutination; tumor-associated

T/A time and amount

T-A toxin-antitoxin

T&A tonsillectomy and adenoidectomy; tonsils and adenoids

Ta tantalum; tarsal

TAA thioacetamide; thoracic aortic aneurysm; total ankle arthroplasty; transverse aortic arch; tumor-associated antigen

TAAF thromboplastic activity of the amniotic fluid

TA-AIDS transfusion-associated acquired immunodeficiency syndrome

TAB total autonomic blockage; typhoid, paratyphoid A, and paratyphoid B [vaccine]

TAb therapeutic abortion

tab tablet

TABC total aerobic bacteria count; typhoid, paratyphoid A, paratyphoid B, and paratyphoid C [vaccine]

TABP type A behavior pattern

Tabs tablets

TABT typhoid, paratyphoid A, paratyphoid B, and tetanus toxoid [vaccine]

TABTD typhoid, paratyphoid A, paratyphoid B, tetanus toxoid, and diphtheria toxoid [vaccine]

TAC tachykinin; terminal antrum contraction; tetracaine, adrenalin, and cocaine; time-activity curve; total abdominal colectomy; total aganglionosis coli; triamcinolone cream

TAC-1 tachykinin-1

TAC-2 tachykinin-2

TACE chlorotrianicene; teichoic acid crude extract

tachy tachycardia

TACR tachykinin receptor

TAD test of auditory discrimination; thoracic asphyxiant dystrophy; transient acantholytic dermatosis

TADAC therapeutic abortion, dilatation, aspiration, curettage

TAE transcatheter arterial embolism

TAF albumose-free tuberculin [Ger. *Tuberculin Albumose frei*]; tissue angiogenesis factor; toxin-antitoxin floccules; toxoid-antitoxin floccules; transabdominal hysterectomy; trypsin-aldehyde-fuchsin; tumor angiogenesis factor

TAG target attaching globulin; technical advisory group; thymine, adenine, and guanine

TAGH triiodothyronine, amino acids, glucagon, and heparin

TAGVHD transfusion-associated graft-versus-host disease

TAH total abdominal hysterectomy; total artificial heart

TAH BSO total abdominal hysterectomy and bilateral salpingo-oophorectomy

TAI Test Anxiety Inventory

TAIS time assessment interview schedule

TAL tendon of Achilles lengthening; thymic alymphoplasia

talc talcum

TALH thick ascending limb of Henle's loop

TALL, T-ALL T-cell acute lymphoblastic leukemia

TALLA T-cell acute lymphoblastic leukemia antigen

TAM tamoxifen; teen-age mother; thermoacidurans agar modified; time-averaged mean; total active motion; toxin-antitoxoid mixture; transient abnormal myelopoiesis

TAME N-alpha-tosyl-1-arginine methyl ester

TAMI thrombolysis and angioplasty in myocardial infarction; transmural anterior myocardial infarction

TAMIS Telemetric Automated Microbial Identification System

TAN total adenine nucleotide; total ammonia nitrogen

tan tandem translocation; tangent

TANI total axial [lymph] node irradiation

TAO thromboangiitis obliterans; triacetyloleandomycin

TAP transesophageal atrial pacing; transluminal angioplasty; transmembrane action potential; transporter associated with antigen presentation

TAPA target of antiproliferative antibody

TAPE temporary atrial pacemaker electrode

TAPS trial assessment procedure scale

TAPVC total anomalous pulmonary venous connection

TAPVD total anomalous pulmonary venous drainage

TAPVR total anomalous pulmonary venous return

TAQW transient abnormal Q wave

TAR thoracic aortic rupture; thrombocytopenia with absent radii [syndrome]; tissue-air ratio; total abortion rate; transanal resection; transaxillary resection; treatment authorization request

TARA total articular replacement arthroplasty; tumor-associated rejection antigen

TAR/PD target nursing hours per patient/day

TARS threonyl-tRNA synthetase

TAS tetanus antitoxin serum; therapeutic activities specialist; thoracoabdominal syndrome; transcription-based amplification system; traumatic apallic syndrome

TASA tumor-associated surface antigen

Tase tryptophan synthetase

TASS thyrotoxicosis-Addison disease-Sjögren syndrome-sarcoidosis [syndrome]

TAT tetanus antitoxin; thematic apperception test; thematic aptitude test; thrombin-antithrombin complex; thromboplastin activation test; total antitryptic activity; toxin-antitoxin; transactivator; transaxial tomography; tray agglutination test; tumor activity test; turnaround time; tyrosine aminotransferase

TATA Pribnow [box]; tumor-associated transplantation antigen

TATR tyrosine aminotransferase regulator

τ Greek lower case letter *tau*; life [of radioisotope]; relaxation time; shear stress; spectral transmittance; transmission coefficient

TATST tetanus antitoxin skin test

TAV trapped air volume

TAVB total atrioventricular block

TAX Taxol

TB Taussig-Bind [syndrome]; terabyte; term birth; terminal bronchiole; terminal bronchus; thromboxane B; thymol blue; toluidine blue; total base; total bilirubin; total body; tracheobronchial; tracheal bronchiolar [region]; tracheobronchitis; trapezoid body; tub bath; tubercle bacillus; tuberculin; tuberculosis; tumor-bearing

Tb Tbilisi [phage]; terbium; tubercle bacillus; tuberculosis

T$_b$ biological half-life; body temperature

tb tuberculosis

TBA tertiary butylacetate; testosterone-binding affinity; tetrabutylammonium; thiobarbituric acid; to be absorbed; to be added; total bile acids; trypsin-binding activity; tubercle bacillus; tumor-bearing animal

TBAB tryptose blood agar base

TBAN transbronchial aspiration needle

TBB transbronchial biopsy

TBBM total body bone minerals

TBC thyroxine-binding coagulin; total body calcium; total body clearance; tuberculosis

Tbc tubercle bacillus; tuberculosis

TBD total body density; Toxicology Data Base

TBE tick-borne encephalitis; tuberculin bacillin emulsion

TBF total body fat

TBFB tracheobronchial foreign body

TBFVL tidal breathing flow-volume loops

TBG beta-thromboglobulin; testosterone-binding globulin; thyroglobulin; thyroid-binding globulin; thyroxine-binding globulin; tracheobronchography; tris-buffered Gey solution

TBGI thyroxine-binding globulin index

TBGP total blood granulocyte pool

TBH total body hematocrit

tBHP terbutyl hydroperoxide

TBHT total-body hyperthermia

TBI thyroid-binding index; thyroxine-binding index; tooth-brushing instruction; total-body irradiation; traumatic brain injury

TBII thyroid-stimulating hormone-binding inhibitory immunoglobulin

T bili total bilirubin

TBK total body potassium

tbl tablet

TBLB transbronchial lung biopsy

TBLC term birth, living child

TBLI term birth, living infant

TBM total body mass; tracheobronchiomegaly; trophoblastic basement membrane; tuberculous meningitis; tubular basement membrane

TBMN thin basement membrane nephropathy

TBN bacillus emulsion; total body nitrogen

TBNA total body neutron activation; treated but not admitted

TBNAA total body neutron activation analysis

TBO total blood out

TBP bithionol; testosterone-binding protein; thyroxine-binding protein; total bypass; tributyl phosphate; tuberculous peritonitis

TBPA thyroxine-binding prealbumin

TBPT total body protein turnover

TBR tumor-bearing rabbit

TB-RD tuberculosis and respiratory disease

TBS total body solids; total body solute; total body surface; total burn size; Townes-Brocks syndrome; tracheobronchial submucosa; tracheobronchoscopy; tribromosalicylanilide; triethanolamine-buffered saline

tbs, tbsp tablespoon

TBSA total body surface area

TBSV tomato bushy stunt virus

TBT tolbutamide test; tracheobronchial toilet; tracheobronchial tree

TBTT tuberculin time test

TBV total blood volume

TBW total body water; total body weight

TBX thromboxane; total body irradiation

TBXA2 thromboxane A2

TBXAS thromboxane A synthase

TBZ tetrabenazine; thiabendazole

TC target cell; taurocholate; temperature compensation; teratocarcinoma; tertiary cleavage; tetracycline; therapeutic community; thermal conductivity; thoracic cage; throat culture; thyrocalcitonin; tissue culture; to contain; total calcium; total capacity; total cholesterol; total colonoscopy; total correction; transcobalamin; transcutaneous; transplant center; transverse colon; Treacher Collins [syndrome]; true channel; true conjugate; tuberculin contagiosum; tubocurarine; tumor cell; tumor of cerebrum; type and crossmatch

T&C turn and cough; type and crossmatch

$T_4(C)$ serum thyroxine measured by column chromatography

TC_{50} medium toxic concentration

Tc correlation time; technetium; tetracycline; transcobalamin

T_c cytotoxic T-cell; the generation time of a cell cycle; tricuspid closure

$t(°C)$ temperature on the Celsius scale

tc transcutaneous; translational control

TCA T-cell A locus; terminal cancer; tetracyclic antidepressant; total cholic acid; total circulating albumin; total circulatory arrest; tricalcium aluminate; tricarboxylic acid; trichloroacetic acid; tricyclic antidepressant; thyrocalcitonin

TCAB 3,3',4,4'-tetrachloroazobenzene

TCABG triple coronary artery bypass graft

TCAD tricyclic antidepressant

TCADA Texas Council on Alcohol and Drug Abuse

TCAG triple coronary artery graft

TCAOB 3,3',4,4'-tetrachloroazoxybenzene

TCAP trimethyl-cetyl-ammonium pentachlorophenate

TCB tetrachlorobiphenyl; total cardiopulmonary bypass transcatheter biopsy; transabdominal chorionic biopsy; tumor cell burden

TCAR T-cell antigen receptor

TCBS thiosulfate-citrate-bile salts-sucrose [agar]

TCC terminal complement complex; thromboplastic cell component; transitional-cell carcinoma; trichlorocarbanilide

Tcc triclocarban

TCCA, TCCAV transitional cell cancer-associated [virus]

TCCD transcranial color-coded Doppler

TCCL T-cell chronic lymphoblastic leukemia

TCCS transcranial color-coded sonography

TCD tapetochoroidal dystrophy; T-cell depletion; thermal conductivity detector; tissue culture dose; transcranial Doppler [sonography]; transverse cardiac diameter; tumor control dose; tumoricidal dose

TCD_{50} median tissue culture dose

TCDB turn, cough, deep breathe

TCDC taurochenodeoxycholate

TCDD 2,3,7,8-tetrachlorodibenzo-p-dioxin

TCE T-cell enriched; tetrachlorodiphenyl ethane; trichloroethylene
T-cell thymus-derived cell

$TCED_{50}$ 50% tissue effective dose

TCES transcutaneous cranial electrical stimulation

TCESOM trichloroethylene-extracted soybean oil meal

TCET transcerebral electrotherapy

TCF tissue coding factor; total coronary flow; transcription factor

T-CFC T-colony forming cell

TCFU tumor colony-forming unit

TCG time-compensated gain

TCGF T-cell growth factor

TCH tanned-cell hemagglutination; thiophen-2-carboxylic acid hydrazide; total circulating hemoglobin; turn, cough, hyperventilate

TC/HDL total cholesterol/high density lipoproteins [ratio]

TChE total cholinesterase

TCI total cerebral ischemia; transient cerebral ischemia; transcobalamin I

TCi teracurie

TCID tissue culture infective dose; tissue culture inoculated dose

$TCID_{50}$ median tissue culture infective dose; 50% tissue culture infective dose

TCIE transient cerebral ischemic episode

TCII transcobalamin II

TCIII transcobalamin III

TCL T-cell leukemia; thermochemiluminescence; total capacity of the lung; transverse carpal ligament

T-CLL T-cell chronic lymphatic leukemia

TC_{Lo} toxic concentration low

TCLP Toxicity Characteristic Leachate Procedure [EPA battery test]

TCM tissue culture medium; transcutaneous monitor

T&CM type and crossmatch

Tc 99m technetium-99m

Tc 99m MDP technetium-99m methylene diphosphonate

TCMA transcortical motor aphasia

TCMP thematic content modification program

TCMZ trichloromethiazide

TCN tetracycline; transcobalamin

TC̄NM tumor with lymph node metastases

TCNS transcutaneous nerve stimulation/stimulator

TCNV terminal contingent negative variation

TCO transcutaneous oximetry

T_{CO_2} total carbon dioxide

TCP T-complex protein; therapeutic continuous penicillin; total circulating protein; transcutaneous pacemaker; transcutaneous pacing; tranylcypromine; tricalcium phosphate; trichlorophenol; tricresyl phosphate; tumor control probability

TCPD$_{50}$ 50% tissue culture protective dose

tcPCO$_2$, tcPCO$_2$ transcutaneous carbon dioxide pressure

tcP$_{O2}$, tcPO$_2$ transcutaneous oxygen pressure

2,4,5-TCPPA 2-(2,4,5-trichlorophenoxy)-propionic acid

TCPA tetrachlorophthalic anhydride

TCP/IP transmission control protocol/Internet protocol

TCPS total cavopulmonary shunt

TCR T-cell reactivity; T-cell receptor; T-cell rosette; thalamocortical relay; total cytoplasmic ribosome; trauma center record; true count rate; turn, cough, and rebreathe

TCRA t-cell receptor alpha

TCRB T-cell receptor beta

TCRD T-cell receptor delta

TCRG T-cell receptor gamma

tcRNA translational control ribonucleic acid

TCRP total cellular receptor pool

TCRZ T-cell receptor Z

TCRV total red cell volume

TCS T-cell supernatant; tethered cord syndrome; total coronary score; Treacher Collins syndrome

TCSA tetrachlorosalicylanilide

TCSF T-colony-stimulating factor

TCT thrombin clotting time; thyrocalcitonin; trachial cytotoxin; transmission computed tomography

Tct tincture

tcTOFA time constrained time-of-flight absorbance

TCU trauma care unit; treatment control unit

TCV thoracic cage volume; three concept view

TD tabes dorsalis; tardive dyskinesia; T-cell dependent; temporary disability; terminal device; tetanus and diphtheria [toxoid]; tetrodotoxin; thanatophoric dwarfism; thanatophoric dysplasia; therapy discontinued; thermal dilution; thoracic duct; three times per day; threshold of detectability; threshold of discomfort; threshold dose; thymus-dependent; timed disintegration; tocopherol deficiency; to deliver; tone decay; torsion dystonia; total disability, total discrimination; totally disabled; total dose; Tourette disorder; toxic dose; tracheal diameter; transdermal; transverse diameter; traveler's diarrhea; treatment discontinued; tumor dose; typhoid dysentery

T/D treatment discontinued

T$_D$ the time required to double the number of cells in a given population; thermal death time

Td doubling time; tetanus-diphtheria toxoid

T$_4$(D) serum thyroxine measured by displacement analysis

TD$_{50}$ median toxic dose

td three times daily [Lat. *ter die*]

TDA thyroid-stimulating hormone-displacing antibody

TDB Toxicology Data Bank

TDC taurodeoxycholic acid; total dietary calories

Td-CIA T-cell-derived colony-inhibiting activity

TDCO thermodilution cardiac output [measurement]

TDD telecommunication device for the deaf; tetradecadiene; thoracic duct drainage; total digitalizing dose; toxic doses of drugs

TDE tetrachlorodiphenylethane; total digestible energy; triethylene glycol diglycidyl

TDF testis-determining factor; thoracic duct fistula; thoracic duct flow; time-dose fractionation; tissue-damaging factor; tumor dose fractionation

TDFA testis-determining factor, autosomal

TDFX testis-determining factor X

TDGF teratocarcinoma-derived growth factor

TDH threonine dehydrogenase

TDI temperature difference integration; three-dimensional interlocking [hip]; toluene 2,4-diisocyanate; total dose infusion; total dose insulin

TDL thoracic duct lymph; thymus-dependent lymphocyte; toxic dose level

TDLU terminal ductal lobular unit

TDM therapeutic drug monitoring

TDN total digestible nutrients

tDNA transfer deoxyribonucleic acid

TDO tricho-dento-osseous [syndrome]; tryptophan 2,3-dioxygenase

TDP thermal death point; thoracic duct pressure; thymidine diphosphate; total degradation products

TdR thymidine

TDS temperature, depth, salinity; thiamine disulfide; transduodenal sphincteroplasty

tds to be taken three times a day [Lat. *ter die sumendum*]

TDSD transient digestive system disorder

TDT terminal deoxynucleotidyltransferase; thermal death time; tone decay test; tumor doubling time

TdT terminal deoxynucleotidyl transferase

TDZ thymus-dependent zone

TE echo-time; expiratory time; tennis elbow; test ear; tetanus; tetracycline; threshold energy; thromboembolism; thymus epithelium; thyrotoxic exophthalmos; tick-borne encephalitis; time estimation; tissue-equivalent; tonsillectomy; tooth extracted; total estrogen; toxic epi-

dermolysis; *Toxoplasma* encephalitis; trace element; tracheoesophageal; transepithelial; treadmill exercise; trial error

T&E testing and evaluation; trial and error

Te effective half-life; tellurium; tetanic contraction; tetanus

T$_E$ exhalation time; expiratory phase time

TEA temporal external artery; tetraethylammonium; thermal energy analyzer; thromboendarterectomy; total elbow arthroplasty; triethanolamine

TEAB tetraethylammonium bromide

TEAC tetraethylammonium chloride

TEAE triethylammonioethyl

TEAM techniques for effective alcohol management; Training in Expanded Auxiliary Management; transfemoral endovascular aneurysm management

teasp teaspoon

TEBG, TeBG testosterone-estradiol-binding globulin

TEC total electron count; total eosinophil count; total exchange capacity; transient erythroblastopenia of childhood; transluminal extraction catheter

T&EC trauma and emergency center

TECV traumatic epiphyseal coxa vara

TED Tasks of Emotional Development; threshold erythema dose; thromboembolic disease

TEDS anti-embolism stockings

TEE thermic effect of exercise; total energy expenditure; transesophageal echocardiography; tyrosine ethyl ester

TEEP tetraethyl pyrophosphate

TEF thermic effect of food; thyrotroph embryonic factor; tracheoesophageal fistula; transcriptional enhancer factor; trunk extension-flexion [unit]

T$_{eff}$ effective half-life

TEFRA Tax Equity and Fiscal Responsibility Act

TEFS transmural electrical field stimulation

TEG thromboelastogram; triethyleneglycol

TEGDMA tetraethylene glycol dimethacrylate

TEHIP Toxicology and Environmental Health Program

TEIB triethyleneiminobenzoquinone

TEL tetraethyl lead

TEM transmission electron microscope/microscopy; triethylenemelamine

temp temperature; temple, temporal

TEN total enteral nutrition; total excretory nitrogen; toxic epidermal necrolysis; transepidermal neurostimulation; Trans-European Network

TENS toxic epidermal necrolysis syndrome; transcutaneous electrical nerve stimulation

TEP tetraethylpyrophosphate; tracheoesophageal puncture; transesophageal pacing

TEPA triethylenephosphamide

TEPP tetraethyl pyrophosphate; triethylene pyrophosphate

TER teratogen; total endoplasmic reticulum; transcapillary escape rate

ter rub [Lat. *tere*]; terminal [end of chromosome]; terminal or end; ternary; tertiary; three times; threefold

term terminal

TERT total end range time

tert tertiary

TES thymic epithelial supernatant; toxic epidemic syndrome; transcutaneous electrical stimulation; transmural electrical stimulation

TESPA thiotepa

TESS treatment emergent symptom scale

TET tetracycline; total ejection time; total exchange thyroxine; treadmill exercise test

Tet tetralogy of Fallot

tet tetanus

TETD tetraethylthiuram disulfide

TETA triethylenetetramine

tet tox tetanus toxoid

TEV tadpole edema virus; talipes equinovarus

TEWL transepidermal water loss

TEZ transthoracic electric impedance respirogram

TF free thyroxine; tactile fremitus; tail flick [reflex]; temperature factor; testicular feminization; tetralogy of Fallot; thymol flocculation; thymus factor; tissue-damaging factor; to follow; total flow; transcription factor; transfer factor; transferrin; transformation frequency; transfrontal; tube feeding; tuberculin filtrate; tubular fluid; tuning fork

t(°F) temperature on the Fahrenheit scale

Tf transferrin

T_f freezing temperature

TFA total fatty acids; transverse fascicular area; triangular fibrocartilage; trifluoroacetic acid

TFC common form of transferrin

TFCC triangular fibrocartilage complex

TFd dialyzable transfer factor

TFE polytetrafluoroethylene; transcription factor for immunoglobulin heavy chain enhancer

TFF tube-fed food

TFI thoracic fluid index

TFM testicular feminization male; testicular feminization mutation; total fluid movement; transmission electron microscopy

TFMPP 1-(trifluoromethylphenyl)-piperazine

TFN total fecal nitrogen; transferrin

TFP tubular fluid plasma

TFPI tissue factor pathway inhibitor

TFPZ trifluoperazine

TFR total fertility rate; total flow resistance; transferrin receptor

TFS testicular feminization syndrome; thyroid function study; tube-fed saline

TFT thin-film transistor; thrombus formation time; thyroid function test; tight filum terminale; trifluorothymidine

TFX toxic effects

TG tendon graft; testosterone glucuronide; tetraglycine; thioglucose; thioglycolate; thioguanine; thromboglobulin; thyroglobulin; tocogram; total gastrectomy; toxic goiter; transmissible gastroenteritis; treated group; triacylglycerol; trigeminal ganglion; triglyceride; tumor growth

Tg generation time; thyroglobulin; *Toxoplasma gondii*

T$_g$ glass transition temperature

6-TG thioguanine

tG$_1$ the time required to complete the G$_1$ phase of the cell cycle

tG$_2$ the time required to complete the G$_2$ phase of the cell cycle

TGA taurocholate gelatin agar; thyroglobulin activity; total glycoalkaloids; total gonadotropin activity; transient global amnesia; transposition of great arteries; tumor glycoprotein assay

TgAb thyroglobulin antibody

TGAR total graft area rejected

TGB thromboglobulin beta

TGBG dimethylglyoxal bis-guanylhydrazone

TGC time pain compensation

TGD thermal-green dye

TGE theoretical growth evaluation; transmissible gastroenteritis; tryptone glucose extract

TGEV transmissible gastroenteritis virus

TGF T-cell growth factor; transforming growth factor; tuboglomerular feedback; tumor growth factor

TG-F transforming growth factor

TGFA transforming growth factor alpha; triglyceride fatty acid

TGFB transforming growth factor beta

TGG turkey gamma globulin

TGL triglyceride; triglyceride lipase

TGP tobacco glycoprotein

6-TGR 6-thioguanine riboside

TGS tincture of green soap

TGT thromboplastin generation test/time; tolbutamide-glucagon test

TGV thoracic gas volume; transposition of great vessels

TGY tryptone glucose yeast [agar]

TGYA tryptone glucose yeast agar

TH tension headache; tetrahydrocortisol; T helper [cell]; theophylline; thorax; thrill; thyrohyoid; thyroid hormone; topical hypothermia; total hysterectomy; triquetrohamate; tyrosine hydrolase; tyrosine hydroxylase

T$_H$, T$_h$, Th T-helper [lymphocyte]; thenar; therapist; therapy; thoracic, thorax; thorium; throat

th thenar; thermie; thoracic; thyroid; transhepatic

THA tacrine; tetrahydroaminoacridine; total hip arthroplasty; total hydroxyapatite; *Treponema* hemagglutination

ThA thoracic aorta

THAL thalassemia

THAM tris(hydroxymethyl)aminomethane

THB thrombocyte B; Todd-Hewitt broth; total heart beats

THb total hemoglobin

THBD thrombomodulin

THBI thyroid hormone binding inhibitor

THBP 7,8,9,10-tetrahydrobenzo[a]-pyrene; thyroid hormone binding protein

THBS thrombospondin

THC terpin hydrate and codeine; tetrahydrocannabinol; tetrahydrocortisol; thiocarbanidin; thrombocytopenia; transhepatic cholangiogram; transplantable hepatocellular carcinoma

THCA alpha-trihydroxy-5-beta-cholestannic acid

THD Thomsen disease; transverse heart diameter

Thd ribothymidine

THDOC tetrahydrodeoxycorticosterone

THE tetrahydrocortisone E; tonic hind limb extension; transhepatic embolization; tropical hypereosinophilia

theor theory, theoretical

ther therapy, therapeutic; thermometer

therap therapy, therapeutic

Θ Greek capital letter *theta*; thermodynamic temperature

θ Greek lower case letter *theta*; an angular coordinate variable; customary temperature; temperature interval

ther ex therapeutic exercise

therm thermal; thermometer

THF tetrahydrocortisone F; tetrahydrofolate; tetrahydrofolic [acid]; tetrahydrofuran; thymic humoral factor

THFA tetrahydrofolic acid; tetrahydrofurfuryl alcohol

Thg thyroglobulin

THH telangiectasia hereditaria haemorrhagica; trichohyalin

THI transient hypogammaglobulinemia of infancy

Thi thiamine

THIP tetrahydroisoxazolopyridinol

Thio-TEPA thiotriethylenephosphamide

THL trichohyalin

THM total heme mass

thor thorax, thoracic

THO titrated water

Thor thoracic

thou thousandth

THP Tamm-Horstall protein; tetrahydropapaveroline; tissue hydrostatic pressure; total hip replacement; total hydroxyproline; transthoracic portography; trihexphenidyl

THPA tetrahydropteric acid

THPP thiamine pyrophosphate; trihydroxy propriophenone

ThPP thiamine pyrophosphate

tHPT tertiary hyperparathyroidism

THPV transhepatic portal vein

THQ tetraquinone

THR targeted heart rate; threonine; thyroid hormone receptor; total hip replacement; transhepatic resistance

Thr thrill; threonine

thr thyroid, thyroidectomy

THRA thyroid hormone receptor alpha

THRF thyrotropic hormone-releasing factor

THRM thrombomodulin

throm, thromb thrombosis, thrombus

THS tetrahydro-compound S; thrombo-hemorrhagic syndrome; Tolosa-Hunt syndrome

THSC totipotent hematopoietic stem cell

THTH thyrotropic hromone

THU tetrahydrouridine

THUG thyroid uptake gradient

THVO terminal hepatic vein obliteration

Thx thromboxane

THY thymosin

Thy thymine

thy thymus, thymectomy

THYB thymosin beta

THz terahertz

TI inversion time; temporal integration; terminal ileum; thalassemia intermedia; therapeutic index; thoracic index; thymus-independent; time interval; tonic immobility; transischial; translational inhibition; transverse inlet; tricuspid incompetence; tricuspid insufficiency; tumor induction

T_I inspiration time

Ti titanium

TIA transient ischemic attack; tumor-induced angiogenesis; turbidimetric immunoassay

TIAH total implantation of artificial heart

TIB tibia; time in bed; tumor immunology bank

TIBC total iron-binding capacity

TIBET Total Ischemic Burden European Trial

TIBS Trends in Biochemical Sciences

TIC Toxicology Information Center; trypsin inhibitory capability; tubulointerstitial cell; tumor-inducing complex

TICC time from cessation of contraception to conception

TICU trauma intensive care unit

TID time interval difference [imaging]; titrated initial dose

tid three times a day [Lat. *ter in die*]

TIDA tuberoinfundibular dopaminergic system

TIE transient ischemic episode

TIF tumor-inducing factor; tumor-inhibiting factor

TIG, Tig tetanus immunoglobulin

TIH time interval histogram

TIIAP technical information infrastructure assistance program

TIL tumor-infiltrating leukocyte; tumor-infiltrating lymphocyte

TIM transthoracic intracardiac monitoring; triose phosphate isomerase

TIMC tumor-induced marrow cytotoxicity

TIMI trhombolysis in myocardial infarction; transmural inferior myocardial infarction

TIMP tissue inhibitor of metalloproteinases

TIN tubulointerstitial nephropathy

tin three times a night [Lat. *ter in nocte*]

tinc, tinct tincture

TINU tubulo-interstitial nephritis- uveitis [syndrome]

TIP thermal inactivation point; Toxicology Information Program; translation-inhibiting protein; tumor-inhibiting principle

TIPI time-insensitive predictive instrument

TIPJ terminal interphalangeal joint

TIPPS tetraiodophenylphthalein sodium

TIPS transjugular intrahepatic portosystemic shunt

TIPSS transjugular intrahepatic portosystemic stent shunt

TIR terminal innervation ratio

TIS tetracycline-induced steatosis; transdermal infusion system; triage illness scale; trypsin-insoluble segment; tumor in situ

TISP total immunoreactive serum pepsinogen

TISS Therapeutic Intervention Scoring System

TIT *Treponema* immobilization test

TIT, TITh triiodothyronine

TIU trypsin-inhibiting unit

TIUV total intrauterine volume

TIV tomographic image visualization

TIVA total intravenous anesthesia

TIVC thoracic inferior vena cava

TJ tetrajoule; thigh junction; triceps jerk

TJA total joint arthroplasty

TJR total joint replacement

TK thymidine kinase; transketolase; triose-kinase; tyrosine kinase

T(°K) absolute temperature on the Kelvin scale

TKA total knee arthroplasty; transketolase activity; trochanter, knee, ankle

TKase thymidine kinase

TKC torticollis-keloids-cryptorchidism [syndrome]

TKCR torticollis-keloids-cryptorchidism-renal dysplasia [syndrome]

TKD thymidine kinase deficiency; tokodynamometer

TKG tokodynagraph

TKLI tachykinin-like immunoreactivity

TKO to keep open

TKR total knee replacement

TKT transketolase

TL temporal lobe; terminal limen; thermolabile; thermoluminescence; threat to life; thymus-leukemia [antigen]; thymus lymphocyte; thymus lymphoma; time lapse; time-limited; total lipids; total lung [capacity]; tubal ligation

T-L thoracolumbar; thymus-dependent lymphocyte

Tl thallium

TLA thymus leukemia antigen; tissue lactase activity; tongue-to-lip adhesion; translaryngeal aspiration; translumbar aortogram; transluminal angioplasty

TLAA T-lymphocyte-associated antigen

TLam thoracic laminectomy

TLC tender loving care; thin-layer chromatography; total L-chain concentration; total lung capacity; total lung compliance; total lymphocyte count; transverse loop colostomy

TLD thermoluminescent dosimeter; thoracic lymphatic duct; tumor lethal dose

T/LD$_{100}$ minimum dose causing 100% deaths or malformations

TLE temporal lobe epilepsy; thin-layer electrophoresis; total lipid extract

TLI thymidine labeling index; total lymphatic irradiation; trypsin-like immune activity; Tucker-Lewis index

TLL T-cell leukemia or lymphoma

TLm median tolerance limit

TLPD thoracolaryngopelvic dysplasia

TLQ total living quotient

TLR tonic labyrinthine reflex

TLS thoracolumbosacral; Tourette-like syndrome

TLSO thoracolumboscral orthosis

TLSSO thoracolumbosacral spinal orthosis

TLT tryptophan load test

TLV threshold limit value; total lung volume

TLW total lung water

TLX trophoblast-lymphocyte cross-reactivity

TM technology management; tectorial membrane; temperature by mouth; temporalis muscle; temporomandibular; tender midline; tendomyopathy; teres major; thalassemia major; Thayer-Martin [medium]; time and materials; time-motion; tobramycin; trademark; traditional medicine; transitional mucosa; transatrial membranotomy; transmediastinal; transmetatarsal; transport mechanism; transport medium; transverse myelitis; tropical medicine; tuberculous meningitis; twitch movement; tympanic membrane

T-M Thayer-Martin [medium]

T&M type and crossmatch

Tm thulium; tubular maximum excretory capacity of kidneys

T$_m$ melting temperature; temperature midpoint; tubular maximum excretory capacity of kidneys

tM the time required to complete the M phase of the cell cycle

tm transport medium; true mean

TMA tetramethylammonium; thrombotic microangiopathy; thyroid microsomal antibody; transcortical mixed aphasia; transmetatarsal amputation; trimellitic anhydride; trimethoxyamphetamine; trimethoxyphenyl aminopropane; trimethylamine

TMACl tetramethylammonium chloride

TMAH trimethylphenylammonium (anilinium) hydroxide

TMAI trimethylphenylammonium (anilinium) iodide

TMAS Taylor Manifest Anxiety Scale

T$_{max}$ maximum threshold; time of maximum concentration

TMB transient monocular blindness

TMBA trimethoxybenzaldehyde

TMBF transmural blood flow

TMC triamcinolone and terramycin capsules

TMD temporomandibular disorder; trimethadione

t-MDS therapy-related myelodysplastic syndrome

TME total metabolizable energy; transmissible mink encephalopathy; transmural enteritis

TMET treadmill exercise test

TMF transformed mink fibroblast; transmitral flow

TM$_g$ maximum tubular reabsorption rate for glucose
TMH tetramethylammonium hydroxide
TM-HSA trimellityl-human serum albumin
TMI testing motor impairment; threatened myocardial infarction; transmural myocardial infarction
TMIC Toxic Materials Information Center
TMIF tumor-cell migratory inhibition factor
TMIS Technicon Medical Information System
TMJ temporomandibular joint; trapeziometacarpal joint
TMJS temporomandibular joint syndrome
TML terminal midline; terminal motor latency; tetramethyl lead
TMN thin membrane nephropathy
TMNST tethered median nerve stress test
TMP thiamine monophosphate; thymidine monophosphate; thymidine-5′-monophosphate; thymolphthalein monophosphate; transmembrane potential; transmembrane pressure; trimethaphan; trimethoprim; trimethylpsoralen
TM$_{PAH}$ maximum tubular excretory capacity for para-aminohippuric acid
TMPD tetramethyl-p-phenylinediamine
TMPDS temporomandibular pain and dysfunction syndrome; thiamine monophosphate disulfide
TMP-SMX trimethoprim-sulfamethaxole; trimethoprim-sulfamethoxazole
TMR tissue maximum ratio; topical magnetic resonance; trainable mentally retarded
TMRM tetramethylrhodamine
TMS thalium myocardial scintigraphy; thread mate system; thymidilate synthase; trapezoidocephaly-multiple synostosis [syndrome]; trimethylsilane

TMST treadmill stem test
TMT tarsometatarsal; Trail-Making Test; trimethyllin
TMTD tetramethylthiuram disulfide
TMTJ tarsometatarsal joint
TMU tetramethyl urea
TMV tobacco mosaic virus
TMX tamoxifen
TMZ transformation zone
TN talonavicular; tarsonavicular; team nursing; temperature normal; tenascin; trigeminal nucleus; total negatives; trigeminal neuralgia; trochlear nucleus; true negative
T/N tar and nicotine
Tn normal intraocular tension; transposon
TNA total nutrient admixture
TNB transnasal butorphanol
TND term normal delivery
t-NE total norepinephrine
TNEE titrated norepinephrine excretion
T$_4$N normal serum thyroxine
TNF true negative fraction; tumor necrosis factor
TNFA tumor necrosis factor alpha
TNFAIP tumor necrosis factor, alpha-induced protein
TNFAR tumor necrosis factor alpha receptor
TNFB tumor necrosis factor beta
TNFBR tumor necrosis factor beta receptor
TNG trinitroglycerin
tng tongue
TNH teaching nursing home; transient neonatal hyperammonemia
T-NHL T-cell-derived non-Hodgkin leukemia
TNHP teaching nursing home program
TNI total nodal irradiation
TNM primary tumor, regional nodes, metastasis [tumor staging]; thyroid node metastases; tumor node metastasis
TNMR tritium nuclear magnetic resonance

TNP total net positive

TNR tonic neck reflex; true negative rate

TNS total nuclear score; transcutaneous nerve stimulation; tumor necrosis serum

TNT tetranitroblue tetrazolium; 2,4,6-trinitrotoluene

TnT troponin T

TNTC too numerous to count

TNV tobacco necrosis virus

TO old tuberculin; oral temperature; original tuberculin; target organ; telephone order; thoracic orthosis; thromboangiitis obliterans; tincture of opium; total obstruction; tracheoesophageal; tubo-ovarian; turnover

T(O) oral temperature

TO$_2$ oxygen transport

T$_o$ tricuspid opening

to tincture of opium

TOA total quality assessment; tubo-ovarian abscess

TOAP thioguanine, oncovin, cytosine arabinoside, and prednisone

TOB tobramycin

TOBEC total body electrical conductivity [test]

TobRV tobacco ringspot virus

TOC total organic carbon

TOCP tri-o-cresyl phosphate

TOCSY total correlation spectroscopy

TOD right eye tension [Lat. *oculus dexter*]; Time-Oriented Data [Bank]; titanium optimized design [plate]

TODS toxic organic dust syndrome

TOE tender on examination; tracheoesophageal; transesophageal echography; transferred nuclear Overhauser effect

TOEFL Test of English as a Foreign Language [for foreign medical graduates]

TOES toxic oil epidemic syndrome

TOF tetralogy of Fallot; time-of-flight; train of four [monitor]; tracheo[o]esophageal fistula

TOFA time-of-flight absorbance

T of F tetralogy of Fallot

TOFHLA test of functional health literacy in adults

TOH transient osteoporosis of hip

TOL trial of labor

tol tolerance, tolerated

TOLB, tolb tolbutamine

TOM toxic oxygen metabolite

TOMHS Treatment of Mild Hypertension Study

Tomo tomography, tomogram

tomos tomograms

TON traumatic optic neuropathy

TONE tilted optimized nonsaturating excitation

tonoc tonight

TOP termination of pregnancy; topoisomerase

top topical

TOPV trivalent oral poliovaccine

TORCH toxoplasmosis, other [congenital syphilis and viruses], rubella, cytomegalovirus, and herpes simplex virus

TORP total ossicular replacement prosthesis

torr mm Hg pressure

TOS thoracic outlet syndrome; toxic oil syndrome

TOT total operating time

TOV trial of voiding

tox toxicity, toxic

TOXICON Toxicology Information Conversational On-Line Network

TOXLINE Toxicology Information On-Line [data bank]

TOXLIT Toxicology Liturature [data bank]

TOXNET Toxicology Network (NLM) [data bank]

TP temperature and pressure; temperature probe; temporal peak; temporoparietal; tension pneumothorax; terminal phalanx; testosterone propionate; thick padding; threshold potential; thrombocytopenic purpura; thrombophlebitis; thymopentin; thymopoietin; thymus polypeptide; thymus protein; torsades de pointes; total positives; total protein; transforming principle; transition point; transverse polarization; transverse process; treatment progress; *Treponema pallidum*; trigger point; triphosphate; true positive; tryptophan; tryptophan pyrrolase; tube precipitin; tuberculin precipitate; tumor protein

6-TP 6-thiopurine

T&P temperature and pressure; temperature and pulse

T+P temperature and pulse

Tp primary transmission; *Treponema pallidum;* tryptophan

T$_p$ physical half-life

TPA tannic acid, polyphosphomolybdic acid, and amino acid; 12-0-tetradecanoyl-phorbol-13-acetate; third-party adnistrator; tissue plasminogen activator; total parenteral alimentation; *Treponema pallidum* agglutination; tumor polypeptide antigen

t-PA tissue plasminogen activator

TPAI tissue plasminogen activator inhibitor

TPase thymidine phosphorylase

TPB tetraphenyl borate; tryptone phosphate broth

TPBF total pulmonary blood flow

TPBG trophoblast glycoprotein

TPBS three-phase radionuclide bone scanning

TPC thromboplastic plasma component; thyroid papillary carcinoma; total patient care; total plasma catecholamines; total plasma cholesterol; *Treponema pallidum* complement

TPCF *Treponema pallidum* complement fixation

TPCV total packed cell volume

TPD temporary partial disability; thiamine propyl disulfide; tripotassium phenolphthalein disulfate; tumor-producing dose

TPDS tropical pancreatic diabetes syndrome

TPE therapeutic plasma exchange; totally protected environment; typhoid-parathyroid enteritis

T^{Pe} expiratory pause time

TPEY tellurite polymyxin egg yolk [agar]

TPF thymus permeability factor; thymus to peak flow; true positive fraction

TPG transmembrane potential gradient; transplacental gradient; tryptophan peptone glucose [broth]

TPGYT trypticase-peptone-glucose-yeast extract-trypsin [medium]

TPH transplacental hemorrhage; tryptophan hydroxylase

TPHA *Treponema pallidum* hemagglutination

TPI time period integrator; treponemal immobilization test; *Treponema pallidum* immobilization; triose phosphate isomerase

T^{Pi} inspiratory pause time

TPIA *Treponema pallidum* immune adherence

TPIIA time of postexpiratory inspiratory activity

TPK tyrosine protein kinase

TPL third party liability; titanium proximal loading; tumor progression locus; tyrosine phenol-lyase

TPLV transient pulmonary vascular lability

TPM temporary pacemaker; thrombophlebitis migrans; total particulate matter; total passive motion; triphenylmethane

TPMT thiopurine methyltransferase

TPN thalamic projection neuron; total parenteral nutrition; transition protein; triphosphopyridine nucleotide

TPNH reduced triphosphopyridine nucleotide

TPO thyroid peroxidase; tryptophan peroxidase

TPP thiamine pyrophosphate; transpulmonary pressure; treadmill performance test; tripeptidyl peptidase; triphenyl phosphite

TPPase thiamine pyrophosphatase

TPPD thoracic-pelvic-phalangeal dystrophy

TPPI time proportional phase incrementation

TPPN total peripheral parenteral nutrition

TPQ Threshold Planning Quantity

TPR temperature, pulse, and respiration; testosterone production rate; third party reimbursement; total peripheral resistance; total pulmonary resistance; true positive rate; tumor potentiating region

TPRI total peripheral resistance index

TPS trypsin; tryptase; tumor polysaccharide substance

TPSE 2-(p-triphenyl)sulfonylethanol

TPST true positive stress test

TPT tetraphenyl tetrazolium; triphalangeal thumb; total protein tuberculin; typhoid-paratyphoid [vaccine]

TPTE 2-(p-triphenyl)thioethanol

TPTX thyro-parathyroidectomized

TPTZ tripyridyltriazine

TPV tetanus-pertussis vaccine

TPVR total peripheral vascular resistance; total pulmonary vascular resistance

TPVS transhepatic portal venous sampling

TPX testis-specific protein

TPZ thioproperazine

TQ tocopherolquinone; tourniquet

TQFCOSY triple-quantum filtered correlated spectroscopy

TQM total quality management

TR recovery time; rectal temperature; repetition time; residual tuberculin; terminal repeat; tetrazolium reduction; therapeutic radiology; therapeutic ratio; time release; thrombin receptor; total resistance; total response; trachea; transfusion reaction; transrectal; tricuspid regurgitation; tuberculin R [new tuberculin]; tuberculin residue; turbidity-reducing; turnover ratio

T&R treated and released

T(°R) absolute temperature on the Rankine scale

Tr trace; tragion; transferrin; trypsin

T$_r$ radiologic half-life; retention time

tr tincture; trace; traction; transaldolase; trauma, traumatic; tremor; triradial

TRA total renin activity; tumor-resistant antigen

tra transfer

TRAb thyrotoxin receptor antibody

TRAC tool for referral assessment of continuity [of health]

trac traction

trach trachea, tracheal, tracheostomy

TRAJ time repetitive ankle jerk

TRALT transfusion-related acute lung injury

TRAM transport remote acquisition monitor; transverse rectus abdominis muscle; Treatment Rating Assessment Matrix; Treatment Response Assessment Method

TRAMPE tricho-rhino-auriculophalangeal multiple exostoses

trans transfer; transference; transverse

trans D transverse diameter

transm transmitted, transmission

transpl transplantation, transplanted

TRAP carpal tunnel syndrome, Raynaud phenomenon, aching muscles, proximal muscle weakness [rheumatic disorders associated with hypothyroidism]; tartrate-resistant acid phosphatase; transport and rapid accessioning for additional procedures; triiodothyronine receptor auxiliary protein

trap trapezius

TRAS transplanted renal artery stenosis

TRASHES tuberculosis, radiotherapy, ankylosing spondylitis, histoplasmosis, extrinsic allergic alveolitis, silicosis [chest x-ray findings]

traum trauma, traumatic

TRB terbutalone

TRBF total renal blood flow

TRC tanned red cell; therapeutic residential center; total renin concentration; total respiratory conductance; total ridge count

TRCA tanned red cell agglutination

TRCH tanned red cell hemagglutination

TRCHI tanned red cell hemagglutination inhibition

TRCV total red cell volume

TRD tongue-retaining device

TRDN transient respiratory distress of the newborn

TRE thymic reticuloendothelial; thyroid hormone response; true radiation emission

TREA triethanolamine

treat treatment

Trend Trendelenburg [position]

Trep Treponema

TRF T-cell replacing factor; thyrotropin-releasing factor; tubular rejection fraction

TRFC total rosette-forming cell

TRG T-cell rearranging tgene; transfer ribonucleic acid glycine

TRH tension-reducing hypothesis; thyrotropin-releasing hormone

TRHR thyrotropin-releasing hormone receptor

TRH-ST thyrotropin-releasing hormone stimulation test

TRI tetrazolium reduction inhibition; Thyroid Research Institute; total response index; toxic chemical release inventory; tubuloreticular inclusion

tri tricentric

T₃RIA, T₃(RIA) triiodothyronine radioimmunoassay

T₄RIA, T₄(RIA) thyroxine radioimmunoassay

TRIC trachoma inclusion conjunctivitis [organism]

TRICB trichlorobiphenyl

Trich Trichomonas

TRIFACTS Toxic Chemical Release Inventory Facts

trig trigger; triglycerides; trigonum

TRIMIS Tri-Service Medical Information System

TRINS totally reversible ischemic neurological symptoms

TRIS tris-(hydroxymethyl)-aminomethane

TRISS trauma and injury severity score

TRIT triiodothyronine

trit triturate

TRITC tetrarhodamine isothiocyanate

TRK transketolase; throsine kinase

TRL transfer ribonucleic acid leucine

TRLP triglyceride-rich lipoprotein

TRMA thiamine-responsive megaloblastic anemia

TRMC trimethylrhodamino-isothiocyanate

TRMI transfer ribonucleic acid initiator methionine

TRML, Trml terminal

TRM-SMX trimethoprim-sulfamethoxazole

TRN tegmental reticular nucleus

tRNA transfer ribonucleic acid

tRNA GLU transfer ribonucleic acid glutamic acid

tRNA-i(met) transfer ribonucleic acid initiator methionine

tRNA-SER transfer ribonucleic acid serine

TRNOE transfer nuclear Overhauser effect

TRNS transfer ribonucleic acid serine

TRO tissue reflectance oximetry

Troch trochanter

TROM torque range of motion

Trop tropical

TRP total refractory period; transfer ribonucleic acid proline; trichorhinophalangeal [syndrome]; tubular reabsorption of phosphate; tyrosine-related protein

Trp tryptophan

TRPA tryptophan-rich prealbumin

TrPl treatment plan

TRPM testosterone-repressed prostate message

TRPO tryptophan oxygenase

TRPS trichorhinophalangeal syndrome

TRPT theoretical renal phosphorus threshold

TRR total respiratory resistance

TRS testicular regression syndrome; total reducing sugars; tubuloreticular structure

TrS trauma surgery

TRSV tobacco ringspot virus

TRT thoracic radiotherapy; transfer ribonucleic acid threonine

TR/TE repetition time/echo time

TRU task-related unit; turbidity-reducing unit

T$_3$RU triiodothyronine resin uptake

TRUS transrectal ultrasonography

TRV tobacco rattle virus

TRVV total right ventricular volume

Tryp tryptophan

TRX thioredoxin

trx traction

TS Takayasu syndrome; Tay-Sachs; temperature sensitivity; temperature, skin; temporal stem; tensile strength; test solution; thermal stability; thoracic surgery; thymidylate synthetase; tissue space; total solids [in urine]; Tourette syndrome; toxic substance; toxic syndrome; tracheal sound; transferrin saturation; transitional sleep; transsexual; transverse section; transverse sinus; trauma score; treadmill score; triceps surae; tricuspid stenosis; triple strength; tropical sprue; trypticase soy [plate]; T suppressor [cell]; tuberous sclerosis; tumor-specific; Turner syndrome; type-specific

T/S transverse section

T+S type and screen

Ts skin temperature; tosylate

T$_s$ T-cell suppressor

tS time required to complete the S phase of the cell cycle

ts temperature sensitivity

ts, tsp teaspoon

TSA technical surgical assistance; toluene sulfonic acid; total shoulder arthroplasty; total solute absorption; toxic shock antigen; transcortical sensory aphasia; trypticase-soy agar; tumor-specific antigen; tumor surface antigen; type-specific antibody

T$_4$SA thyroxine-specific activity

TSAb thyroid-stimulating antibody

TSAP toxic-shock-associated protein

TSAS total severity assessment score

TSAT tube slide agglutination test

TSB total serum bilirubin; trypticase soy broth; tryptone soy broth

TSBA total serum bile acids

TSBB transtracheal selective bronchial brushing

TSC technetium sulfur colloid; thiosemicarbazide; transverse spinal sclerosis; tuberous sclerosis

TSCA Toxic Substances Control Act

TSCS Tennessee Self-Concept Scale

TSD target-skin distance; Tay-Sachs disease; theory of signal detectability

TSE testicular self-examination; tissuespecific extinguisher; total skin examination; trisodium edetate

TSEB total skin electron beam

T sect transverse section

TSEM transmission scanning electron microscopy

TSES Target Symptom Evaluation Scale

T-set tracheotomy set

TSF testicular feminization syndrome; thrombopoiesis-stimulating factor; total systemic flow; triceps skinfold

TSG, TSGP tumor-specific glycoprotein

TSH thyroid-stimulating hormone; transient synovitis of the hip

TSHA thyroid-stimulating hormone, alpha chain

TSHB thyroid-stimulating hormone, beta chain

TSHR thyroid-stimulating hormone receptor

TSH-RF thyroid-stimulating hormone-releasing factor

TSH-RH thyroid-stimulating hormone-releasing hormone

TSI thyroid stimulating immunoglobulin; triple sugar iron [agar]

TSIA total small intestine allotransplantation; triple sugar iron agar

tSIDS totally unexplained sudden infant death syndrome

TSL terminal sensory latency

TSM type-specific M protein

TSP testis-specific protein; thrombin-sensitive protein; thrombospondin; total serum protein; total suspended particulate; trisodium phosphate; tropical spastic paraparesis

tsp teaspoon

TSPA thiotepa

TSPAP total serum prostatic acid phosphatase

TSPL transplant

TSPP tetrasodium pyrophosphate

TSR theophylline sustained release; thyroid to serum ratio; total systemic resistance

TSS toxic shock syndrome; tropical splenomegaly syndrome

TSSA tumor-specific cell surface antigen

TSSE toxic shock syndrome exotoxin

TSST toxic shock syndrome toxin

TST thiosulfate sulfur-transferase; thromboplastin screening test; total sleep time; transforming sequence, thyroid; treadmill stress test; tricipital skinfold thickness; tumor skin test

TSTA toxoplasmin skin test antigen; tumor-specific tissue antigen; tumor-specific transplantation antigen

TSU triple sugar urea [agar]

TSV total stomach volume

TSVR total systemic vascular resistance

TSY trypticase soy yeast

TT tablet triturate; tactile tension; tendon transfer; test tube; testicular torsion; tetanus toxin; tetanus toxoid; tetrathionate; tetrazol; therapeutic touch; thrombin time; thrombolytic therapy; thymol turbidity; tibial tubercle; tilt table; tolerance test; total thyroxine; total time; transient tachypnea; transferred to; transit time; transthoracic; transtracheal; tuberculin test; tuberculoid [in Ridley-Jopling Hansen disease classification]; tube thoracostomy; tumor thrombus; turnover time

T&T time and temperature; touch and tone

TT$_2$ total diiodothyronine

TT$_3$ total triiodothyronine

TT$_4$ total thyroxine

TTA tetanus toxoid antibody; timed therapeutic absence; total toe arthroplasty; transtracheal aspiration

TTAP threaded titanium acetabular prosthesis

TTB third trimester bleeding

TTC triphenyltetrazolium chloride; T-tube cholangiogram

TTD temporary total disability; tissue tolerance dose; transient tic disorder; transverse thoracic diameter; trichothiodystrophy

TTE transthoracic echocardiography

TTFD tetrahydrofurfuryldisulfide

TTG T-cell translocation gene; telethermography; tellurite, taurocholate, and gelatin

TTGA tellurite, taurocholate, and gelatin agar

TTH thyrotropic hormone; tritiated thymidine

TTI tension-time index; time-tension index; timepto-intubation; torque-time interval; transtracheal insufflation

TTIdi tension time index diaphragm
TTIM T-cell tumor invasion and metastasis
T-TIME tourniquet time
TTL total thymus lymphocytes; transistor-transistor logic
TTLC true total lung capacity
TTLD terminal transverse limb defect
TTN titin; transient tachypnea of the newborn
TTNA transthoracic needle aspiration
TTNB transthoracic needle biopsy
TTO time trade-off [method]
TTP thiamine triphosphate; thrombotic thrombocytopenic purpura; thymidine triphosphate; time to peak; tristetraprolin
TTPA triethylene thiophosphoramide
TTR transthoracic resistance; transthyretin; triceps tendon reflex
TTS tarsal tunnel syndrome; temporary threshold shift; through the scope; through the skin; tilt table standing; transdermal therapeutic system; twin transfusion syndrome
TTT thymol turbidity test; tolbutamide tolerance test; total twitch time; tuberculin tine test
TTTT test tube turbidity test
TTV tracheal transport velocity; transfusion-transmitted virus
TTX tetrodotoxin
TU thiouracil; thyroid uptake; Todd unit; toxin unit; transmission unit; transurethral; tuberculin unit; turbidity unit
T₃U T_3U triiodothyronine uptake
TUB tubulin
TUBA tubulin alpha
TUBAL tubulin alpha-like
TUBB tubulin beta
tuberc tuberculosis
TUBG tubulin gamma
TUD total urethral discharge
TUG total urinary gonadotropin
TUGSE traumatic ulcerative granuloma with stromal eosinophilia

TUI transurethral incision
TULIP transurethral ultrasound-guided laser-induced prostatectomy
TUR transurethral resection
TURB, TURBT transurethral resection of bladder [tumor]
turb turbidity, turbid
truboFLASH turbo fast low angle shot
TURP transurethral resection of the prostate
TURS transurethral resection syndrome
TURV transurethral resection of valves
TV talipes varus; television; tetrazolium violet; thoracic vertebra; tickborne virus; tidal volume; total volume; toxic vertigo; transvaginal; transvenous; transverse; trial visit; *Trichomonas vaginalis*; tricuspid valve; trivalent; true vertebra; truncal vagotomy; tuberculin volutin; tubovesicular typhoid vaccine
Tv Trichomonas vaginalis
TVA truncal vagotomy and antrectomy
TVC timed vital capacity; total viable cells; total volume capacity; transvaginal cone; triple voiding cystogram; true vocal cords
TVCV transvenous cardioversion
TVD transmissible virus dementia; triple vessel disease
TVF tactile vocal fremitus
TVG time-varied gain
TVH total vaginal hysterectomy; turkey virus hepatitis
TVI time-velocity integral
TVL tenth value layer; tunica vasculosa lentis
TVMF time varying magnetic field
TVP tensor veli palatini [muscle]; textured vegetable protein; transvenous pacemaker; tricuspid valve prolapse; truncal vagotomy and pyloroplasty
TVR tonic vibratory reflex; total vascular resistance; tricuspid valve replacement
TVRE transvaginal resection or endometrium

TVS transvesical sonography
TVSS transient voltage surge suppressor
TVT transmissible venereal tumor; tunica vaginalis testis
TVU total volume of the urine
TW tap water; terminal web; test weight; total body water; travelling wave
Tw twist
TWA time weighted average
TWBC total white blood cells; total white blood count
TWD total white and differential [cell count]
TWE tap water enema; tepid water enema
TWIST time without symptoms of disease and subjective toxic effects of treatment
TWL transepidermal water loss
TWS tranquilizer withdrawal syndrome
TWs triphasic waves
TWT total waiting time
TWWD tap water wet dressing

TX a derivative of contagious tuberculin; thromboxane; thyroidectomized; transplantation; treatment
T&X type and crossmatch
Tx transplant or transplantation
Tx, T$_x$ treatment; therapy, traction
tx traction
TXA, TxA thromboxane A
TXA2, TXA$_2$ thromboxane A2 (A$_2$)
TXB2, TXB$_2$ thromboxane B2 (B$_2$)
TXDS qualifying toxic dose
TXN thioredoxin
Ty type, typhoid; tyrosine
TYH tyrosine hydrolase
Tymp tympanum, tympanic
TYMS thymidylate synthetase
TYMV turnip yellow mosaic virus
Tyr tyrosine
TyRIA thyroid radioisotope assay
TYRL tyrosinase-like
TYRP tyrosine-related protein
TZ zymoplastic tuberculin [the dried residue which is soluble in alcohol] [Ger. *Tuberculin zymoplastische*]

U congenital limb absence; in electrocardiography, an undulating deflection that follows the T wave; internal energy; International Unit of enzyme activity; Mann-Whitney rank sum statistic; potential difference (in volts); ulcer; ulna; ultralente [insulin]; umbilicus; uncertain; unerupted; unit; universial application [residency]; unknown; unsharpness; upper; uracil; uranium; urea; urethra; uridine; uridylic acid; urinary concentration; urine; urology; uterus; uvula; volume velocity

u unified atomic mass unit; velocity

U/2 upper half

U/3 upper third

UA absorption unsharpness; ultra-audible; ultrasonic arteriography; umbilical artery; unauthorized absence; unit of analysis; unstable angina; upper airways; upper arm; uric acid; uridylic acid; urinalysis; urinary aldosterone; uronic acid; uterine aspiration

U/A urinalysis; uric acid

ua urinalysis

UAC umbilical artery catheter

UA/C uric acid/creatinine [ratio]

U-AMY urinary amylase

UAE unilateral absence of excretion; urine albumin excretion

UAEM University Association for Emergency Medicine

UAI uterine activity interval

UAN uric acid nitrogen

UAO upper airway obstruction

UAP unlicensed assistive personnel; unstable angina pectoris; urinary acid phosphatase; urinary alkaline phosphatase

UAPA unilateral absence of pulmonary artery

UAR upper airway resistance; uric acid riboside

UAS upper abdomen surgery; upstream activation site

UAU uterine activity unit

UB ultimobranchial body; Unna boot; upper back; urinary bladder

UB 82 universal billing document [1982]

UBA undenaturated bacterial antigen

UBB ubiquitin B

UBBC unsaturated vitamin B12 binding capacity

UBC ubiquitin C; University of British Columbia [brace]

UBE ubiquitin-activating enzyme

UBF uterine blood flow

UBG, Ubg urobilinogen

UBI ultraviolet blood irradiation

UBL undifferentiated B-cell lymphoma

UBN urobilin

UBO unidentified bright object

UBP ureteral back pressure

UBS unidentified bright signal

UBW usual body weight

UC ulcerative colitis; ultracentrifugal; umbilical cord; unchanged; unclassifiable; unconscious; undifferentiated cells; unit clerk; unsatisfactory condition; untreated cells; urea clearance; urethral catheterization; urinary catheter; urine concentrate; urine culture; uterine contractions

U&C urethral and cervical; usual and customary

UCB unconjugated bilirubin

UCBC umbilical cord blood culture

UCD urine collection device; usual childhood diseases

UCDS uniform clinical data set

UCE urea cycle enzymopathy

UCG ultrasonic cardiography; urinary chorionic gonadotropin

UCHD usual childhood diseases

UCI unusual childhood illness; urethral catheter in; urinary catheter in

UCL ulnar collateral ligament; upper collateral ligament; upper confidence limit; upper control limit; urea clearance

UCLP unilateral cleft of lip and palate

UCO ultrasonic cardiac output; urethral catheter out; urinary catheter out

UCOD underlying cause of death

UCP uncoupling protein; urinary coproporphyrin; urinary C-peptide

UCPT urinary coproporphyrin test

UCR unconditioned response; usual, customary, and reasonable [fees]

UCS unconditioned stimulus; unconscious; uterine compression syndrome

ucs unconscious

UCT urological care table

UCTD undifferentiated (unclassifiable) connective tissue disease

uCTD undifferentiated connective tissue disease

UCV uncontrolled variable

UD ulcerative dermatosis; ulnar deviation; undetermined; underdeveloped; unit dose; urethral dilatation; urethral discharge; uridine diphosphate; uroporphyrinogen decarboxylase; uterine delivery

UDC usual diseases of childhood

UDCA ursodeoxycholic acid

UDKase uridine diphosphate kinase

UDN ulcerative dermal necrosis

UDO undetermined origin

UDP uridine diphosphate

UDPG uridine diphosphate glucose; urine diphosphoglucose

UDPGA uridine diphosphate glucuronic acid

UDPGT uridine diphosphate glucuronosyl transferase

UDR-BMD ultradistal radius bone mineral density

UDRP urine diribose phosphate

UDS ultrasound Doppler sonography; uniform data system; unscheduled deoxynucleic acid synthesis

UE uncertain etiology; under elbow; uninvolved epidermis; upper esophagus; upper extremity

uE$_s$ unconjugated estriol

UEG ultrasonic encephalography; unifocal eosinophilic granuloma

UEHB uniform effective health benefits

UEL upper explosive limit

UEM universal electron microscope

UEMC unidentified endosteal marrow cell

UES upper esophageal sphincter

u/ext upper extremity

UF film unsharpness; ultrafiltrate; ultrafiltration; ultrafine; ultrasonic frequency; universal feeder; unknown factor; urinary formaldehyde

UFA unesterified fatty acid

UFB urinary fat bodies

UFC urinary free cortisol

UFD ultrasonic flow detector; unilateral facet dislocation

UFFI urea formaldehyde foam insulation

UFL upper flammable limit

UFP ultrafiltration pressure

UFR ultrafiltration rate; urine filtration rate

uFSH urinary follicle-stimulating hormone

UG geometric unsharpness; urogastrone; urogenital

UGD urogenital diaphragm

UGDP University Group Diabetes Project

UGF unidentified growth factor

UGH uveitis-glaucoma-hyphema [syndrome]

UGH+ uveitis-glaucoma-hyphema plus vitreous hemorrhage [syndrome]

UGI upper gastrointestinal [tract]

UGIH upper gastrointestinal hemorrhage

UGIS upper gastrointestinal series

UGME undergraduate medical education

UGP uridyl diphosphate glucose pyrophosphorylase

UGPA undergraduate grade-point average

UGPP uridyl diphosphate glucose pyrophosphorylase

UGS urogenital sinus

UGT uridine diphosphate-glucuronosyltransferase; urogenital tract; urogenital tuberculosis

UH umbilical hernia; uncontrolled hemorrhage; unfavorable histology; upper half

UHD unstable hemoglobin disease

UHDDS uniform hospital discharge data set

UHF ultrahigh frequency

UHL universal hypertrichosis lanuginosa

UHMW ultrahigh molecular weight

UHR underlying heart rhythm

UHS uncontrolled hemorrhagic shock

UHSC university health services clinic

UHT ultrahigh temperature

UI uroporphyrin isomerase

U/I unidentified

UIBC unsaturated iron-binding capacity

UICAO unilateral internal carotid artery occlusion

UID unique image identifier

UIF undegraded insulin factor

UIP usual interstitial pneumonia

UIQ upper inner quadrant

UIS Utilization Information Service

UJT unijunction transistor

UK unknown; uridine kinase; urinary kallikrein

UKa urinary kallikrein

UKAEA United Kingdom Atomic Energy Authority

UKase uridine kinase

UKCCSG United Kingdom Children's Cancer Study Group

UKM urea kinetic modeling

ukn unknown

UL ultrasonic; Underwriters Laboratories; undifferentiated lymphoma; upper limb; upper limit; upper lobe

U&L upper and lower

U/l units per liter

ULBW ultralow birth weight

ULDH urinary lactate dehydrogenase

ULLE upper lid of left eye

ULN upper limits of normal

uln ulna, ulnar

ULP ultra low profile

ULPA ultra low penetration air filter

ULPE upper lobe pulmonary edema

ULQ upper left quadrant

ULRE upper lid of right eye

ULT ultrahigh temperature

ult ultimate

ULTC urban level trauma center

ULV ultralow volume

UM movement unsharpness; upper motor [neuron]; uracil mustard; utilization management

UMA ulcerative mutilating acropathy; upright membrane assay; urinary muramidase activity

Umax maximum urinary osmolality

umb umbilicus, umbilical

UMC unidimensional chromatography; university medical center

UMCV-TO ulnar motor conduction velocity across thoracic outlet

UMDNS Universal Medical Device Nomenclature System

UME undergraduate medical education

UMI urinary meconium index

UMKase uridine monophosphate kinase

UMLS Unified Medical Language System

UMN upper motor neuron

UMNL upper motor neuron lesion

UMNS upper motor neuron syndrome

UMP uridine monophosphate

UMPH uridine 5′-monophosphate phosphohydrolase

UMPK uridine monophosphate kinase
UMPS uridine monophosphate synthase
UMS urethral manipulation syndrome
UMT units of medical time
UN ulnar nerve; undernourished; unilateral neglect; urea nitrogen; urinary nitrogen
UNAI uniform needs assessment for posthospital care
UNa urinary sodium
uncomp uncompensated
uncond unconditioned
UNCV ulnar nerve conduction velocity
undet undetermined
UNDRO United Nations Disaster Relief Organization
UNE urinary norepinephrine
UNFPA United Nations Population Fund
UNG uracil deoxyribonucleic acid glycosylase
UNHCR United Nations High Commission for Refugees
unilat unilateral
UNIS Urological Nursing Information System
univ universal
unk, unkn unknown
UNL upper normal limit
UNLS Unified Nursing Language System
UNOS United Network for Organ Sharing
unsat unsatisfactory; unsaturated
UNT untreated
UNTS unilateral nevoid telangiectasia syndrome
UNX uninephrectomy
UO under observation; undetermined origin; urethral orifice; urinary output
U/O urinary output
u/o under observation
UOP urinary output
UOQ upper outer quadrant
UOsm urinary osmolality
UOV units of variance
UOX urate oxidase

UP parallax unsharpness; ulcerative proctitis; ultrahigh purity; unipolar; upright posture; ureteropelvic; uridine phosphorylase; uroporphyrin
U/P urine to plasma [ratio]
u-PA urinary type plasminogen activator
UPase uridine phosphorylase
UPD urinary production
UPDRS unified Parkinson disease rating scale
UPF universal proximal femur [prosthesis]
UPEP urinary protein electrophoresis; urine protein electrophoresis
UPET urokinase pulmonary embolism trial
UPG uroporphyrinogen
UPGMA unweighted pair group method with averages
UPI uteroplacental insufficiency; uteroplacental ischemia
UPIN universal physician identifier number [HCFA]
UPJ ureteropelvic junction
UPL unusual position of limbs
UPP urethral pressure profile
UPPP uvulopalatopharyngoplasty
UPPRA upright peripheral plasma renin activity
UPS ultraviolet photoelectron spectroscopy; uninterruptible power supply; uroporphyrinogen synthetase; uterine progesterone system
Υ Greek capital letter *upsilon*
υ Greek lower case letter *upsilon*
UPSIT University of Pennsylvania Smell Identification Test
UQ ubiquinone; upper quadrant
UQAC unit quality assurance committee
UQCRC ubiquinol-cytochrome C reductase core
UQS upper quadrant syndrome
UR unconditioned reflex; upper respiratory; uridine; urinal; urology; utilization review

Ur urea; urine, urinary
URA, Ura uracil
URAC Utilization Review Accreditation Commission
URC upper rib cage; utilization review committee
URD unspecified respiratory disease; upper respiratory disease
Urd uridine
ureth urethra
URF unidentified reading frame; uterine relaxing factor
URG urogastrone
URI uniform resource identifier; upper respiratory illness; upper respiratory infection
URK urokinase
URL uniform resource locator
URN uniform resource name
U-RNA uridylic acid ribonucleic acid
URO urology; uroporphyrin; uroporphyrinogen; utilization review organization
UROD uroporphyrinogen decarboxylase
URO-GEN urogenital
Urol urology, urologist
UROS uroporphyrinogen synthase
URQ upper right quadrant
URS ultrasonic renal scanning
URT upper respiratory tract
URTI upper respiratory tract infection
URVD unilateral renovascular disease
US screen unsharpness ultrasonic, ultrasound; ultrasonography; unconditioned stimulus; unique sequence; unit separator; upper segment; upper strength; urinary sugar; Usher syndrome
u/s ultrasonic or ultrasound
USAFH United States Air Force Hospital
USAFRHL United States Air Force Radiological Health Laboratory
USAH United States Army Hospital
USAHC United States Army Health Clinic
USAIDR United States Army Institute of Dental Research

USAMEDS United States Army Medical Service
USAMRIID United States Army Medical Research Institute for Infectious Diseases
USAN United States Adopted Names
USASI United States of America Standards Institute
USB upper sternal border
USBS United States Bureau of Standards
USCG ultrasonic cardiography
USD United States Dispensary
USDA United States Department of Agriculture
USDHEW United States Department of Health, Education, and Welfare
USDHHS United States Department of Health and Human Services
USE ultrasonic echography; ultrasonography
USF upstream stimulatory factor
USFA United States Fire Administration
USFMG United States foreign medical graduate
USFMS United States foreign medical student
USG ultrasonography
USHL United States Hygienic Laboratory
USHMAC United States Health Manpower Advisory Council
USI universal serial interface; urinary stress incontinence
USIA United States Information Agency
USIMG United States citizen international medical school graduate
US/LS upper strength/lower strength [ratio]
USMG United States or Canada medical school graduate
USMH United States Marine Hospital
USMLE United States Medical Licensing Examination

USN ultrasonic nebulizer; unilateral spatial neglect

USNCHS United States National Center for Health Statistics

USNH United States Naval Hospital

USO unilateral salpingo-oophorectomy

USP United States Pharmacopeia

USPC United States Pharmacopeia Convention

USPDI United States Pharmacopeia Drug Information

USPHS United States Public Health Service

USPSTF United States Preventive Services Task Force

USPTA United States Phyical Therapy Association

USR unheated serum reagin

USS ultrasound scanning

USVH United States Veterans Hospital

USVMD urine specimen volume measuring device

USW ultrashort waves

UT total unsharpness; Ullrich-Turner [syndrome]; Unna-Thost [syndrome]; untested; untreated; urinary tract; urticaria

uT unbound testosterone

UTBG unbound thyroxine-binding globulin

UTC upper thoracic compression

UTD up to date

UTI urinary tract infection; urinary trypsin inhibitor

UTO upper tibial osteotomy; urinary tract obstruction

UTP unilateral tension pneumothorax; unshielded twisted pair; uridine triphosphate

UTR untranslated region

UTS Ullrich-Turner syndrome; ulnar tunnel syndrome; ultimate tensile strength

UTZ ultrasound

UU urinary urea; urine urobilinogen

UUN urinary urea nitrogen

UUO unilateral urethral obstruction

UUP urinary uroporphyrin

UV ultraviolet; umbilical vein; ureterovesical; Uppsala virus; urinary volume

UVA ureterovesical angle

UVB ultraviolet B

UVC umbilical venous catheter

UVEB unifocal ventricular ectopic beat

UVER ultraviolet-enhanced reactivation

UVI ultraviolet irradiation

UVJ ureterovesical junction

UVL ultraviolet light

UVO uvomorulin

UVP ultraviolet photometry

UVR ultraviolet radiation

UW unilateral weakness

UWB unit of whole blood

UWD Urbach-Wiethe disease

UWSC unstimulated whole saliva collection

UX uranium X, proactinium

UYP upper yield point

V in cardiography, unipolar chest lead; coefficient of variation; electrical potential (in volts); in electroencephalography, vertex sharp transient; five; a logical binary relation that is true if any argument is true, and false otherwise; luminous efficiency; potential energy (joules); vaccinated, vaccine; vagina; valine; valve; vanadium; variable, variation, varnish; vector; vegetarian; vein [Lat. *vena*]; velocity; ventilation; ventral; ventricular [fibrillation]; verbal comprehension [factor]; vertebra; vertex; vestibular; *Vibrio*; violet; viral [antigen]; virulence; virus; vision; visual acuity; voice; volt; voltage; volume; vomiting

V1 TP V6 ventral 1 to ventral 6 [chest leads in ECG]

v or [Lat. *vel*]; rate of reaction catalyzed by an enzyme; see [Lat. *vide*]; specific volume; valve; vein [Lat. *vena*]; velocity; venous; ventral; ventricular; versus; very; virus; vision; volt; volume

VA vacuum aspiration; valproic acid; vasodilator agent; ventricular aneurysm; ventricular arrhythmia; ventriculoatrial; ventroanterior; vertebral artery; Veterans Administration; Veterans Affairs; vincristine, adriamycin; viral antigen; visual acuity; visual aid; visual axis; volt-ampere; volume-average

V_A alveolar ventilation

V/A volt/ampere

V-A veno-arterial

V_a alveolar ventilation

VAB vincristine, actinomycin D, and bleomycin; violent antisocial behavior

VAB-6 vincristine, actinomycin, bleomycin, cis-platinum, Cytoxan

VABP venoarterial bypass pumping

VAC ventriculoatrial conduction; vincristine, doxorubicin, and cyclophosphamide; virus capsid antigen

vac vacuum

VAcc visual acuity with correction

vacc vaccination

VACO Veterans Affairs Central Office

VACTERL vertebral abnormalities, anal atresia, cardiac abnormalities, tracheoesophageal fistula and/or esophageal atresia, renal agenesis and dysplasia, and limb defects [association]

VAD venous access device; ventricular assist device; vinblastine and dexamethasone; vitamin A deficiency; virus-adjusting diluent

VAE venous air emboli

VAF viral-free antigen

VAG vibroarthrography

vag vagina, vaginal, vaginitis

VAG HYST vaginal hysterectomy

VAH vertebral ankylosing hyperostosis; Veterans Affairs Hospital; virilizing adrenal hyperplasia

VAHS virus-associated hemophagocytic syndrome

VAIN vaginal intraepithelial neoplasm

V_{ak} atrial volume constant

Val valine

val valve

VALE visual acuity, left eye

VAM ventricular arrhythmia monitor

VAMC Veterans Affairs Medical Center

VAMP vincristine, amethopterine, 6-mercaptopurine; and prednisone

VAP vaginal acid phosphatase; variant angina pectoris

vap vapor

VAPS visual analog pain score

V_a/Q alveolar ventilation/perfusion

V_A/Q_C ventilation-perfusion [ratio]

VAR visual-auditory range

Var, var variable; variant, variation, variety

var varicose

VARE visual acuity, right eye

VARS valyl-transfer ribonucleic acid synthetase

VAS vascular; ventriculo-atrial shunt; Verapamil Angioplasty Study; vesicle attachment site; viral arthritis syndrome; Visual Analogue Scale

VASC Verbal Auditory Screen for Children; visual-auditory screening

VAsc visual acuity without correction

vasc vascular

VAS RAD vascular radiology

VAT variable antigen type; ventricular accommodation test; ventricular activation time; vesicular amine transformer; visual action therapy; visual action time; visual apperception test; vocational apperception test

VATER vertebral defects, imperforate anus, tracheoesophageal fistula, and radial and renal dysplasia

VATS Veterans Administration medical center transference syndrome

VATs surface variable antigen

VB vaginal bulb; valence bond; venous blood; ventrobasal; Veronal buffer; vertebrobasilar; viable birth; vinblastine; virus buffer; voided bladder

VBAC vaginal birth after cesarean section

VBAIN vertebrobasilar artery insufficiency nystagmus

VBC vincristine, bleomycin, and cisplatin

VBD vanishing bile duct; Veronal-buffered diluent

VBG vagotomy and Billroth gastroenterostomy; venous blood gases; venous bypass graft; vertical-banded gastroplasty

VBI vertebrobasilar insufficiency; vertebrobasilar ischemia

VBL vinblastine

VBOS Veronal-buffered oxalated saline

VBP vagal body paraganglia; venous blood pressure; ventricular premature beat

VBR ventricular brain ratio

VBS Veronal-buffered saline; vertebrobasilar system

VBS:FBS Veronal-buffered saline-fetal bovine serum

VC color vision; variance cardiography; vascular changes; vasoconstriction; vena cava; venereal case; venous capacitance; ventilatory capacity; ventral column; ventricular contraction; vertebral caval; Veterinary Corps; videocasette; vincristine; vinyl chloride; visual capacity; visual cortex; vital capacity; vocal cord

V/C ventilation/circulation [ratio]

V_C pulmonary capillary blood volume

VCA vancomycin, colistin, and anisomycin; viral capsid antigen

VCAM vascular cell adhesion molecule

VCAP vincristine, cyclophosphamide, Adriamycin, and prednisone

vCBF venous cerebral blood flow

VCC vasoconstrictor center; ventral cell column

VCD vibrational circular dichroism

VCE vagina, ectocervix, and endocervix

VCF velocardiofacial [syndrome]; velocity of circumferential fiber [lengthening]

VCFG volume-cycled flow generator

VCF_{min} minimum velocity of circumferential fiber [lengthening]

VCFS velo-cardio-facial syndrome

VCG vectorcardiogram, vectorcardiography; voiding cystography, voiding cystourethrography

VCL vinculin

VCM vinyl chloride monomer

VCMP vincristine, cyclophosphamide, melphalan, and prednisone

VCN vancomycin, colistomethane, and nystatin; *Vibrio chloreae* neuraminidase

VCO voltage-controlled oscillator

VCO, V_{CO} endogenous production of carbon monoxide

VCO$_2$, V$_{CO2}$ carbon dioxide output

VCP vincristine, cyclophosphamide, and prednisone

VCR vasoconstriction rate; vincristine; volume clearance rate

VCS vasoconstrictor substance; vesico-cervical space

VCSA viral cell surface antigen

VCSF ventricular cerebrospinal fluid

VCT venous clotting time

VCU videocystourethrography; voiding cystourethrogram, voiding cystoure-thrography

VCUG vesicoureterogram; voiding cys-tourethrogram

VD vapor density; vascular disease; va-sodilation, vasodilator; venereal disease; venous dilatation; ventricular dilator; ventrodorsal; vertical deviation; vertical divergence; video-disk; viral diarrhea; voided; volume of dead space; volume of distribution

V&D vomiting and diarrhea

V$_D$ dead space

Vd voided, voiding; volume dead space; volume of distribution

V$_d$ apparent volume of distribution

VDA visual discriminatory acuity

VDAC voltage-dependent anion channel

VdB van der Bergh [test]

VDBR volume of distribution of bilirubin

VDC vasodilator center

VDD atrial synchronous ventricular in-hibited [pacemaker]; vitamin D-depen-dent

VDDR vitamin D-dependent rickets

VDEL Venereal Disease Experimental Laboratory

VDEM vasodepressor material

VDF ventricular diastolic fragmentation

VDG, VD-G venereal disease-gonor-rhea

vdg voiding

VDH valvular disease of the heart

VDI virus defective interfering [parti-cle]

VDL vasodepressor lipid; visual detec-tion level

VDM vasodepressor material

VDP ventricular premature depolariza-tion

VDR venous diameter ratio

VDRG vitamin D-binding alpha-blobu-lin

VDRL Venereal Disease Research Lab-oratory [test for syphilis]

VDRR vitamin D-resistant rickets

VDRS Verdun Depression Rating Scale

VDRT venereal disease reference test

VDS vasodilator substance; vindesine

VDS, VD-S venereal disease-syphilis

VDT vibration disappearance threshold; visual display terminal; visual distortion test

VDU video display unit

VDV ventricular end-diastolic volume

Vd/Vt dead space ventilation/total ven-tilation [ratio]

VDWS van der Woude syndrome

VE vaginal examination; Venezuelan encephalitis; venous emptying; venous extension; ventilation; ventilatory equiv-alent; ventricular elasticity; ventricular extrasystole; vertex; vesicular exan-thema; viral encephalitis; virtual endos-copy; visual efficiency; vitamin E; vol-ume ejection; voluntary effort

V$_E$ environmental variance; respiratory minute volume

Ve ventilation

V&E Vinethine and ether

VEA ventricular ectopic activity; ven-tricular ectopic arrhythmia; viral enve-lope antigen

VEB ventricular ectopic beat

VECG vector electrocardiogram

VEC-MR velocity encoded cine-mag-netic resonance

VECP visually evoked cortical potential

VED vacuum erection device; ventricular ectopic depolarization; vital exhaustion and depression

VEE vagina, ectocervix, endocervix; Venezuelan equine encephalomyelitis

VEF ventricular ejection fraction; visually evoked field

VEG von Egner gland [protein]

VEGAS ventricular enlargement with gait apraxia syndrome

VEGF vascular endothelial growth factor

VEGP von Ebner gland protein

vehic vehicle

vel, veloc velocity

VEM vasoexcitor material

vent ventilation; ventral; ventricle, ventricular

vent fib ventricular fibrillation

ventric ventricle

VEP visual evoked potential

VEPID video-based electronic portal imaging device

VER visual evoked response

Verc vervet (African green monkey) kidney cells

vert vertebra, vertebral

ves bladder [Lat. *vesica*]; vesicular; vessel

vesic a blister [Lat. *vesicula*]

vest vestibular

ves ur urinary bladder [Lat. *vesica urinaria*]

VET ventricular ejection time; vestigial testis

Vet veteran; veterinarian, veterinary

VetMB Bachelor of Veterinary Medicine

Vet Med veterinary medicine

VETS Veterans Adjustment Scale

Vet Sci veterinary science

VEUD virtual emergency and urgency department

VF left leg [electrode]; ventricular fibrillation; ventricular fluid; ventricular flutter; visual field; vitreous fluorophotometry; vocal fremitus

Vf visual frequency

V_f variant frequency

vf visual field

VFA volatile fatty acid

VFC ventricular function curve

VFD visual feedback display

VFI visual field intact

V fib ventricular fibrillation

VFID virtual focus-isocenter-distance

VFL ventricular flutter

VFP ventricular filling pressure; ventricular fluid pressure

VFR voiding flow rate

VFS vascular fragility syndrome

VFT venous filling time; ventricular fibrillation threshold

VF/VT ventricular fibrillation/ventricular tachycardia

VG van Gieson [stain]; ventricular gallop; volume of gas

V_G genetic variance

VGCC voltage-gated calcium channels

VGH very good health

VGM venous graft myringoplasty

VGP viral glycoprotein

VH vaginal hysterectomy; venous hematocrit; ventricular hypertrophy; veterans hospital; viral hepatitis; virtual hospital

V_H variable domain of heavy chain; variable heavy chain

VHA Veterans Health Administration

V/Hallu visual hallucinations

VHAS Verapamil in Hypertension Atherosclerosis Study

VHD valvular heart disease; viral hematodepressive disease

VHDL very high density lipoprotein

VHF very high frequency; viral hemorrhagic fever; visual half-field

VHL von Hippel-Lindau [syndrome]

VHN Vickers hardness number

VHP vaporized hydrogen peroxide

VHR ventricular heart rate

VHS&RA Veterans Health Service and Research Administration

VI Roman numeral six; vaginal irrigation; variable interval; vastus intermedius; virgo intacta; virulence, virulent; viscosity index; visual impairment; visual inspection; vitality index; volume index

Vi virulence, virulent

VIA virus inactivating agent; virus infection-associated antigen

vib vibration

vib & perc vibration and percussion

VIC vasoinhibitory center; visual communication therapy; voice intensity control

VI-CTS vibration-induced carpal tunnel syndrome

VID visible iris diameter

VIF virus-induced interferon

VIG, VIg vaccinia immunoglobulin

VIGRE velocity imaging with gradient-recalled echos

VIIag factor VII antigen

VIIIc factor VIII clotting activity

VIII$_{vwf}$ von Willebrand factor

VIL villin

VIM video-intensification microscopy; vimentin

VIN vulvar intraepithelial neoplasm

vin vinyl

VIP vasoactive intestinal peptide; vasoinhibitory peptide; venous impedance plethysmography; ventricular inotropic parameter; voluntary interruption of pregnancy

VIPoma vasoactive intestinal polypeptide-secreting tumor

VIQ Verbal Intelligence Quotient

VIR virology

Vir virus, viral

vir virulent

VIS vaginal irrigation smear; venous insufficiency syndrome; vertebral irritation syndrome; visible; visual information storage

vis vision, visual

VISC vitreous infusion suction cutter

visc viscera, visceral; viscosity

VISI volar intercalated segment instability

Vit vitamin

vit vital

VITALS vital indicators of teaching and learning success

vit cap vital capacity

VJ ventriculojugular

VJC ventriculojugularcardiac

VK vervet (African green monkey) kidney cells

VKH, VKHS Vogt-Koyanagi-Harada [syndrome]

VL left arm [electrode]; ventralis lateratis [nucleus]; ventrolateral; visceral leishmaniasis; vision, left [eye]

V$_L$ variable domain of the light chain; variable light chain

VLA very late activation [antigen or protein]; virus-like agent

VLAB, VLA-BETA very late activation protein beta

V LACT venous lactate

VLB vinblastine; vincaleukoblastine

VLBR very low birth rate

VLBW very low birth weight

VLCAD very long chain acyl-coenzyme A dehydrogenase

VLCD very low calorie diet

VLCFA very long chain fatty acid

VLD very low density

VLDL, VLDLP very low density lipoprotein

VLDLR very low density lipoprotein receptor

VLF very low frequency

VLG ventral nucleus of the lateral geniculate body

VLH ventrolateral nucleus of the hypothalamus

VLM visceral larva migrans

VLO vastus lateralis obliquus

VLP vincristine, L-asparaginase, and prednisone; virus-like particle

VLR vinleurosine
VLS vascular leak syndrome
VLSI very large scale integration
VM vasomotor; ventralis medialus; ventromedial; ventricular mass; ventriculometry; vestibular membrane; viomycin; viral myocarditis; voltmeter
V/m volts per meter
V_m muscle volume; peak velocity
VMA vanillylmandelic acid
VMAT vesicular monoamine transformer
Vmax maximum velocity
VMC vasomotor center
VMCG vector magnetocardiogram
VMD Doctor of Veterinary Medicine; vitelliform macular dystrophy
vMDV virulent Marek disease virus
VME Volunteers for Medical Engineering
VMF vasomotor flushing
VMGT Visual Motor Gestalt Test
VMH ventromedial hypothalamic [syndrome]
VMI, VMIT visual-motor integration [test]
VMN ventromedial nucleus
VMO vastus medialis obliquus [muscle]; visiting medical officer
VMR vasomotor rhinitis
VMS visual memory span
VMST visual motor sequencing test
VMT vasomotor tonus; ventilatory muscle training; ventromedial tegmentum
VN vesical neck; vestibular nucleus; virus neutralization; visceral nucleus; visiting nurse; vitronectin; vocational nurse; vomeronasal
VNA Visiting Nurse Association
VNDPT visual numerical discrimination pre-test
VNO vomeronasal organ
VNR vitronectin receptor
VNRA vitronectin receptor alpha
VNS visiting nursing service

VNTR variable number of tandem repeats; variable copy number tandem repeats
VO verbal order; volume overload; voluntary opening
Vo standard volume
VO_2, V_{o2} volume of oxygen utilization
VOC volatile organic chemical
VOCC voltage-operated calcium channel
VOD veno-occlusive disease
VOI volume of interest
vol volar; volatile; volume; voluntary, volunteer
VOM volt-ohm-milliammeter
VON Victorian Order of Nurses
V-ONC viral oncogene
VOO ventricular asynchronous (competitive, fixed-rate) [pacemaker]
VOP venous occlusion plethysmography
VOR vestibulo-ocular reflex; volume of regret
VOS vision, left eye [Lat. *visio, oculus sinister*]
VOT voice onset time
VP physiological volume; vapor pressure; variegate porphyria; vascular permeability; vasopressin; velopharyngeal; venipuncture; venous pressure; ventricular pacing; ventricular premature [beat]; ventriculo-peritoneal; ventroposterior; VePepsid; vertex potential; vincristine and prednisone; viral protein; Voges-Proskauer [medium or test]; volume-pressure; vulnerable period
V/P ventilation/perfusion [ratio]
V&P vagotomy and pyloroplasty
Vp peak voltage; phenotype variance; plasma volume; ventricular premature [beat]
vp vapor pressure
VPA valproic acid
VPB ventricular premature beat
VPC vapor-phase chromatography; ventricular premature complex; ventricular

premature contraction; volume-packed cells; volume percent

VPCT ventricular premature contraction threshold

VPD ventricular premature depolarization

VPF vascular permeability factor

VPG velopharyngeal gap

VPGSS venous pressure gradient support stockings

VPI vapor phase inhibitor; velopharyngeal insufficiency

VPL ventroposterolateral

VPM ventilator pressure manometer; ventroposteromedial

vpm vibrations per minute

VPN ventral pontine nucleus

VPO velopharyngeal opening; vertical pendular oscillation

VPP vacuolar proton pump; viral porcine pneumonia

VPR Voges-Proskauer reaction; volume/pressure ratio

VPRBC volume of packed red blood cells

VPRC volume of packed red cells

VPS ventriculoperitoneal shunt; verbal pain scale; virtual point source; visual pleural space; volume performance standard

vps vibrations per second

VPT vibratory perception threshold

V/Q ventilation-perfusion; voice quality

VQE visa qualifying examination [for foreign medical graduates]

VR right arm [electrode]; valve replacement; variable ratio; vascular resistance; venous reflux; venous return; ventilation rate; ventilation ratio; ventral root; ventricular rhythm; vesicular rosette; vision, right [eye]; vital records; vocal resonance; vocational rehabilitation

Vr volume of relaxation

VRA visual reinforcement audiometry

VRBC red blood cell volume

VRC venous renin concentration

VRCP vitreoretinochoroidopathy

VRD ventricular radial dysplasia

VRE vencomycin-resistant enterococcus

VR&E vocational rehabilitation and education

VREF vancomycin-resistant *Enterococcus faecium*

VRI viral respiratory infection; virtual reality imaging

VRL Virus Reference Laboratory

VRML Virtual Reality Modeling Language

VRNA viral ribonucleic acid

VRNI neovascular inflammatory vitreoretinopathy

VROM voluntary range of motion

VRP ventral root potential

VRR ventral root reflex

VRS verbal rating scale; Virchow-Robin space

VRT vehicle rescue technician; volume-rendering technique

VRV ventricular residual volume; viper retrovirus

VS vaccination scar; vaccine serotype; vagal stimulation; vasospasm; venesection; ventricular septum; verapamil shock; vesicular stomatitis; veterinary surgeon; vibration syndrome; visual storage; vital sign; Vogt-Spielmeyer [syndrome]; volatile solid; volumetric solution; voluntary sterilization

Vs venesection

V·s vibration second; volt-second

V x s volts by seconds

vs see above [Lat. *vide supra*]; single vibration; versus; vibration seconds; vital signs

VSA variant-specific surface antigen

VSBE very short below-elbow [cast]

VSC voluntary surgical contraception

VSD ventricular septal defect; virtually safe dose

VSFP venous stop flow pressure

VSG variant surface glycoprotein
VSHD ventricular septal heart defect
VSIE volume surface integral equation [method]
VSINC Virus Subcommittee of the International Nomenclature Committee
VSM vascular smooth muscle
VSMC vascular smooth muscle cell
VSMS Vineland Social Maturity Scale
vsn vision
VSO vertical supranuclear ophthalmoplegia
VSOK vital signs normal
VSP variable spine plating
VSR venous stasis retinopathy
VSS vital signs stable
VST ventral spinothalamic tract; volume-selective excitation
VSV vesicular stomatitis virus
VSW ventricular stroke work
VT tetrazolium violet; total ventilation; vacuum tube; vacuum tuberculin; vasotonin; venous thrombosis; ventricular tachyarrhythmia; ventricular tachycardia; verocytotoxin; verotoxin; vibration threshold
V$_T$ tidal volume; total ventilation
V&T volume and tension
VTA ventral tegmental area
V tach ventricular tachycardia
VTE venous thromboembolism; ventricular tachycardia event
VTEC verotoxin-producing *Escherichia coli*
VTG volume thoracic gas
VTI velocity-time integral; volume thickness index
VTM mechanical tidal volume; virus transport medium
VTN vitronectin
VTOP vaginal termination of pregnancy
VTR variable tandem repeats; videotape recording; vesicular transport system

VTSRS Verdun Target Symptom Rating Scale
VTVM vacuum tube voltmeter
VTX, vtx vertex
VU varicose ulcer; volume unit
vu volume unit
VUJ vesico-ureteral junction
UVO vesico-ureteral orifice
VUR vesicoureteral reflex
VUV vacuum ultraviolet
VV vaccinia virus; varicose veins; veno-venous; viper venom; vulva and vagina
V&V verification and validation
V-V veno-venous [bypass]
vv varicose veins; veins
v/v percent volume in volume
VVAS vertical visual analog scale
VVD vaginal vertex delivery
VVDL venovenous double-lumen [catheter]
VVFR vesicovaginal fistula repair
VVI ventricular inhibited [pacemaker]; vocal velocity index
v$_{vk}$ ventricular volume constant
vvMDV very virulent Marek disease virus
VVS vesicovaginal space; vesicovaginal space; vestibulo-vegetative syndrome
VVT ventricular triggered [pacemaker]
VW vascular wall; vessel wall; von Willebrand's [disease]
v/w volume per weight
vWD von Willebrand disease
VWF velocity waveform; vibration-induced white finger
vWF, vWf von Willebrand factor
VWM ventricular wall motion
vWS van der Woude syndrome; viewing work station; von Willebrand syndrome
Vx vertex
VZ varicella-zoster
VZIG, VZIg varicella zoster immunoglobulin
VZV varicella-zoster virus

W dominant spotting [mouse]; energy; section modulus; a series of small triangular incisions in plastic surgery [plasty]; tryptophan; tungsten [Ger. *Wolfram*]; wakefulness; ward; water; watt; Weber [test]; week; wehnelt; weight; white; widowed; width; wife; Wilcoxson rank sum statistic; Wistar [rat]; with; word fluency; work; wound

W3 World Wide Web

w water; watt; while; with; velocity (m/s)

Wt weakly positive

WA when awake; white adult; Wiskott-Aldrich [syndrome]

W/A watt/ampere

W&A weakness and atrophy

WAB Western Aphasia Battery

WAF weakness, atrophy and fasciculation; white adult female

WAGR Wilms tumor, aniridia, genito-urinary abnormalities, and mental retardation

WAIS Wechsler Adult Intelligence Scale; Western Angiographic and Interventional Society

WAIS-R revised Wechsler Adult Intelligence Scale

WAK wearable artificial kidney

WAM white adult male; worksheet for ambulatory medicine

WAN wide area network

WAP wandering atrial pacemaker

WAR Wasserman antigen reaction; without additional reagents

WARDS Welfare of Animals Used for Research in Drugs and Therapy

WARF warfarin [Wisconsin Alumni Research Foundation]

WAS weekly activities summary; Wiskott-Aldrich syndrome

WASP Weber Advanced Spatial Perception [test]

Wass Wasserman [reaction]

WAT word association test

WB waist belt; washable base; washed bladder; water bottle; Wechsler-Bellevue [Scale]; weight-bearing; well baby; Western blot [assay]; wet bulb; whole blood; whole body; Willowbrook [virus]; Wilson-Blair [agar]

Wb weber; well-being

WBA wax bean agglutinin; whole body activity

Wb/A webers/ampere

WBAPTT whole blood activated partial thromboplastin time

WBC well baby care/clinic; white blood cell; white blood cell count; whole blood cell count

WBCT whole-blood clotting time

WBDC whole-body digital scanner

WBE whole-body extract

WBF whole-blood folate

WBGT wet bulb global temperature

WBH whole-blood hematocrit; whole-body hyperthermia

WBLT Watson-Barker Listening Test

Wb/m² weber per square meter

WBN whole-blood nitrogen

WBPTT whole-blood partial thromboplastin time

WBR whole-body radiation

WBRT whole-blood recalcification time

WBS Wechsler-Bellevue Scale; whole-blood serum; whole-body scan; Wiedemann-Beckwith syndrome; withdrawal body shakes

WBT wet bulb temperature

WC ward clerk; water closet; Weber-Christian [syndrome]; wheel chair; white cell; white cell casts; white cell count; white child; whooping cough;

wild caught [animal]; work capacity; workers' compensation; writer's cramp

WC' whole complement

W/C watch carefully; wheel chair

W3C World Wide Web Consortium

wc wheel chair

WCC Walker carcinosarcoma cells; white cell count

WCD Weber-Christian disease

WCE work capacity evaluation

WCL Wenckebach cycle length; whole cell lysate

w/cm² watts per square centimeter

WCS white clot syndrome; Wisconsin Card Sort [test]

WCST Wisconsin Card Sorting Test

WD wallerian degeneration; well developed; well differentiated; wet dressing; Whitney Damon [dextrose]; Wilson disease; with disease; withdraw or withdrawn; without dyskinesia; Wolman disease; wrist disarticulation

W/D warm and dry

Wd ward

wd well developed; wound, wounded

WDCC well-developed collateral circulation

WDHA watery diarrhea, hypokalemia, achlorhydria [syndrome]

WDHH watery diarrhea, hypokalemia, and hypochlorhydria

WDI warfarin dose index

WDL well-differentiated lymphocytic

WDLL well-differentiated lymphatic lymphoma

WDMF wall-defective microbial forms

WDS watery diarrhea syndrome; wet dog shakes [syndrome]

WDWN, wdwn well developed and well nourished

WE wax ester; Wernicke encephalopathy; western encephalitis; western encephalomyelitis; wound of entry

We weber

WEDI Workshop for Electronic Data Interchange

WEE western equine encephalitis/ encephalomyelitis

WER wheal erythema reaction

WES wall echo sign; work environment scale

WF Weil-Felix reaction; white female; Wistar-Furth [rat]

W/F, wf white female

WFE Williams flexion exercise

WFI water for injection

WFL within function limits

WFOT World Federation of Occupational Therapists

WFR Weil-Felix reaction; wheal-and-flare reaction

WFS Waterhouse-Friederichsen syndrome

WG water gauge; Wegener granulomatosis; Wright-Giemsa [stain]

WGA wheat germ agglutinin

wgt weight

WH well hydrated; Werdnig-Hoffmann [syndrome]; whole homogenate; wound healing

Wh, wh white

w·h watt-hour

WHA warm and humid air

wh ch wheel chair; white child

WHCOA White House Conference on Aging

WHCR Wolf-Hirschhorn chromosome region

WHD Werdnig-Hoffmann disease

WHHHIMP Wernicke encephalopathy/withdrawal, hypertensive encephalopathy, hypoglycemia, hypoxemia, intracranial bleeding/infection, meningitis/encephalitis, poison/medication

WHML Wellcome Historical Medical Library

WHO World Health Organization; wrist-hand orthosis

whp whirlpool

WHR waist:hips girth ratio

whr watt-hour

WHRC World Health Research Centre

WHS Werdnig-Hoffmann syndrome; Wolf-Hirschhorn syndrome

WHV woodchuck hepatic virus

WHVP wedged hepatic venous pressure

WHYMPI West Haven–Yale Multidimensional Pain Inventory

WI human embryonic lung cell line; walk-in [patient]; water ingestion; Wistar [rat]

WIA wounded in action

WIBC Wiggins Interpresonal Behavior Circle

WIC walk-in clinic; women, infants, and children

WICHEN Western Interstate Commission for Higher Education in Nursing

WIPI Word Intelligibility Picture Identification

WIS Wechsler Intelligence Scale

WISC Wechsler Intelligence Scale for Children

WISC-R Wechsler Intelligence Scale for Children-Revised

WIST Whitaker Index of Schizophrenic Thinking

WITT Wittenborn [Psychiatric Rating Scale]

W-J Woodcock-Johnson [Psychoeducational Battery]

WK week; Wernicke-Korsakoff [syndrome]; Wilson-Kimmelstiel [syndrome]

wk weak; week; work

WKD Wilson-Kimmelstiel disease

W/kg watts per kilogram

WKS Wernicke-Korsakoff syndrome

WKY Wistar-Kyoto [rat]

WL waiting list; waterload; wavelength; withdrawal; working level; workload

wl wavelength

WLE wide local excision

WLF whole lymphocytic fraction

WLI weight-length index

WLM white light microscopy; working level month [radon]

WLS wet lung syndrome

WLT whole lung tomography

WM Waldenström macroglobulinemia; ward manager; warm and moist; Wernicke-Mann [hemiplegia]; wet mount; white male; white matter; whole milk; Wilson-Mikity [syndrome]

W-M Weil-Marchesani [syndrome]

W/M white male

wm white male; whole milk; whole mount

w/m² watts per square meter

WMA World Medical Association

WMC weight-matched control

WME Williams' medium E

WMH white matter hyperintensities

WMO ward medical officer

WMP weight management program

WMR work metabolic rate; World Medical Relief

WMS Wechsler Memory Scale; Weill-Marchesani syndrome; Williams syndrome

WMX whirlpool, massage, exercise

WN, wn well nourished

WNE West Nile encephalitis

WNF well-nourished female

WNL within normal limits

WNM well-nourished male

WNPW wide, notched P wave

WNV West Nile virus

WO wash out; will order; written order

W/O water in oil [emulsion]

w/o without

wo weeks old

WOB work of breathing

WOB$_I$ imposed work of breathing

WOB$_P$ physiologic work of breathing

WOB$_T$ total work of breathing (WOB$_P$ plus WOB$_I$)

WOB$_V$ work of breathing performed by ventilator

WOE wound of entry

WONCA World Organization of Family Doctors

WOP without pain
WOU women's outpatient unit
WOWS weak opiate withdrawal scale
WOX wound of exit
WP weakly positive; wedge pressure; wet pack; wettable powder; whirlpool; white pulp; word processor; working point
W/P water/powder ratio
wp wettable powder
WPB whirlpool bath
WPCU weighted patient care unit
Wpf wave at a pilot frequency
WPFM Wright peak flow meter
WPk Ward's pack; wet pack
WPPSI Wechsler Preschool and Primary Scale of Intelligence
WPR written progress report
WPRS Wittenborn Psychiatric Rating Scale
WPS wasting pig syndrome
WPW Wolff-Parkinson-White [syndrome]
WQAC ward quality assurance committee
WR Wassermann reaction; water retention; weakly reactive; weak response; whole response; wiping reaction; work rate
Wr wrist; writhe
WRAIN Walter Reed Army Medical Center Institute of Nursing
WRAMC Walter Reed Army Medical Center
WRAML Wide Range Assessment of Memory and Learning
WRAT Wide Range Achievement Test
WRBC washed red blood cells
WRE wahole ragweed extract
WRC washed red cells; water retention coefficient
WRK Woodward reagent K
WRMT Woodcock Reading Mastery Test
WRN Werner [syndrome]
WRS Ward-Romano syndrome; Wiedemann-Rautenstrauch syndrome

WRVP wedged renal vein pressure
WS Waardenburg syndrome; ward secretary; Warkany syndrome; Warthin-Starry [stain]; water soluble; water swallow; Werner syndrome; West syndrome; Wilder silver [stain]; Williams syndrome; Wolfram syndrome
W·s watt-second
ws water-soluble
WSB wheat-soy blend
w-sec watt-second
WSI Waardenburg syndrome type I
WSA water-soluble antibiotic
WSC water-soluble contrast [medium]
WSL Wesselsbron [virus]
WSP withdrawal seizure prone
WSR Westergren sedimentation rate; withdrawal seizure resistant
W/sr watts per steradian
WSS Weaver-Smith syndrome
WT wall thickness; water temperature; wavelet transform; wild type [strain]; Wilms tumor; wisdom teeth; work therapy
wt weight; white
WTE whole time equivalent
WTF weight transferral frequency
WTP willingness to pay
W/U workup
WV walking ventilation
W/V, w/v percent weight in volume, weight/volume
W^v variable dominant spotting [mouse]
WW Weight Watchers; wet weight
W/W, w/w weight; percent weight
W/wo with or without
WWS Wieacker-Wolff syndrome
WWU weighted work units [of DRGs]
WWW world wide web
WX wound of exit
WxB wax bite
WxP wax pattern
WY women years
WZa wide zone alpha
WZS Weissenbacher-Zweymuller syndrome

X androgenic [zone]; cross; crossbite; exophoria distance; extra; female sex chromosome; ionization exposure; Kienböck's unit of x-ray exposure; magnification; multiplication times; reactance; removal of; respirations [anesthesia chart]; Roman numeral ten; start of anesthesia; "times"; translocation between two X chromosomes; transverse; unknown quantity; X unit; xylene

X̄ sample mean

Ẋ ionization exposure rate

x except; extremity; horizontal axis of a rectangular coordinate system; mole fraction; multiplication times; roentgen [rays]; sample mean; times; unknown factor; xanthine

X3 orientation as to time, place, and person

XA xanthurenic acid; x-ray analysis

X-A xylene and alcohol

Xa chiasma

Xaa unknown amino acid

Xam examination

Xan xanthine

Xanth xanthomatosis

Xao xanthosine

XBP X-box binding protein

XBSN X-linked bulbospinal neuropathy

XC, Xc excretory cystogram

XCE X-chromosome controlling element

X-CGD X-linked chronic granulomatous disease

XD x-ray diffraction

XDH xanthine dehydrogenase

XDP xanthine diphosphate; xeroderma pigmentosum

XDR transducer

Xe electric susceptibility; xenon

XECT xenon-enhanced computed tomography

XEF excess ejection fraction

XES x-ray energy spectrometry

Xfb cross-linked Gibrin

XGP xanthogranulomatous pyelonephritis

XGPT xylosylprotein-4-beta-galactosyltransferase

Ξ Greek capital letter *xi*

ξ Greek lower case letter *xi*

XIC X-inactivation center

XIP x-ray-induced polypeptide

XIST X-inactivation specific transcript

XL excess lactate; X-linked [inheritance]; xylose-lysine [agar base]

XLA, X-LA X-linked agammaglobulinemia

XLAS X-linked aqueductal stenosis

XLCM X-linked dilated cardiomyopathy

XLD xylose-lysine-deoxycholate [agar]

XLH X-linked hypophosphatemia

XLI X-linked ichthyosis

XLMR X-linked mental retardation

XLMTM X-linked myotubular myopathy

XLP X-linked lymphoproliferative [syndrome]

XLPD X-linked lymphoproliferative disease

XLR X-linked recessive

XLS X-linked recessive lymphoproliferative syndrome

XM crossmatch

Xm maternal chromosome X

xma chiasma

X-mas Christmas [factor]

x-mat crossmatch [blood]

X-match crossmatch

XMP xanthine monophosphate

XMR X-linked mental retardation

XN night blindness

XO presence of only one sex chromosome; xanthine oxidase
XOM extraocular movements
XOR exclusive operating room
XP xanthogranulomatous pyelonephritis; xeroderma pigmentosum
Xp paternal chromosome X; short arm of chromosome X
XPA xeroderma pigmentosum group A
XPC xeroderma pigmentosum group C
XPS x-ray photoemission spectroscopy
Xq long arm of chromosome X
XR xeroradiography; X-linked recessive [inheritance]; x-ray
x-rays roentgen rays
XRD x-ray diffraction
XRF x-ray fluorescence
XRMR X-linked recessive mental retardation
XRN X-linked recessive nephrolithiasis
XRS x-ray sensitivity
XRT x-ray therapy
XS cross-section; excessive; xiphisternum
X/S cross-section
xs excess
XSA cross-section area

XSCID X-linked severe combined immunodeficiency [syndrome]
X-sect cross-section
XSP xanthoma striatum palmare
XT exotropia
Xta chiasmata
Xtab cross-tabulating
XTE xeroderma, talipes, and enamel defect [syndrome]
X-TEP crossed immunoelectrophoresis
XTM xanthoma tuberosum multiplex
XTP xanthosine triphosphate
XU excretory urogram; X unit
Xu X-unit
XuMP xylulose monophosphate
Xu5P, Xu5p xylulose-5-phosphate
XX double strength; female chromosome type
46, XX 46 chromosomes, 2 X chromosomes (normal female)
XXL xylocaine
XX/XY sex karyotypes
XY male chromosome type
46, XY 46 chromosomes, 1 X and 1 Y chromosome (normal male)
Xyl xylose

Y a coordinate axis in a plane; male sex chromosome; tyrosine; year; yellow; yield; yttrium; *Yersinia*

y the vertical axis of a rectangular coordinate system

Υ see *upsilon*

υ see *upsilon*

YA *Yersinia* arthritis

Y/A years of age

YAC yeast artificial chromosome

YACP young adult chronic patient

YADH yeast alcohol dehydrogenase

YAG yttrium aluminum garnet [laser]

Yb ytterbium

YBOCS Yale-Brown Obsessive Compulsive Scale

YCB yeast carbon base

yd yard

YDV yeast-derived hepatitis B vaccine

YDYES yin deficiency yang excess syndrome

YE yeast extract; yellow enzyme

YEH$_2$ reduced yellow enzyme

YEI *Yersinia enterocolitica* infection

Yel yellow

YF yellow fever

YFI yellow fever immunization

YFMD yellow fever membrane disease

YLC youngest living child

YLS years of life saved

YM yeast and mannitol

Y$_{max}$ maximum yield

YNB yeast nitrogen base

YNS yellow nail syndrome

y/o years old

YOB year of birth

YP yeast phase; yield pressure

YPA yeast, peptone, and adenine sulfate

YPLL years of potential life lost

yr year

YRD Yangtze River disease

YS yellow spot; yolk sac

ys yellow spot; yolk sac

YST yolk sac tumor

YT, yt yttrium

yWACC younger woman with aggressive cervical cancer

Z acoustic impedance; atomic number; complex impedance; contraction [Ger. *Zuckung*]; the disk that separates sarcomeres [Ger. *Zwischenscheibe*]; glutamine; impedance; ionic charge number; no effect; point formed by a line perpendicular to the nasion-menton line through the anterior nasal spine; proton number; section modulus; standard score; standardized deviate; zero; zone; a Z-shaped incision in plastic surgery

Z',Z'' increasing degrees of contraction

z algebraic unknown or space coordinate; axis of a three-dimensional rectangular coordinate system; catalytic amount; standard normal deviate; zero

ZAG, ZA2G zinc-alpha-2-glycoprotein

ZAP zeta-associated protein zymosan-activated plasma [rabbit]

ZAPF zinc adequate pair-fed

ZAS zymosan-activated autologous serum

ZB zebra body

ZCP zinc chloride poisoning

ZD zero defects; zero discharge; zinc deficiency

Z-D Zamorano-Duchovny [digitizer]

ZDDP zinc dialkyldithiophosphate

Z-DNA zig-zag (left-handed helical) deoxyribonucleic acid

ZDO zero differential overlap

ZDS zinc depletion syndrome

ZDV zidovudine

ZE Zollinger-Ellison [syndrome]

ZEBRA zero blanaced reimbursement account

ZEC Zinsser-Engman-Cole [syndrome]

ZEEP zero end-expiratory pressure

ZEPI zonal echo planar imaging

Z-ERS zeta erythrocyte sedimentation rate

ZES Zollinger-Ellison syndrome

Z Greek capital letter *zeta*

ζ Greek lower case letter *zeta*

ZF zero frequency; zinc finger [protein]; zona fasciculata

ZFF zinc fume fever

ZFP zinc finger protein

ZFX X-linked zinc finger protein

ZG zona glomerulosa

ZGM zinc glycinate marker

ZIFT zygote intrafallopian tube transfer

ZIG, ZIg zoster immunoglobulin

ZIP zoster immune plasma

ZK Zuelzer-Kaplan [syndrome]

ZLS Zimmerman-Laband syndrome

Zm zygomaxillare

ZMA zinc meta-arsenite

Zn zinc

ZNF zinc finger [protein]

ZnOE zinc oxide and eugenol

ZO Zichen-Oppenheim [syndrome]; Zuelzer-Ogden [syndrome]

ZOE zinc oxide-eugenol

ZOL zoladex

Zool zoology

ZP zona pellucida

ZPA zone of polarizing activity

ZPC zero point of change

ZPG zero population growth

ZPO zinc peroxide

ZPP zinc protoporphyrin

ZR zona reticularis

Zr zirconium

ZS Zellweger syndrome

ZSR zeta sedimentation ratio

ZTS zymosan-treated serum

Z-TSP zephiran-trisodium phosphate

ZTT zinc turbidity test

ZVT Zehlenverbindungstest

ZW Zellweger [syndrome]

ZWS Zellweger syndrome

Zy zygion

ZyC zymosan complement

zyg zygotene

Zz ginger [Lat. *zingibar*]